CMSA *Core Curriculum for*

CASE MANAGEMENT

THIRD EDITION

Important Note Regarding the Case Management Society of America

Standards of Practice for Case Management (revised 2016)

A major and new feature of this third edition of the Core Curriculum for Case Management is the integration of the Case Management Society of America (CMSA) Standards of Practice for Case Management. We made an effort to describe in each chapter how the Standards apply into case management practice. At the time we wrote this textbook, the Standards of Practice for Case Management (rev. 2010) was the latest version. As a result, this edition of the Core Curriculum for Case Management references the 2010 Standards. As we went to print, we learned that a revision of the Standards was in process; however, CMSA expected to release this revision in the latter half of 2016. Both editors of the Core Curriculum, among other fellow case management experts, were involved in the revisions. It is important to note that the 2016 Standards of Practice remain substantively similar to and aligned with those released in 2010 and referred to in the Core Curriculum.

For the reader's information, we highlight below select modifications we expect the 2016 revision to reflect. The 2016 CMSA Standards of Practice for Case Management

- Emphasize the practice of *professional* case management in the ever-expanding care settings across the entire continuum of health and human services.
- Include practical updates to the *How Demonstrated* section that accompanies each Standard.
- Reflect legislative and regulatory changes affecting *professional* case management practice.
- Recognize the contribution of scholarship, including research and practice innovations, to the advancement of *professional* case management.
- Reduce the use of stigmatizing language such as problems and issues, reframing these as care needs and opportunities.
- Focus on closure of case management engagement in lieu of termination of services or the case management process.
- Recognize cultural and linguistic appropriateness in all forms of communication with the client and/or client's family caregiver.
- Highlight the value of professional case management practice and the role of the professional case manager.

Questions regarding the Standards of Practice for Case Management (rev. 2016) may be directed to the Case Management Society of America headquartered in Little Rock, Arkansas.

Hussein M. Tahan
Teresa M. Treiger

CMSA *Core Curriculum for*

CASE
MANAGEMENT

THIRD EDITION

Hussein M. Tahan, PhD, RN
System Vice President
Nursing Professional Development and Workforce
    Planning
MedStar Health System Nursing
Columbia, Maryland

**Teresa M. Treiger, RN-BC, MA,
CHCQM-CM/TOC, CCM**
CMSA Past National President (2010–2011)
Principal
Ascent Care Management, LLC
Quincy, Massachusetts

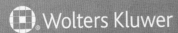

Philadelphia · Baltimore · New York · London
Buenos Aires · Hong Kong · Sydney · Tokyo

Acquisitions Editor: Nicole Dernoski
Product Development Editor: Maria M. McAvey
Production Project Manager: David Saltzberg
Design Coordinator: Holly Reid McLaughlin
Manufacturing Coordinator: Kathleen Brown
Marketing Manager: Tod McKenzie
Prepress Vendor: SPi Global

3rd edition

9 8 7 6 5 4 3 2 1

Printed in China

Library of Congress Cataloging-in-Publication Data
   Names: Tahan, Hussein M., editor. | Treiger, Teresa M., editor. |
Case Management Society of America, issuing body.
   Title: CMSA core curriculum for case management / [edited by] Hussein M.
Tahan, Teresa M. Treiger.
   Other titles: Core curriculum for case management | Case Management Society
of America core curriculum for case management
   Description: Third edition. | Philadelphia : Wolters Kluwer, [2017] |
Includes bibliographical references and index.
   Identifiers: LCCN 2016011171 | ISBN 9781451194302
   Subjects: | MESH: Case Management | Nursing Care—organization &
administration | Outlines
   Classification: LCC RT90.7 | NLM WY 18.2 | DDC 362.1/73068—dc23 LC record
available at http://lccn.loc.gov/2016011171

---

*We, the editors, wish to dedicate this book to
our colleagues, families, and friends who supported us
during the journey of updating the Core Curriculum.
There are some individuals who deserve special recognition
for going above and beyond the call of duty—
to you we are forever grateful!*

*To my parents for always wanting the best for me,
especially for your unconditional love and unwavering
support and encouragement; to Eduardo A.M. for being a
shining light in my life; to Toni and Jane for your love,
friendship, and counsel; and to Bene C.S. and Stavros S.
for always being there for me... Hussein*

*To my wonderful husband Dave for your keen eye and
unfailing support; to my brothers and sisters who are
each a blessing in my life; to R.G. for having confidence
in me; to S.K.P. for being a tremendous role model
and friend; and to my parents LCDR Norman C.
and Eva V. Frates, thank you for unconditional
love and support... Teri*

*We also wish to dedicate this book to professional case
managers past, present, and future...
Thank you for supporting your patients (clients)
and each other, every day, every time ....
Most importantly, we dedicate this third edition
of the Core Curriculum to
Suzanne K. Powell,
Co-editor of the first and second editions.
You are an inspiration to all of us, and a role model
to every case manager. Your contributions to the
professional practice of case management
are palpable everywhere today and for decades to come.
You are the Florence Nightingale of every patient you touch;
the teacher of every case manager you encounter; and
the mentor for all those in your professional world,
including us. We are forever grateful to you ... thank you!*

Contributors

John D. Banja, PhD
Professor
Department of Rehabilitation
Medicine
Medical Ethicist
Center for Ethics
Emory University
Atlanta, Georgia

Jackie Birmingham, BSN, MS, RN
Vice President
Curaspan Health Group
Newton, Massachusetts

Beverly Cunningham, MS, RN
Partner and Consultant
Case Management Concepts

Stefani Daniels, MSNA, RN, CMAC, ACM
President and Managing Director
Phoenix Medical Management, Inc.
Pompano Beach, Florida

Ellen Fink-Samnick, MSW, ACSW, LCSW, CCM, CRP
Principal
EFS Supervision Strategies, LLC
Burke, Virginia

Kathleen Fraser, MSN, MHA, RN-BC, CCM, CRRN
Regional Team Manager of Case
Management
Zurich Services Managed Care
Katy, Texas

Michael B. Garrett, MS, CCM
Principal
Mercer
Seattle, Washington

Deborah Gutteridge, MS, CBIST
Clinical Evaluator and Case Manager
NeuroRestorative
Kansas City, Missouri

Cheri Lattimer, BSN, RN
Executive Director of Case
Management Society of America
Little Rock, Arkansas

Sandra L. Lowery, BSN, RN, CCRN, CCM, CNLCP
President
CCMI Associates, LLC
Francestown, New Hampshire

Mary Jane McKendry, MBA, RN, CCM
Vice President of Quality Management
Neighborhood Health Plan
Boston, Massachusetts

Lynn S. Muller, JD, BA-HCM, RN, CCM
Muller & Muller
Bergenfield, New Jersey

Rebecca Perez, BSN, RN, CCM
Manager of Medical Management
Operations
Centene Corporation
St. Louis, Missouri

Suzanne K. Powell, MBA, RN, CCM, CPHQ
Editor-in-Chief
Professional Case Management
Wolters Kluwer
Philadelphia, Pennsylvania

Karen N. Provine, MS, CRC, CCM, CDMS, LPC
Vocational Rehabilitation and Training Consultant
Albuquerque, New Mexico

Marietta P. Stanton, PhD, RN, C, CNAA, BC, CMAC, CCM
Professor and Director of Graduate Programs
Capstone College of Nursing
University of Alabama
Tuscaloosa, Alabama

Hussein M. Tahan, PhD, RN
System Vice President
Nursing Professional Development and Workforce Planning
MedStar Health System Nursing
Columbia, Maryland

Teresa M. Treiger, RN-BC, MA, CHCQM-CM/TOC, CCM
CMSA Past National President (2010–2011)
Principal
Ascent Care Management, LLC
Quincy, Massachusetts

Reviewers

Stefany H. Almaden, MSN, PhD, RN, CCM, CPUM, CMCN, PHAM, LCP
EVP Consulting, Health Services
The Almaden Group, Inc.
Care Management Consultants
Pasadena, California

Debra Lee Belitter, MBA, RN, CCM
Quality Care Consultant, Care
Delivery–Arizona
Optum Care
Phoenix, Arizona

Margaret P. Chu, BSN, MPA, RN, CCM, CPHQ
President
MPC & Associates
East Williston, New York

Janet Coulter, MSN, MS, RN, CCM
Chair
Breckinridge School of Nursing
ITT Technical Institute
Maineville, Ohio

Foreword

The Case Management Society of America (CMSA), a multidisciplinary organization, dedicated to the support and development of Case Management professionals, is proud to present the *CMSA Core Curriculum for Case Management*, third edition. One outstanding hallmark of Case Management is the willingness of its members to help one another learn and, thereby, improve the services that the profession provides. This textbook is a valuable means of communicating Case Management knowledge, both to the student of case management as well as the seasoned practicing case manager. I want to acknowledge and thank the Core Curriculum authors, Hussein M. Tahan and Teri M. Treiger, for their commitment and support to the advancement of case management, with this revision.

Never before has the role of the case manager been incorporated into so many national mandates and local initiatives. We are called upon to educate and empower patients and their caregivers in order to activate them to truly take responsibility for their own health. Health care, however, is complex and difficult to understand, and patients are searching for assistance in its navigation. Case Managers engage patients and their support systems to problem-solve by exploring options of care, when available, and alternative plans, when necessary, to achieve the best possible outcomes. Through the combined efforts of CMSA, the authors, the contributors, and the editors, the *Core Curriculum* serves as an educational resource, which identifies basic to advanced components, interventions, delivery models, roles, and concepts of case management.

Health care trends and challenges are both energizing and exhausting for case management professionals. We have started to be recognized, moving us from having to battle for our respected place to having it officially written into various models of care. CMSA, just as Case Management itself, transcends *every level of care across the full continuum*. Our discipline is very large yet in many ways continues to be very small. The body of knowledge required to effectively practice Case Management is rapidly growing as this specialty continues to evolve. Modern patient care must be based upon the holistic intertwining of information from a variety of disciplines, from the physical and behavioral sciences, as well as the arts. As our activities become more sophisticated, so must our resources.

Case Management is neither linear nor a one-way exercise. Accountability, facilitation, coordination, and collaboration will occur throughout the patient's (client's) health care encounter. Collaboration among physicians, pharmacists, nurses, case managers, social workers, allied health, and supporting staff is critical to achieving the goals of the interdisciplinary care team, the organization, and changing the way we deliver health care today. A 2012 patient engagement survey identified 14 sources of health information upon which most clients/patients rely. Not surprisingly, the Case Manager ranked third! The primary and the specialist physician ranked first and second, respectively, with only a margin of one percentage point separating the Case

Manager from the specialist physician.[1] I think those findings are incredible yet they are of no surprise to Case Managers. We know who we are, the value of what we do, and the skills we bring to the table. CMSA encourages you to be ready for the opportunities, continues to pursue professional excellence, and maintains your competence in our practice!

Kathleen Fraser, MSN, MHA, RN-BC, CCM, CRRN
National President
Case Management Society of America 2014–2016

---

[1]TCS Healthcare™ Technologies. (2012). Case Management Solutions, 3rd Bi-Annual Health IT Strategy, Trend Report #5: Patient Engagement Strategies. Available at http://www.tcshealthcare.com/Trend-Report-5, Retrieved on November 12, 2015.

Preface

Sixteen years ago, we published the first edition of the Core Curriculum. So much has happened in the practice of case management ever since. Transformation and innovation have been ongoing resulting in a shift in the practice—from being an innovative and unique approach for the betterment of health services and care provision to becoming a necessity today in every setting across the continuum of health and human services. Most importantly, however, case management (or care management, care coordination, transitions of care) has been embedded now in US health care laws and regulations, especially with the advent of the Patient Protection and Affordable Care Act of 2010. This Act has contributed to the legitimization of case management as an essential element of health care delivery—No more raising questions concerning the value of case management.

The US health care system continues to grow in complexity, requiring impactful patient advocacy that ensures the provision of timely, safe, quality, holistic, personalized, and cost-conscious health care and services. The *case manager* is the professional best positioned to work with the patient and patient's family or family caregiver in making the "course" of their care manageable, understandable, familiar, and comfortable. The *case manager* also ensures that access to health care services must happen at the right time, in the most appropriate care setting, through the right provider, to the necessary extent (type and quantity), while the "experience" during the care encounter remains optimal and desirable.

There is enough evidence today that supports the significance of case management (care coordination, care management, transitions of care) and its contribution to efficient, effective, and equitable care provision. Despite its popularity, the practice of case management continues to be primarily learned on-the-job. Academic institutions have not caught on to this evolution, which makes textbooks, such as this Core Curriculum, a go to resource that supports the case manager struggling in determining whether her/his practice is current, exemplary, or effective.

The case management workforce is not based in a specific health discipline or specialty. On the contrary, the practice of case management is diverse. It is interprofessional in nature, with nurses, social workers, vocational rehabilitation counselors, physical and occupational therapists, and other licensed professionals all assuming the role of case manager and often collaborate as a group driven by what makes most sense to the individual patient situation and care setting. This unique diversity makes the practice of case management dynamic, popular, attractive, and influential. Additionally, the Core Curriculum is the one resource that is written for all case managers and their colleagues regardless of their professional backgrounds. Its content also covers the key nuances of the practice in the various care settings.

This Core Curriculum, sponsored by the Case Management Society of America (CMSA), represents a synthesis of the case management evolution and a forecast about its future. The chapters, which have been written by renowned experts in the field, address important topics of case management practice, such as historical perspective; programs and models; practice settings across the continuum of care; roles, responsibilities, qualifications, and competencies of case managers; training, certification, and credentialing; specialty practices; evaluating the effectiveness of case management programs; and legal and ethical obligations.

This third edition of the Core Curriculum expands on the original content and includes new materials, particularly in the areas of practice and ethical standards as they relate to both the general practice and the use of social and digital media; accreditation in case management; professional obligations toward advancing the practice and dissemination of innovations and new knowledge; impact of the Patient Protection and Affordable Care Act on case management practice; value-based purchasing; and primary care and patient-centered medical homes. This additional information is necessary to keep case managers informed about the current state of case management practice and to arm them with the skills, knowledge, and competencies needed for effective delivery of case management services and to meet the increasingly complex demands of our health care system.

It is important to note that what is interesting about this new edition of the Core Curriculum is the integration of CMSA's Standards of Practice for Case Management with an overview in a new introductory chapter and at the beginning of each of the remaining chapters thereafter. We believe this feature adds special value to the Core Curriculum and makes it easier for case managers to apply the standards in their daily practice.

The Core Curriculum is written in an outline format in order to emphasize important information with which a case manager must be familiar in order to ground his/her professional practice. Graphs, tables, boxes, figures, and examples are provided to further highlight useful information for use to enhance one's performance competence and reduce the burden of locating such materials for the ever busy case manager. The broad scope of case management issues presented serves as a teaching tool and reference guide for:

- Clarification of key terms and their relatedness to case management practice (e.g., care management, case management, care coordination)
- Development of degree-granting case management educational programs
- Orientation and training of case managers within an organization or a facility and practice setting
- Preparation (review materials) for case management certification examinations
- Self-study when beginning a "new" case management career or if curious about pursuing one
- Case management program/model design or re-design
- Development of job descriptions, performance appraisals, and essential competencies for case managers
- Evaluation of effectiveness (or return on investment) of case management programs and models
- Value proposition and demonstration
- Adherence to expected practice, ethical, and legal standards

Case management is an important solution to a major economic and humanitarian problem. It will continue to grow in importance, because it works! Current research-based evidence supports it and demonstrates its value. The Core Curriculum reflects the most up-to-date knowledge in case management practice and prevents case managers from having to learn their role solely by "trial and error" on-the-job. It is a "go to" resource for the practicing case manager, the case management executive, the academician, the quality and outcomes management specialist, the provider ultimately responsible for patient care, and others directly or indirectly involved in this practice. It is also a "go to" resource for the various health care professionals across the diverse care settings of our continuum of health and human services, whether a provider, payer, employer, regulator, accreditation agency representative, or consumer.

Hussein M. Tahan
Teresa M. Treiger

Acknowledgments

We, the editors, would like to thank the contributors and reviewers who dedicated so much of their time and expertise to this important work. Your passion for case management practice and devotion for ongoing development of the health care professionals involved is evident in your work. We thank you!

We also would like to thank the Board of Directors of the Case Management Society of America, Executive Director Cheri Lattimer, and President Kathleen Fraser for all of their support, feedback, and encouragement throughout the writing process and for putting their faith in us and our abilities. You are truly a group of special individuals who shared their knowledge for the growth of the case management profession and for the good of health care.

Last, but certainly not least, we would like to thank Executive Editor Shannon Magee and the Wolters Kluwer team for all of their support and guidance during this project. Thank you!

Hussein M. Tahan
Teresa M. Treiger

Contents

Contributors vi
Reviewers viii
Foreword ix
Preface xi
Acknowledgments xiv

SECTION

The Foundation of Case Management Practice

CHAPTER 1

Introduction to the CMSA Core Curriculum for Case Management 2
Hussein M. Tahan
Introduction 3
Descriptions of Key Terms 4
Applicability of the Core Curriculum to CMSA's Standards of Practice for
    Case Management 6
Historical Perspective on CMSA's Standards of Practice for Case
    Management 7
Select Definitions of Case Management 10
Philosophy of Case Management 13
Guiding Principles of Case Management 15
The Case Management Team 18

CHAPTER 2

History and Evolution of Case Management 21
Sandra L. Lowery and Teresa M. Treiger
Introduction 22
Descriptions of Key Terms 24
Applicability to CMSA'S Standards of Practice 26
Factors for the Rapid Growth of Case Management 26
Professional Development of Case Management Practice 28
Purposes and Goals of Case Management 31
Philosophical Tenets of Case Management 32
Case Management Knowledge Domains 33
Case Management Target Populations 33
Case Management Versus Other Job Titles 33

CHAPTER 3

Health Care Insurance, Benefits, and Reimbursement Systems   36

Beverly Cunningham
Introduction   37
Descriptions of Key Terms   38
Applicability to CMSA's Standards of Practice   40
Driving Forces Behind Health Care Reimbursement Systems   41
Types of Insurance   43
Components of Health Care Reimbursement   46
Health Care Delivery Systems   50
Reimbursement Methods   51
Challenges with Health Care Reimbursement   54
Legal Issues Impacting Managed Care   54
Strategies in Managed Care   55
Compliance Considerations for Case Managers   56
Reimbursement Implications for Case Managers   58

CHAPTER 4

Case Management Practice Settings   61

Hussein M. Tahan
Introduction   62
Descriptions of Key Terms   64
Applicability to CMSA's Standards of Practice   66
Case Management Practice Settings   67
Telephonic Case Management   70
Case Management in the Payer-Based Settings or Insurance Companies   73
Case Management in the Community Care Setting   76
Case Management in the Ambulatory Clinic and Outpatient Care
    Setting   77
Case Management in the Patient-Centered Medical Home Care Setting   78
Case Management in the Admitting Department   79
Case Management in the Perioperative Services   82
Independent/Private Case Management   84
Case Management in the Emergency Department   86
Patient Flow, Throughput, and Case Management   88
Transitions of Care and Case Management   93
Role of the Case Manager in Patient Safety and Prevention of
    Medical Errors During Transitions   95

SECTION 2

Case Management and the Health Care Continuum

CHAPTER 5

Case Management in the Acute Care Setting   100

Stefani Daniels
Introduction   101
Descriptions of Key Terms   102
Applicability to CMSA's Standards of Practice   103

Background/Historical Perspective   104
Distinguishing the Hospital Venue   104
Physician Partnerships   106
Designing a Case Management Model for Your Hospital   107
Case Management Program Infrastructure   110
Workflow   113
Program Operations   119
Outcomes   123

CHAPTER   6

Case Management in the Community and Postacute Care Settings   126

Hussein M. Tahan

Introduction   127
Descriptions of Key Terms   130
Applicability to CMSA's Standards of Practice   133
Federally Qualified Health Centers   134
Patient-Centered Medical Home   136
Accountable Care Organizations   139
Roles of Case Managers in FQHCs, PCMHs, and ACOs   142
Long-Term Care   143
Rehabilitation Levels of Care   146
Rehabilitation Services in Non–Inpatient Care Settings   152
Nonmedical Levels of Care   156
Respite Care   159
Financial Aspects of Long-Term and Rehabilitation Care Settings   161
Case Management Roles in Long-Term and Acute Rehabilitation Care
    Settings   162
Resources for the Care of the Elderly   165
The Geriatric and Older Adult Patient   165
Identification of High-Risk Geriatric Patients   172
Comprehensive Geriatric Assessment   174
Geriatric Assessment for Placement of the Geriatric Patient   175

CHAPTER   7

Case Management in the Home Care Setting   178

Hussein M. Tahan

Introduction   179
Descriptions of Key Terms   181
Applicability to CMSA's Standards of Practice   182
The Role of the Hospital-Based Interdisciplinary Health
    Care Team   182
Home Health Care Visits   184
Reimbursement for Home Health Care Services   187
Home Care Nursing Services   188
Home Care Rehabilitation Services   189
Durable Medical Equipment and Other Services   190
Home Care Social Work Services   191

The Role of the Hospital-Based Case Manager   192
The Role of the Community-Based Case Manager   193
Savings, Safety, and Satisfaction   194

CHAPTER 8
Case Management in the Palliative and Hospice Care Settings   195
Hussein M. Tahan
Introduction   196
Descriptions of Key Terms   197
Applicability to CMSA's Standards of Practice   198
Palliative Care   199
Hospice Care   201
Guiding Principles and Goals of Palliative and Hospice Care
    Programs   206
Scope of Palliative and Hospice Care and Services   208
Advance Directives and Health Care Proxies   209
Case Management Services in Palliative and Hospice Care Programs   211

CHAPTER 9
Case Management in the Remote and Rural Care Settings   214
Marietta P. Stanton
Introduction   215
Descriptions of Key Terms   217
Applicability to CMSA's Standards of Practice   218
Understanding Designation of Areas Within United States   219
Rural Culture Health Care Considerations   223
Rural Case Management Programs and Services   225
Behavioral Health Care in Rural Areas   229
The Patient Protection and Affordable Care Act and Rural Case
    Management   230

CHAPTER 10
Transitional Care and Case Management   244
Cheri Lattimer
Introduction   245
Applicability to CMSA's Standards of Practice   245
Descriptions of Key Terms   246
NTOCC Care Transitions Bundle: Seven Essential Intervention
    Categories   250
Legislative and Regulatory Considerations Pertaining to Transitions of
    Care   252
Transition of Care Models and Delivery Systems   254
Transitions of Care and Implications for Case Management Practice   257
Roles and Functions Associated with Transitions of Care   257
Reimbursement Issues   261
Certification and Accreditation in Transitions of Care   262

SECTION ③

Roles, Functions, and Essential Practice Considerations for Case Managers

CHAPTER 11

The Roles, Functions, and Activities of Case Management   268

Hussein M. Tahan
Introduction   269
Descriptions of Key Terms   269
Applicability to CMSA'S Standards of Practice   270
Background   272
Case Management Roles   275
Case Management Functions and Activities   278
Case Management Knowledge for Practice and Qualifications   283
Case Management Knowledge and Skills According to the American Nurses
   Credentialing Center   288
Conclusion   290

CHAPTER 12

The Case Management Process   292

Hussein M. Tahan
Introduction   293
Descriptions of Key Terms   295
Applicability to CMSA's Standards of Practice   296
Steps of the Case Management Process   297
Special Actions Occurring Throughout the Case Management
   Process   309

CHAPTER 13

Transitional Planning and Transitions of Care   312

Jackie Birmingham
Introduction   313
Descriptions of Key Terms   314
Applicability to CMSA's Standards of Practice   317
Transitional Planning as it Relates to Continuity of Care   318
Federal Conditions of Participation that Influence Transitional
   Care From Acute Care Hospitals   321
Other Selected Federal Rules that have Significance in Transition
   Planning   323
Factors that Impact Case Management in Cross-Setting
   Measures   327
Selected Levels of Care to Which Inpatients are Referred   329
The Role of the Case Manager in the Process of Transitional
   Planning   337
Value-Based Purchasing and Impact on Transition Management
   and Readmissions   341
Case Manager and Managing Care Transitions   343

CHAPTER 14

Resource and Utilization Management   349
Michael B. Garrett and Teresa M. Treiger
Introduction   350
Descriptions of Key Terms   350
Applicability to CMSA'S Standards of Practice   353
UM Program and Process   354
UM Team   356
Certifications Related to UM and UR   357
UM Criteria and Strategies   357
UM Clinical Review Criteria and Guidelines   357
Focused UM   358
Denials of Admissions and Services   358
Adverse Review Determination   359
Medical Review Outcomes   359
Appeal Process   360
UM Performance Reporting   363
Key Regulatory and Accreditation Bodies Associated with the UM
    Process   363
UM Regulatory and Accreditation Processes   364
Certification Programs in UR or UM   365

CHAPTER 15

Case Management and Use of Technology   367
Teresa M. Treiger
Introduction   368
Descriptions of Key Terms   369
Applicability to CMSA'S Standards of Practice   371
Health Information Technology and Case Management Information
    Systems   372
Goals, Benefits, and Limitations of Case Management Information System
    (CMIS)   374
CMIS and Case Management Informatics in Support of Consistency and
    Standards of Care   379
Using CMIS to Measure Effectiveness of Case Management
    Intervention   383
The Evolution and Delivery of Telehealth Interventions   383
Telehealth Legislation   385
Barriers to Telehealth   386
Evaluation of Web Sites for Professional and Patient Use   388
HIT Solutions in Support of Case Management   389

CHAPTER 16

Case Manager's Role Leadership and Accountability   392
Suzanne K. Powell and Hussein M. Tahan
Introduction   393
Descriptions of Key Terms   394
Applicability to CMSA's Standards of Practice   395
Accountability   396

Leadership Styles   397
Leadership Skills   400
Negotiation Skills   401
Delegation Skills   403
Communication Skills for Quality and Patient Safety   404
Critical Thinking and Decision-Making   406
The Ethics of Decision-Making   407
Financial/Cost–Benefit Analysis   408
Case Management Outcomes in the Supervisory Role   410
Case Managers as Change Agents   411
Case Managers and Motivational Interviewing   413

C H A P T E R   17

Professional Development, Certification, and Accreditation in Case Management   418

Marietta P. Stanton and Hussein M. Tahan

Introduction   419
Descriptions of Key Terms   420
Applicability to CMSA's Standards of Practice   421
Education and Training of Case Managers   422
Consensus Areas for Case Management Education: Core Components   425
Approaches to Case Management Education and Training   429
Credentialing in Case Management   431
Overview of Certification in Case Management   434
Select Certifications in Case Management   436
URAC Accreditation of Organizations Performing Case Management   443
NCQA Accreditation in Case Management   449
Differentiating Individual from Organizational Certification   452

S E C T I O N   4

Professional Obligations in Case Management

C H A P T E R   18

Ethics and General Case Management Practice   456

John D. Banja

Introduction   457
Descriptions of Key Terms   458
Applicability to CMSA's Standards of Practice   460
Ethical Decision Making and the Case Manager   460
Ethical Theories   462
Ethical Principles and Decision Making   462
Ethical Responsibilities Particularly Affecting Case Managers   466
Strategies for Maintaining Ethical Behavior   467

C H A P T E R   19

Ethical Use of Case Management Technology   471

Ellen Fink-Samnick

Introduction   472

Descriptions of Key Terms   473
Applicability to CMSA'S Standards of Practice   476
Transition in Modes of Patient and Professional Interaction   476
Electronic Communication   478
Social Media   479
To Where Should Your Ethical Compass Point?   483

CHAPTER 20

Legal Considerations in Case Management   491

Lynn S. Muller
Introduction   492
Descriptions of Key Terms   492
Applicability to CMSA'S Standards of Practice   495
Background   496
Regulatory Compliance   504
Contracts   506
The Case Manager and the Legal Community   508
Frequently Asked Questions   511

CHAPTER 21

Use of Effective Case Management Plans   520

Mary Jane McKendry and Teresa M. Treiger
Introduction   521
Descriptions of Key Terms   523
Applicability to CMSA'S Standards of Practice   525
Case Management Care Planning and Plans of Care   525
Case Management Plan Development Begins with Patient
    Assessment   527
Case Management Plan Development—Data Gathering Format   531
Case Management Plan Development Strategies   532
Problem List Identification   535
Case Management Plan Implementation   536
Incorporating Evidence-Based Guidelines in Case Management
    Practice   537
Clinical Pathways   540
Algorithms   541
Evidence-based Decision Support Criteria   542
Benefits of Case Management Plans   542
Case Management and Utilization Management   543

CHAPTER 22

Quality and Outcomes Management in Case Management   547

Michael B. Garrett and Teresa M. Treiger
Introduction   548
Descriptions of Key Terms   550
Applicability to CMSA's Standards of Practice   552
Defining Outcomes Management and Measurement   553
Rationale for Outcomes Management   555
Characteristics of Effective Outcome Measures   556

Outcome Measures Selection and Development   559
Case Management–Specific Outcomes   563
Incorporating Outcomes Measurement into Case Management
   Practice   566
Common Issues in Outcomes Reporting   568

SECTION

Select Specialty Practices in Case Management

CHAPTER 23
Behavioral Health and Integrated Case Management   572
Rebecca Perez and Deborah Gutteridge
Introduction   573
Descriptions of Key Terms   574
Behavioral Health Case Management Models   575
Applicability to CMSA'S Standards of Practice   577
Behavioral Health Care Conditions and Implications for Case
   Management   577
Challenges in Behavioral Health Case Management   589
Treatment Settings and Behavioral Health Case Management   592
Roles and Functions of the Behavioral Health Case Manager   595
How Psychological Factors Impact Medical Conditions
   and Integrated Care Management   595
Reimbursement Issues   596
Integrated Case Management   597
Appendix A—Suicide Practice Protocol   600
Appendix B—Case Management Approaches for Patients with
   Low Self-Care States   600

CHAPTER 24
Workers' Compensation Case Management   605
Hussein M. Tahan and Kathleen Fraser
Introduction   606
Descriptions of Key Terms   607
Applicability to CMSA's Standards of Practice   609
Primary Goals of Workers' Compensation Programs   609
Understanding the Impact of Workers' Compensation Costs   609
Fitting the Pieces Together: Medical Case Management in the Workers'
   Compensation System   611
Key Stakeholders in Workers' Compensation   611
Workers' Compensation Laws That Directly Affect Case Management
   Practice   613
Practicing the Case Management Process Within the Workers'
   Compensation System   615
Requirements for Workers' Compensation Case Managers Roles and
   Employment Settings   619

Scope of Medical Management in Workers' Compensation
    Settings   620
Applying the Case Management Process   621
Workers' Compensation Referrals for Return to Work   628
Ethical Considerations for Workers' Compensation Case Managers   632
Legal Issues for the Workers' Compensation Case Manager   634
Trends in Workers' Compensation Case Management   635
Medical Cost Containment Programs   635
Federal Laws Affecting Workers' Compensation Case Management   636
Documenting Quality of Services Using Outcome Measurements   637

CHAPTER 25

Disability and Occupational Health Case Management   639

Karen N. Provine

Introduction   640
Descriptions of Key Terms   641
Applicability to CMSA's Standards of Practice   645
Perspectives on Disability   646
Components of Disability Case Management Programs   647
Challenges to Disability Case Management   649
The Americans with Disabilities Act (ADA)   650
Resources for Disability Case Management Programs   654
Integrated Disability Case Management Strategies   655
Occupational Health Case Management   656
Role of OH Case Managers   656
Key Concepts of OH Case Management   658
Success Factors for OH Case Management Programs   660
Maximizing Workforce Health and Productivity   664
Models of OH Case Management   665
The Knowledge Base Required for OH and Disability Case
    Managers   668
Return-to-Work Programs   670

CHAPTER 26

Life Care Planning and Case Management   672

Hussein M. Tahan

Introduction   673
Descriptions of Key Terms   675
Applicability to CMSA'S Standards of Practice   675
Aims of Life Care Planning   676
The Process of Life Care Planning   677
Role of the Case Manager as a Life Care Planner   678
The Life Care Plan   681
Development of the Life Care Plan   686
Components of the Life Care Plan   688
Medicare Set Asides: a Life Care Planning Specialty   689
Health and Disability Insurance   691

CHAPTER 27

Suggested Resources and Readings in Case Management   692
Teresa M. Treiger and Hussein M. Tahan

Introduction   692
Descriptions of Key Terms   694
Applicability to CMSA's Standards of Practice   695
Case Management Standards of Practice   696
Case Management Textbooks   696
Case Management Journals   698
History and Evolution of Case Management   698
Healthcare Benefits, Payment, and Reimbursement Systems   699
Case Management Practice Settings and Throughput   700
Case Management in the Acute Care Setting   700
Case Management in the Community and Postacute Care Settings   701
Case Management in the Home Care Setting   701
Case Management in Palliative and Hospice Care Settings   702
Case Management in Remote and Rural Care Settings   702
Case Management and Transitional Care   703
The Roles, Functions, and Activities of Case Management   703
The Case Management Process   704
Transitions of Care and Case Management Practice   704
Resource and Utilization Management   705
Case Management and Use of Technology   705
Case Manager's Role Leadership and Accountability   706
Certification and Accreditation in Case Management   707
Professional Development and Academic Programs in Case
   Management   708
Ethics and General Case Management Practice   709
Ethical Use of Case Management Technology   709
Legal Considerations in Case Management   710
Use of Effective Case Management Plans   710
Quality and Outcomes Management in Case Management Practice   711
Behavioral Health, Substance Use, and Integrated Case Management   712
Workers' Compensation Case Management   712
Disability and Occupational Health Case Management   713
Life Care Planning and Case Management   713

Index   715

The Foundation of Case Management Practice

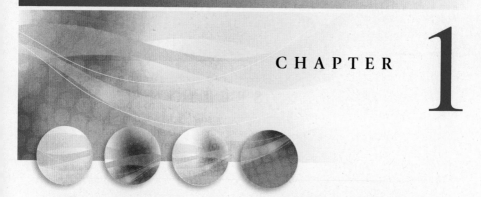

CHAPTER

1

Introduction to the CMSA Core Curriculum for Case Management

Hussein M. Tahan

LEARNING OBJECTIVES

Upon completion of this chapter, the reader will be able to:

1. Describe the relationship between the Core Curriculum for Case Management and the standards of practice of the Case Management Society of America (CMSA).

2. Define case management.

3. Discuss the philosophy and guiding principles of case management according to the Case Management Society of America.

4. Explain the history of the Case Management Society of America's Standards of Practice for Case Management.

5. Describe the meaning of key terms used in the Core Curriculum and CMSA's Standards of Practice for Case Management.

IMPORTANT TERMS AND CONCEPTS

Care Coordination
Care Management
Care Manager
Care Setting
Care Management
Case Management
   Process
Case Manager

Client
Client's Support
   System
Core Curriculum
Guiding Principles
Level of Care
Payer
Philosophy

Philosophy of Case
   Management
Practice Setting
Standards of Practice
Transitions of Care
Work Setting

Introduction

A. The Core Curriculum is written in the format and style of a "detailed topical outline." It highlights current and salient practices and knowledge areas of case management that are useful for all case managers or health care professionals, including those who:
   1. Are new to the field of case management
   2. Have been practicing case management for some time
   3. Are interested in becoming case managers
   4. Interact or collaborate with case managers
B. Similar to the CMSA's Standards of Practice, some adjustments to the content of the Core Curriculum may be necessary before application or incorporation into individual practices or care settings. This may mean using practice setting– or specialty-specific terms instead of the generic ones. For example, in skilled care facilities or nursing homes, the term "resident" may be used instead of "client" or "patient." However, in this Core Curriculum, "client" and "patient" are used as generic reference to the individual receiving health care or case-managed services.
C. Since the terms "client" and/or "patient" do not apply in every setting across the continuum of health and human services, changing the term to another more appropriate is warranted. One may choose to replace the term client and/or patient with:
   1. Resident in skilled care facilities
   2. Consumer in any setting, especially community based
   3. Beneficiary or member in payer-based organizations or health insurance plans
   4. Individual in health and wellness settings
D. The Core Curriculum is intended for voluntary use. It does not replace one's judgment; the relevant legal, ethical, or professional practice requirements; or the policies, procedures, and standards of the organizations where case managers practice.
E. Although it is a helpful resource for preparing for case management certification examinations, the Core Curriculum is not intended as a certification review textbook. Case management professionals are advised to use additional review materials when preparing for certification.
F. The Core Curriculum describes case management programs and models and roles and responsibilities of case managers in the diverse care/practice settings across the continuum of health and human services and the various professional disciplines of those who assume these roles.
G. The Core Curriculum consists of materials that are both directly and indirectly related to the practice of case management.
   1. Examples of directly related materials are descriptions of the roles and functions of case managers, case management models and programs, and transitions of care.
   2. Examples of indirectly related materials are content that pertains to quality and performance improvement, laws and regulations, and ethical standards.
H. Each chapter includes descriptions of some key terms cited in the chapter. These descriptions reflect the way the terms are used in the chapter. They are not necessarily standardized or nationally recognized in the industry;

however, they may be used to establish wide agreement. The descriptions do not necessarily form a glossary of terms. Readers are advised to use their judgment when applying these terms into own practice.

I. Two features are shared at the end of the Core Curriculum. These are as follows:

    1. A list of suggested additional readings; other available materials that may be of interest to case management professionals. These readings are not exhaustive of the available knowledge.

    2. A list of key Web sites and their URL addresses presented by topic. The Web site is cited once and placed in the topic where it is thought to best fit; however, most of the Web sites are of multiple purposes and may belong in more than one category. Similar to the suggested readings, the list of the Web sites is not exhaustive.

J. The Core Curriculum applies certain terms in a generic manner and to refer to other similar terms sometimes used interchangeably in the literature and by health care professionals. For example:

    1. Client also refers to patient, consumer, beneficiary, member, or resident—the recipient of health care services.

    2. Case management also refers to care management, care coordination, and transitional care.

    3. Support system also refers to the client's family member, next of kin, caregiver, health care proxy, or the individual with power of attorney or officially designated by the client to speak on his/her behalf.

    4. Case manager also refers to care manager, care coordinator, transitional care professional, or discharge planner.

    5. Care setting also refers to work setting, practice setting, level of care, case manager's employer, or place where a client accesses health care services.

    6. Health care provider also refers to the individual, agency, or organization responsible to provide care to a client.

    7. Interdisciplinary health care team also refers to multidisciplinary, transdisciplinary, pandisciplinary, interprofessional, and patient-centered health care team.

Descriptions of Key Terms

A. Care Coordination—The deliberate organization of patient care activities between two or more participants (including the patient) involved in a patient's care to facilitate the appropriate delivery of health care services. Organizing care involves the marshaling of personnel and other resources needed to carry out all required patient care activities and is often managed by the exchange of information among participants responsible for different aspects of care (AHRQ, 2007).

B. Care Setting—(Also referred to as *practice site*, practice *setting*, or *work setting*.) The organization or agency at which case managers are employed and execute their roles and responsibilities. The practice of case management extends across all settings of the health and human service continuum. These may include but are not limited to payer, provider, government, employer, community, independent/private, workers' compensation, or a client's home environment.

C. Case Management—"A collaborative process of assessment, planning, facilitation, care coordination, evaluation, and advocacy for options and services to facilitate an individual's and family's comprehensive health needs through communication and available resources to promote quality cost-effective outcomes" (CMSA, 2010, p. 24).

D. Case Manager—(Also referred to as care manager or care coordinator.) The health and human service professional responsible for coordinating and managing the overall care delivered to an individual client or a group of clients. Case manager ensures that care provided is based on the client's health or human service needs, issues, preferences, and interests.

E. Case Management Process—The process through which case management services are offered and case/care managers provide health and human services to clients/support systems. This consists of several phases that are iterative, cyclical, and recursive rather than linear. The phases are applied until clients' needs and interests are met. They may include assessment, problem identification, outcomes identification, planning, implementation (facilitation, advocacy, and coordination), monitoring, evaluation, and follow-up.

F. Client—The recipient of case management and health and human services. "This individual can be a patient, beneficiary, injured worker, claimant, enrollee, member, college student, resident, or health care consumer of any age group." Client can also mean something very different than the end user of case management services. It may "imply the business relationship with a company who contracts, [or pays], for case management services" (CMSA, 2010, p. 24).

G. Client's Support System—Recipients of case management interventions, other than the client. The person or persons identified by each individual client to be directly or indirectly involved in the client's care. This "may include biological relatives [family members], spouses, partners, friends, neighbors, colleagues, or any individual who supports the client [caregivers, volunteers, and clergy or spiritual advisors]" (CMSA, 2010, p. 24).

H. Core Curriculum—An organized package of courses, topics, materials, or areas of content reflective of a particular subject, specialty, or professional practice. These make the essential subject matter and knowledge a professional (e.g., case manager) must possess, or maintain familiarity with, to effectively perform in an area of specialty (e.g., case management).

I. Guiding Principles—Are important concepts or characteristics used to clarify practice and communicate its primary focus and boundaries. They promote a better understanding of the purpose, core values, and objectives of a practice.

J. Level of Care—The intensity and effort of health and human services and care activities required to diagnose, treat, preserve, or maintain a client's health. Level of care may vary from least to most complex, least to most intense, or prevention and wellness to acute care and services.

K. Payer—The person, agency, entity, or organization that assumes responsibility for funding the health and human services and resources consumed by a client while cared for because of an existing health condition or routine checkups and prevention. The payer may be the client himself/herself, a member of the client's support system, an employer, a government benefit program (e.g., Medicare, Medicaid, Tricare), a commercial insurance agency, or a charitable organization.

L. Philosophy—Is a statement of belief that sets forth principles to guide a program and/or an individual in his/her practice of that program.

M. Philosophy of Case Management—Is a statement or belief that sets forth an organization's or individual's practice with special focus on case-managed health care delivery to clients and their support systems or other customers such as employers, payers, regulators, and/or accreditation agencies.

N. Standards of Practice—Authoritative statements agreed upon and recognized by health care professionals and professional organizations and associations as best or ideal practices. Usually based on evidence and assure quality and safe care.

O. Transitions of Care—Is the movement of a client from one health care provider or setting to another as the client's health condition and care needs change. During transitions, case managers facilitate and coordinate care activities and assure that transitioning clients receive the required services to enhance continuity of care and promote safety. Sometimes referred to as care transitions or transitional care (CMSA, 2010).

 ## Applicability of the Core Curriculum to CMSA's Standards of Practice for Case Management

A. The Case Management Society of America (CMSA) developed the Standards of Practice for Case Management to describe the important and current aspects of case management practice. CMSA states that case management today extends across all health care settings (e.g., payer/health insurance plans, providers, government, employers, community, home) and professional disciplines (e.g., nursing, social work, vocational rehabilitation counseling, workers' compensation, disability management, pharmacy).

B. The Core Curriculum for Case Management uses the CMSA Standards of Practice for Case Management as a guide for the essential topics and areas it addresses. It also explains these topics in a way that reflects CMSA's philosophy and guiding principles of case management practice, available knowledge based on published literature, and the opinions of the editors, contributors, and other experts in the field.

C. In the chapters where appropriate, specific content from the CMSA Standards of Practice for Case Management is presented to provide the reader with better understanding of the Core Curriculum and its relevance to case management practice while promoting the standards.

D. The Core Curriculum for Case Management reflects the general and common practice of case management.

  1. It discusses how the practice may vary from one care setting to another (i.e., levels of care) along the continuum of health and human services.

  2. It also explains how the focus of the case manager's role is affected by the professional discipline and background of the person in the role. This is necessary since scopes of practice vary based on the discipline.

  3. Users of the Core Curriculum must consider the differences the care setting and professional discipline impose when they attempt to implement the Core Curriculum's content into the case management programs in their organizations. Individualizing the content where needed before its application into practice is advised.

    a. For example, the Core Curriculum uses the terms "client" and "patient" interchangeably and as generic terms to refer to the recipient of health and human services. These terms are not necessarily used across the various health care settings and organizations.

    b. In health insurance plans, the term "beneficiary" or "enrollee" may be used instead of "client" or "patient."

    c. In workers' compensation arena, the term "injured worker" may be used instead of "patient" or "client."

Historical Perspective on CMSA's Standards of Practice for Case Management

A. The Case Management Society of America (CMSA) first introduced its nationally recognized Standards of Practice for Case Management in 1995. It then revised them in 2002 and most recently in 2010. The revisions were necessary to ensure the standards continue to be current, relevant, and substantiated by the latest changes in the knowledge and practices of case management. The 2010 standards:

    1. Provide voluntary practice guidelines for the case management industry. The Standards of Practice are intended to identify and address important foundational knowledge and skills of the case manager within a spectrum of case management practice settings and specialties.

    2. Reflect many recent changes in the industry, which resonate with current practice today. Some of these changes include, but not limited to, the following:

        a. Minimizing fragmentation in the health care system

        b. Use of evidence-based guidelines in practice

        c. Navigating transitions of care

        d. Incorporating adherence guidelines and other standardized practice tools

        e. Expanding the interdisciplinary health care team in planning care for individuals

        f. Improving care quality and patient safety

    3. Contain information about case management practice, including definition, practice settings, roles, functions, activities, case management process, philosophy, and guiding principles, as well as the standards and how they are demonstrated (CMSA, 2010).

B. The Standards of Practice are intended for voluntary use. They do not replace relevant legal, ethical, or professional practice requirements. CMSA explains that the Standards of Practice for Case Management:

    1. Are offered to standardize the process of case management

    2. Are intended to be realistically attainable by individuals who use appropriate and professional judgment regarding the delivery of case management services to targeted client populations

    3. Present a portrait of the scope of case management practice to both health care consumers and professionals who work in partnership with the case managers

C. A team of case management experts developed the CMSA Standards of Practice. The team included:

    1. A core group of representatives of the case management field from various practice settings and disciplines

    2. A larger reference group that included the CMSA leadership and Board of Directors and legal advisors

    3. Other key representatives of the case management industry

    4. Case managers at large during the public comment period and before the standards were finalized and adopted (CMSA, 2010)

D. Founded in 1990, CMSA is the leading international, nonprofit, interdisciplinary health care association dedicated to the support and development of the profession of case management through educational forums, networking opportunities, and legislative involvement (CMSA, 2015).

E. In its mission, CMSA explains that:

    1. It provides "professional collaboration across the healthcare continuum to advocate for patients' well-being and improved health outcomes through:

        a. Fostering case management growth and development,

        b. Impacting health care policy, and

        c. Providing evidence-based tools and resources" (CMSA, 2015)

    2. Case or "care managers are advocates who help patients understand their current health status, what they can do about it and why those treatments are important. In this way, [case]/care managers are catalysts by guiding patients and providing cohesion to other professionals in the health care delivery team, enabling their clients [and support systems] to achieve goals more effectively and efficiently" (CMSA, 2015).

F. In its strategic vision, CMSA describes "case managers as recognized experts and vital participants in the care coordination team. They empower people to understand and access quality and efficient health care" (CMSA, 2015). Safety is subsumed under quality.

G. To complement the vision, case management practitioners, educators, and leaders have come together to reach consensus regarding the guiding principles and fundamental spirit of the practice of case management (CMSA, 2010).

H. Since the first version, which was published in 1995, the Standards of Practice for Case Management:

    1. Have been based on an understanding that case management is not a specific health care profession rather an advanced practice within the varied health care professions that serves as a foundation for case management

    2. Are not intended to be a structured recipe for the delivery of case management interventions; rather, they present a range of core functions, roles, responsibilities, and relationships that are integral to the practice of case management (CMSA, 2010)

I. The 1995 Standards of Practice for Case Management were recognized as a tool that case management would use within every case management practice arena. They were seen as a guide to move case management practice to excellence.

    1. The Standards explored the planning, monitoring, evaluating, and outcomes phases of case managers' practice, followed by Performance Standards for the practicing case manager.

    2. The Performance Standards addressed how the case manager worked within each of the established Standards and with other disciplines to follow all legal requirements.

BOX

1-1   Changes Evident in the 2002 Standards of Practice for Case Management

- A revision of the definition of case management
- Expansion of the section on Performance Indicators to further define the case manager
- Changes in the purpose of case management to address quality, safety, and cost-effective care as well as to focus upon facilitating appropriate access to care
- More emphasis on the application of the work of case managers to individual clients or to groups of clients, such as in disease management or population health models
- Adding more detail to the facilitation of care section highlighting the importance of communication and collaboration on behalf of the client and the payer
- Increasing the practice settings for case management to capture the evolution of, and the increase in, the number of venues in which case managers worked

From Case Management Society of America (CMSA). (2010). *CMSA standards of practice for case management*. Little Rock, AR: Author.

3. The standards development committee at the time recognized the importance of the case managers basing their individual practice on valid research findings. The committee encouraged case managers to participate in the research process, programs, and development of specific tools for the practice of case management. This was evidenced by key sections of the Standards that highlighted measurement criteria in the collaborative, ethical, and legal sections (CMSA, 2010).

J. In 2001, CMSA's Board of Directors identified the need for a careful and thorough review and, if appropriate, revision of the 1995 Standards of Practice for Case Management. The revised Standards were published in 2002. The new standards included the changes described in Box 1-1.

K. Primary case management functions in the 2002 Standards of Practice for Case Management include those listed in Box 1-2.

BOX

1-2   Primary Case Management Functions Included in the 2002 Standards of Practice for Case Management

- Positive relationship building
- Effective written/verbal communication
- Negotiation skills
- Knowledge of contractual and risk arrangements
- The importance of obtaining consent, confidentiality, and client privacy
- Attention to cultural competency
- Ability to effect change and perform ongoing evaluation
- Use of critical thinking and analysis
- Ability to plan and organize effectively
- Promote client autonomy and self-determination
- Knowledge of:
  - Funding sources
  - Health care services
  - Human behavior dynamics
  - Health care delivery and financing systems
  - Clinical standards and outcomes

From Case Management Society of America (CMSA). (2010). *CMSA standards of practice for case management*. Little Rock, AR: Author.

| BOX 1-3 | Key Areas of Influence in the 2010 Standards of Practice for Case Management |

- Addressing the total individual or client, inclusive of medical, psychosocial, behavioral, socioeconomic, and spiritual needs
- Collaborating efforts that focus upon moving the individual to self-care and self-management whenever possible
- Increasing involvement of the individual client, support system, and/or caregiver in the decision-making process especially regarding care options
- Minimizing fragmentation and duplication of care within the health care delivery system
- Using evidence-based guidelines, as available, in the daily practice of case management
- Focusing on transitions of care, which includes a complete transfer to the next care setting and provider that is effective, safe, timely, and complete
- Improving outcomes by using adherence guidelines, standardized tools, and proven processes to measure a client's understanding and acceptance of the proposed plans, his/her willingness to change, and his/her support to maintain health behavior change
- Expanding the interdisciplinary health care team to include clients and/or their identified support system, health care providers, including community-based and facility-based professionals (i.e., pharmacists, nurse practitioners, holistic care providers, etc.)
- Expanding the case management role to collaborate within one's practice setting to support adherence to regulatory and accreditation standards
- Moving clients to optimal levels of health and well-being
- Improving client safety and satisfaction or experience of care
- Improving medication reconciliation for a client through collaborative efforts with medical and other staff
- Improving adherence to the plan of care for the client, including medication adherence

From Case Management Society of America (CMSA). (2010). *CMSA standards of practice for case management*. Little Rock, AR: Author.

L. The 2010 Standards of Practice for Case Management include topics that influence the practice of case management in today's health care environment (Box 1-3).

M. The 2010 Standards of Practice for Case Management advance case management credibility and complement the current trends and changes in the health care environment. Box 1-4 presents the table of content of the 2010 standards.

N. CMSA expects that future case management Standards of Practice will likely reflect the existing climate of health care and build upon the evidence-based guidelines that are proven successful in the coming years.

Select Definitions of Case Management

A. According to CMSA, the basic concept of case management involves the timely coordination of quality services to address a client's specific needs in a cost-effective manner and in order to promote positive outcomes.

  1. Provision of case management services can occur in a single health care setting or during the client's transitions of care throughout the care continuum.

BOX

1-4   **Table of Content of CMSA's 2010 Standards of Practice for Case Management**

- Introduction
- Evolution of the Standards of Practice for Case Management
  - 1995 Standards of Practice for Case Management
  - 2002 Standards of Practice for Case Management
  - 2010 Standards of Practice for Case Management
- Definition of Case Management
- Philosophy and Guiding Principles
  - Statement of Philosophy
  - Guiding Principles
- Case Management Practice Settings
- Case Management Roles, Functions, and Activities
- Components of the Case Management Process
- Standards of Case Management Practice
  - Client Selection Process for Case Management
  - Client Assessment
  - Problem/Opportunity Identification
  - Planning
  - Monitoring
  - Outcomes
  - Termination of Case Management Services
  - Facilitation, Coordination, and Collaboration
  - Qualifications for Case Managers
  - Legal
    - Confidentiality and Client Privacy
    - Consent for Case Management Services
  - Ethics
  - Advocacy
  - Cultural Competency
  - Resource Management and Stewardship
  - Research and Research Utilization
- Acknowledgments
- Glossary of Important Terms
- References

From Case Management Society of America (CMSA). (2010). *CMSA standards of practice for case management.* Little Rock, AR: Author.

---

  2. The case manager serves as an important facilitator among the client, client's support system (e.g., family, friend, or caregiver), the health care team, the payer, and the community (CMSA, 2010).
B. The definition of case management has evolved over time; it reflects the vibrant and dynamic progression of the standards of practice. The 1995 Standards of Practice for Case Management included a definition of case management that was approved by CMSA's Board of Directors in 1993. The Board of Directors has repeatedly reviewed, analyzed, and revised the definition to ensure its continued application in the dynamic health care environment (Box 1-5). Italics highlight the changes CMSA made to its definition over time.
  1. The definition was modified in 2002 to reflect the process of case management outlined within the Standards.

BOX 1-5 Evolution of CMSA's Definitions of Case Management

1995
Case management is a collaborative process, *which assesses, plans, implements, coordinates, monitors, and evaluates* options and services to meet an individual's health needs through communication and available resources to promote quality cost-effective outcomes.

2002
Case management is a collaborative process of *assessment, planning, facilitation, and advocacy* for options and services to meet an individual's health needs through communication and available resources to promote quality cost-effective outcomes.

2010
Case management is a collaborative process of *assessment, planning, facilitation, care coordination, evaluation, and advocacy* for options and services to meet an individual's *and family's comprehensive* health needs through communication and available resources to promote quality cost-effective outcomes.

From Case Management Society of America (CMSA). (2010). *CMSA standards of practice for case management.* Little Rock, AR: Author.

BOX 1-6 Four Select Definitions of Case Management

Commission for Case Manager Certification (CCMC)
"Case management is a collaborative process that assesses, plans, implements, coordinates, monitors and evaluates options and services required to meet the client's health and human services' needs. It is characterized by advocacy, communication, and resource management and promotes quality and cost-effective interventions and outcomes" (CCMC, 2015, p. 3).

National Association of Social Workers (NASW)
"Case management is a process to plan, seek, advocate for, and monitor services from different social services or health care organizations and staff on behalf of the client. The process enables social workers in an organization, or in different organizations, to coordinate their efforts to serve a given client through professional teamwork, thus expanding the range of needed services offered. Case management limits problems arising from fragmentation of services, staff turnover, and inadequate coordination among providers. Case management can occur within a single, large organization, or within a community program that coordinates services among settings" (NASW, 2013, p. 13).

American Case Management Association (ACMA)
"Case Management in Hospital/Health Care Systems is a collaborative practice model including patients, nurses, social workers, physicians, other practitioners, caregivers and the community. The Case Management process encompasses communication and facilitates care along a continuum through effective resource coordination. The goals of Case Management include the achievement of optimal health, access to care and appropriate utilization of resources, balanced with the patient's right to self-determination" (ACMA, 2002).

URAC
"Case management is a collaborative process that helps consumers manage their comprehensive health needs through communication and available resources to promote quality, cost-effective outcomes. A health professional case manager assesses, plans, implements, coordinates, monitors, and evaluates options for consumers, their families, caregivers, and the health care team, including providers, to promote these outcomes" (URAC, 2015).

    2. The definition was revised in 2009 to further align with the practice of case management known at the time. This revision was then included in the 2010 Standards.

C. Other professional organizations and associations also define case management and contribute to its evolving and dynamic practice. There are more than 30 definitions of case management today. These are as diverse as the organizations that promote them, reflective of the organization's mission, vision, philosophy, and purpose. The increased popularity of case management has contributed to the rise in the number and diversity of the definitions. Four of these definitions are shared in Box 1-6.

Philosophy of Case Management

A. In its philosophy of case management, the CMSA explains that the underlying premise of case management is based in the fact that:
    1. When an individual reaches the optimum level of wellness and functional capability, everyone benefits: the individuals being served, their support systems, the health care delivery systems, and the various reimbursement sources.
    2. It serves as a means for achieving client wellness and autonomy through advocacy, communication, education, identification of service resources, and service facilitation.
    3. Services are best offered in a climate that allows direct communication between the case manager, the client, and appropriate service personnel, in order to optimize the outcome for all concerned (CMSA, 2010).

B. CMSA also underscores in the philosophy statement the recommendation that individuals, particularly those experiencing catastrophic injuries or severe chronic illnesses, be evaluated for case management services. The key philosophical components of case management then address care and services that:
    1. Are holistic and client centered
    2. Focus on the achievement of mutual goals (those of the client/support system and the provider)
    3. Allow stewardship of resources for the client and the health care system
    4. Promote the achievement of health and maintenance of wellness to the highest level possible for each client (CMSA, 2010)

C. It is CMSA's philosophy of case management that when health care is appropriately and efficiently provided, all involved parties or stakeholders benefit.
    1. The provision of case management includes working collaboratively with the health care team in complex situations to identify care options that are acceptable to the client.
    2. Collaborative and client-centered approach to care and services increases the client's adherence to the plan of care and achievement of successful outcomes.
    3. Case management services help prevent or reduce fragmentation of care, which is too often experienced by clients who obtain health care services from multiple providers.

4. The services offered by case managers can enhance client's safety, well-being, and quality of life, while reducing total health care costs. Thus, effective case management can directly and positively affect the health care delivery system (CMSA, 2010).

D. The Commission for Case Manager Certification (CCMC) in its philosophy describes case management as "an area of specialty practice within one's health and human services profession" (CCMC, 2015, p. 3).

E. Similar to CMSA, CCMC also shares the underlying premise that "everyone benefits when clients reach their optimum level of wellness, self-management, and functional capability…[those who benefit include the]:

1. Clients being served
2. Clients' support systems
3. Health care delivery systems and
4. Various payer sources" (CCMC, 2015, p. 3).

F. CCMC explains that case management "facilitates the achievement of client wellness and autonomy through:

1. Advocacy
2. Assessment
3. Planning
4. Communication
5. Education
6. Resource management and
7. Service facilitation" (CCMC, 2015, pp. 3–4).

G. As for case managers, CCMC describes them to play special roles in linking clients/support systems with appropriate providers and resources throughout the continuum of health and human services and care settings while collaborating with other health care providers and ensuring that the care provided meets the Institute of Medicine's recommendation for quality and safe care, that is, safe, effective, client centered, timely, efficient, and equitable (CCMC, 2015).

H. CCMC notes that case managers and other health care professionals may best optimize the services their clients/support systems receive if:

1. The services are offered in an environment that allows direct communication among case managers, clients, payers, primary care providers, and other service delivery professionals.
2. Case managers maintain client's privacy, confidentiality, health, and safety through adherence to ethical, legal accreditation and certification standards and guidelines (CCMC, 2015, p. 4).

I. Unlike CMSA's philosophy of case management, which does not directly discuss certification, CCMC emphasizes that certification in case management determines that a case manager possesses the education, skills, knowledge, and experience required to render appropriate services to clients and their support systems (CCMC, 2015).

J. The National Association of Social Workers (NASW) describes its views on case management in its 2013 standards for social work case management. However, it does not share them explicitly as a philosophy. Case management according to NASW is a "component of many social work jobs." It reports that "significant numbers of social workers…spend more than half of their time on case management" (NASW, 2013, p. 7). NASW explains that:

1. The social work profession is well trained to develop and improve support systems that advance the well-being of individuals, families, and communities.
2. Social workers have long recognized that the therapeutic relationship between the practitioner and the client plays an integral role in case management.
3. The expertise of social workers positions the profession as a leader within the field of case management.
4. Social work case managers operate across the public, nonprofit, and for-profit sectors, in both accredited and nonaccredited organizations, and in urban, suburban, rural, and frontier areas (NASW, 2013).

 ## Guiding Principles of Case Management

A. Guiding principles are important concepts or characteristics used to clarify practice and communicate its primary focus and boundaries. They promote a better understanding of the purpose, core values, and objectives of a practice.
B. CMSA's guiding principles for case management are relevant and meaningful concepts that clarify or guide the practice of case managers within the field and the environment of this practice. The guiding principles for case management practice as described in CMSA's 2010 Standards of Practice include those listed in Box 1-7.
C. The Commission for Case Manager Certification articulates a number of guiding principles for case management practice (Box 1-8). These are

---

BOX 1-7   CMSA's Guiding Principles for Case Management Practice

Case managers, according to CMSA:
- Use a client-centric, collaborative partnership approach.
- Whenever possible, facilitate self-determination and self-care through the tenets of advocacy, shared decision-making, and health instruction or education.
- Apply a comprehensive, holistic approach to care provision.
- Practice cultural competence, with awareness and respect for diversity.
- Promote the use of evidence-based care, as available.
- Promote quality and optimal client safety.
- Promote the integration of behavioral change, science, and principles in care provision.
- Link clients/support systems with community resources.
- Assist clients/support systems in navigating the health care environment to achieve successful care, for example, during transitions from one level of care or provider to another.
- Pursue professional excellence and maintain ongoing knowledge, skills, and competence in practice.
- Promote quality outcomes and measurement of those outcomes.
- Support and maintain adherence to rules and regulations of federal, state, and local governmental agencies and the standards of organizational, accreditation, and certification bodies.

From Case Management Society of America (CMSA). (2010). *CMSA standards of practice for case management.* Little Rock, AR: Author.

BOX 1-8   CCMC's Guiding Principles for Case Management Practice

- Case management:
  - Is not a profession; rather, it is a cross-disciplinary and interdependent specialty practice.
  - Is a means for improving clients' health and promoting wellness and autonomy through advocacy, communication, education, identification of resources, and facilitation of health care services.
  - Is guided by the ethical principles of autonomy, beneficence, nonmaleficence, and justice.
  - Is first and foremost focused on improving clients' clinical, functional, emotional, and psychosocial status (goals).
  - Helps clients achieve wellness and autonomy through advocacy, assessment, planning, communication, education, resource management, service facilitation, and use of evidence-based guidelines or standards.
  - Allows health care organizations to realize lowered health claim costs (if payer based), shorter lengths of stay (if acute care based), or early return to work and reduced absenteeism (if employer based).
  - Is optimized when services are offered in a climate that allows direct, open, and honest communication and collaboration among the case manager, the client/support system, the payer, the primary care provider (PCP), and all other service delivery professionals and paraprofessionals.
- Case managers:
  - Come from different backgrounds within health and human service professions including nursing, medicine, social work, rehabilitation counseling, workers' compensation, and mental and behavioral health.
  - Advocate for clients/support systems (primary function).
  - Understand the importance of achieving quality outcomes for their clients and commit to the appropriate use of resources and empowerment of clients in a manner that is supportive and objective.
  - Coordinate care that is safe, timely, effective, efficient, equitable, and client centered.
  - Approach the provision of case-managed health and human services in a collaborative manner.
  - Enhance the case management services and their associated outcomes by maintaining clients' privacy, confidentiality, health, and safety through advocacy and adherence to ethical, legal, accreditation, certification, and regulatory standards and guidelines, as appropriate to the practice setting.
  - Link clients/support systems with appropriate providers of care and resources throughout the continuum of health and human services and across various care settings.
  - Provide care according to the clients' benefits and as stipulated in their health insurance plans, and based on the cultural beliefs, values, and needs of clients/support systems, while collaborating with other service providers.
  - Possess the education, skills, knowledge, competencies, and experiences needed to effectively render appropriate, safe, and quality services to clients/support systems.
- The Case Management Process is:
  - Centered on clients and their support systems.
  - Holistic in its handling of clients' situations (e.g., addressing medical, physical, emotional, financial, psychosocial, behavioral, and other needs), as well as that of their support systems.
  - Adaptive to case managers' practice settings and the settings where clients receive health and human services.

From the Commission for Case Manager Certification (CCMC). *Case management body of knowledge: Case management knowledge, philosophy and guiding principles.* Mount Laurel, NJ. Retrieved from http://www.cmbodyofknowledge.com/content/case-management-knowledge-2, on July 22, 2015.

communicated through CCMC's Case Management Body of Knowledge (CMBOK), available as a Web portal. These guiding principles are presented here in three groups: case management, case managers, and the case management process.

D. The National Association of Social Workers is another professional organization that promotes the practice of case management. It describes a number of guiding principles for the practice of social work case management in its standards that were published in 2013 (Box 1-9).

BOX 1-9) NASW's Guiding Principles for Case Management Practice

- Goal of case management:
  - Optimize client functioning and well-being by providing and coordinating high-quality services, in the most effective and efficient manner possible, to individuals with multiple complex needs.
- Social work case managers focus their role on the following:
  - Strengthening the developmental, problem-solving, and coping capacities of clients.
  - Enhancing clients' ability to interact with and participate in their communities, with respect for each client's values and goals.
  - Linking people with systems that provide them with resources, services, and opportunities.
  - Increasing the scope and capacity of service delivery systems.
  - Creating and promoting the effective and humane operation of service systems.
  - Contributing to the development and improvement of social policy.
- Characteristics of social work case management:
  - Person-centered services—engaging the client in case management and tailoring services to meet the client's needs, preferences, and goals.
  - Primacy of client–social work case manager relationship—the therapeutic relationship integral to helping the client achieve her or his goals.
  - Person-in-environment framework—understanding that each individual experiences a mutually influential relationship with her or his physical and social environment and cannot be understood outside of that context.
  - Strengths perspective—eliciting, supporting, and building on the resilience and potential for growth and development inherent in each individual.
  - Collaborative teamwork—collaboration with other social workers, disciplines, and organizations is integral to the case management process.
  - Intervention at the micro-, mezzo-, and macro levels—applying a variety of approaches to effect change in individuals, families, groups, communities, organizations, systems, and policies. Advocacy for systemic change plays a key role.
- Core functions to social work case management are executed similar to the case management process:
  - Engagement with clients.
  - Assessment of client priorities, strengths, and challenges.
  - Development and implementation of a care plan.
  - Monitoring of service delivery.
  - Evaluation of outcomes.
  - Closure, including termination or transition follow-up.

From the National Association of Social Workers (NASW). (2013). *NASW standards for social work case management*. Washington, DC: Author.

The Case Management Team

A. Case management is an interdependent function or specialty practice. It cannot happen in isolation of the contributions of other health care professionals to patient/client care provision and patient experience. Thus, case management practice is a team approach. The team is there for the purpose of meeting the patient/client needs and preferences. Therefore, the case management team does not exist without the patient/client and client support system being part of it.

B. Case managers are constantly collaborating and coordinating client's care and services with other health care provider internal and external to the health care organization or care setting that employs them. Together, this is referred to as the case management team.
   1. Health care providers internal to the organization may include, but not limited to, physicians, registered nurses, social workers, physical, occupational and respiratory therapists, pharmacists, speech pathologists, support personnel (e.g., case management associate), discharge planners, utilization review specialists, and registered dietitians.
   2. Those external to the health care organization may include home care nurses, home health aides, and community health workers, in addition to the health care professionals listed above, but happen to be involved in the care of the client when in the community. The external team members may also include paraprofessionals whose involvement is transient and based on the client's needs. The paraprofessionals may include, but not limited to, medical transportation agencies, durable medical equipment vendors, charitable organizations, and clergy/chaplain.

C. Regardless of the type of case management team a health care organization may have, it is always important to include the client and client's support system as part of the team. In fact, the team exists because of the client and the team's goals are what the client/support system agrees upon. The team is then able to provide client-centered care.

D. Often, the case management team is referred to using different terminologies; however, the intent is usually the same, collaborative, client centered, and involves those from the various health disciplines and professions.
   1. The references may include interdisciplinary, multidisciplinary, pandisciplinary, transdisciplinary, interprofessional, and patient-centered health care team.
   2. To avoid confusion and misunderstandings, in the Core Curriculum, the term "interdisciplinary health care team" is used as a generic reference to the various terminologies that may be in use in the diverse care settings.

E. Case management requires the provision of comprehensive health services to clients by multiple health care professionals who work collaboratively to deliver the safest and best quality of care in every health care setting. Therefore, case management is a team effort.

F. The case management team consists of members from multiple health disciplines with diverse knowledge and skills who share an integrated set of goals and who apply interdependent collaboration that involves communication, sharing of knowledge, and coordination of services to provide services to patients/clients and their support systems or caregivers.

G. Being interdisciplinary, interprofessional, or client centered in case management is a means to achieve the Triple Aim of making care affordable, improving population health, and improving the client's experience of care. This plays an important role along the continuum of care, not only for those who live with complex health conditions and psychosocial problems but also to reduce duplication of services across professional silos and to prevent complications.

H. Care coordination helps ensure a patient's needs and preferences for care are understood and that those needs and preferences are shared among health care providers (both professionals and paraprofessionals), patients/clients, and families as the patient moves from one health care setting to another.

I. Teams and teamwork are buzzwords in today's health care organizations. A team may be defined as a small number of people with complementary skills who are committed to a common purpose, performance goals, and approach for which they hold themselves mutually accountable (Box 1-10).

J. There are factors that can influence interprofessional teamwork in health care settings and organizations vary. They may include:

1. *Individual factors*: These are characteristics of each of the health care team members and may consist of the skills of the people involved, the behaviors they model, the extent to which they believe in interdisciplinary teams, and the degree of their collaboration and communication.

BOX 1-10 **Characteristics of the Case Management Interdisciplinary Health Care Team**

- Team members provide care to a common group of patient/clients.
- Team members develop common goals for patient/client outcomes and work toward achieving these goals.
- Appropriate roles and functions are assigned to each member, and each member understands the roles of the other members.
- The team possesses a mechanism for sharing information and to oversee the carrying out of agreed upon plans of care and interventions, to assess outcomes, and to modify the plans based on the outcomes.
- Team members' primary focus is the needs of the patient/client rather than the individual contributions of the members (patient-centeredness).
- Team members engage in timely communication with patient/client, a central principle shared by all health professionals.
- Collaboration of team members requires both depending on others and contributing one's own ideas toward solving a common problem.
- Team members respect, understand roles, and recognize contributions of each other.
- Team members may be from both within and outside the health care organization where the patient/client is being cared for.
- Team outcomes and contributions are also individual outcomes and contributions; value is team based rather than team member specific despite the specialization of each of the members.

2. *Team factors*: These pertain to the evolution of the health care team, which is the stage of the team's development, the goals they set, and the outcomes they achieve.
3. *Organizational factors*: These relate to the practice environment and the extent the health care organization is supportive of team-based practice and what it does to assist the team's growth and development.
4. *Patient or client and support system factors*: These are the characteristics of the patient/client population served and their impact on the team. These also include the way the team members respond to the client/support system and the extent to which they embody client-centered care and practice.

K. Successful interdisciplinary case management teams are able to improve client/patient care experience and outcomes by increasing the coordination of services, integrating health care for the patient's wide range of health needs, and empowering patient/clients as active partners in care.

L. The collaborative team experience enables each health care provider on the interdisciplinary team to learn new skills and approaches to care, provides an environment for innovation, and allows each health care provider (including case manager) to focus on one's own individual areas of expertise and their contribution to the team. Collaboration and cooperation also foster an appreciation and understanding of other disciplines and backgrounds, maximize the potential for more efficient and cost-effective delivery of care, and enhance the appropriate allocation of resources and services.

References

Agency for Healthcare Research and Quality (AHRQ). (2007). Closing the quality gap: A critical analysis of quality improvement strategies. Publication No. 04(07)-0051-7, Volume 7—Care Coordination, June 2007.

American Case Management Association (ACMA). (2002). *Definition of case management*. Little Rock, AR: Author. Retrieved from http://www.acmaweb.org/section.aspx?sID=4, on July 21, 2015.

Case Management Society of America (CMSA). *CMSA's mission and vision*. Little Rock, AR: Author. Retrieved from http://www.cmsa.org/Home/CMSA/OurMissionVision/tabid/226/Default.aspx, on July 21, 2015.

Case Management Society of America (CMSA). (2010). *CMSA standards of practice for case management*. Little Rock, AR: Author.

Commission for Case Manager Certification (CCMC). (2015). *Certification guide to the CCM® examination*. Mount Laurel, NJ: Author.

Commission for Case Manager Certification (CCMC). Case management body of knowledge: Case management knowledge, philosophy and guiding principles. Mount Laurel, NJ. Retrieved from http://www.cmbodyofknowledge.com/content/case-management-knowledge-2, on July 22, 2015.

National Association of Social Workers (NASW). (2013). *NASW standards for social work case management*. Washington, DC: Author.

URAC. *Accreditation programs: Case management*. Washington, DC: Author. Retrieved from https://www.urac.org/accreditation-and-measurement/accreditation-programs/all-programs/case-management/, on July 21, 2015.

CHAPTER *2*

History and Evolution of Case Management

Sandra L. Lowery and Teresa M. Treiger

LEARNING OBJECTIVES

Upon completion of this chapter, the reader will be able to:

1. Recognize the history of case management.
2. Identify the factors for the rapid growth of case management.
3. Identify professional development of case management practice.
4. Identify the sources of national standards of practice and conduct for case managers.
5. List the purposes and goals of case management.
6. Understand the philosophical tenets of case management practice.
7. Define the domains of case management.
8. Describe case management and similar job titles.

IMPORTANT TERMS AND CONCEPTS

American Nurses Association (ANA)
American Nurses Credentialing Center (ANCC)
Association of Rehabilitation Nurses (ARN)
Care coordination
Care management
Case management
Case management certification
Case Management Society of America (CMSA)
Centers for Medicare and Medicaid (CMS)
Certified Case Manager (CCM)
Commission for Case Manager Certification (CCMC)
Domains of case management knowledge

Health Insurance Portability and Accountability Act (HIPAA)

International Association of Rehabilitation Professionals (IARP)

National Association of Social Workers (NASW)

Patient Protection and Affordable Care Act (PPACA)

Primary care case management

Social Security Administration (SSA)

Title V Amendments to the Social Security Act in 1965

Standards of practice

 Introduction

A. History of Case Management
1. Late 1800s–Early 1900—Public health nurses and social workers coordinated services through the Department of Public Health and in settlement houses and charity organizations.
2. 1920s—Psychiatry and social work focused on long-term, chronic illnesses, managed in the outpatient, community setting.
3. 1930s—Public health visiting nurses used community-based case management approaches in their patient care. Passage of the Social Security Act of 1935 provided for general welfare through benefits for the aged, blind, dependent and crippled children, maternal/child health, and old-age benefits.
4. 1943—Liberty Mutual used in-house case management/rehabilitation as a cost management measure for workers' compensation insurance.
5. Post–World War II—Insurance companies employed nurses and social workers to assist with the coordination of care for soldiers returning from the war who suffered complex injuries requiring multidisciplinary intervention.
6. 1960s
   a. The Community Mental Health Act of 1963 was spurred by the federally legislated deinstitutionalization of the mentally ill and developmentally/intellectually disabled (formerly identified as mentally retarded population), and community-based case management was required.
   b. Social Security Act Amendments in 1965 (also referred to as Health Insurance for the Aged Act and Old-Age, Survivors, and Disability Insurance Amendments of 1965) was legislation in which the most important provisions resulted in creation of Medicare and Medicaid. Providing the elderly (over 65) and for poor families.
   c. Medicaid and Medicare demonstration projects employed social workers and human service workers to arrange for and coordinate medical and social services to defined patient populations in the community, particularly the elderly.
   d. In 1966, the Insurance Company of North America (INA, now CIGNA) led by George Welch developed an in-house program that incorporated vocational rehabilitation and nurse case management, which later became known as Intracorp.

7. 1970s
   a. Due to the success of Liberty Mutual and INA in managing medical costs and returning workers to work, other workers' compensation insurers developed case management programs.
   b. Amendments to The Older Americans Act authorized case management for elders through area agencies on aging throughout the United States.
   c. Health Maintenance Act of 1973 was government response to growth in health care delivery and cost to consumers establishing federal standards for structure and operational requirements.
   d. National Long Term Care Channeling Demonstration Projects began in 1978. These government-funded community-based programs, focused on the low-income and frail elderly, were designed to maintain this population in the community.
8. 1980s
   a. Health insurers developed case management programs, targeted at the catastrophically injured and ill population. Focus was on cost containment due to the double-digit inflation rate for medical costs.
   b. Some programs were designed similarly to the workers' compensation insurance models, with a focus on quality and cost of care to achieve results. Others implemented a utilization management approach, with a focus on cost outcomes.
9. 1980s–2000s
   a. Provider-based case management programs implemented in acute care hospitals, home care agencies, rehabilitation facilities, and skilled nursing facilities. Growth of provider-based case management was spurred by the shifting of financial risk to provider organizations, as well as by external quality and cost demands by payers and accreditation bodies.
   b. Case management models frequently combined utilization review and discharge planning functions into a case management role. Both nurses and social workers were hired for provider-based case management positions.
   c. First CMSA Standard of Practice for Case Management released in 1995.
   d. The number of case managers increased to an estimate of greater than 100,000, with significant growth in Medicare and Medicaid managed care plans.
   e. Cost containment remained important, with the realization that quality care is essential to achieve this.
   f. Health Insurance Portability and Accountability Act (HIPAA) passage in 1996 provided additional protections for maintaining health insurance coverage when transitioning between employers or as an individual. Also addressed confidentiality issues pertaining to protected health information and coordination of benefits.
   g. Second revision of the CMSA Standards of Practice for Case Management released in 2002.

10. 2010s
    a. The 21st century has witnessed significant expansion of case management with passage of the Patient Protection and Affordable Care Act (PPACA). This legislation will ultimately lead to health coverage for 32 million uninsured Americans with provisions that continually highlight the focus on improving coordination and transitions of care through support of initiatives and pilot projects focused on patient-centered medical homes and accountable care organizations.
    b. In 2010, the third revision of the CMSA Standards of Practice for Case Management released.
    c. In 2012, the Supreme Court of the United States (SCOTUS) ruled that the individual mandate within the PPACA is a valid tax. "Although the federal government does not have the power to order people to buy health insurance, it does have the power to impose a tax on those without health insurance" (Cable News Network, 2012).
    d. In 2015, SCOTUS ruled that tax subsidies under PPACA are available to all Americans, even those who reside in states that have not established their own health insurance exchanges (Becker's Hospital Review, 2015).

Descriptions of Key Terms

The understanding of these terms is important to case management practice but may not be expanded upon within this chapter's content.

A. ADLs—Activities of Daily Living include activities carried out for personal hygiene and health.
B. Assessment—The process of collecting in-depth information about a person's health and functioning to identify needs in order to develop a comprehensive case management plan that will address those needs. In addition to client contact, information gathered should be from all relevant sources.
C. Autonomy—A form of personal liberty in which the client holds the right and freedom to make decisions regarding his or her own treatment and course of action and take control for his or her health, fostering independence and self-determination.
D. Case Manager—A health care professional who is responsible for applying the case management process in the care of individuals with health-related needs (e.g., biopsychosocial, physical, functional, cognitive, emotional, financial, etc.) with the goal of maximizing their wellness, autonomy, safety, appropriate use of resources, and maintenance of health condition. The case manager applies the process in collaboration with the patient/family or caregiver and other health care providers.
E. Catastrophic Case—Any medical condition that has heightened medical, social, financial, and functional consequences.
F. Continuum of Care—The continuum of care matches ongoing needs of the individuals being served by the case management process with the appropriate level and type of health, medical, financial, legal,

and psychosocial care for services within a setting or across multiple settings.

G. Coordination—The process of organizing, securing, integrating, and modifying the resources necessary to accomplish the goals set forth in the case management plan.

H. Developmental Disability—Any mental and/or physical disability that has an onset before age 22 and may continue indefinitely. It can limit major life activities.

I. Disability Case Management—A process of managing occupational and nonoccupational health conditions with the goal of returning the disabled employee to health, productivity, and employment.

J. Discharge Planning—The process of assessing an individual's health care needs upon discharge from a health care facility or agency and ensuring that the necessary services are in place before discharge.

K. Disease Management—A system of coordinated health care intervention and communication aimed at populations with chronic conditions in which the patient's self-care efforts and day-to-day living are significantly affected.

L. Implementation—The process of executing specific case management activities and/or interventions that will lead to accomplishing the goals identified in the case management plan.

M. Integrated Delivery System (IDS)—A single organization, or group of affiliated organizations, providing a wide spectrum of ambulatory and tertiary care and services. Care may also be provided across various settings of the health care continuum.

N. Intellectual Disability—Refers to the below-average general intellectual functioning manifested during the developmental period and existing concurrently with impairment in adaptive behavior. This was previously referred to as mental retardation.

O. Monitoring—The ongoing process of gathering sufficient information from all relevant sources regarding the effectiveness of the case management plan implemented.

P. Outcome Indicators—Measures of quality and cost of care. Metrics used to examine and evaluate the results of the care delivered.

Q. Outcomes Management—The use of information and knowledge gained from outcomes monitoring to achieve optimal patient outcomes through improved clinical decision making and service delivery.

R. Outcomes Measurement—The systematic, quantitative observation, at a point in time, of outcome indicators.

S. Planning—The process of determining specific needs, goals, and actions designed to meet the client's needs as identified through the assessment process.

T. Primary Care—A process of assessing, planning, coordinating, and providing health care from a consistent practitioner who serves as the central point of contact for all other practitioners.

U. Provider—A person, facility, or agency that provides health care services.

V. Social Work—Social work is a practice-based profession and an academic discipline that promotes social change and development, social cohesion, and the empowerment and liberation of people. Principles of social justice, human rights, collective responsibility, and respect for diversity are central to social work. Underpinned by theories of social work, social sciences, humanities, and indigenous knowledge, social work engages people and structures to address life challenges and enhance well-being (International Federation of Social Workers, 2014). Social workers usually collaborate with case managers and other members of the interdisciplinary health care team in the care of individuals, especially in the coordination of needed community resources and health and human services.

W. Standards of Practice—Statements of acceptable level of performance or expectation for professional intervention or behavior associated with a professional practice.

X. Transition Planning—The process case managers apply to ensure that appropriate resources and services are provided to patients and that these services are provided in the most appropriate setting or level of care.

Y. Utilization Review—A mechanism used by some insurers and employers to evaluate health care on the basis of medical appropriateness, necessity, and quality. Typically, this is used to determine access to an insurance benefit.

Z. Vocational Rehabilitation—A process whereby a skilled professional utilizes the case management process to address the medical and vocational services necessary to facilitate a disabled individual's expedient return to suitable employment.

 ## Applicability to CMSA'S Standards of Practice

A. The Case Management Society of America (CMSA) describes in its standards of practice for case management (CMSA, 2010) that case management practice extends across all health care settings, including payer, provider, government, employer, community, and home environment. It also explains that the role of a case manager may be assumed by individuals from a variety of professional disciplines including nursing, social work, and vocational rehabilitation counseling.

B. It is known that the roots of case management are about a century old. The practice, however, has evolved over time and gained increased attention based on the sociopolitical dynamics of the health care environment in the United States. Understanding the historical background of this practice by case managers is essential for professional standing in society and the health care industry. The CMSA's standards of practice also evolved over time and have been affected by the changes in the health care environment, which have occurred over the past three decades.

C. This chapter contains historical background, which outlines the underpinnings of modern case management practice. The CMSA Standards of Practice highlights pertinent to this chapter include the following: Philosophy and Guiding Principles, Definition of Case Management, and Client Selection Process for Case Management Standard.

 ## Factors for the Rapid Growth of Case Management

A. Cost of health care—Increasing amount of the gross domestic product (GDP) that goes toward health care. In the early 1990s, one-seventh of the U.S. GDP went toward the payment for health care (Cohen, 1996).

The U.S. health care spending grew 3.6% in 2013, reaching $2.9 trillion or $9,255 per person. As a share of the nation's GDP, health spending accounted for 17.4% (Centers for Medicare and Medicaid Services, 2015).

B. Increasing consumerism secondary to more accessible information, increased expectations of patient involvement on the part of health plans, shift of health care onto financing onto consumers, and negative repercussions of managed care.

C. New emphasis on evidence-based health care reimbursement by health plans.

D. Information explosion through expansive use of electronic communication technology, digital tools, and social media.

E. Rapid development of genetic and medical advances.

F. Growing emphasis on results, the value of health care dollars, and accountability for end outcomes, not just process.

G. Rapid and significant changes in the health care delivery system and reimbursement for care.
  1. Increased fragmentation of care delivery
  2. Increased level of consumer financial responsibility with decreased benefits, higher co-pays, and deductibles
  3. Multiple levels and settings of care delivery developed, leading to much confusion, poorly coordinated care, poor care accountability, and cost shifting
  4. Health information exchanges
  5. Health insurance marketplaces

H. Public awareness of the fallibility of the health care system.
  1. National reports (e.g., To Err is Human: Building a Safer Health System, Crossing the Quality Chasm: A New Health System for the 21st Century) by the Institute of Medicine identified safety problems from medical errors and ways to improve health care delivery and quality
  2. Increased accessibility to public report cards on providers and to comparative quality and cost data (e.g., Hospital Compare, Agency for Healthcare Research, and Quality's Effective Health Care Program)
  3. Published data showing great variability in treatment and inconsistent application of medical evidence (e.g., Dartmouth Atlas of Health Care, Institute for Healthcare Improvement)

I. Demands for quality care as well as cost-effectiveness by private and public payers, though accreditation, pay-for-performance measures, and value-based purchasing.

J. Increased recognition of case management as beneficial for cost and quality outcomes.

K. Demographic changes (e.g., increasing longevity, geographic separation of extended families, increased reliance on institutions for long-term care).

L. Awareness of the prevalence and cost of chronic diseases and conditions, and the most preventable of all health problems. As of 2012, about half of all adults have one or more chronic health conditions. One of four adults has two or more chronic health conditions. Seven of the top ten causes of death in 2010 were chronic diseases (Ward, Schiller, & Goodman, 2014).

M. PPACA incentivized care coordination as a means of financing new programs and health care models.

N. Chronic care management and transitional care billing codes provide a mechanism for claims submission to payers relative to case management services (Centers for Medicare and Medicaid, 2013).

O. Legislation and Regulation
   1. Private Sector
      a. Workers' compensation insurance regulations
      b. State-specific regulations governing managed care, accountable care organizations, and utilization review
   2. Public Sector
      a. Medicare and Medicaid demonstration and waiver programs
      b. Community human service agencies serving the mentally ill, intellectually and developmentally disabled population
      c. Community-based Care Transition Program
      d. Dual eligibility (Medicare + Medicaid population) programs

Professional Development of Case Management Practice

A. Practice Acts
   1. Each jurisdiction (e.g., state, commonwealth, territory) maintains individual practice acts, which define one's scope of practice.
   2. When individual licensure is not granted, regulations define scope and limitations of practice.

B. Standards of Professional Practice and Codes of Conduct for the Individual Case Manager Practitioner
   1. Standards of practice are intended to identify and address important foundational knowledge and skills of the case manager within a spectrum of case management practice settings and specialties (CMSA, 2010).
   2. Separate standards of practice also apply depending upon one's professional educational background (e.g., registered nursing, social work).
   3. Box 2-1 lists examples of organizations and associations that issue practice standards and/or codes of conduct for case management.

BOX 2-1   Sample Organizations that Affect Case Management Practice

- Case Management Society of America (CMSA)
- National Association of Social Workers (NASW)
- American Nurses Association (ANA)
- International Association of Rehabilitation Professionals (IARP)
- Association of Rehabilitation Nurses (ARN)
- Aging Life Care Association (ALCA). This organization was formerly known as National Association of Professional Geriatric Care Managers
- American Case Management Association (ACMA)
- Commission for Case Management Certification (CCMC) Code of Professional Conduct
  - The Code prescribes a level of conduct required of individuals who have attained the CCM credential.
  - Compliance with the Code is considered mandatory for certificants.

C. Accreditation Sources for Organizations
1. URAC (formerly known as the Utilization Review Accreditation Commission)
2. Commission on Accreditation of Rehabilitation Facilities (CARF)
3. National Committee for Quality Assurance (NCQA)
4. The Joint Commission (TJC)
D. Case Management Certification Sources
There are over 16 case management–related credentials offered by a variety of health care organizations (Table 2-1).
E. Model Legislation
A model act is a draft proposal for legislation or regulation. It is put forth by an organization to be used as a framework for state or federal legislatures or regulatory agencies.
1. CMSA Case Management Model Act
a. The Case Management Model Act (CMSA, 2009) was written to establish the key elements of a comprehensive case management program. CMSA developed the Model Act and encourages public policymakers to review and use its provisions for legislative and regulatory matters relating to health care case management.
b. The model act includes a number of sections such as those summarized in Box 2-2.

TABLE 2-1 Case Management Certifications and Sponsoring Organizations

Certification	Sponsoring Organization
ABDA	American Board of Disability Analysts
ACM	American Case Management Association
C-ACSWCM	National Association of Social Workers
C-SWCM	National Association of Social Workers
CCM	Commission for Case Manager Certification
CDMS	Certified Disability Management Specialists
CHCQM	American Board of Quality Assurance & Utilization Review Physicians
CMAC	Center for Case Management
CMCN	American Board of Managed Care Nursing
COHN-CM	American Board for Occupational Health Nurses
CPDM	Insurance Educational Association
CPHQ	National Association for Healthcare Quality
CRC	Commission on Rehabilitation Counselor Certification
CRRN	Rehabilitation Nursing Certification Board
CRRN-A	Rehabilitation Nursing Certification Board
NACCM	National Academy of Certified Case Managers
PAHM	Academy for Healthcare Management/American Health Insurance Professionals
FAHM	Academy for Healthcare Management/American Health Insurance Professionals
RN-BC	American Nurses Credentialing Center

BOX 2-2   Important Sections of the Case Management Model Act

1. Definitions
2. Staff Qualifications
3. Case Management Functions
4. Authorized Scope of Services
5. Payment of Services
6. Other Program Requirements
7. Training
8. Quality Management
9. Antifraud & Consumer Protections
10. Complaints
11. Regulatory Oversight and Implementation

    2. Association of Social Work Boards (ASWB) Model Social Work Practice Act (2012)
       a. This model act establishes standards of minimal social work competence, methods of fairly and objectively addressing consumer complaints, and means of removing incompetent and/or unethical practitioners from practice.
  F. National journals, magazines, and newsletters
    1. Professional Case Management
    2. Case Management Today
    3. Care Management
    4. Case Management Advisor
    5. Journal of Case Management
    6. Case in Point
  G. Education
    1. Continuing Education and Academic Advancement
       a. Certificate programs may provide overview exposure to case management. Usually do not provide college credit and do not equate with certification.
       b. Baccalaureate degree programs provide general grounding and serve as an educational baseline recognized in the CMSA Case Management Model Act.
       c. Graduate degree programs, usually in Nursing, specialize in case management and are offered by a number of colleges and universities.
       d. Core curriculum for baccalaureate social work degree includes the core principles of case management.
       e. Online education courses provide learner flexibility to self-pace and complete coursework at convenient times.
          i. CMSA's Career and Knowledge Pathways
          ii. PRIME
          iii. Athena Forum
          iv. Contemporary Forums
          v. American Academy of Ambulatory Care Nursing
          vi. Publishers such as Lippincott Williams and Wilkins

      f. Live conferences and educational meetings provide traditional face-to-face learning and networking opportunities.
          i. CMSA Annual Conference and Regional Events
          ii. CMSA Chapter Conferences and Education Meetings
          iii. Dorland Healthcare Summits
          iv. American Association of Managed Care Nurses Forums

H. Professional Associations, including commonly known abbreviations
    1. Case Management Society of America (CMSA)
    2. Aging Life Care Association (ALCA)
    3. International Association of Rehabilitation Providers (IARP)
    4. Association of Certified Case Managers (ACCM)
    5. American Case Management Association (ACMA)

I. Professional Recognition Awards
    1. CMSA Achievement and Recognition awards
      a. Lifetime Achievement Award
      b. Case Manager of the Year
      c. Award of Service Excellence
      d. Chapter Excellence Awards
    2. Dorland Health Platinum awards

Purposes and Goals of Case Management

A. Purposes of Case Management.
    1. Case management interjects objectivity and information where it is lacking to promote informed decision making by the client and others; maximizes efficiency in use of available resources; work collaboratively with patient, family/significant other, and the health care team to implement a plan of care that meets the individual's needs; and serves as a means for achieving client wellness and autonomy through advocacy, communication, education, identification of service resources and service facilitation (CMSA, 2010).
    2. Case management facilitates the achievement of client wellness and autonomy through advocacy, assessment, planning, communication, education, resource management, and service facilitation.
      a. Based on the needs and values of the client, and in collaboration with all service providers, the case manager links clients with appropriate providers and resources throughout the continuum of health and human services and care settings, while ensuring that the care provided is safe, effective, client centered, timely, efficient, and equitable.
      b. This approach achieves optimum value and desirable outcomes for all—the clients, their support systems, the providers, and the payers (CCMC, 2015).
    3. The purpose of case management services is to help patients handle aspects of their lives that are not necessarily related to substance abuse but that might impact whether the patient remains in treatment or has successful treatment outcomes.
      a. These services provide assessment, planning, coordination, monitoring, and evaluation of options and resources to meet

2-3   Goals of Case Management

1. To enhance client safety, productivity, satisfaction, and quality of life; to assist clients to appropriately self-direct care, self-advocate, and make informed and timely health care decisions (CMSA, 2010).
2. Through early assessment, ensure that services are generated in a timely and cost-effective manner.
3. Assist patients to achieve an optimal level of wellness and function by facilitating and coordinating timely and appropriate health services.
4. Assist patients to self-direct care appropriately, self-advocate, and make informed decisions to the degree possible.
5. The goal was then as it is now—to ensure that patients received safe care, at the right time, in the right place, and for the most cost-effective price (ANCC, 2012).
6. The ultimate goal of both vocational and medical case management is to return the "client or individual with a physical, mental, and/or emotional impairment" to his or her highest level of functioning in the areas of work, home life, school, and society in general in the most efficacious, ethical, and cost-effective manner (International Association of Rehabilitation Professionals, 2015).
7. Return the patient to work or assess the patient's ability to return to work and develop a plan that will assist the patient in returning to work or becoming employable.
8. Optimize client functioning and well-being by providing and coordinating high-quality services, in the most effective and efficient manner possible, to individuals with multiple complex needs (NASW, 2013).

an individual's specific needs (Illinois Department of Human Services, 2015).

4. The purpose of care coordination is to work directly with clients and families over time to assist them in arranging and managing the complex set of resources that the client requires to maintain health and independent functioning.
   a. Care coordination seeks to achieve the maximum cost-effective use of scarce resources by helping clients get the health, social, and support services most appropriate for their needs at a given time.
   b. It guides the client and family through the maze of services, matches service needs with funding authorization, and coordinates with clinician and provider organizations (Williams & Torrens, 1993).
5. The purpose is to move the client toward successful meeting of planned outcomes where interventions are tied to a sense of movement, and constant evaluation occurs to measure progress (Cohen, 1996).

B. Goals: Regardless of practice setting, the goals of case management are to simultaneously promote the client's wellness, autonomy, and appropriate use of service and financial resources (Box 2-3).

Philosophical Tenets of Case Management

A. The underlying premise of case management is based on the fact that when an individual reaches the optimum level of wellness and functional capability, everyone benefits: the individuals being served, their support systems, the health care delivery systems, and the various reimbursement sources.

  1. The case manager helps identify appropriate providers and facilities throughout the continuum of services, while ensuring that available resources are being used in a timely and cost-effective manner in order to obtain optimum value for both the client and the reimbursement source.

  2. Case management services are best served in a climate that allows direct communication between the case manager, the client, and the appropriate service personnel, in order to optimize the outcome for all concerned (CMSA, 2010).

B. Case management is an area of specialty practice within one's health and human services profession.

  1. Its underlying premise is that everyone benefits when clients reach their optimum level of wellness, self-management, and functional capability: the clients being served, their support systems, the health care delivery systems, and the various payer sources (CMSA, 2010).

C. The primary mission of the social work profession is to enhance human well-being and to help meet the basic needs of all people, with particular attention to the needs of individuals and communities who are vulnerable and oppressed (NASW, 2013).

 ## Case Management Knowledge Domains

Encompassing the case management process are seven knowledge domains, which contribute to the value of case management, which are as follows:

A. Case Management Concepts
B. Principles of Practice
C. Healthcare Management & Delivery
D. Healthcare Reimbursement
E. Psychosocial Aspects of Care
F. Rehabilitation
G. Professional Development & Advancement (CCMC, 2011)

 ## Case Management Target Populations

A. Identification and selection of clients who may benefit the most from case management services is an essential standard of practice (CMSA, 2010).

  1. High-risk screening criteria to assess appropriateness for case management services (Box 2-4).

B. Client selection criteria are determined by the state (e.g., Worker's Compensation regulation), purchaser, or employer of the case manager.

 ## Case Management Versus Other Job Titles

A. Case manager, care manager, guided care nurse, patient navigator, patient advocate, and care coordinator are terms used loosely and interchangeably; however, there are fundamental differences between them. Continuing to view these jobs as being equivalent perpetuates confusion across the health care spectrum.

BOX 2-4   High-Risk Screening Criteria for Case Management Services

1. Advanced age or prematurity
2. History of mental illness or substance abuse, suicide risk, or crisis intervention
3. Social issues (e.g., homelessness, abuse, neglect, absence of social support, financial risk or poverty)
4. Multiple chronic illnesses
5. Catastrophic illness or injury
6. Multiple inpatient acute admissions within a specific time frame
7. Multiple emergency room visits for the same or related condition
8. Cognitive or functional impairment causing a high-risk living situation
9. Multiple home health or durable medical equipment needs
10. Large consumption of health care resources
11. Work-related illness or injury requiring sustained time off and return-to-work needs
12. Absence or primary care provider or medical/health home care team.

B. In order to ensure job title accuracy, the position's roles, functions, and activities, the job description must be assembled carefully and regularly updated to ensure it is a bona fide case management position.

C. Care management is sometimes used as the department title that includes multiple functions such as case management, utilization review, benefit denial management, quality management, or others.

D. Care management, as well as other terms such as care coordination, evolved in recent years to provide some distance from the managed care backlash, where case management was often perceived to be a negative component.

E. Care management is often used instead of case management for chronic, elderly, and long-term care client populations.

F. Branding of terms and job descriptions has been used to distinguish an organization's products and services. These proprietary terms must be examined to understand the qualifications, roles, and responsibilities associated with the position.

G. Examples of other job titles include the following:
   1. Guided Care is a model of case management targeting the complex needs of patients with multiple chronic conditions. A trained nurse works with patients, physicians, and others to provide coordinated, patient-centered care.
   2. Patient Advocate is a nurse and other professional who works with a client to help navigate the health care system, provide the necessary resources to understand the condition and to offer support.
   3. Patient Navigator provides individualized service for clinical advocacy, care coordination, medical research, and insurance resolution.

H. Primary Care Case Management involves dual roles: caregiving and case management. This may create potential ethical and conceptual conflict influenced by the care setting and involvement in benefit determinations, "Severe conflicts of interest can emerge when case managers are also service providers rather than relatively disinterested allocators of service" (Kane, 1988). This is a federally legislated model of case management for Medicaid risk plans. This is a model frequently used in home care agencies, ambulatory care settings, and skilled nursing facilities.

References

American Nurses Credentialing Center. (2012). *Clinical case management practice. Nursing case management review and resource manual* (4th ed.). Retrieved from http://www.nursecredentialing. org/documents/certification/reviewmanuals/nursecasemgmtsamplechap.aspx, on June 26, 2015.

Association of Social Work Boards (ASWB) Model Social Work Practice Act. (2012). *Association of social work boards.* Retrieved from https://www.aswb.org/wp-content/uploads/2013/10/ Model_law.pdf, on June 30, 2015.

Becker's Hospital Review. (2015). *Supreme Court upholds PPACA subsidies in King v. Burwell: 10 things to know.* Retrieved from http://www.beckershospitalreview.com/legal-regulatory-issues/supreme-court-upholds-ppaca-subsidies-in-king-v-burwell-10-things-to-know.html, on July 1, 2015.

Cable News Network. (2012). *Emotions high after Supreme Court upholds Health Care Law.* Received from http://www.cnn.com/2012/06/28/politics/supreme-court-health-ruling, on July 1, 2015.

Case Management Society of America. (2009). *Case Management Model Act.* Retrieved from http:// www.cmsa.org/PolicyMaker/HealthCareReform/tabid/446/Default.aspx, on July 1, 2015.

Case Management Society of America. (2010). *Standards of practice for case management.* Little Rock, AR: Author.

Centers for Medicare and Medicaid. (2013). *Frequently asked questions about billing Medicare for transitional care management services.* Retrieved from http://www.cms.gov/Medicare/Medicare-Fee-for-Service-Payment/PhysicianFeeSched/Downloads/FAQ-tcms.pdf, on June 30, 2015.

Centers for Medicare and Medicaid. (2015). *Historical national health expenditure data.* Retrieved from http://www.cms.gov/Research-Statistics-Data-and-Systems/Statistics-Trends-and-Reports/ NationalHealthExpendData/NationalHealthAccountsHistorical.html, on June 30, 2015.

Cohen, E. (1996). *Nurse case management in the 21st century.* St. Louis, MO: Mosby Year Book.

Commission for Case Management Certification. (2011). *Case Management Body of Knowledge—Case Management Knowledge Domains.* Retrieved from http://www.cmbodyofknowledge. com on June 29, 2015.

Commission for Case Management Certification. (2015). *Philosophy of case management.* Retrieved from http://ccmcertification.org/about-us/about-case-management/definition-and-philosophy-case-management, on June 29, 2915.

Illinois Department of Human Services. (2015). *What is the purpose of case management?* Retrieved from https://www.dhs.state.il.us/page.aspx?item=33612, on June 25, 2015.

International Association of Rehabilitation Professionals. (2015). *Case management—What's it all about?* Retrieved from http://www.rehabpro.org/sections/rehab-disability-case-management/ cmdm-resources/case-management-whats-it-all-about, on June 26, 2015.

International Federation of Social Workers. (2014). *Social work.* Retrieved from http://ifsw.org/ policies/definition-of-social-work, on August 23, 2015.

Kane, R. (1988). Case management: Ethical pitfalls on the road to high-quality managed care. *QRB Quality Review Bulletin, 14*(5), 161–166.

National Association of Social Workers. (2013). *NASW's standards for social work case management.* Retrieved from https://www.socialworkers.org/practice/naswstandards/CaseManagement Standards2013.pdf, on June 26, 2015.

Ward, B. W., Schiller, J. S., & Goodman, R. A. (2014). Multiple chronic conditions among US adults: A 2012 update. *Preventing Chronic Disease, 11,* 130389. Retrieved from http://dx.doi. org/10.5888/pcd11.130389, on June 30, 2015.

Williams, S. J., & Torrens P. R. (1993). *Introduction to health services,* (4th ed.). Albany, NY: Delmar.

CHAPTER 3

Health Care Insurance, Benefits, and Reimbursement Systems

Beverly Cunningham

LEARNING OBJECTIVES

Upon completion of this chapter, the reader will be able to:

1. Define important terms and concepts related to the health care delivery system, health care insurance, and reimbursement.
2. Name four types of health care delivery systems.
3. Name three challenges facing managed care and health care delivery systems.
4. Name the different types of reimbursement methods and describe each.
5. Name the types of insurance.
6. Identify the role of the case manager in health care reimbursement.

IMPORTANT TERMS AND CONCEPTS

Accountable Care
  Organization (ACO)
All Patient-Related
  Diagnosis-Related
  Group (APR-DRG)
Ambulatory Payment
  Classification (APC)
Capitation Carve-Out
Coinsurance
Commercial Insurance
Concurrent Review

Continuum of Care
Co-pay
Deductible
Denial of Payment
Diagnosis-Related
  Group (DRG)
Gatekeeper
Health Care
  Reimbursement
Health Care Savings
  Account (HSA)

Health Maintenance
  Organization (HMO)
Indemnity/Fee
  for Service
Lifetime Maximum
Local Coverage
  Determination (LCD)
Managed Care
Medicaid
Medical Necessity
Medicare

Medicare Shared
  Savings Program
  (MSSP)
Minimum Data
  Set (MDS)
National Coverage
  Determination
  (NCD)
Out-of-Pocket
Patient Protection
  and Affordable Care
  Act (PPACA)
Per Diem

Point of Service Plan
Preauthorization
Predictive Modeling
Preferred Provider
  Organization (PPO)
Primary Care
  Physician (PCP)
Prospective Payment
  System (PPS)—
  Inpatient, IPPS;
  Outpatient, OPPS
Quality Improvement
  Organization (QIO)

Resource Utilization
  Groups (RUGs)
Retrospective Review
Risk Sharing
Stop Loss
Third-Party
  Administrator (TPA)
Utilization Review
  and Management
Value-Based
  Purchasing (VBP)

 # Introduction

A. Increased costs of health care services, as well as consumer demand for high quality and safe care, have given rise to ever-changing methods of health care reimbursement. Quality of care has become an essential factor in reimbursement equations.

B. Changes in payment structures continue to take place in almost every sector of the health care industry. In the past, the most dominant driver for these changes was cost containment. Now, costs are coupled with quality processes and outcomes, as payers and the public are looking for value in health care delivery.

1. Managed care health plans became popular over past decades, and regulatory attempts to contain health care costs continue to evolve through the use of more aggressive cost containment strategies and federally funded demonstration projects.

2. The Centers for Medicare and Medicaid Services (CMS) extended the prospective payment system (PPS) methods to almost all care settings of health care delivery. In addition to acute care, PPS is now applied in ambulatory, long-term, and home care settings, among others. IPPS is the inpatient prospective system, and OPPS is the outpatient prospective system.

3. Additionally, CMS has transformed reimbursement from prospective, based on DRG or outpatient payments, to conditional reimbursement based on quality indicators (e.g., readmissions, hospital-acquired conditions, patient safety indicators, patient satisfaction, spending per Medicare beneficiary) (2014a).

4. Insurance is now mandated for every person with penalties for those not covered. Coverage is both offered and governed through the Patient Protection and Affordable Care Act (PPACA) with costs for coverage based on the finances of the individual applying for coverage. This legislation is also referred to as the Affordable Care Act (ACA) (Kaiser Family Foundation, 2012).

5. Employers and other independent groups are offering high-deductible plans, featuring higher deductibles, co-pays, and coinsurance. This attempts to shift cost-related decisions to the consumer and also moves more financial liability to the consumer.

C. Reimbursement methodologies for health care services vary widely. They are determined by the reimbursement source/payer: PPS, managed care, capitation, fee for service, and so on.

D. Managed care encompasses a wide variety of terms and concepts, from the structure and purpose of the health care organization itself to the tools used in a health care delivery system or insurance plan.

E. Government-based insurers/payers (e.g., Medicare and Medicaid) programs often influence the processes used by managed care organizations and plans. For example, managed care is adopting many of the CMS quality metrics, such as readmissions and hospital-acquired conditions, as a part of their reimbursement methodology.

F. Benefit systems and reimbursement amounts are determined by payer source, which can be classified into two broad groups: commercial insurance and government payers.
   1. Benefits are usually received only by those who are covered by a health insurance plan.
   2. Federal government assumes health care responsibility for older citizens and those with specified long-term disabilities.
   3. State government assumes health care responsibility for children and indigent adults meeting specific state guidelines.

G. Health care responsibility varies by state policies. For example, federal and state programs may offer responsibility for management of health care benefits to a third party, known as Medicare Advantage and managed Medicaid plans. These plans contract with federal and state programs to deliver cost-effective, quality care.

H. The case manager's involvement with health care reimbursement varies based on the degree and complexity of the:
   1. Health care services offered
   2. Needs of the patient and family served
   3. Benefits as defined in the health insurance plan
   4. The payer/insurer and its contract
   5. Value restrictions
   6. Compliance requirements

Often, the case manager works for the payer and interacts with case managers in working across the care continuum. In some instances, the payer case manager is the only individual aside from the patient who continues to be involved in the patient care team throughout the episode of illness.

 ## Descriptions of Key Terms

A. Accountable Care Organization (ACO)—A healthcare organization characterized by a payment and care delivery model seeking to link provider reimbursements to quality metrics and reductions in the total cost of care for an assigned population of patients. The goal of an ACO is to coordinate care among the providers in the organization. Providers may include hospitals, physicians, and other health care providers.

B. Affordable Care Act (ACA)—Officially known as the Patient Protection and Affordable Care Act of 2010 (PPACA). In 2011, the Congressional Budget Office projected that it would lower both future deficits and Medicare spending. Its initial goal was to increase the quality and affordability of health insurance, lower the uninsured rate by expanding public and private insurance coverage, and reduce the costs of health care for individuals and the government. It introduced mechanisms like mandates, subsidies, and insurance exchanges. Many regulations for insurance companies and employers were included in the act (Department of Health and Human Services, 2014a).

C. Capitation—Often seen in an HMO, capitation pays a set amount paid to a provider (e.g., individual, facility, agency) on the basis of per member per month (or other interval). Regardless of the type or amount of care or service provided or not provided, rates vary based on member demographics (e.g., age, gender). Amount is predetermined and stipulated in the managed care contract between the payer and the health care provider.

D. Coinsurance—Payment by an insured member who pays a share of the payment made against a claim.

E. Commercial insurance—Payers that are not government (e.g., Medicare, Medicaid).

F. Co-pay or co-payment—Predetermined dollar amount for which a member of a health plan is responsible to pay each time a service is rendered (e.g., office visit, emergency department visit, prescription, specialist visit, hospitalization).

G. Deductible—Fixed amount of money a member in a health plan must pay each year before benefits are paid by the insurance company.

H. Diagnosis-related groups—The DRG system is an inpatient classification method providing a means of relating the type of patient being treated (e.g., the medical/clinical condition, acuity, diagnosis) to the costs incurred by the hospital during care provision (e.g., resource utilization and intensity).

I. Gatekeeper—A primary care provider (usually a family practitioner, internist, pediatrician, or nurse practitioner) chosen by or assigned to a health plan's member. This is most frequently seen within the managed care and patient-centered medical home environments. The provider is responsible for managing all care needs and referrals used by the member.

J. Government payers—Payers that are related to, or sponsored by, state or federal health insurance programs (e.g., Medicare, Medicaid).

K. Health care delivery system—An organizational, comprehensive model or structure used in the delivery of health care services to individuals or target.

L. Health care reimbursement—Payment for health care and services provided by a physician, medical professional, facility, or agency to individuals in need of such services.

M. Managed care—A system of health care delivery that aims to provide a generalized structure and focus when managing the use, access, cost, quality, and effectiveness of health care services.

N. Medicare Shared Savings Program (MSSP)—A key component of the Medicare delivery system reform initiatives that is included in the Patient Protection and Affordable Care Act of 2010. It is a new approach to the delivery of health care. Created to facilitate coordination and cooperation among health care providers to improve the quality of care for Medicare fee-for-service (FFS) beneficiaries and reduce unnecessary costs. Eligible providers, hospitals, and suppliers may participate in the MSSP program by creating or participating in an Accountable Care Organization (ACO).

O. Minimum data set (MDS)—The assessment tool used in long-term care facility settings as a primary screening and assessment tool. The MDS places a patient in a resource utilization group (RUG), which determines the facility's reimbursement rate. Measures include physician, psychological, and psychosocial functioning.

P. Network model—A group of physicians and related health care providers (e.g., individual, institutional), contracted with a health insurance plan, from which a member should seek services. In this model, members have the option to go out of network for services. However, in most cases should the member elect to go to an out-of-network provider, his/her out-of-pocket expenses will be higher than those incurred had an in-network provider been seen.

Q. Out-of-pocket—Refers to expenses for health care for which the consumer is responsible. Coinsurance, deductible, and co-payments may be included in the out-of-pocket as well as services not covered by a payer.

R. Predictive modeling—A process used by managed care organizations, ACOs, and population health models to identify which of their members will have the highest future medical costs and will be in need of an increased amount of health care services. This tends to be based on clinical and demographic patient information and past expenditures.

S. Prospective payment system (PPS)—A health care payment system used by the federal government for reimbursing health care providers and agencies for medical care provided to individuals who belong to a governmental insurance plan.

T. Reinsurance—Insurance to cover losses incurred while covering claims that exceed a specified dollar threshold. This is most frequently purchased by health maintenance organization (HMO)-type plans.

U. Value-based purchasing—A demand strategy to measure, report, and reward excellence in health care delivery. CMS uses a penalty and reward strategy based on clinical and financial outcomes that change annually. The penalty and reward for hospitals are based on a percentage of the DRG payment and the hospital's ability to provide the utmost outcomes compared to other IPPS hospitals.

V. Physician Quality Reporting System (PQRS)—Quality reporting program that encourages individual eligible professionals and group practices to report information on the quality of care to CMS. It is likely that ultimately, the PQRS results will drive physician reimbursement.

Applicability to CMSA's Standards of Practice

A. The Case Management Society of America (CMSA) describes in its standards of practice for case management (CMSA, 2010) that case management practice extends across all health care settings, including payer, provider, government, employer, community, and home environment. It also explains that case managers are involved in the allocation of resources and the utilization review and management where it is necessary for them to be knowledgeable in health care payment and reimbursement methods.

B. This chapter describes the various payment systems found across the health care continuum as well as case management practice in payer (e.g., private insurance, managed care organizations, Medicare, Medicaid) and nonpayer settings.

C. This chapter addresses case management practice knowledge of and proficiency in payer systems, benefits, and reimbursement. The following practice standards described in the CMSA standards of practice are most applicable to this chapter: advocacy, resource management, and stewardship.

D. Case managers apply the knowledge of payment systems and skills of utilization review and management, resource management, cost reduction, and reimbursement-related denials and appeals when executing their roles taking care of patients and their families. They use such knowledge and skills in every step of the case management process.

Driving Forces Behind Health Care Reimbursement Systems

A. There are several factors that impact the nature of the health care delivery system and its reimbursement structures. As the health care industry continues its dynamic evolution, and innovations in diagnostics and therapeutics occur, the cost of health care services will continue to increase prompting modifications in the reimbursement and delivery systems. Important factors will affect such changes.

B. Commercial payers
   1. Technology and innovations are more popular today in the health care market than ever before.
      a. Are evident in the increased use of Web-based products, including systems used for verification, authorization, approval of benefits, and claims payments or denials
      b. Are used to improve the efficiency and effectiveness of health care services
      c. Have resulted in a surge of expensive and complex technological advances in health care services, including diagnostic and therapeutic modalities
      d. Also include clinical trials, especially in the area of pharmaceuticals
   2. Need to reduce the increased costs of care. Some of the reasons behind the increased costs are described in Box 3-1.
   3. Consumer demand for lower costs and higher quality.
   4. Malpractice insurance claims.
   5. Insurance premiums—For insurance plans, single individuals, and employers.
   6. Opportunity for managed care to administer federal or state plans, such as ACA plans (e.g., insurance exchanges), Medicare Managed Care, Medicaid Managed Care, Children Health Insurance Plan, and Family Health Plus.
   7. The Leapfrog Group initiatives—A coalition of public and private organizations (including employers and insurance plans) setting quality standards for hospitals to avoid preventable patient care errors; examples of such standards include the use of intensivists and computerized order entry systems (The Leapfrog Group, 2015).

- Aging population
- Complexity and chronicity of patients' health conditions, including the increased number of comorbidities and need for polypharmacy
- Need for postacute medical care management; for example, durable medical equipment (DME), home health services, and posthospital services, such as long-term acute care, subacute rehabilitation care, and skilled nursing care
- Pharmaceutical costs
- Implants and prostheses costs
- Inpatient versus outpatient medical management
- Fraud and abuse
- Non–value-adding care processes
- Duplication and fragmentation in care activities and services

8. Accreditation agencies—Agencies that set health care standards and expectations and recognize those that meet the standards (Box 3-2).
9. Federal rules, laws, and regulations.
10. Employer costs.
11. Influence of Accountable Care Act regulations and plans for individuals and small businesses.

C. Government payers
   1. Are affected by the Balanced Budget Act (BBA) of 1997, which was a response to concern of potential insolvency of the Medicare Hospital Insurance Trust Fund. The primary goal of BBA was to reduce Medicare spending as follows:
      a. Reduced Medicare beneficiary health care benefits
      b. Eliminated cost-based reimbursement for postacute care services (CMS, n.d.a)
   2. Desire to balance cost with payment
      a. Value-based purchasing and health care reform strategies
      b. Move from payment by DRG to payment using the MS-DRG reimbursement system

- National Committee for Quality Assurance (NCQA)
- Hospital accreditation agencies: The Joint Commission (TJC), Healthcare Facilities Accreditation Program (HFAP), and Det Norske Veritas Healthcare, Inc. (DNV), being the most common
- URAC (formerly Utilization Review Accreditation Commission)
- Commission on Accreditation of Rehabilitation Facilities (CARF)
- Accreditation Association for Ambulatory Health Care (AAAHC)
- Community Health Accreditation Program (CHAP)
- RadSite
- Additionally, there are many disease-specific certifications offered by various accreditation agencies, for example, bariatric surgery, stroke, chest pain, ventricular assist device, and joint replacement

   c. Transition from ICD-9 patient classification codes to ICD-10, the 10th revision of the International Statistical Classification of Diseases and Related Health Problems, a medical classification list used by the World Health Organization (WHO)

 3. The prospective payment system (PPS), which was originally defined by Social Security Act amendment of 1983 and focused on reimbursement for hospital care (CMS, 2015a)

   a. Uses the diagnosis-related group (DRG), a financial tool, as the reimbursement method for health care services rendered in the hospital setting and is characterized by the following:

     i. Payment is fixed and based on the operating costs of the patient's diagnosis.

     ii. Predetermined case rate that is paid regardless of the actual costs incurred by the provider of services.

     iii. Uses the DRG to establish amount of reimbursement.

   b. DRGs demonstrate groups of patients using similar resources and experiencing similar length of hospital stay.

 4. The APC system, which was implemented in 2000

   a. Prospective payment fee schedule for bundled outpatient services.

   b. An encounter-based outpatient reimbursement system that is similar in philosophy to the DRG system.

   c. Unlike DRG, a single outpatient encounter may result in the payment of one or more APC.

   d. Used more frequently with the increase in the use of observation services (driven initially by CMS, but now adopted by all payers) for short-stay hospital patients (Department of Health and Human Services, 2014b).

 5. Rehabilitation prospective payment system

   a. A prospective payment system for rehabilitation facilities, similar to that of acute care/hospital-based care (e.g., DRG system).

   b. Includes a patient assessment instrument (PAI) that captures a score that is used to place a patient in a Case Mix Group (CMG) to establish the reimbursement rate.

   c. CMG functions similar to the DRG and APC systems.

   d. In CMG, a rehabilitation patient is classified into groups based upon clinical/medical characteristics and expected resource consumption.

 6. Resource utilization group

   a. A prospective payment system for long-term nursing facilities, similar to that of the DRG system.

   b. Classifies long-term nursing facility patients into groups based on information from the minimum data set.

   c. Reimbursement is based on the assigned hierarchy and RUG (The Hilltop Institute, 2009).

Types of Insurance

A. Commercial programs

 1. Liability insurance—Benefits paid for bodily injury, property damage, or both

2. Workers' compensation
   a. Insurance program that may provide medical benefits and replacement of lost wages for persons suffering from injury or illness that is caused by or occurred in the workplace
   b. An insurance system for industrial- and work-related injury and is regulated primarily by the state
   c. Often requires the employee to follow a specific process/procedure for the medical services and benefits to be paid
   d. Is a heavy user of the case manager's role
   e. Focuses on timely return to work to minimize outlay of lost wages
3. Accident and health insurance
   a. Includes payment for health care–related costs
   b. May have an annual and/or lifetime maximum benefit
   c. May include long-term or short-term disability insurance to provide replacement of salary when the member is unable to work, due to illness or injury
4. Insurance plans
   a. Indemnity—Security against possible loss or damages. Reimbursement for loss that is paid in a predetermined amount in the event of covered loss.
   b. Group medical—Insurance plan providing health care coverage to a select group of people. Group health insurance plans are one of the major benefits offered by many employers. Generally, plans offer the same benefits to all employees or members of the group. The plan may have optional coverages that can be purchased, such as disability (either short or long term) and vision or dental coverages.
   c. Consumer driven—Health insurance plans that allow members to use health savings accounts (HSAs), Health Reimbursement Accounts (HRAs), or similar medical payment products to pay routine health care expenses directly, while a high-deductible health plan (HDHP) protects them from catastrophic medical expenses. HSAs and HRAs can be self-funded, pretax benefit, or tax benefit. It is important for individuals including health care professionals to be aware of and understand this benefit.
   d. Diagnosis-specific benefits
      i. Additional funding by regulatory agencies (state, federal, local)
      ii. Examples: cystic fibrosis, premature babies, crippled children, Easter Seals, Shriners
      iii. Variation in funding from private sector and regulatory agencies
   e. Stop loss insurance—Takes effect after a certain high dollar amount has been paid in claims
   f. Managed care organization
      i. A generic term applied to a managed care plan, which is inclusive of plans that do not conform to strict health maintenance organization definition but still manage the care received by its members (Kongstvedt, 2013).
      ii. A system designed to maintain the quality of health care in a cost-effective manner with a focus on delivery of health care services and payment for those services.
      iii. Also refers to both an organization that coordinates the purchase and/or delivery of health care services and a set of

        techniques used to ensure the efficiency and effectiveness of the use of these services.

    iv. The primary goal is to have a system that delivers value by giving access to quality, cost-effective health care.

B. Government programs
  1. Medicare
     a. Created in 1966, Title 18 of the Social Security Act, the official name of this piece of legislation is Health Insurance for the Aged and Disabled. Intended to finance medical care for persons aged 65 years or older and the disabled who are entitled to social security benefits (Social Security Administration, 2015)
     b. Under the administrative oversight of CMS, within the U.S. Department of Health and Human Services
     c. Identifies mandated hospital services through conditions of participation for hospitals
     d. Traditional Medicare
        i. Part A covers hospitalization, skilled nursing care, nursing home care (as long as custodial care isn't the only care required), and hospice and home health care.
        ii. Part B covers physician services, outpatient services, ambulance transport, clinical research, and mental health.
        iii. Part D covers prescription drugs.
     e. Medicare Advantage (e.g., Medicare Choice, Managed Medicare, Part C)
        i. Created by the Balanced Budget Act of 1997.
        ii. An option afforded to Medicare enrollees provided by private insurance plans.
        iii. Provides many services that a Medicare recipient would normally receive under traditional Medicare coverage.
        iv. Network may be narrow, based on contracts by plan.
        v. CMS oversees compliance of plans to federal regulations.
     f. Secondary Medicare Insurance (Medicare as Secondary Payer or MSP)
        i. Insurance provided to a Medicare beneficiary who does not select a Medicare Advantage Plan
        ii. Covers much of the co-pay and other financial responsibilities not covered by traditional Medicare
  2. Medicaid
     a. Created in 1966, Title 19 of the Social Security Act, to finance health care of the indigent and other special designated groups.
     b. Jointly financed by federal and state governments through the tax structure.
     c. States may impose nominal deductibles and co-payments on Medicaid recipients for certain services.
     d. Eligibility criteria vary from state to state and are based on the person's income, assets, and dependents.
     e. Managed Medicaid
        i. Similar to Managed Medicare, afforded to the recipients of Medicaid benefits.
        ii. Focuses on cost containment, improved access to care, and quality of care.
        iii. Provides many services that a Medicaid recipient would normally receive.
        iv. Provides health care services on a prepaid capitation basis.

   v. Many states now mandate that Medicaid beneficiaries select a
      managed Medicaid plan.
  vi. Networks may be narrow, based on plan's contracts.
 vii. State oversees compliance of plan to state regulations (CMS,
      2009).
3. Military insurance
   a. Tricare—Managed care insurance plan for active duty and retired
      members of the military, their families, and survivors
   b. CHAMPVA—Medical program with the Department of Veterans
      Affairs helping pay the cost of medical services for eligible
      veterans, veteran's dependents, and survivors of veterans
   c. Veteran Administration—Insurance plan for eligible veterans

 Components of Health Care Reimbursement

A. Limits
   1. Defines access to care for many plans including types of services
      covered.
   2. Includes list of providers an enrollee may use for health care services.
   3. Delineates consumer choice for services, for example, within or out of
      network.
   4. Cost and premiums, with patient responsibility varying significantly.
   5. Benefits vary by plan and often by plan period.
B. Reimbursement mechanism—The method applied for payment for care
   rendered. This could be in the form of case rate, capitated rate, fee for
   service, discounted, per diem, percent of charges, or others.
C. Quality management program/model
   1. A formal and planned, systematic, organization-wide (or network-
      wide) approach to the monitoring, analysis, and improvement of the
      organization's performance; focus and goal is to continually improve
      the extent to which providers conform to defined standards, the
      quality of patient care and services provided, and the likelihood of
      achieving desired outcomes.
   2. May focus on measuring outcomes on certain quality metrics (e.g.,
      immunization rates, mammography and cervical cancer rates, and so
      on), provider profiles on resource utilization, diabetics' blood sugar
      management, utilization, and enrollee satisfaction with care.
   3. Government payers such as Medicare and Medicaid examine
      quality improvement through the use of a Quality Improvement
      Organization (QIO). In some states, although rare, QIOs are still
      referred to as peer review organizations (PROs).
      a. Medicare and Medicaid oversight for appropriateness and quality
         of care. CMS has increased focus on appropriateness of care,
         including inpatient and outpatient procedures and tests.
         i. National Coverage Determinations—appropriateness of
            care established by CMS to assure no procedure or testing is
            provided without appropriate reason/indication, appropriate
            pretreatment, and/or appropriate documentation
         ii. Local Coverage Determinations—appropriateness of care
             established by Medicare contractors to assure no procedure
             or testing is provided without appropriate reason/indication,
             appropriate treatment, and/or documentation

    b. The QIO agency is also the agency that Medicare beneficiaries, both fee-for-service and Medicare Advantage plans, appeal or exercise their rights (e.g., Important Message) when being discharged from a facility while they feel they are not ready or being discharged too early.

    c. Establish and monitor medical necessity criteria.

    d. Tie financial risk to quality of care.

    e. Focus on measuring outcomes on specific metrics with outcomes linked to reimbursement through value-based purchasing program.

    f. Health care reform designated penalties for specific outcomes, such as readmissions, when the hospital is in the highest quartile for readmissions.

D. Risk sharing—The process whereby an HMO and contracted provider each accepts partial responsibility for the financial risk and rewards involved in cost-effectively caring for the members enrolled in the plan and assigned to a specific provider.

E. Credentialing—The review process applied to approve a health care professional, such as a physician as a provider of care and participant in a health plan.

F. Continuum of care—Integrated system of care that guides and tracks patients over time through a comprehensive array of health services spanning all levels of care; matches the needs of the patient with their needs and their resources.

G. Medical management—Includes case management, disease management, population management, and patient-centered medical home (PCMH).

    1. Case management—Defined by the Case Management Society of America as "a collaborative process of assessment, planning, facilitation, care coordination, evaluation, and advocacy for options and services to meet an individual's and family's comprehensive health needs through communication and available resources to promote quality, cost-effective outcomes" (2010).

        a. Other definitions exist and often differ from this definition by a few words.

        b. The CMSA definition is the one used by accreditation organizations (e.g., NCQA, URAC).

    2. High-risk screening criteria, which may indicate need for case management and/or medical management, include, but are not limited to, those listed in Box 3-3 (CMSA, 2010).

    3. Disease management—A system of coordinated health care interventions and communications for populations with chronic conditions in which patient's self-care and self-management efforts are significant. Currently these programs are referred to more as chronic care management programs (Box 3-4).

    4. Population health management program—A population health management program "strives to address health needs at all points along the continuum of health and well-being through participation of, engagement with and targeted interventions for the population" (Care Continuum Alliance, 2015). The goal for PHM is to "maintain or improve the physical and psychosocial well-being of individuals through cost-effective and tailored health solutions" (Care Continuum Alliance, 2015).

3-3 High-Risk Screening Criteria for Case Management

- Age
- Poor pain control
- Low functional status or cognitive deficits
- Previous home health and durable medical equipment usage
- History of mental illness or substance abuse, suicide risk, or crisis intervention
- Chronic, catastrophic, or terminal illness
- Social issues such as a history of abuse, neglect, no known social support, or lives alone
- Repeated emergency department visits
- Repeated admissions
- Need for admission or transition to a postacute facility
- Poor nutritional status
- Financial issues

     a. Mortality and health-related quality of life are common metrics.

     b. Policies and programs impacted by disparity and determinate factors.

         i. Disparities include race or ethnicity, sex, sexual identity, age, disability, socioeconomic status, and geography.

        ii. Determinate factors include health care, individual behavior, social environment, physical environment, and genetics.

      iii. Example focus areas include precise patient registries, determine patient–provider attribution, define precise numerators in the patient registries, monitor and measure clinical and cost metrics, adhere to basic clinical practice guidelines, engage in risk management outreach, communicate with patients, educate patients and engage with them, establish and adhere to complex clinical practice guidelines, coordinate effectively between care team and patient, and track specific outcomes.

    5. Patient-Centered Medical Home (PCMH)—A primary care organization with an emphasis on care coordination and communication to transform primary care. The American

3-4 Key Characteristics of Disease Management Programs

- Supports the physician or practitioner/patient relationship
- Uses disease management plans of care that emphasize prevention of exacerbations and complications of medical condition
- Employs evidence-based practice guidelines
- Focuses on patient empowerment strategies with the goal of improving overall health
- Focuses mainly on chronic disorders
- May include risk assessment of members
- Population management
- Management of acute phase of disease, with a focus on disease-specific complication management

College of Physicians notes, "The Patient Centered Medical Home is a care delivery model whereby patient treatment is coordinated through their primary care physician to ensure they receive the necessary care when and where they need it, in a manner they can understand" (2015). The goal of the PCMH is higher quality and lower costs, with improved patient and provider experience of care.

H. Utilization management (UM)—Review and management of health care products and services to ensure that they are medically necessary, provided in the most appropriate care setting, and at or above quality standards.
   1. Should be active and not passive.
   2. Prior approval requirements for specific procedures, such as transplants, potentially cosmetic procedures, and investigational procedures; as time goes on, more and more prior approval is required by payers.
   3. Precertification, most often related to medical necessity.
      a. Focus may be primarily on inpatient versus outpatient.
      b. Goal by payer is to reduce inpatient/hospital days to only those medically necessary.
      c. Hospital days per member per month reports are reviewed by the plan's oversight group as a measure of utilization and resource consumption.
      d. Seen most in higher cost procedures, treatments, and prescriptions.
   4. Concurrent review (continued stay review)—Reviews to approve continued treatments (e.g., inpatient hospitalization, rehabilitation, home care, DME, long-term care).
   5. Retrospective review—A form of review of a patient's medical record, conducted after health care services (including hospital stay) have been rendered and the patient is released; used to track appropriateness of care and consumption of resources.
   6. Transitional/discharge planning—Transitioning patients from one level of care to another, usually from most to least acute; however, the reverse may also happen.
   7. Based on the conditions of participation, CMS expects hospitals to provide utilization management.

I. Outcomes reporting
   1. Outcome metrics compare providers with other providers and may include:
      a. Physician practice patterns
      b. Hospital length of stay, complication rate, mortality rate, and readmission rate
      c. Home care outcomes
      d. CMS metrics, such as value-based metrics. Often includes benchmarking
   2. Health Plan Employer Data and Information Set (HEDIS)
      a. Performance measurement set for managed care organizations; focuses on the quality of the systems, processes, and services offered by the plan to enrollees. Also includes access to services and effectiveness of care.
      b. Maintained by NCQA.
      c. Data are made available to both consumers and providers.
   3. Benchmark opportunity for plans, providers, and facilities

J. Pharmaceutical services—Medication-related services and options offered by the health insurance plan
   1. Mail-order services for 90-day prescriptions at lower costs.
   2. Prescription cards for decreased costs for formulary medications (members are generally responsible for a co-pay, coinsurance, or both).
   3. Medicare Advantage (MA) Plans (Part C) provide pharmacy coverage for covered beneficiaries who are members of a given plan. Medicare Advantage Plans also cover Part B pharmaceuticals for MA members while these members still have Part D coverage on certain pharmaceuticals that are classified as Part D.
   4. Medicare Part D provides pharmacy coverage for traditional Medicare beneficiaries.
   5. Many pharmacy companies provide prescription services at a discounted rate for patients with financial limitations; these plans are usually based on a financial screen and are often referred to as Prescription or Pharmacy Assistance Programs.
K. Centers of Excellence
   1. Service lines—Location where the member, if receiving care by the provider, receives discounted services (e.g., cardiology, oncology)
   2. Encourages best practice outcomes (e.g., length of stay, readmission rates, cost per case, clinical outcomes, member satisfaction)
   3. Directs member to center with best volumes, outcomes, and lower costs
   4. Differs according to health plan

Health Care Delivery Systems

A. Health maintenance organization (HMO)—An organization that provides or arranges for coverage of designated health services needed by plan members for a fixed prepaid premium
   1. Four basic models of HMO exist, but variations on the types of plans change over time.
      a. Group model
      b. Individual practice association (IPA)
      c. Network model
      d. Staff model
   2. Under the Health Maintenance Organization Act of 1973, an organization must possess the following to call itself a health maintenance organization (HMO).
      a. Deliver a more comprehensive package of benefits
      b. Be made available to more broadly representative population
      c. Be offered on a more equitable basis
      d. More participation of consumers
      e. All at the same or lower price than traditional forms of insurance coverage
   3. Set of designated health care providers who receive a predetermined payment.
   4. Special attention is paid to access to specialists' care to influence appropriate utilization of specialty care or services (e.g., those necessary due to patient's condition and choice of the most relevant treatment approach).
   5. Primary care provider serves as gatekeeper.

6. Coverage for services out of network is limited and carefully determined.
7. May be combined with health care delivery system and various insurance plans such as a preferred provider organization.

B. Preferred provider organization (PPO)
   1. Insurance structure in which contracts are established with providers of medical care.
   2. Providers under a PPO contract are referred to as preferred providers.
   3. Usually, the contract provides significantly better benefits for services received from preferred providers, thus encouraging members to use these providers.
   4. Allows self-referral.
   5. May be higher co-pay for out-of-network referrals.

C. Point of service (POS)
   1. A type of health plan allowing the covered person to choose to receive a service from a participating or a nonparticipating provider.
   2. Different benefit levels associated with the use of participating providers.
   3. Members usually pay substantially higher costs in terms of increased premiums, deductibles, and coinsurance.
   4. Allows a blend of HMO and PPO.

D. Integrated delivery system (IDS)
   1. Partnership formed among physicians, physician groups, hospitals, and other providers to manage health care and often involves contract with payer organization.
   2. Provides services across the continuum of care and settings.
   3. May be a group that becomes an Accountable Care Organization.
   4. IDS has become increasingly popular today in light of financial risk and assurance of market share. Most common is an academic medical center partnering with other health care organizations from across the continuum of care to create vertical integration opportunity. These may include community hospitals, home care, skilled care facility, physician practices/primary care, and so on.

Reimbursement Methods

A. Fee for service (FFS)
   1. Providers are paid for each service performed.
   2. Set fee for service provided.
   3. Fee schedules are an example of fee for service.
   4. No discounts given.

B. Discounted fee for service—providers are paid set fee for specific service, but at a previously agreed-upon discount.

C. Per diem
   1. All services provided for a specific amount per day regardless of actual costs
   2. Based on averaging costs and number of days of service
   3. Often have strong oversight by payer, as each hospital day must be authorized by the plan for reimbursement to occur

D. Percent of charges
   1. Fixed percentage of charges paid to hospitals, based on charges on patient's bill.
   2. Percent may vary based on contractual agreements.

E. Risk sharing—commercial health insurance plans
   1. The process whereby an HMO and contracted provider each accepts partial responsibility for the financial risks and rewards involved in caring for the members enrolled in the plan.
   2. Focuses on target payment for health care costs per member per month between a plan and a provider or a network of providers.
   3. The payer uses a withhold process in which payment for services is reduced by a specified amount. At year end, calculations determine that the percent of the withheld amount will be returned to the provider.
F. Medicare Shared Savings Program, established as part of the Patient Protection and Affordable Care Act of 2010 (CMS, 2015c)
   1. Medicare has risk-sharing contracts such as the MSSP plan tier 3 along with the Medicare ACOs (e.g., Pioneer, NextGen). There are upside and downside risks for these contracts.
   2. Accountable Care Organizations are groups of doctors, hospitals, and other health care providers, who come together voluntarily to give coordinated high-quality care to a predetermined group of Medicare beneficiaries.
      a. The goal of coordinated care is to ensure that patients, especially the chronically ill, receive the right care at the right time while avoiding unnecessary duplication of services and preventing medical errors.
      b. When an ACO succeeds both in delivering high-quality care and spending health care dollars more wisely, it will share in the savings it achieves for the Medicare program (CMS, 2015c).
   3. Participation in the Medicare Shared Savings Program (Shared Savings Program) is voluntary. Program participants are required to collect and report on 33 quality measures, including:
      a. Patient experience survey measures
      b. Claims-based measures
      c. The Electronic Health Record (EHR) Incentive Program measure
      d. Twenty-two measures reported via the ACO GPRO Web interface
   4. ACOs, on behalf of their ACO provider/suppliers who are eligible professionals, must submit the measures determined under §425.500 using an online/Web interface–established mechanism (CMS, 2015c).
G. DRG/case rate: Traditional Medicare payment system that has also been adopted by Medicaid, MA Plans, and some commercial insurance plans
   1. Rate of reimbursement that packages pricing for a certain category of services.
   2. Specific dollar amount paid based on classification of illness, diagnosis, or procedure.
   3. Audits may be done to ensure accurate coding.
H. Capitation
   1. A fixed amount of money, determined on a per member per month (PMPM) basis, paid to a care provider for covered services rather than based on specific services provided
   2. The typical reimbursement method used by HMOs
   3. Whether a member uses the health service once or more than once, a provider who is capitated receives the same payment

I. Carve-out services
   1. Services excluded from a provider contract that may be covered through arrangements with other providers; usually refers to a specific service provided
   2. Separate negotiations for unusually complex or high-cost services, such as organ transplant or bone marrow transplant
   3. Could be services required in a complicated case, such as additional home care services that exceed expected care, such as additional physical therapy services
J. Pay-for-performance (P4P), also known today as value-based purchasing
   1. Pay based on outcomes of specific diseases or DRGs.
   2. May be managed through a center of excellence, such as cardiovascular or orthopedic.
   3. Outcomes may include mortality and morbidity rates, core measures, clinical outcomes, patient/family health-related teaching, length of stay, costs, readmission and complication rates, and satisfaction with care.
   4. Medicare is using P4P in its contracting with Medicare Shared Savings Programs (MSSPs) and Accountable Care Organizations (ACOs).
K. Global payment or bundled payment
   1. A predetermined all-inclusive payment structure for a specific set of related services, treated as a single unit for billing or reimbursement purposes
   2. Combines reimbursement for both facility and professional services into one lump sum payment
   3. Commonly seen in transplants
   4. Usually includes services or procedures with any related postcare included
   5. Increased focus by CMS with both demonstration projects and proposed mandatory involvement by specifically identified geographic areas
L. Stop loss
   1. Used to share risk in complex patients.
   2. Payment may increase to a provider after a specified dollar threshold is met. For example, the hospital payment converts from DRG payment to percent of charges once a specified dollar threshold is reached.
   3. Stop loss can be first dollar after the specific dollar amount is reached or can be the first dollar of an entire episode of care or hospital stay.
M. Managed government plans
   1. Payment by a plan that agrees to pay health care benefits for specific populations, such as Medicare or Medicaid.
   2. Managed Medicare plans are selected by patients and are optional.
   3. Managed Medicaid plans may be either selected by patients or, most frequently, mandated by a state.
   4. Provider follows government rules and regulations for these payment groups; that is, at a minimum, providers must offer the same services offered under the government plans (mainly Medicare and Medicaid).
   5. Plan assumes risk for member, who relinquishes traditional coverage (either voluntary or assigned, depending on state regulations).

N. Third-party administrator/administration (TPA)
   1. Administration of a group insurance plan by some person or firm other than the insurer of the policyholder
   2. Organization outside of the insuring organization that handles only administrative functions, such as utilization review and processing of claims
   3. Used by organizations that directly fund the health benefits but do not find it cost-effective to administer the day-to-day operation of their own plan
O. Government payers
   1. Medicare and Medicaid benefit plans
   2. Future plans for reimbursement
      a. Continued Medicare demonstration projects including ACOs and MSSPs
      b. ICD-10
      c. Mandatory bundled payment
      d. Reimbursement only for quality
      e. Additional national and local coverage determinations
      f. Additional billing compliance requirements
      g. Value-based purchasing
      h. Quality outcomes–based payment

Challenges with Health Care Reimbursement

A. Financial—Concern that financial incentives may compromise quality of care.
B. Patient choice of physicians/care providers and facilities limited unless patient pays out-of-network fees or has PPO.
C. Benefits mandated by various state regulations.
D. Patient and provider education are essential.
E. Increased requirement for electronic communication.
F. Often minimum flexibility, especially when it comes to:
   1. Nontraditional treatments
   2. Uncovered benefits
   3. Postacute levels of care
G. Focus on technical/administrative denials rather than payment for services provided.
H. Uninsured and underinsured patients.
I. Medicare demonstration projects and their effects on reimbursement systems will result in renewed reimbursement methods such as pay-for-performance or global funding for certain procedures or diseases.
J. Continued contraction of payer market (e.g., mergers) and increased power to control health care service delivery and reimbursement may limit consumer choice.

Legal Issues Impacting Managed Care

A. Government and legislative issues
   1. Employee Retirement Income Security Act (ERISA)—Federal law sets minimum standards for most voluntarily established pension and

health plans in private industry to provide protection for individuals in these plans. Increased concern about ethical decisions impacting patient care (Department of Labor, n.d.a).
2. Consolidated Omnibus Budget Reconciliation Act of 1986 (COBRA)—Law requires certain employers to allow qualified employees, spouses, and dependents to continue health insurance coverage when it would otherwise stop (e.g., upon leaving employment) (Department of Labor, n.d.b).
3. Health Insurance Portability and Accountability Act of 1996 (HIPAA)
    a. Came about with the advent of electronic medical records and the transfer of information electronically from one health plan to another or care provider to another.
    b. Privacy rule protects individual medical records and personal health information (PHI).
    c. Limits the release of information to the minimum reasonably needed for the purpose of disclosure.
    d. Includes a variety of regulations, such as fraud and abuse.
    e. Gives patients the right to obtain copies of their own health records (Department of Health and Human Services, n.d.).

Strategies in Managed Care

A. Managed care practices have resulted in the addition or reinforcement of many strategies that ensure quality of care and assist in controlling health care costs. Some of the strategies case managers must be aware of the following:
1. Medical management practices that are part and parcel of managed care—utilization management, case management, quality management, disease management, and population management
2. Claims processing and the use of information systems
3. Keeping costs at a minimum by applying the following strategies:
    a. Complying with the procedures and practices stipulated in the contractual agreement between health plans and providers/agencies
    b. Ensuring that bed days in hospitals are appropriate and as indicated by the patient's conditions
    c. Using the case management services offered by the plan
    d. Employing health promotion and illness prevention strategies such as patient and family education, risk reduction programs, etc.
4. Managed care/insurance contracts that are specific about reimbursement, utilization management, and the denials and appeal processes/procedures
    a. Utilization management practices: precertification, authorization, level of care and status for services, and denial and appeal processes
    b. Definitions of medical necessity for care and treatment applying evidence-based guidelines and protocols
    c. Reimbursement methods, such as per diem or case rate
    d. May be very detailed, including reimbursement terms and criteria by service line or time of day for communication requirements
    e. Often stipulate billing mechanism and process
    f. Quality metrics impacting reimbursement

3-5 HEDIS Main Areas of Measurement

- Effectiveness of care
- Access to and availability of services
- Consumer satisfaction/experience with care
- Health plan stability
- Consumer health choice
- Cost of services
- Utilization management
- Credentialing of health care professionals

5. Shifting from inpatient care to outpatient care, when possible
   a. Insurance plans may try to decrease hospital bed days by shifting inpatients to observation.
   b. Decisions regarding best care setting for treatment are made based on the clinical condition of the patient and the treatment options to be implemented.
6. Tracking the duration/length of treatment, especially length of hospital stay; lifetime maximum, episode-of-care maximum payment
7. Complying with NCQA standards and the HEDIS national indicators and performance measures
   a. NCQA—National organization comprised of health care quality management professionals.
      i. Offers an accreditation program for managed health care plans
      ii. Focus on the quality of the systems, processes, and services a managed care/health plan delivers to its enrollees
   b. HEDIS measures of health plan performance are in the public domain and accessible to health care consumers; measures vary in focus but include clinical, financial, and experience of care (Box 3-5).

 Compliance Considerations for Case Managers

A. Bill only for the level of care that is provided.
   1. When in the hospital, level of care is driven by medical necessity of care delivered, not by the location of patient in a facility.
   2. For example, a patient in an ICU bed who is not receiving ICU level of care should not be billed for ICU care.
B. Follow CMS rules and regulations for hospital billing.
   1. The Two Midnight Rule.
      a. Guides billing and documentation for short-stay patients as either inpatients or patients in observation service
         i. Appropriate order for admission, if inpatient.
         ii. Indicate if patient expected to be in hospital at least two midnights.
         iii. Document requirement for hospital services, if inpatient.
         iv. Discuss discharge plan in record.
         v. Authenticate order before discharge.
         vi. Perform self-audit on all short stays (CMS, 2015b).

2. Patients who are admitted as inpatient but do not meet medical necessity must not be billed as inpatient.
   a. Must follow Condition Code 44 process if billing Condition Code 44 (CMS, n.d.b).
      i. Must refer case to Utilization Management (UM) Committee.
      ii. UM Committee must discuss case with physician of case.
      iii. If physician agrees with UM Committee, notation of agreement with UM Committee is made in medical record.
      iv. If physician disagrees, cannot bill Condition Code 44.
      v. To bill Condition Code 44, patient must not be discharged from hospital before process completed.
   b. If patient has been discharged from hospital before completion of process, provider liable is billed.
3. Conditions of participation requirement for utilization management plan and committee.
   a. Utilization Management Committee
      i. Staff committee of institution or outsourced approved by a hospital committee
      ii. Must consist of two or more practitioners who carry out the UR function and at least two of the members of the committee must be doctors of medicine or osteopathy.
      iii. Committee or group's reviews may not be conducted by any individual who has a direct financial interest (e.g., an ownership interest) in that hospital or was professionally involved in the care of the patient whose case is being reviewed.
      iv. Must conduct reviews of duration of stays and review of professional services.
      v. In hospitals paid under the prospective payment system, the UR committee must review all cases reasonably assumed by the hospital to be outlier cases because the extended length of stay exceeds the threshold criteria for the diagnosis.
   b. Utilization review plan
      i. Having a utilization review plan is required.
      ii. Must address review for Medicare and Medicaid beneficiaries with respect to the medical necessity of admissions to the institution, duration of stays, and professional services furnished, including drugs and biologic agents.
4. Important Message (IM)—Allows for a beneficiary to appeal inpatient discharge. The first IM notice is usually given to the patient/family upon admission to the hospital. The second IM notice must be delivered within 2 days of discharge and not at the time of discharge. The beneficiary must have the opportunity to appeal if he/she chooses to do so. The appeal is done through the regional QIO (CMS, n.d.c).
5. Advanced beneficiary notice (ABN) or hospital-issued notice of noncoverage (HINN) must be given to beneficiary per regulations for services not covered by Medicare to be billed to patient (CMS, 2014b, 2014c).

Reimbursement Implications for Case Managers

A. For effective practice and performance, case managers must be knowledgeable in the following areas:
   1. The health plan or the managed care contract
      a. Payer contact information
      b. Reimbursement method(s)
      c. Utilization review and management requirements, including medical necessity criteria used by plan
      d. Postacute care–approved panel of providers (individuals and facilities/agencies)
      e. Denials and appeal processes/procedures
   2. The relationships with the insurance-based case manager
      a. Be aware of the implications of the role of the case manager in insurance companies and the complexity of the said role, especially when there is a need for plan dollars to be utilized in a nontraditional fashion.
      b. Provide advocacy when patients' needs may not be considered in the typical premium structure; these situations result in the need for case managers to ensure advocacy for their patients' benefits.
      c. Be aware of the layers of fiduciaries, administrators, and claims adjustors involved in approval processes.
      d. Special attention should be paid to untimely decisions, which delay case manager interventions and patient treatment; case manager must be aware of the contractual and legislative time frames required.
      e. Size of insured groups can impact the timeliness of appropriate cost-effective care.
      f. Case managers must know state regulations for plan coverage to ensure timely coordination of benefits.
      g. Optimize communication opportunities with insurance company staff.
   3. Use of medical necessity and appropriateness of services criteria to ensure approval of benefits and reimbursement
      a. Be knowledgeable of the utilization review/management criteria used by payers.
      b. Gain a comprehensive understanding of benefits based on specific health plans, for example, lifetime maximums and use of Medicare days for hospitalized patients.
      c. Be able to develop effective plans of care for patients and broker appropriate services as needed and across the continuum of care.
      d. Ensure optimal use of available benefits.
      e. Coordinate care and services with patients, families, and other care providers.
   4. Building partnerships with physicians
      a. Function as an effective leader or facilitator of the multidisciplinary team.
      b. Work closely with physicians on establishing appropriate and timely plans of care for patients, including discharge plans, reimbursement plans, and procurement of resources.

      c. Collaborate with physicians when addressing reimbursement denials.

      d. Educate physicians about the dynamics of health care delivery systems, including the various types of health plans and their related utilization management procedures.

5. Identifying nonmedical challenges that influence patient care outcomes and transitions of care

      a. Understand the impact of underinsurance (and lack of insurance altogether) on patient care delivery, access to services, and outcomes of care.

      b. Identify the presence of psychosocial and financial barriers that impact care delivery, decision making regarding treatment options, and patient's adherence to treatment regimen.

      c. Be aware of the reasons that patients may exhibit behaviors of noncompliance with the plan of care, identify such behaviors, and address them to prevent undesired outcomes.

      d. Be sensitive to cultural factors that may negatively or positively affect patient's behaviors and adherence to the plan of care.

6. Managing conflict and resolving problems as they arise

      a. Coordinate patient care activities when patient choices do not match recommendations by health care providers, such as the patient or family who chooses to take a patient home when a skilled nursing facility is recommended and necessary.

      b. Hold a case conference when conflicts regarding the development of the plan of care or making decisions regarding treatment options arise between patients and their families or between patients and their health care providers.

      c. Be able to assume the role of the patient advocate when needed.

      d. Seek the counsel of a third party, such as a patient representative, when unable to resolve conflict.

      e. Call for an ethics consult when the need arises.

      f. Actively participate in multidisciplinary rounds, both in the inpatient and outpatient settings.

References

American College of Physicians. (2015). *What is the patient-centered medical home?* Retrieved from http://www.acponline.org/running_practice/delivery_and_payment_models/pcmh/understanding/what.htm, on July 30, 2015.

Care Continuum Alliance. (2015). *Understanding population health.* Retrieved from http://www.populationhealthalliance.org/research/understanding-population-health.html, on July 30, 2015.

Case Management Society of America. (2010). *CMSA standards of practice for case management.* Little Rock, AR: Author.

Centers for Medicare and Medicaid Services. (2009). *Brief summaries of Medicare and Medicaid.* Retrieved from http://www.cms.gov/Research-Statistics-Data-and-Systems/Statistics-Trends-and-Reports/MedicareProgramRatesStats/downloads/MedicareMedicaidSummaries2009.pdf, on July 30, 2015.

Centers for Medicare and Medicaid Services. (2014a). *Conditional payment information.* Retrieved from http://www.cms.gov/Medicare/Coordination-of-Benefits-and-Recovery/Attorney-Services/Conditional-Payment-Information/Conditional-Payment-Information.html, on July 30, 2015.

Centers for Medicare and Medicaid Services. (2014b). *FFS HINNS.* Retrieved from http://www.cms.gov/Medicare/Medicare-General-Information/BNI/HINNs.html, on July 30, 2015.

Centers for Medicare and Medicaid Services. (2014c). *FFS ABN.* Retrieved from http://www.cms.gov/Medicare/Medicare-General-Information/BNI/ABN.html, on July 30, 2015.

Centers for Medicare and Medicaid Services. (2015a). *Prospective payment systems—General information.* Retrieved from http://www.cms.gov/Medicare/Medicare-Fee-for-Service-Payment/ProspMedicareFeeSvcPmtGen/index.html?redirect=/ProspMedicareFeeSvcPmtGen, on July 30, 2015.

Centers for Medicare and Medicaid Services. (2015b). *Fact sheet: Two midnight rule.* Retrieved from http://www.cms.gov/Newsroom/MediaReleaseDatabase/Fact-sheets/2015-Fact-sheets-items/2015-07-01-2.html, on July 30, 2015.

Centers for Medicare and Medicaid Services. (2015c). *Medicare: Shared savings program.* Retrieved from https://www.cms.gov/Medicare/Medicare-Fee-for-Service-Payment/sharedsavings-program/index.html, on September 7, 2015.

Centers for Medicare and Medicaid Services. (n.d.a). *Legislative summary: Balanced Budget Act of 1997 Medicare and Medicaid provisions.* Retrieved from https://www.cms.gov/Medicare/Demonstration-Projects/DemoProjectsEvalRpts/downloads/cc_section4016_bba_1997.pdf, on July 30, 2015.

Centers for Medicare and Medicaid Services. (n.d.b). *Frequently asked questions: Using Condition Code 44.* Retrieved from https://questions.cms.gov/faq.php?id=5005&faqId=9742, on July 30, 2015.

Centers for Medicare and Medicaid Services. (n.d.c). *An important message from Medicare about your rights.* Retrieved from http://www.cms.gov/Medicare/Medicare-General-Information/BNI/downloads/RevisedImportantMessageFromMedicare05_2007.pdf, on July 30, 2015.

Department of Health and Human Services. (2014a). *About the law.* Retrieved from http://www.hhs.gov/healthcare/rights, on July 30, 2015.

Department of Health and Human Services. (2014b). *Hospital outpatient prospective payment system.* Retrieved from http://www.cms.gov/Outreach-and-Education/Medicare-Learning-Network-MLN/MLNProducts/downloads/HospitalOutpaysysfctsht.pdf, on July 30, 2015.

Department of Health and Human Services. (n.d.). *Health information privacy.* Retrieved from http://www.hhs.gov/ocr/privacy, on July 30, 2015.

Department of Labor. (n.d.a). *Employee Retirement Income Security Act.* Retrieved from http://www.dol.gov/dol/topic/health-plans/erisa.htm, on July 30, 2015.

Department of Labor. (n.d.b). *Frequently asked questions—COBRA continuing health coverage.* Retrieved from http://www.dol.gov/ebsa/faqs/faq_compliance_cobra.html, on July 30, 2015.

Kaiser Family Foundation. (2012). *Summary of coverage provisions in the Patient Protection and Affordable Care Act.* Retrieved from http://kff.org/health-costs/issue-brief/summary-of-coverage-provisions-in-the-patient, on July 30, 2015.

Kongstvedt, P. R. (2013). *Essentials of managed health care* (6th ed.). Burlington, VT: Jones & Bartlett.

Social Security Administration. (2015). *Compilation of Social Security Laws.* Retrieved from http://www.ssa.gov/OP_Home/ssact/title18/1800.htm, on July 30, 2015.

The Hilltop Institute. (2009). *Resource utilization groups.* Retrieved from http://www.hilltopinstitute.org/publications/ResourceUtilizationGroups-RUGs-September2009.pdf, on July 30, 2015.

The Leapfrog Group. (2015). *Who we are.* Retrieved from http://www.leapfroggroup.org, on July 30, 2015.

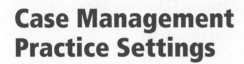

CHAPTER 4

Case Management Practice Settings

Hussein M. Tahan

LEARNING OBJECTIVES

Upon completion of this chapter, the reader will be able to:

1. Identify the various health care settings that constitute the continuum of care/continuum of health and human services.
2. Define the continuum of care/continuum of health and human services.
3. List the practice settings of case management.
4. Describe the role of the case manager in relation to the continuum of care and practice settings.
5. Define patient flow and throughput and describe their relationships with case management.
6. Describe the role of the case manager in throughput and patient flow.

IMPORTANT TERMS AND CONCEPTS

Beyond-the-Walls Case Management
Continuum of Care
Continuum of Health and Human Services
Independent Case Management
Input
Level of Care
Outcome

Output
Patient Flow
Patient-Centered Medical Home
Payer-Based Case Management
Practice Setting
Private Case Management
Process

Structure
Telephonic Case Management
Throughput
Transition of Care
Within-the-Walls Case Management

Introduction

A. Case management has been applied as a strategy, process, system, or a model for care delivery in every setting of the health care continuum.
B. There are many reasons for the implementation of case management models in various care settings across the continuum of health and human services. Some of these are shared in Box 4-1.
C. Case management is not a new approach to managing patient care. It has reached every health care setting across the continuum.
   1. 1880s: Outpatient and community settings, particularly the care of the poor
   2. 1920s: Outpatient and community care settings, particularly the care of psychiatric patients and individuals with chronic and long-term illnesses
   3. 1930s: Public health/community care settings

BOX 4-1 Reasons for Implementation of Case Management Models

- Rising number of the elderly, especially those with multiple chronic and complex health conditions
- Use of innovative and sophisticated health care technology that tends to be costly, including biomedical informatics, social media and Internet-based tools, and remote monitoring
- Increase in the use of minimally invasive and robotic surgery and the likelihood of performing surgical procedures in the ambulatory care setting
- Rising number of newer and rare diseases especially those that are infectious in nature and that require costly health care resources
- Popularity of life-prolonging treatments such as organ transplantation and life-sustaining measures
- Changes in health care reimbursement methods, particularly those that place the provider of care or the consumer at higher financial risk. For example, managed care, capitation, and bundled and prospective payment methods
- Prospective payment systems being applied by federal and state governments that have reached almost all settings of care delivery such as long-term care, home care, acute care, subacute care, rehabilitation, and skilled care environments
- Recent legal and regulatory changes including the Patient Protection and Affordable Care Act of 2010 and Value Based Purchasing programs
- Educated consumers of health care
- Pressures to cut the forever rising cost of health care services
- Shortages in health care workforces including nursing, pharmacy, primary care providers, and physical, occupational, and respiratory therapy
- Rising ethical concerns and legal liability resulting in the practice of defensive medicine
- Shift of health care delivery and services from the acute to the non–acute care settings such as home care, patient-centered medical home, long-term care, and rehabilitation care settings
- Increased demand for quality of care that is supported or evidenced by measurable outcomes
- Changes in the standards of accreditation and regulatory agencies, particularly those that impact on case management practice, such as those that address continuity of care, care across the continuum, discharge and transitional planning, safety, and patients' rights and self-management

4. 1950s: Behavioral health across the continuum of care, especially deinstitutionalization of patients with mental health issues
5. 1970s and 1980s: Long-term care settings through demonstration projects funded by Medicare and Medicaid waivers
6. 1985s: Acute care settings, particularly as nursing case management programs
7. 1990s: Virtually all health care settings including health insurance plans and managed care organizations
8. 2000s: Changes in health care laws and regulations as a result of health care reform resulting in more insured individuals and increased financial risk on the provider of care. Also shift in reimbursement for care to a value-based purchasing model where financial penalties are imposed on the providers by the Centers of Medicare and Medicaid Services when outcomes (i.e., quality, safety, and cost) are not considered meeting targets or expectations
9. 2010s: Shift from reimbursement based on volume to value of care and proliferation of community-based (e.g., patient-centered medical home) and nontraditional sites of care such as Walgreens and CVS

D. The use of case management varies from one practice setting to another, with its identifying characteristics dependent on the discipline that applies it, the professional who assumes the role of the case manager, the staffing mix, and the context of the setting where it is implemented including its related reimbursement method(s).
E. The main characteristics of case management, regardless of care or practice setting, include those listed in Box 4-2.
F. Case management allows the integration and coordination of health care services across consumers of health care, providers of care, payers for

BOX 4-2   Characteristics of Case Management Programs or Models

- Outcomes-oriented care delivery that focuses on monitoring and measurement of patient safety, continuity, cost, and quality of care
- Appropriate resource allocation and utilization that is justified by the patient's condition and the required treatment, using nationally recognized medical necessity criteria, with cost-effectiveness as the ultimate outcome
- Comprehensive care planning including early assessment, intervention, and linking patients and their families to needed services, to be offered by the right provider, at the right time, in the right quantity, and in the most appropriate level of care
- Integration and coordination of care delivery to eliminate fragmentation, duplication, and/or wastes
- Collaboration across care providers, disciplines, care settings, and nontraditional care providers
- Advocacy to ensure that needed services are obtained and expected outcomes are met
- Use of a licensed professional as the case manager with support from unlicensed personnel functioning in case manager's associate role (e.g., community health worker)
- Adherence to the standards of accreditation and regulatory agencies
- Open lines of communication and sharing of important information across care providers, care settings, and the patient/family
- Consumers' experience of care and staff's job satisfaction

services, and care settings; that is, across persons, space, and time. This is most effective because case management

1. Opens lines of communication about needed and important information among providers, consumers, and payers.
2. Facilitates an environment of collaboration among providers, consumers, and payers regardless of space and time. Such is most evident in the presence of shared goals, effective communication, handoff communications during transitions of care, and shared decision making.
3. Promotes a patient-centered approach to care by meeting all of the patient's and family's needs, preferences, and interests.
4. Ensures continuity of care over time and across care settings or providers.

G. Case management gained more momentum when the health care delivery system began to gradually shift away from the inpatient care setting (hospital). Owing to numerous technological advances in diagnostics, medications, and procedures, and the evolution of reimbursement plans that limit inpatient hospital stays (e.g., Medicare's prospective payment system and managed care health plans), most health care needs can be handled on an outpatient basis.

H. Case management has been described as "within the walls" and "beyond the walls" (Cohen & Cesta, 2005).
1. Within the walls—Case management models in the acute care/hospital settings
2. Beyond the walls—Case management models in the outpatient, community, long-term, and payer-based settings

I. Case management has also been implemented as a core strategy of population-based disease management and population health programs.

J. Recently, case management became an essential strategy for ensuring care quality and patient safety, especially in reducing or preventing the risk for medical errors during transitions of care (handoffs), patient flow through the system of health care services and throughput, and core measures of the value-based purchasing programs such as low to no avoidable hospital readmissions.

Descriptions of Key Terms

A. Beyond-the-walls case management—Models of case management that are implemented outside the acute care/hospital setting; that is, in the community, outpatient clinics and physician practices, long-term care, ambulatory surgery centers, and payer settings.

B. Boarding patients—Occurs as a result of situations when a patient remains in an area such as the emergency department (ED) or postanesthesia care unit for a period of time, usually 2 hours or longer, after a decision has been made to admit the patient to an inpatient bed. Sometimes, this term is used when a patient is temporarily admitted to a specialty other than the one needed based on condition and care needs due to lack of beds in the appropriate setting; for example, surgical instead of a medical unit.

C. Crowding—Increased number of patients who are awaiting care or are in the process of receiving care in an area (i.e., care setting such as the ED) beyond the capacity the area can handle. An example is ED crowding as a result of inability to move patients out of the ED and into inpatient beds when these patients must be admitted rather than released.

D. Diversion—Occurs when hospitals request that ambulances bypass their EDs and transport patients to other health care facilities who otherwise would have been cared for at these EDs. This event happens as a result of ED crowding and situations where EDs cannot safely handle additional ambulance patients.

E. Handoff—The act of transferring the care of a patient from one provider to another, from one care setting to another, or from one level of care to another.

F. Health care continuum—Care settings that vary across a continuum based on levels of care that are also characterized by complexity and intensity of resources and services. Sometimes, it is referred to as the continuum of health and human services; in this case, the focus is more on the type of services available across the care settings, which include those that address socioeconomic and psychosocial issues rather than just medical care.

G. Input—Elements or characteristics taken into consideration when providing care to a patient. It also may mean the patient's condition at the time he or she presents for care in a particular care setting such as a clinic, emergency department, or hospital. Examples may include age, gender, health status, social network, reason for accessing health care services, or insurance status.

H. Left before a medical evaluation—Occurs when a patient who presents to the ED for care, but leaves the ED after triage and before receiving a medical evaluation. Generally, this happens with nonemergent conditions where patients need to wait for treatment of lowest type of urgency, usually nonlife sustaining.

I. Level of care—The intensity of resources and services required to diagnose, treat, preserve, or maintain an individual's physical and/or emotional health and functioning. Levels of care vary across a continuum of least to most complex resources and/or services—that is, from prevention and wellness, to nonacute, rehabilitative, subacute, and acute, to critical.

J. Level of service—The delivery of services and use of resources that are dependent on the patient's condition and the needed level of care. Assessment of the level of service is used to ensure that the patient is receiving care at the appropriate level.

K. Outcome—The result, output, or consequence of a health care process. It may be the result of care received or not received. It also represents the cumulative effects of one or more care processes on an individual at a defined point in time. Outcome can also mean the goal or objective of the care rendered.

L. Output—Results or outcomes of care provision. It also may mean the patient's condition at the time he or she exits a health care setting, an episode of care, or transitions to another level of care, location, or provider. Examples may include death, discharge to home with home care or no services, or discharge to a skilled nursing facility.

M. Patient flow—The movement of patients through a set of locations in a health care facility. These locations are the levels of care required by the patient based on health condition and clinical treatment. Patient flow entails the transitioning of an individual from point A to point B of a health care facility or setting; that is, from the patient's entry point to the checkout point of the health care facility where care is being provided.

N. Practice setting—A care setting in which a case manager is employed and is able to execute his or her role functions and responsibilities. Care settings (and therefore practice settings) vary across homogeneous populations of patients such as organ transplant, pediatrics, and geriatric or across physical care delivery areas such as ambulatory clinics; acute hospital; long-term, skilled care facilities; subacute rehabilitation; or payer organizations.

O. Process—The methods, procedures, styles, and techniques rendered in the delivery of health care services. These relate to the roles, responsibilities, and functions of the various health care providers, including case managers, and how they go about fulfilling them.

P. Structure—The characteristics of the system/environment of care or health care organization including those associated with the providers of care and the patients/families who are the recipients of care. It relates to the level of care or setting, the nature of the care delivery model, the health and socioeconomic status of the patients, and the skills, knowledge, education, and competencies of the health care providers.

Q. Throughput—The actual operations of a care setting. It also refers to the clinical and administrative processes applied in the setting to deliver quality patient care and services. Processes may include the use of a case manager; availability of ancillary services such as pharmacy, laboratory, and radiology; and the type of treatments implemented for the care of a patient.

R. Transition of care—The process of moving patients from one level of care or provider to another, usually from most to least complex or from generalist to specialty care provider; however, depending on the patient's health condition and needed treatments, the transition can occur from least to most complex.

S. Within-the-walls case management—Models of case management that are implemented in the acute care/hospital-based setting.

Applicability to CMSA's Standards of Practice

A. The Case Management Society of America (CMSA) describes in its standards of practice for case management (CMSA, 2010) that case management practice extends across all health care settings, including payer, provider, government, employer, community, and home environment.

B. CMSA explains that case management practice varies in degrees of complexity and comprehensiveness based on four factors:
1. The context of the care setting (e.g., wellness and prevention, acute, subacute, rehabilitative, or end of life)
2. The health conditions and needs of the patient population(s) served including those of the patients' families
3. The reimbursement method applied for services rendered (payment), such as managed care, workers' compensation, Medicare, or Medicaid
4. The health care professional discipline assuming the role of the case manager such as registered nurse, social worker, or rehabilitation counselor

| 4-3 | **Various Case Management Practice/Care Settings** |

- Hospitals and integrated care delivery systems, including acute care, subacute care, long-term acute care (LTAC) facilities, skilled nursing facilities (SNF), and rehabilitation facilities
- Ambulatory care clinics and community-based organizations, including student/university counseling and health care centers
- Corporations
- Public health insurance programs, for example, Medicare, Medicaid, and state-funded programs
- Private health insurance programs, for example, workers' compensation, occupational health, disability, liability, accident and health, long-term care insurance, group health insurance, and managed care organizations
- Independent and private case management companies
- Government-sponsored programs, for example, correctional facilities, military health care/Veterans Administration, and public health
- Provider agencies and community facilities, that is, mental health centers, home health services, and ambulatory and day care facilities
- Geriatric services, including residential and assisted living facilities
- Long-term care services, including home and community-based services
- Hospice, palliative, and respite care programs
- Physician and medical group practices, including patient-centered medical home
- Life care planning programs

C. This chapter describes the various care settings across the continuum of health and human services with special focus on the role of the case manager in these settings and the case management services provided.

D. CMSA identifies case management practice settings (Box 4-3) to include but not limited to those listed below. This chapter describes these settings based on the complexity of the services offered and the acuity of the health conditions of the patients cared for in these settings. The care settings are grouped into preacute, acute, and postacute types.

E. Although CMSA describes practice settings of case managers, these settings also may be viewed as patient care settings across the continuum.

 ## Case Management Practice Settings

A. Case management is practiced across all settings of the health care continuum in varying degrees of complexity and intensity and is dependent on five factors (Box 4-4).

B. The role of the case manager also varies based on the care/practice setting and the above five factors. It tends to be more complex as the needs and services a patient requires intensify. The role also is more necessary and valuable when a multidisciplinary team of providers is involved in the care of a patient compared to a single or primary care provider alone.

C. The best and most effective models of case management are those that focus on the continuum of care and settings. Regardless of the setting in which the model is implemented, it is most beneficial if

BOX
4-4

Factors That Impact the Complexity and Intensity of Case Management

1. The context of the care setting (e.g., ambulatory or community based vs. acute or hospital based)
2. The patient's health condition and needs (e.g., critical or acute episode of illness vs. long-term and chronic condition)
3. The reimbursement method applied (e.g., managed care, capitation, or bundled vs. prospective payment system)
4. The type of care provider(s) needed for care provision (e.g., generalist vs. specialist physician and individual provider vs. an interdisciplinary team)
5. The intensity of the resources and services needed to meet the care and health needs of the patient; for example, prevention and wellness, life-saving or life-sustaining measures, rehabilitative, or screening for disease risk factors and early diagnosis

it facilitates (specifically in the role of the case manager) open lines of communication and collaborations/partnerships with health care providers practicing within and outside the setting where the patient is being cared for, emphasizes a patient- and family-centered approach to care provision, and ensures that the patient/family needs are addressed even beyond the setting the patient accesses for care.

D. According to Cesta and Tahan (2003), the health care continuum can be divided into three major settings based on the scope, type, and cost of services provided. These are preacute, acute, and postacute (Box 4-5).

E. The preacute case management practice settings include the following:
1. Telephonic
2. Payer-based or managed care organization
3. Ambulatory or clinic/outpatient/patient-centered medical or health home
4. Community care
5. Disease management
6. Population health management.

F. The acute case management practice settings include the following:
1. Hospital
2. Acute rehabilitation
3. Emergency department
4. Transitional hospitals, also known as subacute care facilities
5. Disease management
6. Surgical centers.

G. The postacute case management practice settings include the following:
1. Subacute
2. Home care
3. Long-term care
4. Palliative, hospice, or end of life
5. Respite care
6. Residential
7. Custodial
8. Assisted living
9. Day care

BOX 4-5 Three Major Settings of the Health Care Continuum

1. Preacute setting
   a. Focus is on the prevention of illness or deterioration in an individual's health condition.
   b. Least complex services; primarily proactive approach to care provision that can be self-directed or that may not require the attention of a health care provider.
   c. Cost is low and, in some instances, may be free.
   d. Examples may include primary prevention of illness in the form of health promotion, risk assessment, and screening, fitness, counseling, lifestyle changes, and behavior modification.
   e. Provision of care does not require admission to a health care facility; care may be limited to a clinic or outpatient setting including a physician's office, a managed care organization, and community-based health centers.
   f. Case management services are minimal and include telephonic health promotion services and advice lines, health appraisals, and risk reduction strategies.
2. Acute setting
   a. Focus is on treating an acute episode of illness such as medical or surgical management and trauma or emergency care.
   b. Most complex services; primarily reactive approach to care provision and requires the attention of a health care provider.
   c. Cost is high; care provision may require the authorization of the payer or insurer.
   d. Examples may include secondary and tertiary prevention of illness, major diagnostic and therapeutic modalities, surgical/operative procedures, medical management, acute or intensive/critical care, emergency care, and specialty care.
   e. Provision of care requires admission to an acute care facility/hospital, acute rehabilitation facility, postanesthesia and intensive care area, or emergency department.
   f. Case management services are intensive and comprehensive in nature including primarily care coordination and management.
3. Postacute setting
   a. Focus is on the provision of services needed by patients after an acute episode of illness that may have required an acute care/hospital admission.
   b. Moderate complexity services; primarily reactive approach to care provision and requires the attention of multiple health care professionals such as physical and occupational therapists.
   c. Cost is moderate to high; care provision may require the authorization of the payer or insurer.
   d. Examples may include home care, palliative and end-of-life care, rehabilitative and restorative services, and long-term care including custodial and skilled care.
   e. Provision of care may occur in the home or community setting, ambulatory clinic, and patient-centered medical home or may require admission to a health care facility such as a subacute rehabilitation or nursing home, assisted living, hospice, or day care centers.
   f. Case management services are moderate to complex including primarily transitional planning activities such as placement of patients in appropriate level of care setting.

10. Independent or private case management agency
11. Workers' compensation
12. Disability management
13. Occupational health
14. Life care planning
15. Disease management and population health
16. Patient-centered medical or health home.

Telephonic Case Management

A. *Telephonic* case management is defined as the delivery of health care services to patients and their families or caregivers over the telephone or via the use of various forms of telecommunication methods such as fax, e-mail, or other forms of electronic communication methods and digital technologies such as remote monitoring.

B. Most commonly used in the commercial health insurance or managed care organization (MCO) setting. It takes place in the form of communication between the MCO representatives (mostly MCO-based case managers) and its members.

C. Became more popular in the 1990s with the increased infiltration of managed care health plans. It was viewed as an essential strategy for cost containment. Today, this approach is also used in workers' compensation and disability management.

D. Commercial health insurance plans and MCOs provide telephonic case management services as an additional benefit to their members. Through this strategy, telephonic triage and the provision of health advice have become more common. Through these approaches, case managers ensure the appropriate use of health care resources and allocated such resources based on the needs of the individual member.

E. Telephonic case management is considered a cost-effective, easily accessible, and proactive approach to preventing catastrophic health outcomes or deterioration in a patient's condition that requires acute care or a hospital stay.

F. Case managers in the telephonic case management practice setting are available 24 hours per day, 7 days a week. The main focus of this access is triage services and utilization management of health care resources.

G. Case managers in the telephonic case management practice setting engage in specific case management activities such as those listed in Box 4-6.

H. Case managers in the telephonic case management practice setting also apply the case management process, however, without a face-to-face interaction with the patient or family. In this process, they
   1. Interview the patient and/or family member/caregiver.
   2. Complete an assessment or evaluation of the patient's condition, situation, and the reason for reaching out to the case manager.
   3. Analyze the assessment findings using an algorithm or a guideline (usually automated).
   4. Determine the urgency of the situation and plan care (i.e., triage or advice) accordingly.

4-6   Examples of Telephonic Case Management Activities

- Telephonic triage
- Easing the access of patients to appropriate health care services and settings
- Facilitating the access of the patient to the appropriate level of care, health care provider, and service
- Intervening in a timely manner and sharing real-time information
- Empowering the patient/family/caregiver to assume responsibility for self-care/ self-management and health management
- Identifying the patient's health risk and instituting appropriate action or referral for services
- Engaging in cost reduction activities by promoting access to health services that are appropriate to the patient's condition; for example, preventing the provision of care in the emergency department setting when the patient's condition does not warrant such services, rather directing the patient to seek health services by the primary care provider
- Educating patients and their families about health regimen, including medications, and encouraging them to adhere to it
- Following up with patients and/or their families postdischarge from an episode of care (e.g., hospital, surgical center, or ED) to ensure safety, postdischarge services are in place, comfort in using durable medical equipment, and adherence to medical regimen, to answer their questions, and to provide counseling and emotional support
- Coordinating and integrating services using evidence-based algorithms, protocols, or guidelines, which include decision trees that are based on certain criteria or assessment cues/data
- Assessing and evaluating the patient's condition over the telephone, identifying problems, and directing appropriate action. The assessment is guided by the relevant protocol. Depending on the findings, the case manager determines the urgency of the situation and decides on the necessary type of intervention or advice and the best way to arrange for the needed services
- Counseling patients regarding their health benefits and answering their questions
- Providing health advice
- Explaining claims or care invoices
- Authorizing services
- Brokering services or directing other case managers to arrange for community-based services with participating agencies or providers

5. Implement necessary action or care strategy (e.g., refer to ED or the primary care provider).
6. Evaluate outcomes.
7. Follow up after the interaction and check that patient is safe and concern is resolving.
8. Document the episode of service.
9. Complete any value-based purchasing program activities such as monitoring of performance on core measures (e.g., quality, safety, and cost indicators).

I. Telephonic case management is known to apply two main strategies to ensure cost-effectiveness and the provision of care in the most appropriate setting and by the necessary care provider. These are as follows:

1. Demand management
   a. The main focus is on the appropriate utilization of resources and services.
   b. Case managers provide patients with information about their disease and health condition, disease process, medical regimen, prescribed medications, use of durable medical equipment, and desired outcomes.
   c. Case managers also encourage patients to participate in self-care and self-management and in making decisions regarding their health care needs and options.
   d. The primary outcome is reduction in unnecessary use of EDs, urgent care settings, or acute care facilities.
2. Telephone triage
   a. The main focus is sorting out requests for health care services based on need, severity, urgency, and complexity.

J. In deciding on the urgency of need for access to health care services, case managers place patients into three categories based on the findings of the telephonic assessment and evaluation. These are emergent, urgent, and nonurgent (Box 4-7).

K. In making triage decisions, case managers also use other information such as age, gender, past medical history and recent episodes of care, medication intake, allergies, and primary care provider. In addition, they may ask for health insurance plan–related information such as plan/account number, location of residence, and so on.

L. A rule of thumb for the case manager in telephonic triage is referring those who require care to the appropriate care provider and optimal setting.

BOX 4-7 Three Categories of Urgency for Health Care Services

1. Emergent
   a. Need to be seen by a health care provider immediately (e.g., acute chest pain or possible stroke).
   b. Usually, the patient is referred to the ED.
   c. May need the help of emergency medical services personnel.
2. Urgent
   a. Need to be seen within 8 to 24 hours (e.g., vomiting).
   b. Usually, the patient is referred to the primary care provider.
   c. Health advice may be given to be followed while the patient is waiting to see the primary care provider (e.g., drink extra fluids).
3. Nonurgent
   a. Can be seen routinely by a primary care provider or treated at home with appropriate follow-up (e.g., minor bruise or abrasion).
   b. Health advice is given and the patient is directed to see the primary care provider within a certain number of days if symptoms are not improved.

Case Management in the Payer-Based Settings or Insurance Companies

A. Case managers in the payer-based setting are employees of the insurance company (i.e., health maintenance and managed care organizations).

B. In this setting, the main focus of case management is the health and wellness of the enrollee and the role of the case manager as a liaison between the providers of care—whether an individual or an agency/facility—and the insurance company.

C. Case managers are not the "claims police" despite the fact that they ensure cost-effective treatment plans. Rather, they are as follows:
   1. Coordinators of care, problem solvers, advocates, and educators
   2. Professionals who collaborate with physicians and other care providers (including the provider-based case manager) to ensure the provision of appropriate, quality, cost-effective, and safe care
   3. Negotiators of services such as home care, durable medical equipment, consults with specialty care providers, and physical therapy;
   4. Counselors; they ensure that the patient follows the prescribed treatment plan; and
   5. Liaisons with insurance claims staff. In this regard, they clarify insurance claims information.

D. In the payer-based setting, case managers build programs or systems that make it feasible to identify enrollees who are at risk for illness or avoidable disease progression, and those who are considered the "high-risk, high-cost" cases.
   1. Examples of such cases are cancer, AIDS, organ transplantation, head/brain injury, spinal cord injury, severe burns, high-risk pregnancy, neuromuscular problems, and others.
   2. High-cost cases often are those with multiple chronic and complex conditions and are on high volume of medications (polypharmacy).
   3. Case managers work closely with these types of enrollees to ensure they receive the services they need in a timely fashion, in the appropriate level of care/setting and by the necessary provider(s).
   4. The main goal is provision of quality, safe, timely, and cost-effective care.

E. Mullahy (2014) identified four major areas of activities for case managers in the health insurance/managed care or payer-based practice settings. Some of these activities are applied based on the need and the situation or the job description designed by the insurance company for the case manager (Box 4-8).
   1. Medical activities—to ensure that the enrollee receives the most effective medical/health care
   2. Financial activities—to ensure timely, cost-effective treatments
   3. Behavioral/motivational activities—to ensure adherence to medical regimen, self-management, and to reduce stress or frustration
   4. Vocational activities—to ensure continued employment and facilitate return to work

F. The insurance company–based case manager may engage in activities either telephonically or face to face/on site in the health care provider organization where an enrollee is being treated.

BOX
4-8

Four Main Case Management Activities in the Payer-Based Care Settings (Mullahy, 2014)

1. Medical activities
   a. Keeping contact with the patient while at home or in a health care facility receiving care
   b. Assessing the patient's condition and working closely with the health care team to discuss the enrollee's course of treatment, progress, and needs
   c. Arranging for services required or working closely with the internal or hospital-based case manager on such. Services may include transportation, home care, durable medical equipment, care supplies, home utilities, psychosocial counseling, and therapy
   d. Coordinating activities closely with the health care team (especially the case manager and the social worker of the facility where an enrollee is being treated) to eliminate duplication or fragmentation of services and to conserve health insurance benefit dollars
   e. Providing health education and psychosocial counseling services to the enrollee and family
   f. Assisting in obtaining payer authorizations for modalities of treatment recommended or indicated
   g. Acting as a liaison between the insurance company and the health care team including the physician or primary care provider
2. Financial activities
   a. Assessing the enrollee's medical benefits plan for coverage, out-of-pocket expenses, out-of-plan coverage, and other limitations
   b. Suggesting to the health care team medically appropriate alternative treatment settings and options
   c. Counseling the enrollee and family about benefits and budgeting and sorting out bills
   d. Educating the insurance company about the risk of noncompliant, untreated, or unmanaged cases
3. Behavioral/motivational activities
   a. Exploring the enrollee's (and family's) feelings about self and the illness or injury
   b. Supporting the enrollee and family in dealing with the illness and the treatment by providing psychosocial counseling and behavioral modification activities
   c. Offering reassurance and information about the enrollee's illness and treatment
   d. Encouraging the enrollee to pursue a healthy lifestyle—smoke cessation, exercise, and healthy eating
   e. Referring the patient for counseling by a specialist (psychologist or psychiatrist)
4. Vocational activities
   a. Overseeing psychovocational testing, work evaluation, and on-the-job training as appropriate
   b. Assessing the enrollee's past education, employment history, work experiences, job skills, and vocational interests
   c. Assisting the enrollee in using the recuperative period in a constructive manner
   d. Communicating with the enrollee's employer or employment supervisor especially to discuss expectations, options, and the enrollee's needs
   e. Completing a job analysis and discussing the possibility of returning to the same job/work setting or another modified job/work setting

From Mullahy, C. (2014). *The case manager's handbook* (5th ed.). Sudbury, MA: Jones and Bartlett Learning.

BOX 4-9   Examples of Utilization Management Activities in Payer-Based Case Management

1. Notification of service or access to care
2. Authorizations or certifications for services
3. Preadmission, concurrent, continued, and retrospective reviews
4. Denials and appeals management
5. Reporting on utilization management activities and outcomes

G. Many insurance companies employ case managers to assume responsibility for their utilization management programs. Examples of utilization management activities are available in Box 4-9.
H. Payer-based case managers may execute their roles either onsite where the provider of care is or via the telephone in the form of telephonic case management.
I. The telephone-based case manager's role is necessary for the following:
   1. Maintaining open lines of communication between the enrollee/family, the provider (individual or agency), the provider-based case manager, and the payer staff
   2. Triage for timely access to services and reduction of cost
   3. Prevention of inappropriate access to health care services
   4. Screening of enrollees and tracking of low-intensity patients and those who have improved and no longer require in-person case management services
J. Onsite case management is common when a large number of individuals from one insurance company (especially a managed care organization) tend to seek care at the same contracted provider agency (e.g., a hospital). In this context, the onsite case manager's role is necessary and focuses on activities such as those listed in Box 4-10.

BOX 4-10   Focus of the Onsite Case Manager's Role

- Timely access to care by enrollees
- Bridging the gaps, especially those related to communication, between the patient, the payer, and the provider agency
- Expediting the process of utilization review and management; that is, timely communication between the provider-based and payer-based case managers regarding treatment plans, treatment options, discharge and transition plans, required postdischarge services, and patients' progress
- Coordination of discharge/transitional planning activities such as identifying the preferred provider of home care services, transportation services, skilled nursing facility, or durable medical equipment vendor
- Discussing posthospital care, services, and options with the patient and family as needed
- Providing health education services to patients and their families for the purpose of enhancing self-management abilities
- Explaining the health plan and benefits to patients and their families
- Solving problems and conflicts as they arise and in a timely manner

Case Management in the Community Care Setting

A. Designed to support and empower patients and their families in achieving or maintaining an optimal level of wellness and functioning by accessing and using community-based health care services and resources.

B. Programs focus on primary care, health promotion and prevention, and/ or management of chronic illness and avoidance of disease progression.

C. Target individuals who are healthy, but may be at risk for certain illnesses or needing to access health care services. In some settings such as the patient-centered medical home, accountable care organizations, and Federally Qualified Health Centers, focus is on prevention of disease progression, adherence to medical and health regimen, and self-management.

D. Work through outreach programs such as screening for illness (e.g., mammography, prostate cancer, cholesterol, diabetes, and blood pressure screening). These programs identify individuals who are predisposed for illness and enroll them in specific care programs or refer them to other care providers.

E. Other examples of primary prevention include wellness programs such as yearly physical examinations, well-baby care, and immunizations.

F. Work closely with individuals to prevent illness or a sudden change in one's condition to a state that may require hospitalization.

G. In addition to screening, case managers offer health education services to those at risk and others who are interested. They also offer psychosocial and financial counseling and advice, especially to those who are poor, uninsured, or underinsured.

H. Programs also may focus on secondary disease prevention or progression of illness.

I. Case managers work closely with individuals who have already experienced certain illnesses, have been hospitalized in an acute care setting, and need to maintain optimal health and functioning.

J. Services offered may include health education, lifestyle changes and behavior modification (e.g., smoke cessation; diet and exercise counseling), psychosocial counseling, financial counseling, assessment and monitoring of health condition (e.g., home care services; laboratory testing such as blood sugar and coagulation profile), telephonic advice and counseling, and medication adherence.

K. A special focus here is on prevention of readmission to the acute care setting or ED or exacerbation of one's health condition/disease state.

L. Case managers in the community care setting coordinate medical as well as social services and provide care to patients in their homes, day care centers, or ambulatory clinics with the goal of enhancing self-care management skills and patient-directed decision making and empowerment.

M. Case managers assess the patient's condition (health, physical, psychosocial, emotional, functional, and financial), plan and implement appropriate interventions, evaluate the patient's responses to treatment, provide patient and family education, and monitor the patient's use of necessary medical technologies, such as glucose monitoring devices, scales, and blood pressure machines, for self-monitoring of health condition.

N. Case managers may incorporate health education and promotion activities into existing settings such as day care, youth and adult recreation programs, summer camps, schools, support groups, meals for elders, churches, charitable organizations/agencies, and other community development efforts.

O. Case managers may also be involved in value-based purchasing program-related activities such as monitoring of performance on specific core measures (e.g., quality, safety, and cost indicators).

Case Management in the Ambulatory Clinic and Outpatient Care Setting

A. Community-based case management services also can be provided in walk-in clinics (scheduled and unscheduled visits), urgicare centers, home visits, day care centers, assisted living facilities, and telephonically. Urgicare centers are available to offer care to walk-in patients in a setting that is more acute than a routine physician's office or clinic but less intense than an emergency department.

B. Case management in the ambulatory clinic or outpatient care setting may focus on the following:

1. Patient access to care, scheduling appointments, documenting key information relevant to each visit, and answering patient/family questions

2. Provision of care for specific populations with chronic illnesses and ensuring that treatment plans are oriented to the continuum of care; that is, including well care, acute care, chronic care, rehabilitative care, and terminal care. Case management in these cases is most beneficial if it encompasses the context of disease management and chronic care management

3. Reducing or preventing the demand for acute, complex, or expensive care. This is best accomplished by applying the strategy of demand management; for example, using nurse advice lines, call centers, telephone triage, health risk assessments, and outreach programs

4. Use of long-term plans of care that apply evidence-based practice guidelines and protocols

5. Reviewing results of laboratory and radiological tests and procedures, identifying any abnormalities, and intervening accordingly; for example, calling the patient about a change in dosage of a medication or frequency, asking a patient to come back for an early ambulatory care visit, or referring a patient to a specialist type care provider

6. Keeping a vital link between the patient/family, the medical team, and the payer company

7. Measuring outcomes of care (e.g., clinical and financial issues and processes of care outcomes), quality and safety, and reporting on such to appropriate parties including regulators. This function is tied to the value-based purchasing program as it applies to the ambulatory care setting

8. Ensuring that the patient and family are satisfied with care delivery and service

9. Referring the patient for admission to the acute care setting when needed and securing transportation and inpatient bed availability

10. Notifying the health insurance plan of the patient's need for hospitalization or surgical procedure and obtaining authorizations for care as indicated and based on the payer's policies and procedures
11. Ensuring compliance with standards of regulatory and accreditation agencies

Case Management in the Patient-Centered Medical Home Care Setting

A. Patient-centered medical home (PCMH) is also referred to as primary care medical home or patient-centered health home. Regardless of the terminology used, it refers to a community-based clinic, physician group, or physician-hospital practice that provides ambulatory care services with special focus on the provision of primary care offered by a primary care clinician (a doctor of medicine or doctor of osteopathy or advanced practice registered nurse or physician assistant).
B. PCMH is a way of organizing the delivery of comprehensive primary care services with special focus on care coordination, open and timely communication among health care providers and patient/family, access to care and services, and patient engagement and self-management, with the ultimate goal being higher quality, safety, and lower cost.
C. Characteristics of effective PCMH practice include the following:
   1. A clearly identified provider to assume primary accountability for care and to function as the leader of the health care team involved in the care of the individual patient
   2. Focus on the patient in a holistic manner (patient centered); provision of comprehensive care, including acute care, chronic care, preventive services, and end-of-life care, at all stages of life
   3. Integrated and coordinated culturally sensitive care and services
   4. Focus on quality, safety, and timely access to care as well as use of evidence-based practice guidelines
   5. Technology and digital tools to enhance delivery of high-quality and safe care, electronic communication among providers and with patients/families, and tracking of outcomes.
D. Case managers are integral members of the PCMH teams and are usually responsible for a variety of functions such as those described in Box 4-11.

BOX

4-11   Sample Responsibilities of Case Managers in the PCMH

- Coordination of care and services
- Facilitation of patient's timely access to services
- Engaging patients/families in decision making about care options
- Health education and self-care management
- Remotely monitoring patients' conditions and adherence to care regimen
- Following up on tests, procedures, and consults with specialty providers
- Facilitating interdisciplinary care rounds for long-term care planning
- Coordinating transition of care activities
- Assuring patients show up to follow-up appointments and they bring all the necessary information with them

E. Currently, most PCMHs have moved in the direction of focusing on population health. In this regard, they identify the common chronic illnesses prevalent in their market share and the community they serve, assess and monitor the quality measures (e.g., hemoglobin A1C for diabetes) appropriate for each of the chronic illnesses, and implement improvement plans in these measures to ultimately enhance the quality and safety of the patients and the health of the population.

F. Other areas of focus in PCMHs are similar to those usually are characteristic of ambulatory clinic and outpatient care settings.

G. Federally Qualified Health Centers (FQHCs) and Accountable Care Organizations employ the concepts, model, purpose, and focus of the PCMH.

1. These settings or types of health care organizations have adopted the role of the case manager with special focus on improvement in population health, lowering health care costs, and prevention of need for access to acute care or emergency services.

2. These organizations either are federally funded as part of a demonstration project or have committed to financial risk agreement with the Centers for Medicare and Medicaid Services. Agreements include commitment to specific quality, safety, and cost targets.

3. Although they have started as a result of the Patient Protection and Affordable Care Act of 2010 and are available for the care of Medicare and Medicaid beneficiaries, some commercial health insurance plans have adopted similar approaches and have begun to engage in financial risk agreements with providers.

Case Management in the Admitting Department

A. Case management in the hospital-based admitting department has gained increased attention because of concerns regarding patient flow, throughput, and bed capacity, particularly in the acute care setting. It has also become a necessary function due to the need for adherence to the utilization management standards of health insurance plans and payers, including MCOs.

B. Case management in the admitting department takes the form of gatekeeping, including the following:

1. Management and control of who gets admitted to the acute care setting
2. Securing authorizations and precertifications for care from MCOs or other payers as needed
3. Communicating with the payer organization regarding patient conditions and the need for acute care stay (hospitalization).

C. The case manager in the admitting department may assume responsibility for activities and functions such as those described in Box 4-12.

D. Case managers in the admitting office also review patients' need for admissions to the hospital setting. They determine appropriateness of the admission based on pre-established criteria and reimbursement for such. In this case, they ensure that the admission is warranted based on the patient's condition. The intensity of service and the severity of condition are the main determining factors.

1. An important factor in deciding on the appropriateness of the admission to the acute care setting is reimbursement, especially in

BOX
4-12   **Examples of Roles and Functions of Admitting Office Case Managers**

- Screening patients who are presented for admission to the acute care setting using specific criteria such as those described in InterQual or Milliman Care Guidelines.
- Evaluating the patient's condition to determine medical necessity for acute care; that is, examining the severity of illness and the intensity of needed resources or services. Based on these two factors, the case manager determines whether the acute care setting is the best level of care needed by the patient.
- Communicating with the admitting physician regarding medical necessity for acute care and negotiating the best level of care for the patient if hospitalization was not indicated based on the patient's presenting condition and care needs.
- Providing the physician with an alternative level of care (e.g., ambulatory surgery, outpatient clinic, home care) as necessary when it is determined that admission to the inpatient/hospital care setting is not appropriate and is denied.
- Engaging in timely communication with the physician, patient/family, and payer regarding the decision is important to prevent problems or delays in care.
- Communicating with the admitting department staff the decisions made by the case manager regarding the potential admissions reviewed.
- Keeping in touch with payer-based case managers and other staff.
- Consulting with other staff (e.g., finance, managed care office) and health care professionals (e.g., social worker, physician, patient representative or advocate) to eliminate barriers to care or delays in treatment or services.
- Documenting activities, interventions, assessment, and communications.
- Educating health care professionals and allied health staff about admitting office case management structure and functions.
- Providing patients and their families with health education, promotion, and prevention activities.
- Ensuring compliance with standards of regulatory and accreditation agencies.
- Review of patients who are transferred from another hospital or facility for appropriateness of admission and adherence to EMTALA law.

the case of the MCO where preauthorization for hospital admission is expected. Timely communication with the payer is an important function of case managers in the admitting office.

2. Reviewing all surgical admissions to the hospital, especially those who are admitted a day or more prior to surgery. In this case, the case manager ensures that the admission is warranted based on the patient's condition. Some surgical patients may require hospitalization for medical management or further diagnostic testing prior to surgery.

3. Under certain circumstances, the patient is still approved for admission to the hospital prior to the day of surgery regardless of lack of reimbursement (e.g., a patient who is unable to complete a bowel preparation for major abdominal surgery in the home setting prior to surgery).

4. Reviewing admissions to ensure the patient's condition and needed care potentially meets the two-midnight rule requirement of the Centers for Medicare and Medicaid Services (CMS), where appropriate.

   a. The "two-midnight" rule is a condition CMS imposed on hospitals regarding when inpatient admissions are appropriate for payment under Medicare Part A.

b. The rule emphasizes the importance of a physician's medical judgment in meeting the needs of Medicare beneficiaries.

c. Generally speaking, the rule states that inpatient admissions is reimbursable under Medicare Part A if the admitting practitioner expected the patient to require a hospital stay that crossed two midnights and the medical record documentation supports that reasonable expectation. Thus, Medicare Part A payment is considered not appropriate for hospital stays not expected to span at least two midnights and therefore may need to be billed as observation following the Hospital Outpatient Prospective Payment System (OPPS).

5. Reviewing the medical records of patients who are admitted to the hospital and released within 24 or 48 hours. This is an important function and assists in avoiding reimbursement denials. For example, if the case manager determines that the admission is not justified, he or she will convert the admission to an ambulatory encounter or observation status, only where deemed appropriate.

E. Case managers also review interhospital transfers for appropriateness and that the transfer meets the MCO's standards and Medicare guidelines; that is, to avoid noncompliance with the Emergency Medical Treatment and Active Labor Act (EMTALA).

1. For the transfer to be appropriate and necessary the transferring organization must not be able to provide the level of care required by the patient and the receiving organization must have the capacity to provide the level of service needed.

2. EMTALA was established to ensure that individuals are able to access emergency services regardless of their ability to pay.

3. Section 1867 of the Social Security Act imposes specific obligations on Medicare-participating hospitals that offer emergency services to provide a medical screening examination (MSE) when a request is made for examination or treatment for an emergency medical condition (EMC), including active labor, regardless of the ability to pay.

4. Hospitals are required to provide stabilizing treatment for patients with EMCs. If a hospital is unable to stabilize a patient within its capability, or if the patient requests, an appropriate transfer can then be implemented.

F. When admitting office-based case managers complete a preliminary assessment of the patient's condition, they focus on the following:

1. Appropriateness of the admission
2. Appropriateness of the setting or level of care
3. Type of patient—observation, outpatient, and acute/admission
4. Potential discharge planning needs
5. Need for care facilitation/coordination
6. Psychosocial situation.

G. Admitting office case managers also notify the inpatient case managers of the admission and the findings of the preliminary assessment, including the following:

1. Coverage limitations of health insurance plan; for example, sharing the outcome of conversations with the payer entity
2. Special patient/family circumstances; for example, lack of family support, availability of next of kin/caregiver, health care proxy, advance directive, or do-not-resuscitate status

3. Potentially avoidable days; for example, presurgical days and preprocedure days
4. Other issues as appropriate; for example, recipient of home care services prior to admission and skilled nursing facility transfer.

 Case Management in the Perioperative Services

A. Case management in the perioperative services has become increasingly popular due to concern about patient flow and throughput in the acute care setting/hospital. It is also viewed as necessary because it represents a route of entry to an ambulatory or acute care setting, making it necessary for the case manager to ensure appropriateness of the admission and reimbursement and that care is provided at the relevant level or setting.
B. The main focus of case management here is the care of the surgical patient—pre-, intra-, and postsurgery. The process of case management is applied in the preadmission testing area, continues in the immediate preoperative and intraoperative periods, and terminates postoperatively in the postanesthesia care unit (PACU) upon recovery and discharge of the patient to home or transfer to an inpatient care setting.
C. A major interest in case management in the perioperative services setting is the provision of care for patients that is relevant to their needs and according to regulatory and accreditation standards. Another is the focus on efficiency and efficacy of care and services.
D. Select case management functions in the preadmission testing area are sometimes assumed by the admitting department case manager, the dedicated preadmission testing area case manager, or the perioperative services case manager. Regardless of who assumes responsibility, the preadmission case management role focuses on the functions shared in Box 4-13.
E. Select case management functions in the immediate preoperative period may include the following:
   1. Assessing the patient's readiness for surgery.
   2. Reviewing the medical record and completing the following activities:
      a. Evaluating results of laboratory and radiological tests and procedures
      b. Securing the availability of blood and blood products if required
      c. Ensuring that medical and surgical clearances have been obtained, including the history and physical and anesthesia evaluation
      d. Ensuring that the surgical and blood and blood products consents have been completed.
   3. Communicating any abnormal results or other concerns to the physician (anesthesiologist and/or surgeon) in a timely manner. This task is important because abnormalities may delay surgery.
   4. Confirming that certification for surgery by the payer (if needed) has been secured and documented.
   5. Ensuring appropriateness of the level of care; that is, those scheduled for an ambulatory or same-day surgery meet the criteria for ambulatory or same-day surgery, and those who are to be admitted also meet the inpatient intensity of service and severity of illness criteria.

BOX 4-13   Example of Roles and Functions of the Perioperative Services Case Manager

- Interviewing the patient and family to evaluate condition (medical, physical, psychosocial, emotional, and financial) and identify any preadmission or preoperative issues or concerns that might affect the postsurgical period including discharge to home
- Exploring discharge planning options and services. For example, determining the need for home care services if the patient or family is unable to assume responsibility for self-care management
- Educating the patient/family regarding the surgical procedure and course of treatment and recovery
- Referring for psychosocial counseling as necessary based on the patient's and family's situation; consulting with a social worker if needed
- Evaluating the patient's readiness for surgery; for example, reviewing results of laboratory and radiological tests and procedures and past medical history; securing the availability of blood and blood products if required, medical and surgical clearance, and consent for surgery
- Confirming the date and time of surgery and availability of the surgical team
- Keeping open communication with members of the health care team, especially the surgeon and the anesthesiologist, as well as inpatient and admitting office case managers
- Initiating the discharge planning process, especially in the case of a surgical procedure where it is clear in advance that the patient will require a transfer to a subacute or acute rehabilitation facility or postdischarge services in the home setting
- Communicating with the payer-based case manager to secure authorization for surgery, admission to the hospital, or postdischarge services
- Documenting in the patient's medical record all assessments, interventions, communication, outcomes, and services arranged for

F. Select case management functions in the intraoperative period may include the following:
   1. Ensuring operating room efficiency; that is, maximizing the operating room utilization. This may entail specific activities such as the following:
      a. Tracking housekeeping turnaround time, first patient out–next patient in time, delays in surgery and reasons for delays, and so on
      b. Communicating with the surgical team about any actual or potential delays and intervening as necessary
      c. Ensuring availability of surgical equipment, trays, and supplies to maximize operating room readiness
      d. Changing operating room schedule to avoid waste, especially when the patient or surgical team is not ready
   2. Addressing quality and risk management issues as they arise
   3. Maintaining a vital link between the patient/family, the surgical/medical team, and the perioperative services staff
   4. Securing inpatient or PACU beds for patients as needed
   5. Ensuring timely patient transfer to the next phase of care or next level of care/setting

G. Select case management functions during the postanesthesia care period may include the following:

1. Arranging for admission to an inpatient bed (regular and intensive care–type bed based on the patient's condition and care needs); securing bed and medical, surgical, or critical care team availability; and expediting transfer out of the PACU
2. Securing authorizations for care and treatment plans
3. Identifying and addressing, or preventing, delays in care
4. Reviewing appropriateness of level of care/setting and the involvement of relevant care providers
5. Obtaining authorizations for care from the payers (insurers) as needed to ensure reimbursement; also, providing them with progress reports and completing concurrent and retrospective review activities
6. Addressing quality, safety, and risk management issues as they arise
7. Maintaining a vital link between the patient/family, the surgical/medical team, the inpatient care team, the PACU team, and the perioperative services staff
8. Ensuring timely patient transfer to the next phase of care or next level of care/setting (i.e., the inpatient care unit)
9. Complete any value-based purchasing program activities such as monitoring of performance on core measures (e.g., quality, safety, and cost indicators) as they apply to the perioperative areas

Independent/Private Case Management

A. Independent or private case management is also known as *external* case management compared to the hospital-based case management, which is known as *internal* case management.
B. Defined as the provision of case management services by self-employed case managers or those who are employees of a privately owned company.
C. The term *independent* or *private* refers to the absence of oversight by a third party such as a payer (e.g., MCO) or a health care provider organization.
D. Independent and private case management services emerged as a cost-effective approach to the care of
1. An increased number of the elderly population with multiple complex and chronic illnesses
2. Disabled individuals who require coordination of expensive and intense services (medical, social, financial, and mental or behavioral health) for an extended period of time—sometimes for a number of years
3. Workers' compensation or occupational health cases that have resulted in chronic, catastrophic, or permanent injury and that are known to consume expensive and complex health care resources
E. Independent and private case management are similar in relation to the structure and type of services they provide to patients; however, subtle differences between the two do exist. They are usually used interchangeably; however, as an expert, the case manager must be able to differentiate between these two terms and use them appropriately.
1. Private case management refers to the services provided by an independent case manager privately contracted or hired by a

chronically ill individual or family member to manage the complex care and services needed.

2. Independent case management refers to services offered by a case manager who is hired by an independent case management firm and contracted by a health care organization (usually a managed care company, an employer, or a health care provider or facility) to provide case management services on a long- or short-term basis to certain individuals, especially those who are disabled.

F. Case managers in the independent or private case management practice settings represent the health care organization or insurance company that hires them unless they are hired directly by the patient or family, in which case they represent the patient/family.

G. Independent and private case management focuses on the following:
   1. Enabling the patient and family to transition along the health care continuum
   2. Assisting the patient and family in successfully navigating the health care delivery system and the continuum of health and human services
   3. Monitoring services and resource utilization
   4. Evaluating quality outcomes; for example, clinical, physical functioning, emotional, safety, and financial
   5. Managing cost of care and services and health benefits
   6. Ensuring the provision of quality and safe care and services, which may include the following:
      a. Retirement planning
      b. Home health care; homemaker and companion services
      c. Respite care
      d. Transportation
      e. Family and legal counseling
      f. Physical and occupational therapy
      g. Psychosocial counseling and crisis intervention
      h. Referrals to specialty providers
      i. Durable medical equipment and medical/surgical supplies
   7. Ensuring patient and family satisfaction and content with the experience of care
   8. Advocating for the patient/family
   9. Assisting patient/family to develop self-management skills and knowledge

H. The goals of independent and private case management are similar to those of other models or practice settings of case management. They may include, but are not limited to, the following:
   1. Coordination and facilitation of complex medical, psychosocial, functional, and financial services
   2. Provision of timely, quality, safe, and appropriate services
   3. Patient advocacy
   4. Cost-effectiveness
   5. Provision of one-to-one individualized and personalized relationship between a health care provider and the patient/family
   6. Integration of health care services and resources including mental health assessment and counseling and referrals to specialty providers.

I. MCOs and employers are more likely to subcontract with an independent or private case management agency for services such as rehabilitation and disability case management.

J. Although they may be hired by an insurance company (payer), private and independent case managers are expected to adhere to the utilization management procedures followed by the insurance company. They seek authorization for services, provide concurrent and ongoing utilization review and progress reports, and ensure the provision of services that are satisfactory to both the patient/family and the insurer.

K. Reimbursement for private and independent case management services is either on an hourly, daily, or case rate basis. Sometimes, sliding fee schedules are used.

L. Private and independent case management practice settings allow the case manager to function independently and autonomously, especially in decision making, achieve greater income, and attain professional satisfaction.

M. Private and independent case management practice settings provide the case manager with the opportunity to manage a personal/private business with all its aspects including hiring and firing staff, marketing, budgeting and financial management, accounting, public relations, purchasing, sales, and so on.

N. Private and independent case managers engage in cost–benefit activities about treatment options, complete reports about patient's progress on regular basis and share with the entity or individual who engaged them, and summarize the care provided and its outcomes at the end of the engagement as a termination of care summary.

Case Management in the Emergency Department

A. The emergency department (ED) is a common route of entry to the acute care hospital setting. Issues of ED overcrowding have resulted in a dire need for case management services to ensure efficient, safe, and effective patient flow and throughput.

B. The primary benefits of ED case management are as follows (Tahan & Cesta, 2005):
1. Cost-effectiveness
2. Provision of efficient, effective, timely, safe, and quality care
3. Patient and family satisfaction with the care experience
4. Reduction in diversion hours and frequency
5. Elimination of unnecessary admissions to the hospital setting
6. Expeditious admissions to inpatient beds/hospital setting
7. Prevention of lost revenues due to diversions and inappropriate admissions
8. Linking the patient/family to community-based services and resources in an effort to avoid improper admissions to the hospital setting
9. Reduction in the number of patients "left without seen."

C. The ED case manager provides an important gatekeeping function for the hospital and ensures that patients are either appropriately admitted to the hospital or treated in and released from the ED.

D. The ED case manager facilitates care processes from the time of the patient's arrival in the ED, through registration and triage, assessment and treatment, until discharge from the ED or admission to the hospital

setting (Tahan & Cesta, 2005). Activities may include the facilitation of the following:
1. Timely triage and initiation of treatment according to urgency of the situation
2. Diagnostic tests and procedures (e.g., laboratory, radiology)
3. Therapeutic procedures (e.g., insertion of a gastric tube for feeding)
4. Discharge and transitional planning
5. Patient and family education
6. Transfers to inpatient beds or other facilities.

E. ED case managers are active members of interdisciplinary teams that include physicians, nurses, social workers, patient representatives, navigators, admitting office staff, and other personnel. Examples of ED case manager's role functions are in Box 4-14.

F. Traditional admission and discharge/transitional planning responsibilities of the case manager in an acute care setting may be extended to the ED case manager. This role allows for timely

BOX 4-14   Examples of Roles and Functions of ED Case Managers

- Act as a liaison between the ED, hospital, and community case management programs and personnel, particularly to improve continuity and efficiency of care.
- Ensure and expedite appropriate patient disposition—hospital admission, transfer to another facility or level of care, discharge home with visiting nurse services, and alternative placements.
- Evaluate the decision to admit a patient to a hospital setting based on specific criteria (intensity of service and severity of illness).
- Coordinate appropriate use of efficient services and resources.
- Evaluate outcomes and examine system efficiency and effectiveness.
- Arrange for postdischarge care such as visiting nurse services.
- Ensure adherence to standards of regulatory and accreditation agencies.
- Communicating with the patient's primary care provider to share information about patient's condition, plan of care, and assure that a postdischarge follow-up appointment has been secured.
- Assisting indigent patients who need community services such as shelter and charity care.
- Engaging in financial screening activities and the necessary utilization management processes such as securing certifications for treatment and postdischarge services from health insurance plans and MCOs.
- Coordinating the patient's admission to the hospital setting and facilitating the transfer of patients from the ED to the assigned inpatient beds; also assuring that a medical team has been secured to care for the patient upon admission to an inpatient bed.
- Securing medications and durable medical equipment for those in need.
- Ensuring provision of health education services to patients and families.
- Facilitating the patient's release after treatment and arranging for necessary transportation.
- Preventing unsafe discharges from the ED.
- Obtaining follow-up appointments for those discharged from the ED who require such care.
- Facilitating the exchange of information among physicians, social workers, nurses, other hospital staff, patient and family, and community providers.

assessment of patients' needs (current and forecasted postdischarge) and intervention accordingly.

G. Case managers in the ED make sure that patients who can be treated on an outpatient basis or in another level of care are not inappropriately admitted to an acute inpatient care setting. They work with physicians and others to avoid "social admissions." Social admissions refer to patients who are admitted to the acute care setting not for medical necessity reasons, rather a social support reason such as family/caregiver is asking for a break.

H. Case managers in the ED participate in the monitoring ED patient flow metrics and evaluation of performance, especially related to ED crowding. National indicators for ED crowding may include the following:
   1. Diversion—Number of hours the ED is unable to receive and care for patients who need transportation by the emergency medical services (EMS) personnel
   2. Boarding—Number of patients remaining in the ED after a decision has been made to admit them to an inpatient bed
   3. Left before a medical evaluation (left before seen or treatment)—Number of patients who leave the ED after triage but before receiving medical evaluation
   4. Length of time in ED—Total, time intervals of each phase of care such as arrival to triage, triage to seen by physician, seen by physician to decision to admit or discharge, decision to release or to admission to inpatient bed
   5. Turnaround time for tests and procedures (e.g., laboratory or radiologic)
   6. Volume of patients seen in the ED by triage category and breakdown by admitted (regular bed vs. critical care bed) and treated and released.

I. Ensuring compliance with EMTALA regulations (Wilson et al., 2005):
   1. All patients seen in the ED must receive the following:
      a. Appropriate medical screening examination within the capability of the ED.
      b. No delay in care on account of insurance or reimbursement.
      c. Transfer to another facility should be because of the patient's request or due to inability of the ED to provide the needed service.
   2. It essentially established a universal federal right to ED care without earmarking payment for this care.
   3. EDs must provide open access to individuals who may not have real or perceived open choices for care.

Patient Flow, Throughput, and Case Management

A. Patient flow focuses on the clinical and operational processes of care that facilitate the movement of the patient from point A to point B within the health care system (i.e., from one location/level of care to another). Usually, these movements are necessary and required by the patient based on his or her condition, treatment plan, and related services.

B. Throughput encompasses the actual operations/activities of a care provision that are essential for effective delivery of care. Conceptually, throughput is "part and parcel" of patient flow; without it, patients may not transition effectively and efficiently from one place to another as their conditions require.

C. For throughput to be efficient and effective, it must focus on the structure, processes, and expected outcomes of care delivery.

1. Structure—Characteristics of the care setting and the patient population served. Examples may include type of care setting (e.g., acute, ambulatory, patient-centered medical home, ED), type and number of care providers (e.g., nurses, physicians, case managers, social workers), services available (e.g., laboratory, pharmacy, physical therapy), or credentials and qualifications of the care providers (educational preparation, skills, abilities, competencies, specialty certifications).

2. Processes—The steps to be followed to ensure the completion of care activities. Examples may include the process of medications management, triage, obtaining a blood sample and running a test, insertion of an intravenous access, and transfer of a patient from an ED to an inpatient unit.

3. Outcomes—End results or outputs of a process. Examples are discharge of a patient to home, relief of symptoms, and experience of care.

D. Patient flow and throughput are terms that have often been used in reference to the hospital-based care setting as a result of ED crowding and inefficiency in moving patients from an ambulatory or procedural setting into inpatient beds.

E. Patient flow and throughput tend to be used interchangeably. In this section, they will be addressed as if they are the same because both terms denote the way patients are transitioned across a set of locations (levels of care) within the hospital; however, implicit in that are the treatments they receive and the types of services and resources they use.

F. Examining the hospital's efficiency in patient flow and throughput focuses on careful evaluation of the operations of areas known to experience bottlenecks, increased traffic, and process variations. These may include the following:

1. EDs
2. PACUs
3. Intensive care units (ICUs)
4. Procedure areas such as intervention cardiology laboratories, bronchoscopy and endoscopy suites, and operating rooms.

G. Case managers are professionals best prepared to assume an integral role in coordination, facilitation, or management of patient flow and throughput activities. With their leadership skills and knowledge of utilization management, medical necessity criteria, and patient care services/resources across the continuum of care, they are able to ensure the efficiency and effectiveness of the health care facility operations.

H. The 2005 patient flow standard from The Joint Commission (TJC, then known as the Joint Commission on Accreditation of Healthcare Organizations [JCAHO]) called for hospital leadership staff to have a process in place for managing patient flow and throughput, especially in the EDs and PACUs. This expectation then was incorporated in the already-existing leadership standard. The standard requires hospitals to have a process in place for managing patient flow throughout the hospital. In 2012, TJC expanded this standard to also include language about boarding patients in the ED or another location while awaiting admission to an inpatient bed (TJC, 2014). Case managers, especially those in the ED, can play an integral role in meeting the expectations of this standard.

I. The patient flow standard requires hospitals to measure and set goals for mitigating and managing the boarding of patients in the ED or another location while awaiting admissions and that boarding time set at 4 hours as a guideline but not a requirement, to assure patient quality and safety.

J. Case managers in the ED and other throughput and inpatient areas may contribute to adherence to TJC standard on patient flow as follows:
   1. Engage in an ongoing evaluation of patient flow practices.
   2. Develop and implement plans to identify and mitigate impediments to efficient patient flow throughout the hospital as a result of overcrowding:
      a. Patients who are admitted through the admitting office (elective admissions)
      b. Patients who are admitted postsurgery through the PACUs (elective and emergency admissions)
      c. Patients who are admitted through the ED (emergency admissions)
   3. Implement strategies for process improvement with a main focus on patient access to care (efficiency, effectiveness, and timeliness).
   4. Review all patients who are boarding in the ED, PACU, or another temporary location and facilitate their expeditious transfer to the appropriate location
   5. Manage overcrowding of patients in the ED, because this population is particularly vulnerable to experiencing negative effects of inefficiency.

K. Inefficient patient flow can affect patient safety and quality of care, as well as the hospital's bottom line. It may increase the number of reimbursement denials and avoidable days and therefore impacts negatively on revenue.

L. Patient flow can be viewed from two perspectives—clinical and operational.
   1. Clinically, patient flow represents the progression of a patient's health status as it relates to disease, treatment, and recovery progression.
   2. Operationally, patient flow means the transition of a patient through a set of locations in a health care facility or across facilities.

M. Patient flow is determined based on clinical needs (i.e., level of care needed, medical necessity, intensity of service, and severity of illness) of the patient and the best place that necessary health care services are available.

N. Patient flow is important today more than ever because of current reimbursement methods (e.g., managed care, capitation, federal prospective payment systems, bundled payment, observation status, value-based purchasing) that place the provider of care at financial risk or that place the patient at risk (e.g., risk for medical errors and unsafe experiences) as he or she transitions across the continuum of care.

O. Case managers may take the lead in their hospitals in ensuring efficient patient flow and throughput. They may collaborate with multidisciplinary health care teams, including administrators and staff from the admitting office, ED, medicine, surgery, nursing, social work, environmental services, information technology, and others, to

1. Oversee patient flow processes.
2. Measure outcomes of patient flow processes and practices. Examples of measures, according to TJC (2014) may include the following:
    a. Available supply of inpatient beds
    b. Available supply of medical/surgical teams
    c. Efficiency of patient care, treatment, and service areas; for example, turnaround time on tests and procedures
    d. Safety of patient care, treatment, and service areas
    e. Support service processes that impact patient flow
    f. Number of patients boarding in an area other than their appropriate care destination
3. Examine relevant data that evaluate performance such as measures: door-to-door time, time from admission order to arrival in inpatient room, number of patients leaving before being seen by the physician or licensed independent practitioner, time from discharge order written to patient actually leaves the inpatient bed, and turnaround time for bed cleaning and readiness for a new admission.
4. Execute actions for improvement.
5. Ensure compliance with regulatory and accreditation patient flow standards.

P. The multidisciplinary patient flow team allows a better understanding of the issues of patient volume, demand for inpatient beds, bed capacity and supply, and necessary resources (staff and otherwise).

Q. The patient flow standard requires that patients access services as soon as they are in the system (e.g., ED, admitting office, clinic, PACU, or other area of the hospital system) and that there is no delay in admission to an inpatient bed or in receiving diagnostic and therapeutic tests and treatments.

R. Case managers can facilitate timely patient flow and throughput by
    1. Making sure that those in the ED are triaged in a timely manner and treated accordingly.
    2. Expediting delivery of care.
    3. Coordinating the completion of tests and procedures.
    4. Ensuring that the results of tests and procedures are available to physicians and other clinicians/staff so they can make decisions about the plan of care and care progression.
    5. Securing inpatient beds for those who require admission to the hospital care setting.
    6. Facilitating a safe transfer process from one location to another, internal or external to a health care facility, especially as the patient's condition requires a transition from one level of care (or setting) to another.
    7. Evaluating the patient's health insurance plans or lack thereof.

S. Case managers not only check the appropriateness of admissions to the hospital setting, but also make sure that patients receive the care they need as well, in a timely manner and while in the ED awaiting admission or in the PACU awaiting transfer, as if they already were in an inpatient bed.

T. For any patient flow process, there always exists an entry point (input), an exit or checkout point (output), and a path connecting the two points together. The path is in essence what throughput is all about. Therefore, generally speaking, patient flow can be described as a model of "entry–path–exit" or "input–throughput–output."

U. Using the "input–throughput–output" model as an approach for improving the efficiency of ED operations has merits for other care settings across an organization or among organizations. Therefore, one can apply this model to managing and improving any patient flow and throughput issue in an organization. This model provides a structure for examining the factors that impact on patient flow in the ED (Box 4-15).

BOX 4-15 Applicability of the Input–Throughput–Output Model in the ED

Examples of input factors:
- The reasons why people present to the ED for care
- Patients' demographics
- Patients' health status
- Health insurance status and type; benefit coverage
- Availability of alternative sites of care such as "fast track," urgicare
- Perceptions of quality
- Skills and knowledge of clinicians
- ED space and capacity
- Patient's desire for immediate care
- Ambulance diversion

Examples of throughput factors:
- Actual processes of care in the ED
- Registration
- Triage
- Authorization for care (certification)
- Level of service
- Treatment
- Availability of staff
- Availability of specialists
- Diagnostic services
- Information systems and technology
- Communication channels
- Staff assignments and caseloads
- Case management services
- Physician's practice
- Equipment and therapeutic approaches
- Bed management and capacity
- Care rounds
- Boarding

Examples of output factors:
- The ability to move the patient to his or her next disposition
- Discharge decision/order
- Available care/services in the community
- Patient's discharge
- Boarding patients
- Transfer to other facilities
- Bed tracking and availability
- Availability of transportation services
- Availability of housekeeping/environmental services
- Access to follow-up care and follow-up appointments

V. For an organization attempting to improve the efficiency of its patient flow operations, it is important to evaluate the above factors to identify issues that result in undesirable performance and to address them accordingly.

W. Understanding the input–throughput–output model and the patient flow operations in a facility allow health care professionals, including case managers, to improve its performance. Case managers may assist in identifying the important metrics that must be used for measuring the system's efficiency and monitoring of these metrics. Case managers may also bring patient flow data and reports to the hospital utilization review committee for performance improvement action planning.

Transitions of Care and Case Management

A. The provision of quality and safe health care services to patients requires them to receive care in multiple settings and from varied providers. This is even more so in the case of individuals with multiple chronic and complex illnesses, regardless of age.

B. Transitions from one care setting to the next or from one provider to the next often parallel changes (transitions or progression) in patients' health status and care needs. For example, patients who are transferred from a skilled nursing facility to an acute care hospital undergo such activity because of a change in condition that requires care (or the attention of a specialist health care provider) that is not available at the skilled nursing facility and usually at a higher acuity and intensity.

C. The health care system in the United States is not equipped with one single health care professional or team that assumes full responsibility for the coordination of care across settings or care providers during transitions of care.

D. Transitions of care occur during a time when patients journey the health care system. This journey may result in vulnerable situations and require an increased need for coordination, communication, and continuity of care.

E. Case management is most important during transitions of care where inefficiencies may occur leaving the patient at risk for poor quality, unsafe experiences, or negative and unexpected outcomes.

F. The National Quality Forum (NQF, 2006, p. D-9) describes care transition as a "change or interruption of patient care such as a discharge, a change in medications, a transfer among care units, a referral to services such as physical or occupational therapy, and the use of emergency services."

G. NQF also describes care coordination (a core aspect of case management) as the "synchronization of patient care and services during care transitions" (NQF, 2006, p. D-9). Care transitions may compromise patient safety and increase the likelihood for medical errors to occur primarily as a result of miscommunications.

H. Care transition is also described by the HMO Workgroup on Care Management (2004, p. 1) as "patient transfers from one care setting to another." This group focused its report on the improvement of the quality of care transitions for members of MCOs. However, the lessons learned from this report have been beneficial to all other care settings.

I. The report describes a transition of care as occurring when there is a change in necessary care or services as follows:
   1. Transfer of responsibility of care from one health care professional to another such as from a primary care to a specialist physician or from one nurse to another
   2. Change in the environment of care (care setting or level of care) within a health care facility; that is, a transfer from an intensive care to a regular unit or ED to an inpatient bed
   3. Change in care environment from one facility to another including hospitals, skilled nursing facilities, the patient's home, outpatient primary care and specialty clinics, and assisted living and other long-term care facilities.
J. The HMO Workgroup on Care Management (2004) proposed six specific strategies for care of patients during transitions. These are as follows:
   1. Ensuring that someone on the health care team assumes accountability for the patients' transitions
   2. Facilitating the effective transfer of information
   3. Enhancing health care practitioners' skills and support systems
   4. Enabling patients and caregivers to play a more active role in their transitions
   5. Aligning financial and structural incentives to improve patient flow across care settings, providers, and facilities
   6. Initiating a quality improvement/management strategy for care transitions.
K. The Workgroup emphasized the importance of other aspects of care during the time when a patient transitions from one health care provider or care setting to another, including, but not limited, to those described in Box 4-16.
L. The risk for suboptimal or unsafe care presented during transitions of care provides an excellent opportunity for case management.
M. In this regard, case managers may:
   1. Assume the role of the "single" professional on the health care team responsible and accountable for the essential activities that ought to occur during patients' transitions.
   2. Speak up and act on behalf of the multidisciplinary team and the organization for which he or she works.
   3. Incorporate the "lessons learned" from the HMO Workgroup on Care Management report into their own practice in the care settings where they work.
   4. Focus on patient safety and error prevention (discussed in next section) as they assist patients, families, and other health care providers during care transitions.
N. NQF (2006, p. D-9) identified transitions of care as one of four domains that constitute the framework for assessing the quality of care coordination in the hospital setting, a core aspect of case management. In fact, these four domains are integral to case management practice in any care setting:
   1. Transitions of care, including transfer among units within a hospital as well as admission to and discharge from the hospital; discharge includes transfer to other facilities such as acute or subacute rehabilitation.
   2. Communications among providers.

4-16 Important Aspects of Patient Care During Transitions

- Both entities assuming responsibilities in maintaining continuity of care and ensuring patient safety by controlling the risk for medical error.
- Keeping the patients informed about their plans of care, especially their transitional plans and what to expect during the transitions. Health care professionals must answer the patients' questions and alleviate their anxiety.
- Transfer of timely and accurate information, especially clinical. Such practice ensures effective and safe transitions. Information may include these described below:
  - Goals and plan of care
  - Patient's baseline functional status (physical and cognitive)
  - Active medical and behavioral health problems
  - Medications regimen
  - Social support network and support resources
  - Durable medical equipment needs and life-sustaining equipment use such as oxygen therapy
  - Ability for self-care management
  - Health care proxy, advance directive, and resuscitation status
  - Financial status such as type of insurance and benefits.
- Use of transfer note or summary that provides a comprehensive picture of the patient's status and the course of treatment followed prior to the transition.
- Making sure that enough time and attention are spent by health care professionals on patient transitions, similar amount compared to that exerted at the time of the patient's entry into the system.
- Making appropriate resources available—staff, equipment, space, etc.
- Shifting the perspective/framework of care provision from that of "discharge planning" to "transitions to continuous care."
- Collaboration in and integration of care provision across settings and disciplines.
- Using "transitional care managers."

3. Information, including the availability of health information when needed and the provision of information to patients about their condition and plan of care.
4. Capacity for services, including the availability of specialized services, waiting time for care, and the need for transfer to another facility or care setting when necessary services are unavailable.
O. The above domains cover aspects of care coordination that occur within a facility or setting (internal) and those that require collaboration with other facilities or settings (external).

Role of the Case Manager in Patient Safety and Prevention of Medical Errors During Transitions

A. Across the health care continuum, patients are routinely transferred from one provider to another, one service to another specialty, or one practice/care setting to another. With such activity, risk for suboptimal (or poor) quality of care may exist.
B. At each juncture, there is a handoff and a necessary exchange of information that requires close attention to ensure safety, eliminate the likelihood of medical errors, and maintain continuity of care.

C. The case manager may assume responsibility for professional, legal, and ethical practices that extend beyond the patient's discharge from a practice/care setting.

D. If the transitions of care were not handled properly and with caution, the patient's health condition will be placed at risk for unsafe situation (e.g., deterioration), which may result in serious negative outcomes.

E. From assessment and planning to evaluation and outcomes, the case management process must provide a proactive approach to safety by ensuring access to quality, safe, effective, and timely care. Each step in the case management process provides an added and significant benefit; that is, the potential to reduce or prevent risk of medical errors.

F. The case management process provides numerous opportunities along the continuum of care and across providers to identify and address potential risks for errors and ensure patient safety. Tahan (2005a) described how essential activities of case management can enhance patient safety. For example:

1. An appropriate assessment of the patient's needs focusing on the "total patient," not just the medical condition at hand that provides a step toward proactively preventing errors by being comprehensive in identifying the patient's concerns, interests, and health-related problems.

2. The design of a comprehensive case management plan of care that is patient and family centered, from the onset of the injury or illness through treatment and recovery or rehabilitation, and one that is based on the patient's individualized needs and desires will ensure safety.

3. Obtaining authorization for care from the payer (as needed) and advocating for the needs of patients and their families expedites access to care.

4. Understanding and communicating all facets of the patient's treatment plan to the patient/family and the members of the health care team and agreeing on the plan can also help prevent medical errors from occurring.

G. Through advocacy, the case manager is able to ensure that the care plan is closely followed by all health care providers. He or she ensures that specialty providers are consulted as indicated by the patient's condition and treatment plan including transitional planning. To avoid errors, this may involve open communication with all care providers, who may not necessarily have the same "global view" of the plan of care as the case manager.

H. Focusing on care across the continuum, the case manager can ensure that information is shared appropriately regarding such things as medications, diet, prior and future treatment, follow-up appointments, physical activity, and so on. Maintaining continuity of care through this sharing of information can reduce or prevent errors.

I. Monitoring of the delivery of care throughout the case management process and adjustment of the treatment plan as needed enhance safety. For example, when there is a delay or variance in the provision of care (e.g., an important diagnostic test is delayed), the case manager identifies the cause of the delay and immediately institutes appropriate corrective actions.

J. Close monitoring and management of the patient's plan of care, progress, outcomes, as well as the behaviors of the care providers expedite patient's care and progression. Such actions can prevent undesirable events from occurring or delay in meeting the patient's interests and treatment goals.

K. Comprehensive view of the patient's case management plan of care and desired outcomes and evaluation of the overall plan for appropriateness, relevancy to the patient/family's interests, and timeliness of care activities identifies situations where the patient is not progressing according to expectations. This prompts the case manager to implement necessary actions and to ensure safety.

L. Collecting and analyzing outcomes data can help determine elements of the care plan that are not successful or have not been carried out according to plan. This may help determine whether a medical error did occur and provide for appropriate corrective action and help prevent similar errors from reoccurring in the future.

M. The role of the case manager in ensuring patient safety during transitions of care is integral to the health care system and essential in case management practice (Tahan, 2005b).

N. Individuals with chronic health conditions—and often more than one—frequently receive their care from a variety of health care professionals and across varied care settings across the continuum of care leaving the patient unsure of which primary provider is accountable for coordinating the plan of care and treatment options and who possesses ultimate responsibility for outcomes.

O. Hospital stays have become shorter. Thus, more patients with serious and/or complicated chronic health conditions are being treated in non–acute (e.g., outpatient and home) care settings and perhaps by less specialized providers.

P. There continues to be an element of increased fragmentation in the provision of health care services, ultimately leading to increased risk for medical errors.

Q. Case managers have a very clear role, regardless of practice settings, in improving patient safety whether in preventing, reporting, acknowledging, or correcting a situation. No matter where they work, they may
   1. Advocate for patients and their families/caregivers.
   2. Promote health education of individuals and their families or other caregivers.
   3. Improve communication and coordination among care providers.
   4. Ensure continuity in patient care (Tahan, 2005b).

R. Case managers may assume a special focus on patient safety in their roles in five main areas. These are (Tahan, 2005b):
   1. Transitions or handoffs of care when a patient is transferred from one level of care or practice setting to another.
   2. Medical regimen (including medications and other treatments) reconciliation. A special focus is on medications, including a complete listing of all medications—prescription drugs, over-the-counter drugs, and herbal treatments—that have been prescribed and/or a patient is taking.
   3. Patient/caregiver education, to empower and educate patients and their caregivers on self-care management skills and compliance with medical regimens.

4. Access to services through a plan of care that provides access to the right amount and type of care and treatment at the right time, with the right provider, and to achieve the right outcome.

5. Communication among providers to make sure that all treating physicians, specialists, and other care providers are aware of the latest treatment plan and to maintain timely communication and exchange of information.

S. When medical errors occur, health care providers including case managers are ethically, morally, and legally obligated to disclose them.

T. The case manager might not be the right person to disclose a medical error, if one has occurred; however, he or she can be the right person to make sure the health care team is aware of its duty to disclose to the patient that an error has occurred, how it will be handled, what the patient can expect to do himself or herself, and what he or she can expect the team to do to rectify the error.

References

Case Management Society of America (CMSA). (2010). *CMSA standards of practice for case management*. Little Rock, AR: Author.

Cesta, T., & Tahan, H. (2003). *The case manager's survival guide: Winning strategies for clinical practice* (2nd ed.). St. Louis, MO: Mosby.

Cohen, E., & Cesta, T. (2005). *Nursing case management: From essentials to advanced practice applications* (4th ed.). St. Louis, MO: Elsevier Mosby.

HMO Workgroup on Care Management. (2004). *One patient, many places: Managing health care transitions*. Washington, DC: AAHP-HIAA Foundation.

Mullahy, C. (2014). *The case manager's handbook* (5th ed.). Sudbury, MA: Jones and Bartlett Learning.

National Quality Forum (NQF). (2006). *National voluntary consensus standards for hospital care: Additional priority areas—2005–2006: A consensus report*. Washington, DC: Author.

Tahan, H. (2005a). Identifying and reducing the risk for medical errors. *The Case Manager*, *16*(3), 80–82.

Tahan, H. (2005b). Enhancing patient safety: The role of the case manager. *Care Management*, *11*(5), 19–26.

Tahan, H., & Cesta, T. (2005). Managing emergency department overload. *Nurse Leader*, *3*(6), 40–43.

The Joint Commission (TJC). (2014). *Comprehensive accreditation manual for hospitals*. Chicago, IL: Author.

Wilson, M., Siegel, B., & Williams, M. (2005). *Perfecting patient flow: America's safety net hospitals and emergency department crowding*. Washington, DC: National Association of Public Hospitals and Health Systems.

Case Management and the Health Care Continuum

CHAPTER 5

Case Management in the Acute Care Setting

Stefani Daniels

IMPORTANT TERMS AND CONCEPTS

Advocacy
Centers for Medicare and Medicaid Services (CMS)
Congruency
Coordination of Care
Discharge Planning (DP)

Fee for service (FFS)
Hospital Case Manager (HCM)
Hospital Readmissions Reduction Program (HRRP)
Infrastructure

Progression of Care (PoC)
Prospective Payment System (PPS)
The Triple Aim
Transitional Planning
Utilization Management (UM)

Utilization Review (UR)   Value-Based   Workflow Processes
Value-based care   Purchasing Program
  (VBC)   (VBP)

Introduction

A. Rapid change is dominating the health care landscape, and acute care case management programs are feeling the pinch. Hospital case management is on a rapid evolutionary track as hospital programs respond to the changes in the marketplace, the same dominant marketplace that prompted its origins back in the early 1980s.

B. The market shift toward value-based care (VBC) presents unprecedented opportunities and challenges for the US health care system. Instead of rewarding volume, new value-based payment models reward better results in terms of cost, quality, safety, patient experience of care, and other outcome measures.

C. To keep up with demands for better outcomes, hospital case management (HCM) programs are moving to more contemporary models, and they are exploring opportunities to extend care management beyond the traditional walls of the hospital and across the full care continuum for selected high-risk patients. In adapting to new expectations, the traditional, functional case manager role as a utilization reviewer and discharge planner is disappearing. New blended roles of case managers are evolving and supported by other members of the case management team assuming specialized focus on utilization review and discharge planning.

D. Today, successful HCM programs are the orchestra leaders helping the various musicians stay in tune and keep up the tempo as the patient progresses through the acute episode of care. In keeping with the Institute of Healthcare Improvement's (IHI's) Triple Aim (better care, better health, and lower cost), today's case management programs are designing infrastructures and workflow process to promote the right care, in the right place, at the right time—every time. This ultimately is improving the quality of patient care, reducing the costs of care, and enhancing an optimal patient's experience of care.

E. The practice of hospital case management is no longer defined by UR and discharge planning functions. Today's models are more reflective of the actual definitions promulgated by the professional case management societies and are designed to achieve desired outcomes in the current fee-for-service environment while preparing for the leap "from the first curve, or volume-based environment, to the second curve, building value-based systems and business models."

F. According to industry observers, hospitals will succeed in the current environmental chaos by establishing partnerships with their stakeholders and postacute care partners to develop solutions tailored to selected patient populations.

G. From the perspective of many hospital executives who are preparing their organizations for a future of bundled payment methods, capitation, shared savings plans, medical homes, and accountable care organizations, HCMs are now challenged to achieve three major outcomes for selected patients:

1. Identify and overcome system and process obstacles that impede the patients' progression of care and delay discharge
2. Prevent or, at least, minimize the occurrence of unwanted operational events or inappropriate clinical interventions that add unnecessary clinical or financial risk to the organization's multiple stakeholders
3. Orchestrate the coordination and transitions of care to meet the needs and preferences of selected patient populations

H. The new generation of hospital case management programs is typically structured and operationalized to rapidly achieve these three goals. Within these programs, there are many features that should be integrated into every hospital's program no matter where they are on the evolutionary scale (Daniels & Ramey, 2005).

Descriptions of Key Terms

The understanding of these terms is important to case management practice but may not be expanded upon within this chapter's content.

A. Advocacy—A proactive process that promotes beneficence, justice, and autonomy for clients. To the extent possible, advocacy in the acute care setting aims to foster the client's engagement in decisions affecting the goals of their treatment plan. It involves educating clients about their rights, resources available, and insurance benefits. Advocacy facilitates appropriate and informed decision making and includes considerations for the client's values, beliefs, and interests (Gilpin, 2005).

B. Congruency—Congruency refers to the "fit" between the case management program and its environment. The environment includes the unique cultural climate that is internal to the organization and the external pressures of the marketplace.

C. Coordination of care—Organizing activities and sharing information among the care team to achieve safer and more effective care outcomes in accordance with the patients' needs and preferences.

D. Discharge planning—The process of assessing the patient's needs after leaving the acute care/hospital setting or another health care facility and ensuring that these services are in place for the patient before leaving.

E. Infrastructure—Relates to the alignment of hospital case management within the organizational structure; the composition and positions of team members; and the assignment, staffing, and scheduling of case management team positions.

F. Progression of care (PoC)—Encompasses a diverse set of activities designed to influence the efficient and effective movement of selected patients through the acute episode of care leading to a safe and timely transition to another level of care including home.

G. Transitional planning—A process applied to ensure that necessary resources and services are provided to a patient and that these services are delivered in the most appropriate level of care based on the patient's health condition and needs and in consideration with applicable laws and regulations or standards.

H. Utilization management—A process that focuses on the review of services and resources offered to patients on the basis of medical necessity, in the most relevant care setting/level of care, and in concert with quality and safety standards. A special focus here is cost-effective allocation of resources.

I. Utilization review—A mechanism used by some health insurance plans/payers to evaluate health care services provided (or about to) to a patient on the basis of necessity, appropriateness, and quality.

J. Workflow processes—Day-to-day case manager activities specifically designed to deliver the scope of practice to a selected patient population.

Applicability to CMSA's Standards of Practice

A. The Case Management Society of America (CMSA) describes in its standards of practice for case management that case management extends across all health care settings (CMSA, 2010). This without a doubt includes acute care/hospital levels of care, the subject of this chapter.

B. Case managers, according to CMSA, are recognized as expert clinicians and vital participants in the case management team. They empower people to understand and access quality, safe, cost-effective, and efficient health care services in the various care settings across the continuum and by diverse providers; acute care is one of these settings (CMSA, 2010).

C. Case managers in acute care settings focus on a variety of roles and functions described in CMSA's standards of practice for case management. Of special importance are care coordination, transitions of care, utilization management, and discharge/transitional planning. These are even more important considering the type of patients case managers care for in the acute care setting: individuals with multiple chronic illnesses and of various age groups especially the elderly.

D. CMSA's standards of practice highlight special activities that are pertinent to this chapter. These include client selection process for case management services, client assessment, problem or opportunity identification, planning care, monitoring of progress, evaluation of outcomes, facilitation and coordination of care and services, collaboration with other health care professionals, resource management, and stewardship (CMSA, 2010).

E. Case managers according to CMSA's standards conduct a comprehensive assessment of the client's health and psychosocial needs and develop a case management plan collaboratively with other members of the interdisciplinary health care team but most importantly with the client and family or caregiver. Focus of these activities is the movement of the patient to the most appropriate level of care. These functions are integral to the role of case managers in the acute care setting.

F. The acute care settings are characterized by higher complexity and intensity of services and resources compared to other care settings. It is highly important for acute care case managers to facilitate communication and coordination among the various members of the health care team and involve the patient/family or caregiver in the decision-making process about their care options, especially those needed postdischarge from acute care.

G. CMSA in its standards of practice for case management highlights the importance of advocacy in case management practice (CMSA, 2010). Case managers advocate for both the client and the payer in an effort to facilitate positive outcomes for the client, the health care team, and the payer, while keeping the needs of the client as the primary priority. This chapter describes the role case managers play in this regard.

Background/Historical Perspective

A. Hospital case management has its roots in the expanded role of the clinical nurse at Massachusetts' New England Medical Center (Zander, 1988). A "nurse case manager" followed a patient throughout the episode of care to overcome obstacles that may delay discharge. It was conceived as a strategy to lower lengths of stay at the time when the new PPS was introduced and to increase revenue or reduce financial risk.

B. Following the introduction of the PPS in the early 1980s, more than 1,000 hospitals went bankrupt and were closed or acquired, and there was a scramble to quickly reduce costs. Management engineers collapsed social work and UR departments and created case management programs. The concept of progressing the patient's care got lost in the shuffle, and we've been living with variations of this functional model ever since.

C. With the publication of Institute of Medicine's (IOM's) report, *To Err Is Human* (1999), the marketplace shifted once again and demanded improved outcomes in care and costs. Hospital case management programs responded by returning to its roots, focusing on progression of care to improve outcomes. At the same time, the UR function expanded exponentially with the growing list of regulatory oversight agencies demanding appropriate use of hospital level of care services. This leads to the creation of dedicated teams of UR specialists skilled in navigating the morass of rules and regulations governing medical necessity.

D. As the US hospital industry continues to change in structure, delivery of care, and payment models, the case manager has emerged as an important part of the workforce and a key driver of managing access to care, coordination of care, and cost/quality outcomes of across the entire health care continuum.

E. Delivering patient-centered care and services is one of the goals CMSA describes in its standards of practice. This is especially synergistic with the demands imposed on the health care delivery system by the Patient Protection and Affordable Care Act of 2010. It is also a requirement in acute care settings and necessary focus of the role of the case manager in these settings.

Distinguishing the Hospital Venue

A. The primary purposes of case management—to advocate on behalf of the patient and facilitate access to and the delivery of safe, appropriate care in a cost-effective manner, while seeking to promote positive health care outcomes—remain constant regardless of the practice venue. However, the practice of case management in a hospital looks quite different from case management practiced in a community health program or a health insurance company.

B. There are three key dimensions that distinguish case management in the hospital from those in other practice venues, and each dimension reflects the changing marketplace. These include designation of the program, congruency, and leverage.

C. Designation of the program:

1. Today's hospital case management programs straddle both sides of the value chasm and bridge the knowledge gap between the business and the clinical components of health care.

2. Hospital case management is often characterized in the literature as a clinical program despite the fact that case managers do not provide clinical, hands-on services. Rather, HCMs supplement the clinical expertise of the care team by providing information related to the business of managing care and the timely progression of effective patient's care.

3. Hospitals are under more scrutiny than any other practice venue to lower costs and remove progression of care inefficiencies while enhancing safe, high-quality care.

4. In 2011, only 7% of noninstitutionalized civilian population had an inpatient hospital stay; however, the spending associated with those stays accounted for 29% of all health care expenses (Gonsalez, 2013).

5. The share of the economy devoted to health spending has remained at 17.4% since 2009 as health spending and the gross domestic product increased at similar rates for 2010 to 2013 (CMS, 2013a). These statistics indicate that for every dollar spent on health care, over $0.40 was spent on personal hospital care.

D. Congruency

1. Within the larger context of the political, structural, economical, and cultural forces of the hospital, HCM must find a balance between its goals and the operational challenges of the traditional hospital organization.

2. Physicians are predominantly paid under FFS, which rewards them for the volume of services provided. Under the current payment system, physicians do not suffer any consequences if the care they prescribe is deemed not medically necessity resulting in a payment denial for the hospital. Therefore, there is no economic incentive for them to adhere to evidence-based protocols, algorithms, or order sets that specify best practice interventions.

3. Hospitals, on the other hand, are typically paid a fixed rate or discounted FFS or are experimenting in bundled payments that may include professional and facility fees.

4. Hospitals are employing physicians using incentive compensation packages that reward optimal clinical and financial performance.

5. Hospitals suffer financial penalties if predetermined performance expectations are not achieved.

E. Leverage

1. Unlike their counterparts in payer case management programs, HCMs have neither the positional authority nor the economic leverage to muster the support needed to overcome delivery of care inefficiencies

or medical practice decisions, both of which influence the patient's progression of care and timely transition. Leverage and influence must, therefore, be created.

2. To create leverage and influence, hospital case management must consider its customer base and shift problem solving to the perspective of that customer.

3. Spending on physician and clinical services increased 3.8% in 2013 to $586.7 billion, from 4.5% growth in 2012 (CMS, 2013a). As the second highest component in national health expenditures at 20%, physician/clinical services have captured everyone's attention (The Physicians Foundation, 2012).

4. Medical culture still dominates many hospital organizations, and without physician buy-in, hospital case management will not achieve the level of success envisioned by planners. Arguably, physicians are the hospital case management's primary customer in the acute care setting. By influencing physician practice decisions, without impinging on their medical judgment, every stakeholder benefits—especially the patient.

5. Addressing these operational tensions requires a case management structure and activities, which are aligned with these realities to the extent feasible.

Physician Partnerships

A. Hospital case management operates within a supply-driven market. It is generally the provider (the physician) rather than the consumer (the patient) who determines the type and extent of treatment, care, or services required.

B. To a modest degree, the explosion of the baby boomers, transparency in public reporting, the Internet, and direct-to-consumer advertising have eroded a portion of this market. Nevertheless, within the acute care environment, it is safe to say that, for the most part, the physicians' practice choices drive resource consumption, costs, and clinical outcomes.

C. To influence the type and extent of practice choices and promote appropriate and cost-effective interventions, a collaborative partnership between the case manager and the physician must be nurtured. Aligned with such partnership is another between the case manager and the patient/family/caregiver.

D. Case manager–physician partnerships are not forged overnight. While community-based primary care providers (PCPs) are generationally more resistant to partnerships, the presence of hospitalists has positively shifted the landscape since they are often working under incentive-based contracts and will seek the support of an HCM to navigate the system and achieve aligned goals.

E. Working in partnership with the physician may mean adopting new styles of communication or a new attitude. It means that the case manager will probably be making rounds with the physician partner whenever feasible, questioning practice decisions and offering alternatives, and coaching the physician on the "business" of managing the patients' care. Optimal patient advocacy requires continual diligence during the patient's progression of care to minimize the patient's exposure to unnecessary risk. Successful case managers work *with* the physician not *around* him/her.

F. Despite the case manager's level of clinical competence, the case manager's role is not to exercise clinical skills, but rather to apply critical thinking and clinical judgment skills, knowledge of health care treatments, familiarity with evidence-based interventions, and erudition of the health care system to influence the physician's medical decision making. To promote a safe, cost-effective episode of acute care, forging a relationship with the physician and provider team is essential (Commission for Case Manager Certification, 2010).

G. To influence a physician so that treatment decisions are made timely, appropriately, and in the patient's best interest, a conceptual shift to problem solving from the customer's perspective must occur and become second nature to the hospital case manager. If the case manager can recognize what is important to the physician, that insight can be used to offer a trade, or exchange, that brings value to the physician in practical terms.

H. Generally, physicians want help in effectively managing their time while in the hospital. They are interested in having:
  1. An advocate to make sure the patient receives prescribed treatments
  2. Information to stay up to date and to make sound decisions that are in their patient's best interest
  3. Relief from the business transactions they see as obstacles to care and a challenge to their autonomy.

I. By and large, physicians will not buy into a case management program, and acceptance will never occur if the physician perceives the role of the case manager as being simply to police his/her patients' charts, reduce length of stay, cut costs for the hospital, or challenge his/her medical judgment.

Designing a Case Management Model for Your Hospital

A. As programs continued to evolve, no single "reference model" of acute care case management has emerged. As a result, hospital case management today is often a reactive conglomeration of activities without a coherent vision or rational intent.

B. Envisioning the future—Given the chaos in the current hospital environment, coupled with the lack of a reference model for hospital case management, every successful program planner first creates a vision for the model.
  1. Visioning is a collective process of imagining the future.
  2. When a group of individuals get together to brainstorm about a case management model, creative juices start to flow and "why can't we" ideas surface.
  3. Through the visioning process, the purpose and intent of a program can be defined, along with its philosophy, values, core competencies, operational focus, and principles.
  4. When vision and intent are neglected, there is dissonance and confusion and the case managers feel the push and pull of multiple constituencies.

     5. Considering CMSA's standards of practice for case management can be helpful when engaged in a visioning exercise. It also can guide the discussion about what makes most sense in the design of the acute care case management model for your hospital.

C. While determining the purpose and intent of the hospital's case management program, important and sensitive outcomes are articulated. Knowledge at the outset on how hospital case management will be evaluated gives planners information to help design a relevant infrastructure and operations.

     1. Each program goal should be translated into measurable objectives.

     2. Aggregate objectives into a program scorecard to demonstrate the value of the hospital case management program.

     3. Large hospitals have a dedicated informatics analyst to generate actionable outcomes.

D. While many hospitals continue to use functional, second-generation, task-oriented models, outcome models represent the current best practice in many hospitals that are preparing for the future of VBC where appropriate resource utilization management is critical and where care coordination across the continuum has been initiated.

     1. Case managers follow selected patients through the acute progression of care facilitation, coordination, and collaboration (Box 5-1).

     2. To achieve the desired outcomes, case management activities focus on access processes, the nature and appropriateness of treatment, and alternatives for timely transition to a postacute venue.

     3. Outcome achievement capitalizes on the critical thinking skills of a well-rounded, business savvy case manager. They eschew task completion in favor of outcome achievement.

BOX 5-1　Case Managers Follow Select Patients

- Hospital case management is too expensive for all and not needed by most.
- Efforts must be made to accurately segment the acute care population and identify patients at risk.
- Absent of any real-time predictive modeling applications, the patient's initial assessments completed by health care team members and the potential obstacles identified concerning progression of care and timely discharge may be used to select patients in need for and benefiting from case management oversight.
- Case management oversight includes comanaging the progression of care (with the physicians and health care team) and removing obstacles that may delay transition.
- Following selected patients from access to transition reduces handoffs and gaps in communications, which, according to The Joint Commission, are the leading cause of sentinel events.
- Routine tasks associated with transition plan arrangements are typically delegated to support team members working in a centralized resource center, thereby freeing up the patient's nurse or case manager to remain engaged with the patient and as they navigate through the system in the safest, most cost-efficient manner.
- A team of UR specialists complement the HCM with payer-specific medical necessity information.

4. Case managers collaborate with the physicians and consider patient preferences and evidence-based protocols to drive effective progression of care.
5. The HCM monitors resource utilization on a real-time basis to avoid excessive, wasteful, and possibly harmful interventions.
6. Patients with chronic illnesses, such as heart failure, renal failure, asthma, diabetes, and others, are either followed by their case manager into the community or a seamless handoff to a transitional coach or community case manager is affected.

E. Outcome models are heavily data driven.
1. To drive improvement in patient care outcomes, anecdotal information is inadequate. Contemporary case management programs rely on data to drive improvement and demonstrate success.
   a. Whenever available, case managers rely on evidence-based care protocols or order sets to keep treatment plan on track.
   b. Delays resulting from undocumented noncompliance with evidence-based protocols that may add clinical or financial risk are captured, quantified, and reported.
   c. Inefficiencies in delivery of care processes, which delay progression of care, are captured, quantified, and reported.
   d. Executive leaders use these objective data to hold process owners responsible for delays and avoidable days.

F. There are different approaches to role integration for the case manager. Some models have designated the case manager to be responsible for the various case management functions; others have not. Those who have not integrated the role have identified other members of the case management team to assume responsibilities for specific functions such as discharge planning support and utilization review or management.
1. Regardless of who assumes which role, the case management functions tend to include clinical care management, discharge/transitional planning, utilization review and management, delays/variance management, and outcomes evaluation.
2. Contemporary case management programs place the case manager (a registered professional nurse) as the leader of the case management team and have designated a utilization management specialist and discharge planning associate to support the case manager.
3. Contemporary case management programs have also designated social workers in supportive role where case managers refer patients with complex discharge needs to the social worker for follow-up. Specific criteria for referrals are identified, which may include need for Medicaid application or charity care, crisis intervention and counseling, and placement in rehabilitation facilities or nursing homes.
4. Contemporary case management programs also allocate case management associate staff to function in a supportive role and focus primarily on clerical or administrative transactions such as arranging for patient's transportation upon discharge, scheduling of follow-up care appointments, ordering durable medical equipment, and transmitting of paperwork and other information to care providers internal or external to the hospital as necessary.

Case Management Program Infrastructure

A. Infrastructure relates to the alignment of hospital case management within the organizational structure; the nature of the team and the positions within the hospital case management program; and the assignment, staffing, and scheduling of case management team positions.

B. There is no one best way to structure hospital case management. Nevertheless, there are features that define the successful programs.
   1. Case management programs in acute care settings typically report to the Chief Medical Officer (CMO) or the Chief Operations Officer (COO), less frequently with the Chief Financial Officer (CFO) and rarely with the Chief Nursing Officer (CNO) or the Chief Quality Officer (CQO). Some organizations have the program reporting jointly to the CMO and CNO.
      a. The choice of an executive sponsor plays a key role in setting the image of the program, the rules that guide behaviors, and the responsiveness of stakeholders to the program. It also has the capability of changing or perpetuating mental models of behaviors.
      b. A mental model is a set of perceptions that color the images, assumptions, and stories that individuals carry in their minds about how things work.
      c. Simply put, the accountability relationships and mental models of behavior that the table of organization represents will affect how people perceive case management (Daniels & Ramey, 2005).
   2. Horizontal alignment refers to the way hospital programs are separated or combined under a single administrator.
      a. The richest path for sharing information and ideas is often a lateral trail that includes case management, psychosocial counseling, UR, medical necessity appeal activities, and clinical documentation improvement (CDI).
      b. Assignment of responsibility refers to the manner in which the case management workforce is distributed. There are pros and cons to every method.
         i. Geographic assignment is prevalent in hospitals using functional models where HCMs conduct chart audits for UR, serve as the primary discharge planners, and are responsible for the clerical activities associated with transition logistics.
         ii. Anecdotally, HCMs prefer physician or service line assignment models because they can exercise greater influence by working with a consistent group of physicians.
   3. Staffing of hospital case management programs refers to the plan for how many case management personnel are needed and of what classification.
      a. For several reasons, there is no staffing "best practice." Box 5-2 describes three important reasons.
      b. The four different issues described in Box 5-2 are why there are no set staffing standards—nor should there be.
   4. Caseloads refer to the entire scope of service that the assigned population represents. In reality, case management services may only be needed by 40% to 50% of the client list.

BOX 5-2 **Reasons for Lack of Standardized Staffing Patterns in Acute Care Case Management Models**

1. No two hospital case management programs are the same, and every hospital case management program has a scope of practice and scope of service unique to its facility. Case management expectations in one hospital will not necessarily parallel the expectations in another hospital.
2. The degree of support staff is a major variable. In some hospitals, case managers are expected to perform clerical as well as professional activities, while others have "back room" support personnel.
3. The nature of the patient populations and the character of the case management assignment are additional variables that must be considered. Case managers working exclusively with physicians caring for orthopedic patients, for example, will be able to oversee progression of care for more patients than a colleague who is partnered with the internal medicine doctors caring for patients with multiple diagnoses.
4. Staffing depends on the chosen model of practice, the relationships that the case manager is expected to nurture, the payer mix, the managed care contractual obligations, and the availability of data (Daniels & Ramey, 2005).

---

   a. Best advice—Look beyond caseload statistics and ask yourself what you are trying to achieve and who needs the services of the case manager to drive progression of care beyond that for which the patient's nurse is responsible.
5. Scheduling refers to the most productive pattern of staff presence to achieve the best outcomes. It should be predicated on an aggregate of several factors.
   a. Needs of primary customers.
   b. Pattern of presence based on scope of service (ambulatory surgery may not require weekend case management, while emergency department case management may require 7-day coverage).
   c. Hospital service availability. Many large and small community hospitals do not offer 7-day service access.
      i. While case management may not be essential on the weekends, UR specialists and the centralized Resource Center team charged with arranging transition plans are typically open 7 days a week.
   d. Contextual issues including scope of practice and available resources.
   e. Level of preparation and experience of the case managers.
C. Competency of the case management staff is a product of professional training, experience, mentorship, and exposure to new information. Critical thinking skills are vital for every case manager, but in the high-risk hospital environment where case managers lack any positional authority, failure to exercise critical thinking skills on behalf of the patient could be a matter of life or death.
   1. Other basic skills of a successful hospital case manager include:
      a. Outstanding communication skills—Able to easily use language to present a position and build more productive relationships with key business partners

      b. Essential negotiation skills—Able to tackle difficult people situations effectively and improve collaboration with colleagues

      c. Self-confidence and assertiveness—Able to get message across in a secure manner.

  2. A mountain of anecdotal evidence suggests that a real-time, physician-centric partnership results in better outcomes for all stakeholders.

  3. Activities that diminish the case managers' role or remove the case manager from the center of action and easy access to physicians will undermine the case managers' efforts to influence outcomes.

  4. Case manager–physician–pharmacist–nurse manager rounds represent the latest iteration of a simple but highly effective strategy to promote the partnership building process.

D. The case management infrastructure typically includes a physician advisor (PA).

  1. Today's PA role differs significantly from the advisor of the past, an individual who was viewed as the "hatchet man" for utilization problems. Today, the PAs serve as a resource and recourse to the case management and UR teams, and they understand and interact with the systems related to patient safety and resource management.

      a. Depending upon the size of the institution, the PA may provide advisory services for all the hospital's performance improvement initiatives or for specific programs such as quality, documentation, UR, or UM (Daniels & Hirsch, 2015).

      b. PAs serve as a champion for the case management program supporting activities to promote safety, quality, and reductions in cost of care.

      c. PAs further the case managers' clinical knowledge, adding to their credibility when interacting with their physician partners.

      d. Effective PAs also coach case managers on approaches that will be best received by a physician colleague.

  2. Since case managers are typically functioning in a fast-paced and high-pressure environment, PAs can mitigate some of the daily chaos associated with the role and provide a sense of organizational support (Smith, 2003).

      a. Serve as liaison between payers and providers

      b. Work with executive team and medical staff leadership to develop processes and guidelines to improve quality of care

      c. Direct interactions with medical staff to resolve issues that affect resource utilization or quality of care

      d. Educate medical staff on issues affecting the business of managing care

E. With the migration of health care to the ambulatory setting, today's inpatient populations tend to be more in need of psychosocial–spiritual support.

  1. Often, a diverse group of master's prepared professionals can meet the diverse needs of the patient populations. Counselors, behavioral health specialists, social workers, and others who specialize in public health, addictive behaviors, family dynamics, AIDS/HIV, and other challenging areas are appropriate in various situations dependent upon patient population.

2. Counselors are best positioned as consultants to the case managers to avoid redundancy in case finding and overlap as well as help to minimize professional tension.

   a. With some exceptions in larger hospitals or academic teaching facilities, social work departments have virtually disappeared and counseling positions are incorporated under the case management umbrella.

   b. The relationship between the case manager and the counselor is reinforced through a referral process that recognizes the special expertise that the counselor brings to a situation.

   c. When the case manager determines that psychosocial–spiritual issues could potentially obstruct the patient's safe and efficient navigation through the acute episode of care, a referral to a counselor may help save the day.

      i. Referrals by case managers avoid independent case finding, which serves to confuse patients, confound physicians, and other staff, and are often the root cause of case manager–social work tension (Daniels & Ramey, 2005).

Workflow

A. In an era where duplication of work and overlapping responsibilities are financially indefensible and coordination of services is highly desirable, the performance of the case manager includes activities that are meant to optimally integrate effective progression of care initiatives, efficient resource management to minimize patient risk, and timely transition.

B. There is a direct link between case management workflow activities and the goals cited above.

   1. Advocacy is the hospital case manager's primary ethical obligation. All activities related to facilitating the patient's progression of care, influencing efficient use of resources, and supporting a timely transition are based on the case manager's advocacy role to minimize the patients' iatrogenic risk of hospitalization. This is and should always be the "prime objective" of the hospital case manager and, within the context of describing the hospital case manager role, is the primary motivating factor.

   2. "Advocacy must be viewed as an unwritten contract between the case manager and the patient. To fulfill the terms of the contract, hospital case managers must revisit their day-to-day practice and identify activities to boost their value as navigators, facilitators, and advocates. Leaders must set conditions and promote expectations for advocacy that each case manager must meet. Job descriptions must be changed, and case management plans incorporating scopes of practice that underscore the advocacy role must be created" (Daniels, 2009).

   3. More than any other practice environment, the hospital represents the highest-risk setting for the patient and demands an assertive, self-confident case manager to guard the patient's exposure to unnecessary clinical, financial, and operational risks. In terms of day-to-day practice, this means that the case manager must question any decision or delay that may negatively impact the patient or his/her progression of care.

4. The proliferation of high deductible and co-pay insurance plans warrants the case manager's attention to avoid inappropriate, repeated, or excessive medical interventions that add to the patients' anxiety over their ability to pay.

5. In the hospital environment, the case manager's persuasive involvement in clinical and resource management activities reflects the supremacy of the advocacy role.

C. There are several resources and tools that the HCM can use to further the intent of the case management program:

1. Evidence-based protocols, endorsed by the medical staff, are powerful guidelines for best practice care. If the physician strays from the guidelines, the HCM can inquire the reason, suggest documentation to defend the deviation and medical decision, and provide alternative considerations, if warranted.

   a. In some HCM programs, a utilization review specialist may be involved. Such person may be responsible for the review of clinical care and practice based on already established evidence-based care guidelines and address the identified deviations (also known as variance) while considering medical necessity criteria and utilization review guidelines.

   b. A real-time, point-of-care interaction is the single most effective activity where a combination of a case manager, physician, and the application of an evidence-based guideline could favorably affect the cost and quality of medical care.

   c. Evidence-based protocols are not immutable mandates. They are guidelines that are developed through a consensus of research found in the literature.

2. Comparative physician practice profiles are objective measures to draw attention to the cost of rendering care and the wide variation in medical practice.

   a. Severity adjusted practice profiles are constructed using a collection of empirical data on demographics, diagnoses, procedures, and treatments. They can be generated by the data analytic team in the hospital, or hospital data can be transmitted and processed by a third-party vendor.

   b. Profiles cite all prescribed resources used in the course of providing inpatient care to the patient and are a direct result of the physician's practice decisions.

   c. Because CMS is not able to attribute resource utilization to specific physicians, profiles include all resources provided to the patient during a single episode of care by every physician including the ED physicians and any consultants brought in on the case by the attending of record.

   d. Each intervention has an associated revenue code, and each revenue code is converted to an associated cost. Thus, when a physician's order for a chest x-ray is entered into the order entry system, it is typically translated into a revenue code with a price tag attached to it for billing.

   e. For the purposes of practice profile reporting, all the claims data are organized by diagnosis and formatted so that the resources are categorized into major resource categories.

    f. All Patient Refined Diagnostic Related Group (APR DRG) software is the best application for this purpose because its severity adjusts all patients in a given population, not just Medicare patients.

    g. As an example, a single report will identify all APR DRG 140, Chronic Obstructive Pulmonary Disease (COPD) patients. All the resources reported under each attending physician's National Provider Identification (NPI) number caring for APR DRG 140 patients are listed in bucket columns such as respiratory services, medications, lab-hematology, lab-chemistry, intravenous medications, etc. In this manner, comparisons of the resources used are made among different physicians caring for COPD patients. These reports come in many formats though the best practice is a simple spreadsheet format where physicians can see their profile in comparison with their peers and no interpretative explanation is required.

    h. Data is transparent; blinding physician names is a legacy holdover and has little use in today's environment considering that a physician's Medicare earnings is posted online and publically available.

    i. Data must be adjusted for severity to dispute physician claims of "I use more resources because my patients are sicker."

    j. Severity adjustment profiles level the playing field to ensure that apples are being measured against other apples and are widely used by state, federal, and payer agencies to evaluate medical practice patterns.

    k. These profiles serve as a resource to advance the case manager's efforts to motivate and influence physician decisions to achieve expected outcomes.

3. Discharge planning has always been a nursing responsibility. The Conditions of Participation (CoP) are clear that every inpatient must be screened for discharge planning needs. The operative word is "screened."

    a. Without the benefit of a real-time predictive modeling application, screening is most efficiently achieved using the patient's initial assessment, which is completed by the clinical nurse.

        i. Case managers and staff nurses collaborate to ensure that the assessment tool incorporates indicators that will identify a progression of care issue that may delay a timely transition and any readmission risk factors. Many organizations incorporate bona fide readmission risk scoring systems (e.g., Society of Hospital Medicine 8P Risk Assessment).

        ii. Each indicator is given a numerical score. If the tool is embedded within the electronic health record (EHR), the information technicians can map the nurse's responses to electronically and automatically generate a referral directly to the case management office if the cumulative score meets predefined criteria.

        iii. If a paper assessment tool is used, each indicator contains a value—if the values of all the checked indicators reached a sum greater than a predetermined amount, a phone call or face-to-face referral is made to the case manager.

    b. Using the practical Pareto approach, the case manager can concentrate on those patients at most risk for progression of care obstacles that may delay transition and add readmission risk.

    c. Readiness for transition is not a discrete activity. It is the end product of the progression of care activities.

    d. The professional nurse owns his or her patient's discharge, plan but arranging the logistics of the discharge plan is a distinct activity and does not require a professional license. A discharge planning associate may assist in this process and assume responsibility for the clerical aspects of the discharge plan such as arranging for transport or ordering durable medical equipment.

    e. Once the nurse, in collaboration with the patient, family, physician, and members of the health care team, endorses a discharge plan, the nurse makes the referral to the personnel in the Resource Center to facilitate the associated logistics.

    f. It is anticipated that a well-designed and fully completed initial patient assessment tool will identify patients with complex needs and generate a referral to an HCM who will collaborate with the physician and the care team on what postacute resources will work best for the patient.

    g. Patients needing home care return to a nursing home, or other straightforward arrangement can be referred by their nurse to the Resource Center.

D. Crossing the acute care continuum

    1. Access management is generally defined as the entry into the acute care environment and includes the essential activities necessary to obtain services at the acute hospital level of care (Box 5-3).

    2. Throughput refers to the patient's progression of care and the various touchpoints that impact efficiency. Throughput is a product of the

---

BOX

5-3 Access Management

1. Access management includes a robust UR component applicable to all requests for direct admissions, transfers, and ED to determine whether:
   a. The patient's medical condition requires hospital level of care.
   b. The admission to the hospital meets evidence-based acute care screening criteria.
2. If screening indicators confirm hospital level of care needs are met, does the physician anticipate that the patient requires two midnights to provide care and address patient needs? The following is of importance as decisions are made:
   a. If care requires a hospital stay extending over two midnights, the patient is admitted as an inpatient.
   b. If it is anticipated that care will not require a hospital stay over two midnights, the patient should remain as an outpatient and placed on observation status.
   c. Medical documentation should be available and supports above determinations.
3. Only if the three items in point number 2 above are present, patients are then registered for hospital care.
4. If the three items are absent, a referral to the physician advisor is required unless the Access UR Specialist is able to offer the admitting physician acceptable alternatives (Daniels & Hirsch, 2015).

services, treatments, interventions ordered for the patient, and the efficiency in which those services, treatment, and interventions are delivered. Inefficient throughput is a product of excessive, wasteful, duplicative, and repeated testing or services ordered, which are not related to the reason for the patient's hospital admission, and inefficient delivery of care processes.

a. Case managers have no positional authority so they have to rely on other means to influence improvement in delivery of care. One of the more popular strategies hospital case managers use is the capture and quantification of information on the touchpoint obstacles encountered that result in a delay of progression-of-care day (PoCD) or a potentially avoidable day (PAD).

b. Data on avoidable days are not intended to play "gotcha" or to point a finger or placing blame.

c. PoCD and PAD may be a cost issue to hospital administration, but it is a quality issue for the physician, the patient, and the hospital case manager. This distinction must be clearly understood.

i. The effectiveness of the case manager's efforts to reduce PoCD and/or PAD and move the patient efficiently through the episode of care will suffer if the case manager connects these impediments to the loss of revenue to the hospital.

d. To create a system of capture and quantification of PoCD and/or PAD, consider the key points described in Box 5-4.

3. Transition is the movement of the patient from one level of care to another, generally in diminishing order, and one setting to another.

a. Hospital specialty beds are scarce and expensive. They should be used judiciously for patients who need critical care interventions to recover from an acute episode of illness or major invasive procedures.

i. Criteria for use of specialty beds are developed by the medical staff and reflect best practice as evidenced in the medical literature.

ii. Oversight of the use of critical care beds is generally in the hands of an intensivist or as otherwise indicated in the medical staff bylaws.

iii. With enforced criteria in place, the role of the HCM may be to monitor the progression of care and confer with the team to identify milestones for transition to a lower level of care.

iv. Oftentimes, the presence of a counselor in the critical care areas is of greater value than a case manager since critical care nurses are oftentimes very diligent about progressing their patients' care when milestones are met.

b. Hospitals are required to "screen all inpatients to determine which ones are at risk of adverse health consequences post-discharge if they lack discharge planning" (CMS, 2013b). Patients and families, no matter how well adjusted, often need considerable consultation to help them explore and evaluate all the options regarding postacute needs.

c. Ongoing evaluation of transition needs is the responsibility of the entire clinical team and is documented by the patient's nurse.

BOX 5-4   Capture and Quantification of PoCD and PAD

- Identify the full range of care delay variables. It's not unusual to identify over 100 items that contribute to the interruption or delay of the patient's progression of care. Each item should be clearly attributable, for example, "Test delay" versus "Radiology test delay."
- Categorize the items by source: patient, physician, system, community, and other practitioners.
- Create a form (e.g., paper or digital) listing each of the items with room for two check boxes. Or use electronic tools for the gathering, tracking, trending, analysis, and reporting of such data. Today, many acute care hospitals are using case management software applications for electronic documentation and to capture these data.
- PoCD and PADs do not have to be justified but simply captured by every member of the case management team.
- Consistently capture each occurrence with a check in one box; if the CM or UR staff has acted in some capacity to overcome or prevent the PoCD/PAD, then have a related check box available indicative of an intervention.
- When the patient is discharged, submit the captured information to clerical staff who handles data entry into a database making sure that there are fields for attending physician's name, attributable physician, admission date, date of occurrence, diagnosis, and payer.
- Confer with the Chief Finance Officer to determine a metric, which financially quantifies the results; average cost per patient day is the most frequently used.
- Clerical staff should be responsible to generate pertinent reports of all the PoCD/PADs, the associated costs of the delay, and the savings on a regular basis (e.g., bi-weekly).
- As trends emerge, narrow the list of variables down to the most frequently occurring items.
- Whenever available, eliminate the manual process and convert delay item tracking to an electronic capture system.
- At regular intervals (e.g., monthly, quarterly), distribute the report of findings to the UR Committee, the respective delivery of care process owners, and attributed members of the medical staff.

    d. Routine transitions to home without services or to home with home care are generally handled between the patient, the family, the physician, and the case manager. In some models, the patient's nurse is involved in the coordination of home care services, often in collaboration with support staff functioning in what is known as Discharge Resource Center.

        i. The case manager (or the nurse where applicable) provides the patient/family with a brochure listing all the available home care agencies and gives the Discharge Resource Center the patient's preferences so that staff in the Center can make the arrangements.

        ii. There are different approaches to patient's discharge with home care services. Some have the case manager responsible for coordinating such services. Others may have the clinical nurse responsible for the coordination of home care services for patients with less complex conditions and needs.

      iii. With home care regulations being increasingly stringent, it is probably best for home care referrals to require the involvement of a case manager or discharge planning specialist to efficiently coordinate the process, avoid any concerns, and assure adherence to regulatory and accreditation standards.

      iv. Some HCM programs use a Discharge Resource Center as a forum where support staff work in the capacity of case management associates and collaborate with case managers and social workers.

        a. Staff in this Center are usually responsible for clerical or administrative functions such as arranging for durable medical equipment for patients based on a request from the case manager or social worker, coordinating patient's transportation upon discharge from the hospital (taxi or ambulance), and sharing of certain paperwork or care summaries with external providers or agencies as required.

        b. Availability of such Center and associates relieves case managers from clerical functions and maximizes their availability to patients at the bedside.

   e. If the patient is being managed by a case manager, there is a high probability that the patient may be advised to transition to rehab services, or LTACH, or SNF. In these cases, it is essential that the family has the opportunity to review service providers.

      i. Medicare patients must be given choice of available resources. It is essential that the Resource Center understands the plan as quickly as possible so they can determine availability within the anticipated time frame.

      ii. Once availability is determined, the patient has a choice among providers. If the patient is medically stable, but his/her preferred choice is not available and the patient refuses the transfer, the patient is given a Hospital-Issued Notices of Noncoverage (HINN) letting him/her know that she/he will be responsible for the costs of the days in the hospital.

Program Operations

A. Coordination of care describes the assistance needed to ensure the effective organization of, and access to, services and resources that are appropriate to the needs of the patients and their families.

  1. Coordination can be categorized into five primary advocacy accountabilities:

    a. Advanced communication among clinical team members

    b. Organization of multidisciplinary teamwork

    c. Liaison with payers and business team members

    d. Initiation of referrals to internal and external resources

    e. Fueling the progress of the patient's transition to the next level of care

  2. Coordination is often best effectuated with the presence of a single consistent resource throughout the patient's acute episode of care.

    a. This is not an easily obtainable goal in large hospitals where the physical distance between patient care areas can be considerable.

b. In those situations, case management teams design mechanisms for a seamless handoff from one case manager to another to minimize communication gaps and to avoid one of the biggest patient dissatisfiers: asking the same questions over again.

B. Coordination of care is strengthened through the interactions of the multiple providers involved in the patient's progression of care. Structured interactions ensure sharing essential information, while informal interactions are generally topic specific.

1. Every hospital has scheduled meetings meant to share patient information among providers and discuss care progression and case management plans. Some are more valuable than others. Key to the value of interdisciplinary meetings is the presence of medical representation. Since time is their most valuable commodity, physicians will attend if they perceive the meeting to be time well spent.

2. There is no one best model of interdisciplinary meetings, though some of the more valuable are comprised of three levels: morning, midday, and weekly (Box 5-5).

C. The revenue cycle is a series of financial processes that begin when the patient comes into the system and includes all of those activities that have to occur in order for the hospital to bill for services and collect revenue at the end of the process.

1. The revenue cycle cuts across every area/department in the hospital from registration's responsibilities to generate an accurate and complete face sheet to medical necessity for services and from charge capture by clinicians to medical record documentation.

2. Revenue cycle activities are now viewed as an enterprise-wide process rather than a series of disconnected department activities.

3. Representatives from the hospital case management program are members of the revenue cycle team because of their participation in the episode of acute care and their knowledge of navigational breakdowns that may result in a delay or avoidable day, ultimately leading to a payer denial.

4. Patient Financial Service (PFS) departments are the keepers of denial information. The information is shared with the case managers and UR specialists to target opportunities to prevent denials from occurring in the first place. Important information is that related to the 835 payment remittance (Box 5-6).

5. PFS refers denials for reasons other than physician practices to the attributable source. For example, denials arising from a delay in treatment are referred to the department head for that treatment area. Similarly, denial due to the lack or delay of precertification is forwarded to the access management department (admissions and registration). However, a denial for a quality of care issue is followed up by the case manager.

D. UR is mandated through the Conditions of Participation for regular FFS Medicare and Medicaid patients.

1. It is also a compulsory obligation under the terms of the insurer's contract.

2. The process typically uses a method of chart review to evaluate the medical necessity and appropriateness of an admission and duration of stay, level of care, procedures/services consumed, and readiness for discharge.

BOX 5-5   Interdisciplinary Care Management Meetings/Forums

1. Morning handoff rounds. If the hospital has the presence of residents and/or hospitalists, the most valuable time to share information is during the morning handoff rounds. This is the time many hospitalists/residents "run the list" and review the:
   a. "Plan for the stay"—Why the patient was admitted and the treatment goals.
   b. "Plan for the day"—What is being done today to advance the treatment plan.
   c. "Plan for the way"—What probable postacute needs will the patient need and are there resources to pay for them. Sometimes this is referred to as "plan for the post stay."
   d. "Plan for the pay"—Are we providing services that may put the patient or the organization at financial risk? What can we do about it? (Zander, 2003).
   e. These meetings are generally attended by the key players in the patients' progression of care including the case manager, nurse manager, pharmacist, therapists, clinical documentation improvement specialist, and a UR specialist.
   f. These meetings are concise with little sideline discussions. Some tasks are completed, for example, writing scripts for patients being discharged, and changes in the treatment plan may result from the input of the participants (e.g., test results).
   g. It's also a good time to remind the medical team about any documentation improvement opportunities or payer concerns.
2. Midday huddles, also known as flash rounds, table top rounds, and many other designations. These are typically update meetings early in the afternoon to keep everyone on the team apprised of any changes or new information about some or all of the patients, depending upon the size of the hospital.
   a. The latest iteration of these meetings is the room-to-room patient rounds where the physician accompanied by key team members visits selected or all the patients on that physician's service.
   b. Room rounds have the advantage of motivating patient involvement in care decisions as well as influencing physician practice decisions at the point of care.
3. The weekly meeting is formally structured and focused on select patients who present unusual or long-standing challenges for progression of care or transition to another care setting. Some features of successful weekly meetings include:
   a. Administrative leadership—sends a loud endorsement by the executive staff of the importance of team-based care.
   b. Held in boardrooms—sends a subliminal message about the importance of the meeting.
   c. Representatives of clinical and business departments are present and all are active participants.
   d. Representatives of affiliated postacute service providers attend to offer immediate options for transition.
   e. Presence of an ethicist to address end-of-life care issues or family concerns regarding patient's prognosis and terminal stage of illness.
4. The morning handoff rounds and midday huddles serve multiple purposes:
   a. Avoid intrusive follow-up phone calls questioning the physician's decisions
   b. Allow each member of the interdisciplinary care team to leave the meeting room with clear priorities
   c. Keep everyone current about the population being served by the care team
   d. Promote patient/family engagement, which is a major contributor to patient and family satisfaction

BOX 5-6 Payment Remittance Information and the Case Manager

- PFS provides information from the payer remittances (835 electronic remittances from the payer) explaining the reason for nonpayment. These remittances tell the story of what the payer is denying.
- The information from the 835 is integrated into the billing system so that a record is maintained and action can be taken to respond to the payer, to provide any requested documentation to avoid the denial, or to overturn the denial through an appeal.
- The total of all the 835s is the gross revenue loss to the hospital *unless* PFS takes action to override the payers' decision.
- To reduce that amount of potential loss, any initial denials or payment holds contingent on further information about clinical or medical necessity issues are generally referred to the appeal team to determine whether an appeal is feasible.
- Knowledge of the 835 information is important to prevent denials in the future.
- A monthly report is prepared by PFS citing all the 835 denials related to clinical quality and absence of medical necessity.
- The monthly report may include several data elements so that action can be taken to avoid denials in the future: the payer, the physician, the reason codes (the 835 software generally uses hundreds of reason codes explaining the cause of the denial), the DRG/diagnosis, and the amount involved.
- Armed with this information, the case manager can target opportunities with certain patients or physicians to avoid future denials and minimize all the back end fixes and rework that has to be done at a great cost and loss of productivity.

3. The growing presence of automated and interactive software application often belies the need for a professional to conduct the chart audit.
4. It is important to distinguish contractual obligations from regulatory requirements for UR.
    a. For the most part, contracts are quite explicit about their procedures and policies regarding the review process. In contrast, regulatory agencies (e.g., Centers for Medicare and Medicaid Services, State Departments of Health and Human Services) generally promulgate a set of guidelines but leave it to each hospital to determine its own procedures and processes.
    b. The predominant chart review process of UR is generally a retrospective activity. With the exception of the decision to admit, which is more and more becoming a concurrent process, continuing stay review and readiness for discharge is generally a retrospective process.
    c. Commercial contracts establish the UR requirements by referring to the terms contained in its provider manual (Box 5-7).
E. Documentation drives revenue for both the physician and the hospital.
    1. Specifically, doctors complete their charting responsibilities, the chart flows to the health information management (HIM) department for the coder to abstract essential information and assign related codes.
        a. The information captured as part of the abstracting and coding process is converted to the UB-92 format so that the patient accounting office can generate a bill.

5-7 **UR Requirements in Commercial Insurance Plans**

- Contracts are typically endorsed by the Chief Financial Officer, managed care department, and chief executive officer once fees are negotiated.
- The terms of UR are typically contained in boilerplate language that invariably favors the payer. The terms should be reviewed by the director of case management to avoid placing the hospital in a defensive posture (Daniels & Hirsch, 2015).
- While some provisions will inevitably favor one side or the other, overall balance is a key to more harmonious payer–provider relationships.
- Contract addendums are not unusual anymore. The director should review the utilization language prior to each contract renewal and recommend addendums that level the playing field.
- Every case manager should have knowledge of the payers' reimbursement methods. Case management or UR activities and priorities may hinge on knowledge that reimbursement is per diem versus fixed rate versus discounted FFS versus bundled payment.
- In areas with aggressive managed payer contracts (e.g., Medicare Advantage, Managed Medicaid), physician contracts may be capitated or they may be participating in a bundled payment arrangement. Case manager knowledge of this information will prove beneficial in helping the physician efficiently manage the patient's treatment plan.

   b. Neither physicians nor case managers are knowledgeable about coding and would find it difficult to master the time-consuming and technically tricky coding functions. However, since documentation drives the coding process, a clinical documentation improvement specialist would be beneficial to the team.

   c. The implementation of the ICD-10 coding process, which demands more specificity than its ICD-9 predecessor, has prompted the creation of several web-based and user-friendly CDI programs that can be viewed on smartphones and iPads during multidisciplinary meetings. These applications make the documentation improvement process much simpler than in the past.

 Outcomes

A. The value of case management is a product of its contribution to the organization's clinical and financial bottom lines. Therefore, the case manager's performance goals must be aligned with the goals of the organization, and case management activities must reflect the strategic outcomes the hospital desires to achieve on behalf of its many stakeholders.

   1. Outcomes measurement can be quite complicated especially if data are not easily accessible. Fortunately, the use of informatics has dramatically changed the face of the health care industry and has enabled case management to more easily demonstrate its influence.

2. Case management outcomes are the end results of the case managers' work activities that objectively measure the program's effectiveness and demonstrate a positive correlation between its interventions and the outcomes being measured.
3. Case management outcome indicators are surrogate measures of the case manager's sphere of influence.
4. Outcomes generally fall into four major categories:
   a. Clinical outcomes reflect improvement in patient care. For example, data may show that more patients are getting beta-blockers as a result of point-of-care reminders by the case manager.
   b. Cost outcomes measure the costs of resources being consumed in the care of the patient.
   c. Noncontributory medical interventions add clinical and financial risks per patient day and should result in lower costs per case.
   d. It is not accidental that CMS chose Medical Spending Per Beneficiary (MSPB) as its efficiency indicator. It is more relevant than the persistent focus on hospital length of stay.
   e. Revenue outcomes measure the gains as a result of the case manager's activities. An example would be an increase in payments due to a decrease in denials.
5. A case management outcomes scorecard often begins by aligning program objectives with organizational goals.
   a. If one of the hospital's objectives is to improve revenue, then case management may develop objective indicators to demonstrate that as a result of their proactive denial prevention initiatives, the volume and amount of denials decreased a certain percentage over a given period.
   b. If one of the hospital objectives is operational excellence, then case management may identify a metric to demonstrate that PoCD and PADs due to delays in imaging procedure scheduling delays were reduced by 11% over the last month.
6. Outcomes require objective information, which is recorded and stored in department repositories.
   a. Case management leaders must work with data analytic specialists to set up systems that benchmark their performance and contributions.
   b. Integration of data and production of information from disparate systems is now possible because of the availability of interface engines, data warehouses, data mining software, and decision support services.
   c. Case management outcomes are essential to monitor progression of care quality, and hospital executives are often willing to dedicate an informatics resource to the department for outcomes reporting.
   d. Outcomes of case management must incorporate the core measures of the value-based purchasing program, the Hospital Readmissions Reduction Program, and the patient experience using the Hospital Consumer Assessment of Healthcare Providers and Systems (HCAHPS).
7. For the purposes of case management, ROI is the profit or loss resulting from the hospital's investment in case management.
   a. Calculating the ROI requires a comparison of the costs of case management resources against the benefits it provides and is expressed in the following formula: [(benefits − costs)/costs] × 100% = % ROI.

References

Case Management Society of America. (2010). *Standards of Practice for Case Management.* Little Rock, AR: Author.

Centers for Medicare and Medicaid Services. (2013a). *National health expenditures 2013 highlights.* Retrieved from http://www.cms.gov/Research-Statistics-Data-and-Systems/Statistics-Trends-and-Reports/NationalHealthExpendData/downloads/highlights.pdf, on July 2, 2015.

Centers for Medicare and Medicaid Services. (2013b). *Revision to state operations manual (SOM), hospital appendix A—Interpretive guidelines for 42 CFR 482.43, discharge planning.*

Commission for Case Manager Certification. (2010). *Care Coordination: Case managers "connect the dots" in new delivery models.* Issue Brief, Volume 1, Issue 2. Retrieved from http://ccm-certification.org/sites/default/files/downloads/2011/4.%20Care%20coordination%2C%20 case%20managers%20connect%20the%20dots%20-%20volume%201%2C%20 issue%202.pdf, on July 2, 2015.

Daniels, S. (2009). Advocacy and the hospital case manager. *Professional Case Management, 14*(1), 48–51.

Daniels, S., & Hirsch, R. (2015). *The hospital guide to contemporary utilization review.* Danvers, MA: HCPro.

Daniels, S., & Ramey, M. (2005). *The leader's guide to hospital case management.* Sudbury, MA: Jones and Bartlett.

Gilpin, S. (2005). Advocacy and case management. *Care Management, 11*(1), 28.

Gonsalez, J. M. (2013). *National health care expenses in the U.S. civilian noninstitutionalized population, 2011* (Statistical Brief #425). Rockville, MD: Agency for Healthcare Research and Quality. Retrieved from http://meps.ahrq.gov/mepsweb/data_files/publications/st425/stat425.shtml, on July 2, 2015.

Institute of Medicine. (1999). To Err is Human: Building a Safer Health System. In L. T. Cohn, J. M. Corrigan, & M. S. Donaldson (Eds.). Retrieved from https://www.iom.edu/~/media/Files/Report%20Files/1999/To-Err-isHuman/To%20Err%20is%20Human%201999%20%20report%20brief.pdf, on March 2015.

Smith, A. P. (2003). Case management: Key to access, quality, and financial success. *Nursing Economics, 21*(5), 237–240, 244.

The Physicians Foundation. (2012). *Drivers of healthcare costs: A physicians foundation white paper.* Retrieved from http://www.physiciansfoundation.org/uploads/default/Drivers_of_Health_Care_Costs_-_November_2012.pdf, on July 2, 2015.

Zander, K. (1988). Managed care within an acute care setting: Design and implementation via nursing case management. *Health Care Supervisor, 6*(2), 27–43.

Zander, K. (2003). Planning for the day, the pay, the stay, and the way. *Center for Case Management, The Definition, 18*(2), 1–3.

CHAPTER 6

Case Management in the Community and Postacute Care Settings

Hussein M. Tahan

LEARNING OBJECTIVES

Upon completion of this chapter, the reader will be able to:

1. Identify the community-based care settings available for clients especially the elderly and older adult persons, including rehabilitation, skilled nursing, long-term, and nonmedical levels of care.

2. Determine criteria for placement of the elderly and older adults in various levels of care.

3. Describe the use of respite care.

4. Determine critical questions to ask when completing a financial assessment.

5. Describe the role of the case manager in community-based care settings including rehabilitation and long-term care.

6. Describe the impact of the Patient Protection and Affordable Care Act on ambulatory and primary care.

7. Assess for and identify common problems the elderly or geriatric patient faces.

8. Identify steps case managers may take to place a geriatric patient in long-term care.

IMPORTANT TERMS AND CONCEPTS

Activities of Daily
  Living (ADLs)
Aging in Place
Assisted Living
Comprehensive Geriatrics
  Assessment (CGA)
Comprehensive
  Outpatient
  Rehabilitation Facility
  (CORF)
Custodial Care
Elder Abuse

Elder Neglect
Inpatient
  Rehabilitation
  Facility (IRF)
Instrumental Activities
  of Daily Living
  (IADLs)
Limitation of Activity
Long-Term Care
Long-Term Care
  Insurance
Nonskilled Care

Reasonable and
  Necessary Care
Personal Care Services
Rehabilitation
Respite Care
Restorative Nursing
  Services (NRS)
Skilled Nursing Care
Skilled Nursing Facility
  (SNF)
Speech and Language
  Pathology (SLP)

 Introduction

A. Case management in community care settings may include ambulatory-based/clinic-based care, health care centers (both federally and nonfederally qualified or privately operated), physician group practices, accountable care organizations, patient-centered medical homes, and hospital-based clinics.

B. Case management in the postacute settings or levels of care may include acute and subacute rehabilitation hospitals/facilities, skilled care and nursing homes, "aging in place" (Fig. 6-1), and long-term care.

C. Most of the frail elderly in the United States require at some point or another community and long-term care or rehabilitation services in acute or subacute care facilities. This is mostly due to deconditioning after an acute care hospitalization or injury.

D. Today's older adults and elderly patients who seek health care services encounter a variety of providers and organizations, including primary care physicians (ambulatory- and clinic-based care), specialists, acute care hospitals, skilled nursing facilities (SNFs), nursing homes, rehabilitation facilities, and home health care.

E. Assessment for placement of the clients/patients in a specific level of care should:
   1. Yield the *least* restrictive level of care possible for safe care.
   2. Meet the care needs of the client and support system.
   3. Be financially feasible and sustainable for the patient/client and family.
   4. Meet the conditions stipulated in either laws and regulations or health insurance policies.
   5. Ensure a reimbursable episode of care.

NOTE: This chapter is a revised version of Chapters 6 and 22 in the second edition of *CMSA Core Curriculum for Case Management*. The contributor wishes to acknowledge the work of Linda N. Schoenbeck and Suzanne K. Powell, as some of the timeless material was retained from the previous version.

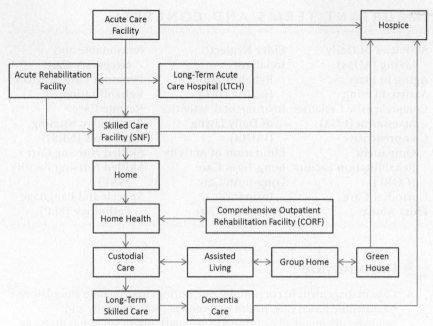

FIGURE 6-1. Postacute levels of care.

F. Health insurance plans usually pay for "medically reasonable and necessary" care. However, each insurance company has its own rules and definitions of "medical necessity" and "skilled" versus "unskilled" services that play an integral role in deciding whether to reimburse for care or not.

G. The prospective payment system (PPS) has resulted in patients' early discharge or transition from the acute care/hospital setting to another less complex or restrictive level of care. This has increased the need for follow-up care in settings such as the patient's home, provider's clinic, and patient-centered medical home but most commonly in the long-term care and rehabilitation settings.

H. As integrated care delivery systems have become more common, new approaches to care, especially for the elderly, disabled, or functionally impaired, have been created. A common approach is subacute care, which is a level of care that blends acute and long-term care skills and philosophies.

I. Recent changes in health care delivery systems (e.g., Patient Protection and Affordable Care Act of 2010 and value-based purchasing programs) have resulted in an increased demand for case management and the role of the case manager in settings beyond the acute care/hospital, that is, long-term care, rehabilitation, patient-centered medical homes (PCMHs), federally qualified health centers (FQHCs), or accountable care organizations (ACOs).

J. Care of the older adult, elderly, and pediatric or young adult patients with one or more chronic illnesses requires the services of interdisciplinary teams of health care professionals including geriatricians, nurses, social workers, dieticians, physical therapists,

6-1   Aspects of the Patient's Assessment for Better Care Provision

- Functional and medical assessments to develop a full understanding of the patient's needs
- Physical and mental status examination
- Balance and gait test
- Nutritional/dietary assessment
- Psychosocial and socioeconomic history including health insurance plan and benefits
- Home safety
- Battery of laboratory and x-ray (radiologic) tests as necessary
- Other tests as indicated by the patient's condition
- Self-management ability and adherence to health regimen including medications
- Use of assistive devices and technology
- Availability of support system and involvement in patient's care
- Risk category or class (e.g., low, moderate, high, very high) especially if suffering one or more chronic illnesses

occupational therapists, speech and language therapists, and pharmacists, but especially case managers.

K. To ensure effective care of the elderly and chronically ill, the interdisciplinary team must assess specific aspects of the patient situation, health condition, and plan of care (Box 6-1).

L. Care for the aged, chronically sick, and mentally ill has been affected by specific milestones in laws and regulations in the United States (Box 6-2).

6-2   Examples of Laws that Affected Care of the Chronically Ill

- Almshouses: Institutions to house the poor, aged, and mentally ill; regulation in 1873.
- County homes: Result of regulation; historically, terrible conditions for the older adult.
- 1935—Social Security Act: Provided catalyst for privately funded institutions for the aged.
- 1965—Medicare and Medicaid reimbursement: Allowed expansion of this industry.
- 1965—Older Americans Act: Created primary vehicle for organizing, coordinating, and providing community-based services and opportunities for older Americans and their families.
- Office of Nursing Home Affairs of 1971 and Nursing Reform Act of 1987: Established minimum requirements for nursing assistants, created a resident rights statement, and implemented a single standard for 24-hour care for all residents in nursing homes.
- Mid-1980s: Inpatient Prospective Payment System went into effect.
- 1991: Federally funded health centers for care provision for the underserved, immigrant, and rural population.
- Late 1990s and early 2000s: Prospective Payment System expansion to nonacute care settings such as long-term care, rehabilitation, and home care.
- 2010: The Patient Protection and Affordable Care Act (PPACA) went into effect.
- 2011: Expansion of federally funded health centers as a result of the PPACA and increased popularity of Federally Qualified Health Centers.

M. This chapter does not discuss provision of care in the ambulatory- and clinic-based settings. This is addressed in Chapter 4. However, the role case management plays in the ambulatory care setting is similar to that in PCMHs, ACOs, and FQHCs.

 ## Descriptions of Key Terms

A. Activities of daily living (ADLs)—Activities related to personal care include bathing or showering, dressing, getting in or out of bed or a chair, using the toilet, and eating. If a person has any difficulty performing an activity by himself or herself and without special equipment, or did not perform the activity at all because of health problems (physical, mental, or emotional), the person is categorized as having a limitation in that activity. The limitation may be temporary or chronic.

B. Aging in place—Process by which a person chooses to remain in his or her living environment (home) and to remain as independent as possible despite the physical or mental decline.

C. Assisted living—A type of living arrangement in which personal care services such as meals, housekeeping, transportation, and assistance with activities of daily living are available as needed to people who still live on their own in a residential facility. In most cases, the assisted living residents pay a regular monthly rent and an additional fee for the services they receive.

D. Comprehensive outpatient rehabilitation facility (CORF)—A facility that provides coordinated outpatient diagnostic, therapeutic, and restorative services, at a single fixed location, to outpatients for the rehabilitation of injured, disabled, or sick individuals.

E. Continuing care retirement community (CCRC)—A housing community that provides different levels of care based on what each resident needs over time. This is sometimes called *life care* and can range from independent living in an apartment, to assisted living, to full-time care in a nursing home. Residents move from one setting to another based on their needs but continue to live as part of the community. Care in CCRCs is usually expensive. Generally, CCRCs require a large payment before an individual moves in and then a certain monthly fee.

F. Custodial care—The provision of services that can be safely and reasonably given by individuals who are neither skilled nor licensed medical personnel. These may include personal care, such as help with activities of daily living (bathing, dressing, eating, getting in or out of a bed or chair, moving around, and toileting). It may also include care that most people do themselves, like administering eye drops. In most cases, Medicare does not pay for custodial care unless if it is provided in a skilled care setting and under a skilled plan of care.

G. Custodial care facility—A facility that provides room, board, and other personal assistance services, generally on a long-term basis, which does not include a medical component.

H. Elder abuse—The willful infliction of injury, unreasonable confinement, intimidation, or cruel punishment with resulting pain or mental anguish or the willful depreciation by a caretaker of goods or services that is necessary to avoid physical harm, mental anguish, or mental illness.

I. Elder neglect—The failure to provide the goods or services that are necessary to avoid physical harm, mental anguish, or mental illness.

J. Independent living—A service delivery concept that encourages the maintenance of control over one's life based on the choice of acceptable options that minimize reliance on others performing everyday activities.

K. Inpatient rehabilitation facility (IRF)—A freestanding rehabilitation hospital or rehabilitation unit(s) in an acute care hospital that provides intensive rehabilitation programs; patients who are admitted to such facilities must be able to tolerate 3 hours of intense rehabilitation services per day.

L. Instrumental activities of daily living (IADLs)—Activities related to independent living, including preparing meals, managing money, shopping for groceries or personal items, performing light or heavy housework, and using a telephone. If a person has any difficulty performing an activity by himself or herself and without special equipment, or does not perform the activity at all because of health problems, the person is categorized as having a limitation in that activity. The limitation may be temporary or chronic.

M. Limitation of activity—Refers to a long-term reduction in a person's capacity to perform the usual kind or amount of activities associated with his or her age group due to a chronic condition. This may include a limitation in activities of daily living, instrumental activities of daily living, play, school, work, difficulty in walking or remembering, or any other.

N. Long-term care—A variety of services that help people with health or personal needs and activities of daily living over a period of time. Long-term care can be provided at home, in the community, or in various types of facilities, including nursing homes and assisted living facilities. Most long-term care is custodial care, which few (if any) insurance companies will pay for if skilled care is also not required, with the exception of long-term care insurance.

O. Long-term care insurance—A private insurance policy to help pay for some long-term medical and nonmedical care. Some long-term care insurance policies offer tax benefits; these are called *tax-qualified policies.*

P. Multidimensional assessment or comprehensive geriatric assessment (CGA)—A comprehensive assessment that includes evaluation of an elderly patient in several domains: physical, mental, socioeconomic, functional, and environmental status.

Q. Noncovered services—These services are not considered skilled and do not meet the requirements of a Medicare benefit category, are statutorily excluded from coverage on grounds other than 1862(a)(1), or are not considered reasonable and necessary under 1862(a)(1).

R. Nursing home—A residence that provides individuals with a room and meals and assists with activities of daily living and recreation. Generally, nursing home residents have physical or mental problems that keep them from living on their own. They usually require daily assistance.

S. Occupational therapy (OT)—Structured activity focused on activities of daily living skills (feeding, dressing, bathing, grooming), arm flexibility and strengthening, neck control and posture, perceptual and cognitive skills, and using adaptive equipment to facilitate activities of daily living.

T. Outpatient care—Medical, behavioral, or surgical care that is provided in a clinic/ambulatory setting and does not include an overnight hospital stay.

U. Personal care services—Nonskilled assistance (e.g., bathing, dressing, light housework) provided to individuals in their homes.

V. Physical therapy (PT)—Structured activity focused on mobility skills (bed and chair transfers, wheelchair use, walking), leg flexibility and strengthening, trunk or gait control and balance, endurance training, and use of adaptive equipment to facilitate mobility and physical functioning.

W. Predictor of repeat admissions (PRA)—A valid and reliable tool for identifying high-risk seniors (age 65 years or greater) who have a statistically higher probability of repeat hospital admission; developed by Chad Boult and associates from the University of Minnesota.

X. Reasonable and necessary care—Health care or services that are required by Medicare recipients and that is considered important for their medical condition. The Medicare program generally covers only items or services that are "reasonable and necessary" for the diagnosis or treatment of illness or injury or "to improve the functioning of a malformed body member." This "reasonable and necessary" language is the basis for most Medicare coverage policies, but its meaning remains ill defined and controversial.

Y. Rehabilitation—A restorative process through which an individual with a complex, chronic, or terminal illness develops and maintains self-sufficient functioning consistent with his/her capability. Usually provided by licensed health care professionals such as nurses and physical, occupational, and speech therapists.

Z. Respite care—Temporary or periodic care provided in a nursing home, assisted living residence, or other type of long-term care program so that the usual caregiver can rest or take some time off.

AA. Restorative nursing services (NRS)—Replication of activities initiated by a physical therapist (PT), occupational therapist (OT), or a speech–language pathologist (SLP) and then performed and maintained by the nursing staff. These may include services such as range-of-motion exercises, dressing, personal hygiene, walking, and feeding.

BB. Skilled care—The provision of services that can be given only by or under the supervision of skilled and licensed medical personnel/health care professionals, that is, skilled and competent staff such as registered nurses; social workers; physical, occupational, and speech therapists; rehabilitation counselors; and registered dietitians/nutritionists. These staff are required to manage, observe, and evaluate the skilled care activities.

CC. Skilled nursing care—A level of care that includes services that can only be performed safely and correctly by a licensed nurse (either a registered nurse or a licensed practical nurse).

DD. Skilled nursing facility (SNF)—A facility (which meets specific regulatory certification requirements) that primarily provides inpatient skilled nursing care and related services to patients who require medical, nursing, or rehabilitative services but does not provide the level of care or treatment available in a hospital. Sometimes referred to as nursing facility.

EE. Skilled nursing facility care—A level of care that requires the daily involvement of skilled nursing or rehabilitation staff. Examples of skilled nursing facility care include intravenous injections, wound care, and physical therapy. The need for custodial care (e.g., assistance with activities of daily living, like bathing and dressing) cannot, in itself, qualify for Medicare coverage in a skilled nursing facility.

FF. SNF coinsurance—For day 21 through 100 of extended care services in a benefit period, a daily amount for which the beneficiary is responsible, equal to one eighth of the inpatient hospital deductible.

GG. Speech and language pathology (SLP)—Structured activity focused on communication skills, perceptual and cognitive skills, and swallowing.

HH. Federal Qualified Health Center (FQHC)—Are outpatient clinics that qualify for specific reimbursement systems under Medicare and Medicaid. Original FQHCs from the early 1990s were grant-funded programs under Section 330 of the Public Health Services Act. They functioned as "safety net" providers such as community health centers, public housing centers, outpatient health programs funded by the Indian Health Service, and programs serving migrants and the homeless. The main purpose of the FQHC Program is to enhance the provision of primary care services in underserved urban and rural communities. FQHCs expanded as a result of the Patient Protection and Affordable Care Act of 2010 to also function as patient-centered medical homes.

II. FQHC Look-Alike (FQHC LA)—Are health centers that have been certified by the federal government as meeting all the Health Center Program requirements, but do not receive funding under the Health Center Program or Section 330 of the Public Health Services Act.

JJ. Community Health Center (CHC)—A general term not defined in Section 330 of the Public Health Services Act that is used to describe community-based clinics, ambulatory care provider practices, or care centers.

 ## Applicability to CMSA's Standards of Practice

A. The Case Management Society of America (CMSA) describes in its standards of practice for case management that case management extends across all health care settings (CMSA, 2010). This includes community-based levels of care, long-term care, and rehabilitation, the focus of this chapter. For example:
   1. Provider agencies and community facilities (i.e., mental health facilities, ambulatory and day care facilities)
   2. Geriatric services, including rehabilitation, residential, and assisted living facilities
   3. Long-term care services, including community-based primary care centers
   4. Physician and medical group practices

B. Case managers, according to CMSA, are recognized as expert clinicians and vital participants in the case management and care coordination team. They empower people to understand and access quality, safe, cost-effective, and efficient health care services (CMSA, 2010). These characteristics of the case manager are especially important when dealing with vulnerable patients/clients such as the elderly and older adult at a time of most need such as when suffering multiple complex illnesses or requiring placement in a long-term care facility.

C. Delivering patient-centered care and services is one of the goals CMSA describes in its standards of practice. This is especially synergistic with the demands imposed on the health care delivery system by the Patient

Protection and Affordable Care Act of 2010, which resulted in the proliferation of care settings such as the patient-centered medical home and accountable care organizations, known to improve primary care and advance the roles case managers play today.

D. The various roles and responsibilities case managers assume in the diverse health care settings described by CMSA in its standards for case management (CMSA, 2010) are all important and apply to the roles of case managers in the community and long-term care settings. However, of special importance are the following when case managers care for the elderly and older adult patient who is often vulnerable and at risk of receiving suboptimal care and services.

1. Conducting a comprehensive assessment of the client's health and psychosocial needs and developing a case management plan collaboratively with the client and family or caregiver that focuses on placing the client in the most appropriate level of care

2. Planning with the client, family, or caregiver, the primary care physician/provider, other health care providers, the payer, and the community to assure the achievement of quality, safety, and cost-effective outcomes

3. Facilitating communication and coordination among the various members of the health care team and involving the client in the decision-making process about their care options, especially those needed postdischarge from an acute care facility

4. Educating the client, the family or caregiver, and members of the health care delivery team about available community resources, insurance benefits, case management services, and levels of care available to the elderly and older adults

5. Empowering the client to explore options of care and decide on alternative plans, when necessary, to meet care and personal needs

6. Assisting the client and health care team in the safe transition of client's care to the next most appropriate level or provider

7. Promoting client's self-advocacy and self-determination

8. Advocating for both the client and the payer to facilitate positive outcomes for the client, the health care team, and the payer while keeping the needs of the client as the primary priority

Federally Qualified Health Centers

A. Federally Qualified Health Centers (FQHCs) have existed for more than 25 years. They are community-based health care providers that receive funds from the Health Resources and Services Administration (HRSA) Health Center Program to provide primary care services in underserved and rural areas (USDHHS, 2013).

1. FQHCs must meet a specific set of requirements, which consist of those described in Box 6-3 (USDHHS, 2015).

2. FQHCs have traditionally existed to provide care in the community (i.e., in ambulatory or clinic care settings) to migrants, homeless, residents of public housing or rural areas, and other impoverished or uninsured individuals (USDHHS, 2013).

B. The original defining legislation for Federally Qualified Health Centers is Section 1905(l)(2)(B) of the Social Security Act. FQHCs' benefit under Medicare became effective in October, 1991, when Section 1861(aa) of

6-3   Requirements of FQHCs

- Use of a sliding scale fee schedule based on the client's ability to pay
- Operations under a governing board that includes patients as members
- Being a public and private nonprofit health care organizations that comply with federal requirements
- Serving underserved populations
- Demonstrating sound clinical and financial management
- Employing an ongoing quality assurance and improvement program
- Providing the following health care services:
  - Primary care
  - Preventive health services such as immunizations, visual acuity, and hearing screenings
  - Prenatal and postpartum care
  - Mental and behavioral health
  - Substance abuse counseling
  - Acute or hospital-based care either directly or through contractual arrangements with other providers
  - Diagnostic and therapeutic tests and procedures

the Social Security Act was amended by Section 4161 of the Omnibus Budget Reconciliation Act of 1990 (USDHHS, 2013).

C. In June 2011, the Department of Health and Human Services announced the FQHC Advanced Primary Care Practice (FQHC-APCP) demonstration project as part of the PPACA and under the authority of Section 1115A of the Social Security Act, and upon the establishment of the Center for Medicare and Medicaid Innovation (CMI).

1. This initiative resulted in funding of over 500 FQHCs where more than $40 million was invested as part of the PPACA over 3 years.

2. The demonstration project was designed to evaluate the impact of the advanced primary care practice (APCP) model, also referred to as the patient-centered medical home (PCMH) on improving health, quality of care and lowering the cost of care provided to Medicare beneficiaries.

3. Participating FQHCs agreed to adopt care coordination practices set by the National Committee for Quality Assurance (NCQA) and were expected to achieve level 3 patient-centered medical home recognition.

4. The health center program's annual federal funding has grown from $1.16 billion in fiscal year 2001 to $1.99 billion in fiscal year 2007. The passage of the PPACA in March 2010 resulted in provisions that increased federal funding to FQHCs to help them meet the anticipated health care demand of millions of Americans who will gain health care coverage as result of the health reform law. The PPACA set aside $11 billion for community health centers over a period of 5 years to meet this goal (USDHHS, 2015).

5. Overall, since the passage of the PPACA, health centers have increased the total number of patients served on an annual basis by nearly 5 million people: from 19.5 million in 2010 to an estimate of 24 million in 2014.

D. Reimbursement for care provided by FQHCs changed to the prospective payment system (PPS) method in October 2014, under Medicare Part B. Prior to PPS, Medicare paid FQHCs directly based on an all-inclusive per visit payment.
   1. Based on the statutory requirements of Section 10501 of the Patient Protection and Affordable Care Act of 2010, Medicare pays FQHCs a national encounter-based rate per beneficiary per day, set at 80% of either the PPS rate of $160.60 or the total charges for services furnished on same day of an in person visit for care, whichever is less, effective January 1, 2016 (CMS, 2014).
   2. FQHCs can bill separately for a mental health visit when it occurs on the same day as a medical visit (CMS, 2015a).
   3. The FQHC PPS rate is adjusted for geographic differences in the cost of services (CMS, 2015a).
   4. The PPS visit rate is increased by 34% when an FQHC furnishes care to a patient that is new to the FQHC or to a beneficiary receiving a comprehensive initial Medicare visit or an annual wellness visit (CMS, 2015a).
E. The quality of the care provided in FQHCs equals and often surpasses that provided by other primary care providers or settings.
   1. FQHCs emphasize the provision of coordinated, comprehensive, and integrated primary and preventive services, which also includes behavioral and mental health services. This approach to care employs the "medical home" care approach, which promotes reductions in health disparities for low-income individuals, racial and ethnic minorities, rural communities, and other underserved populations.
   2. Despite serving a population that is often sicker and more at risk than the general population (e.g., patients with multiple chronic illnesses), FQHCs are also able to lower the costs of services and enhance both the patient and provider experience of care.
F. FQHCs play an essential role in the implementation of the PPACA. They use quality improvement practices, health information technology (e.g., electronic health records, digital tools), patient-centered and culturally appropriate care, and case management services to ensure better quality, desirable outcomes, and safer care.
G. FQHCs' model of care overcomes geographic, cultural, linguistic, and other barriers by employing a team-based approach to care. The team consists of physicians, other advanced providers (e.g., nurse practitioners, physician assistants, certified nurse midwives), case managers, clinical nurses, dental providers, social workers, behavioral health care providers, health educators, community health workers, pharmacists, and many others.

Patient-Centered Medical Home

A. The Agency for Healthcare Research and Quality (AHRQ) recognizes that revitalizing the primary care delivery system is foundational to achieving high-quality, accessible, efficient health care for all Americans. It also believes that the primary care medical home is a promising model for transforming the organization and delivery of primary care (AHRQ, 2015).
B. The primary care medical home is also known as the patient-centered medical home (PCMH), advanced primary care, the health care home,

or patient-centered health home. Regardless of the terminology used, it refers to a primary care transformational model that exists in a community-based clinic, physician group, or physician–hospital practice. It provides ambulatory care services with special focus on the provision of holistic care by a primary care clinician (a doctor of medicine or doctor of osteopathy or advanced practice registered nurse or physician assistant).

C. AHRQ defines a medical home not simply as a place but as a model of the organization of primary care that delivers the core functions of primary health care. The medical home encompasses five functions and attributes (Box 6-4).

D. The PCMH is accountable for meeting each patient's physical and mental health care needs, including prevention and wellness, acute care, and chronic care.

    1. A clearly identified provider to assume primary accountability for care and to function as the leader of the health care team involved in the care of the individual patient; usually, the primary care provider is supported by a team of health professionals including case managers.

BOX 6-4 Characteristics of the PCMH

- Comprehensive health care services:
  - Serving patient with complex needs and conditions
  - Integration of mental health and substance use in medical care
  - Coordination of care for patients with complex needs and chronic illnesses using interdisciplinary health care teams
- Patient-centered and holistic care:
  - Focus on health literacy tools
  - Capitalization on patient and family engagement for self-management
  - Health instruction and adherence
- Coordinated care:
  - Case management approach to provision of comprehensive care and services
  - Use of navigators and case managers in care facilitation and promotion of adherence
  - Communication among health care providers, case managers, and patient/family
  - Planning and providing care based on the individual patient's health risk category or class
- Accessibility to health care services and resources:
  - Access to specialty and preventive care
  - Health risk assessment and outreach
  - Prevention of unnecessary acute and emergency care
- Quality and safety:
  - Long-term care planning (year long rather than visit focus)
  - Transitions of care/handoff communication
  - Health condition–related outcomes
  - Lower cost
  - Use of health information technology

From Agency for Healthcare Research and Quality (AHRQ). (2015). *Patient centered medical home (PCMH)*. Rockville, MD: AHRQ. Available at https://pcmh.ahrq.gov/page/tools-resources, retrieved on July 28, 2015.

2. Providing comprehensive care requires an interdisciplinary team of health care providers. The team may include physicians, advanced practice nurses, physician assistants, nurses, pharmacists, nutritionists, social workers, educators, and care coordinators or case managers.

3. PCMHs may not always bring together diverse teams of care providers to meet the needs of their patients. Some, especially smaller practices, may use virtual teams instead and link themselves and their patients to other providers and services in their communities (AHRQ, 2015).

E. The PCMH provides primary health care that is patient centered and relationship based with an orientation toward the whole person.

1. Patient-centered care allows a special focus on patients and their families and promotes the understanding and respect of each patient's unique needs, culture, values, and preferences.

2. The medical home practice actively supports patients in learning to manage and organize their own care at the level the patient chooses. Recognizing that patients and families are core members of the care team, medical home practices ensure that they are fully informed partners in establishing their plans of care and health goals.

3. The approach to care and services focuses on the patient in a holistic manner (patient centered) and assures provision of comprehensive care, including acute care, chronic care, preventive services, and end-of-life care at all stages of life (AHRQ, 2015).

F. The patient-centered medical home coordinates care across all elements of the broader health care system, including specialty care, hospitals, home health care, and community services and supports.

1. Such coordination is particularly critical during transitions between sites of care, such as when patients are being discharged from the hospital.

2. Medical home practices also excel at building clear and open communication among patients and families, the medical home, and members of the broader care team (AHRQ, 2015).

G. The patient-centered medical home delivers accessible services with shorter waiting times for urgent needs, enhanced in-person hours, around-the-clock telephone, or electronic access to a member of the care team.

1. It applies alternative methods of communication such as e-mail and telephone care.

2. It is responsive to patients' needs, interests, and preferences, especially regarding how best to access necessary services.

H. The PCMH demonstrates a commitment to quality and safety including quality improvement.

1. It engages in ongoing quality improvement activities such as using evidence-based guidelines and clinical decision support tools to guide shared decision making with patients and families.

2. It focuses on performance measurement and improvement. In this regard, it measures and responds to patient experiences and patient satisfaction and practices population health management.

3. Sharing robust quality and safety data and improvement activities publicly is also an important marker of a system-level commitment to quality.

BOX

6-5   Focus of Outcomes Used to Measure Impact of the PCMH

Patient experiences:
- Global/overall patient experiences
- Coordination of care (as perceived by patients)
- Patient–provider interaction/communication

Staff experiences:
- Global/overall staff experiences
- Staff retention rates
- Staff burnout

Processes of care:
- Preventive services
- Chronic illness care services

Clinical outcomes:
- Patient's health status
- Physiologic parameters
- Mortality
- Complications
- Medical errors

Economic outcomes:
- Inpatient use
- Emergency department use
- Overall costs
- Unintended consequences or other harms

---

4. Use of health information technology (HIT) and digital tools to enhance delivery of high quality and safe care, electronic communication among providers and with patients/families, clinical decision making, and patient self-management. HIT can also support the collection, storage, aggregation, and management of important data for the purpose of processes improvement and outcomes evaluation (AHRQ, 2015) (Box 6-5).

I. Currently, most PCMHs have moved in the direction of focusing on population health. In this regard, they identify the common chronic illnesses prevalent in their market share and the community they serve, assess and monitor the quality of care measures (e.g., hemoglobin A1C for diabetes) appropriate for each of the chronic illnesses, and implement improvement plans in these measures to ultimately enhance the quality and safety of the patients and the health of the population.

Accountable Care Organizations

A. Accountable Care Organizations (ACOs) are groups of physicians, hospitals, and other health care providers, who come together voluntarily to provide coordinated and high-quality care to Medicare beneficiaries. ACOs resulted from the enactment of the Patient Protection and Affordable Care Act in 2010, under the CMS Center for Innovation (CMS, 2015b).

1. The main purpose of ACOs is to improve beneficiary outcomes and increase value of care by providing better care for individuals, better health for populations, and lowering growth in expenditures.
2. The goal of coordinated care is to ensure that patients, especially the chronically ill, access the right care at the right time while avoiding unnecessary duplication of services, preventing medical errors, and putting patients first.
3. When an ACO succeeds both in delivering high-quality, safe care and lowering health care costs, it shares in the savings it achieves for the Medicare program.
4. Participation in an ACO is voluntary for health care providers (physicians and/or organizations) (CMS, 2015b).

B. Medicare offers three types of ACO programs. They are according to CMS as follows:

1. *Medicare Shared Savings Program*: Helps a Medicare fee-for-service program providers become ACOs. This program facilitates coordination and cooperation among health care providers to improve the quality of care for Medicare fee-for-service (FFS) beneficiaries and reduce unnecessary costs.
   • *Advance Payment ACO Model*: a physician-based and rural providers program who joint efforts voluntarily to provide coordinated high-quality care to the Medicare patients they serve. It offers supplementary incentive for selected participants in the shared savings program; amount is determined based on the number of Medicare beneficiaries served. Financial support may be offered upfront or as monthly payments for participants to use in making important investments in their care coordination infrastructure.
2. *Pioneer ACO Model*: Designed for early adopters of coordinated care. This type has been discontinued and was designed for health care organizations and providers that are already experienced in coordinating care for patients across care settings and provided opportunity for testing the ACO initiative (CMS, 2015b).
3. CMS allocates the Medicare beneficiaries an ACO care for based on a review of the beneficiary's past health resource utilization. The review results in identifying the place (care provider and organization) the patient has received majority of the health services needed and zip code of residence. The most common provider is likely to be assigned responsibility for patient's care as the ACO.

C. Fee-for-service Medicare patients who see providers who are participating in Medicare ACOs maintain all their Medicare rights, including the right to choose any doctors and providers who accept Medicare. Whether a provider chooses to participate in an ACO or not, their patients with Medicare may continue to see them.

D. The Pioneer ACO Model allowed the experienced provider group participants to move more rapidly from a shared savings payment model to a population-based payment model on a track consistent with, but separate from, the Medicare Shared Services Program (CMS, 2015b).

1. This was designed to work in coordination with private payers by aligning provider incentives, which improve quality and health

6-6 **CMS Criteria for Admission to SNF**

- Medically stability.
- Confirmed diagnoses (e.g., patient does not have conditions that require further testing for proper diagnosis).
- Inpatient hospital evaluation or treatment is not required.
- Identified skilled nursing or rehabilitation need that cannot be provided on an outpatient basis or through home health services.

outcomes for patients across the ACO and achieve cost savings for Medicare, employers, and patients.
2. Those who moved to a population-based payment model receive a per-beneficiary per month payment amount that replaces some or all of the ACO's fee-for-service (FFS) payments with a prospective monthly payment.
3. Pioneer ACOs receive a waiver of the 3-day inpatient stay requirement prior to admission to a skilled nursing facility (SNF) or acute care hospital with swing-bed approval for SNF services.
   a. This benefit enhancement allows Medicare beneficiaries to be admitted to qualified Pioneer SNF affiliates either directly or with an inpatient stay of fewer than 3 days.
   b. An aligned beneficiary is eligible for admission in accordance with this waiver if the beneficiary does not reside in a nursing home or SNF for long-term custodial care at the time of the decision to admit to an SNF; and the beneficiary meets all other CMS criteria for SNF admission (Box 6-6) (CMS, 2015b).
E. CMS is moving to a *Next Generation ACO Model*, which applies refined benchmarking methods that reward the attainment and improvement in cost containment. In this model, it transitions away from comparisons to an ACO's historical expenditures.
   1. The model offers a selection of payment mechanisms to enable a shift from fee-for-service (FFS) reimbursements to capitation.
   2. The model includes several "benefit enhancement" tools to help ACOs improve their engagement with beneficiaries (Box 6-7) (CMS, 2015b).

6-7 **Enhancements in ACO Model to Improve Patient Engagement**

- Greater access to home care visits, telehealth services, and skilled nursing facility services
- Opportunities for beneficiaries to receive a reward payment for receiving care from the ACO and certain affiliated providers
- A process that allows beneficiaries to confirm their care relationship with ACO providers
- Greater collaboration between CMS and ACOs to improve communication with beneficiaries about the characteristics and potential benefits of ACOs in relation to patient care

Roles of Case Managers in FQHCs, PCMHs, and ACOs

A. Case managers are integral members of the health care teams responsible for provision of care in FQHCs, PCMHs, and ACOs. The role of the case manager is similar in these care settings (Box 6-8).
B. Case managers assume the role of care coordination and management for a caseload of patients cared for in the FQHC, PCMH, or ACO. They complete a comprehensive assessment of each individual they care for to identify their health and social support needs. They periodically reassess the patient and update available information, including when new medical problems or other changes in health or functional status arise. The assessment may include the following:
   1. Standard medical, surgical, family, and medication history
   2. Physical function
   3. Family and other social support systems
   4. Care needs, goals, and preferences of both the patient and the caregivers that can be used to formulate the individualized care plan
   5. Health care professionals involved
   6. Financial situation and health insurance benefits.
C. Assessment of patient for health risk stratification using predictive modeling methods and techniques is common in the FQHCs, PCMHs, and ACOs. Case managers play an essential role in the assessment and classification or stratification of patients into a risk category: low, moderate, high, or very high.
   1. The stratification is completed based on a number of important factors including but not limited to age, gender, past use of health

BOX 6-8   Sample Responsibilities of Case Managers in FQHCs, PCMHs, and ACOs

- Assessment of patient needs and establishing care goals and plans of care
- Determining the patient's health risk assessment category or class (low, moderate, high, very high)
- Coordination of care and services
- Facilitation of patient's timely access to services including hospitalization when necessary
- Engaging patients/families in decision making about care options
- Health education and self-care management
- Remotely monitoring patients' conditions and adherence to care regimen
- Following up on tests, procedures, and consults with specialty providers
- Facilitating interdisciplinary care rounds for long-term care planning
- Coordinating safe transition of care activities
- Assuring patients show up to follow-up appointments and they bring all the necessary information with them
- Communication and information sharing with patient/family and health care team members
- Aligning resources with patient and population needs
- Responding to changes in patient's condition
- Evaluating the quality, cost, and safety outcomes of care

care services, socioeconomic status, availability of social support system, and use of medications.

2. Case managers stratify patients into risk categories; however, if a risk assessment and category already exist, confirming or updating the category becomes the focus.

3. Case managers plan care and comprehensive case management services for their patients based on the risk category identified.

4. Use of a very high-risk class has recently become more common to allow special focus on prevention of the use of avoidable health care services such as emergency visits and acute care hospital admissions. This risk class reflects the 1% to 2% of patients in the highest-risk class but presents the most quality, safety, and financial risk to the provider.

D. Case managers may be allocated to specific primary care provider teams or based on patient populations; regardless however, the role does not vary.

E. Case managers make themselves available as a resource in these settings to patients, families, and other health care providers.

Long-Term Care

A. Long-term care is necessary when individuals require someone else to help them with their physical and/or emotional needs. This help may be required for many of the activities or needs healthy and active people take for granted.

B. Long-term care and assistance may be necessary as a result of a chronic or terminal condition, disability, illness, injury, or merely old age.

C. The need for long-term care may last for a few weeks, months, or years. The length of time needed depends on the underlying reasons and medical/health condition.

D. Long-term care may take the form of temporary or ongoing care (Box 6-9).

1. Temporary long-term care—Need for care for a limited period of time, usually for only a few weeks or months

2. Ongoing long-term care—Need for care for an extended period of time, usually many months or years

BOX 6-9 Long-Term Care Conditions

Temporary Condition
• Rehabilitation from a hospital stay
• Recovery from illness
• Recovery from injury
• Recovery from surgery
• Terminal medical condition

Ongoing Conditions
• Chronic medical illness
• Chronic severe pain
• Permanent disability
• Dementia
• Ongoing need for help with ADLs
• Need for supervision
• Behavioral, emotional, or mental health concern

   E. Long-term services are provided in varied care settings such as:
  1. Home (either the patient's or that of a family member)
  2. Adult day care center
  3. Assisted living facility
  4. Board-and-care home
  5. Hospice facility
  6. Nursing home
   F. Case management in the home care setting is discussed in Chapter 7 and case management in the palliative care and hospice settings is discussed in Chapter 8. Other settings are discussed in this chapter.
   G. Health care services provided in the long-term care settings are of two types: custodial and skilled (Box 6-10).

BOX
6-10   Custodial and Skilled Care

Custodial care and services may include any or all of the following activities:
- Walking
- Bathing, personal hygiene, and grooming
- Dressing
- Feeding and providing meals
- Toileting and helping with incontinence
- Managing pain
- Preventing unsafe behavior such as wandering around aimlessly
- Providing comfort and assurance
- Providing physical or occupational therapy
- Attending to medical needs
- Counseling
- Answering the phone
- Meeting doctors' appointments
- Maintaining the household
- Shopping and running errands
- Providing transportation
- Administering medications
- Managing money
- Paying bills
- Doing the laundry
- Writing letters or notes
- Maintaining a yard
- Removing snow

Skilled care and services may include any or all of the following activities:
- Monitoring vital signs
- Ordering medical tests
- Diagnosing problems
- Administering intravenous medications
- Administering intravenous fluids/nutritional support
- Dispensing medications, including injections
- Drawing blood
- Wound care and dressing changes
- Psychosocial counseling and therapy
- Physical therapy and exercise
- Occupational therapy
- Speech therapy

1. *Custodial services*—The provision of services that can be safely and reasonably given by individuals who are neither skilled nor licensed medical personnel.
   a. Services may include personal care such as help with ADLs (bathing, dressing, eating, getting in or out of a bed or chair, moving around, and toileting). It may also include care that most people do themselves, like administering eye drops.
   b. In most cases, Medicare does not pay for custodial care, unless it is provided in combination with skilled services and as part of a skilled plan of care.
2. *Skilled services*—The provision of services that can be given only by or under the supervision of skilled and licensed medical personnel/health care professionals.
   a. Services provided by knowledgeable and competent staff such as registered nurses; social workers; physical, occupational, and speech therapists; rehabilitation counselors; and registered dietitians/nutritionists.
   b. Members of the professional staff are required to manage, observe, supervise, and evaluate the skilled care activities.
H. The individual who requires custodial services is someone who:
   1. Can no longer perform daily tasks necessary to maintain health and safety
   2. Cannot safely perform ADLs or preserve health from further decline
   3. By choice or circumstance has decided to reside in the nursing home as primary residence
   4. Receives nonskilled physical therapy services (restorative nursing by nursing assistants) to maintain function.
I. The individual who requires skilled services is someone who:
   1. May have exhausted Medicare Part A benefit period or is not eligible for benefits
   2. Can no longer care for himself or herself
   3. Requires assistance in ADLs, IADLs, taking medication, or skilled treatments.
J. Skilled and custodial services do not refer to a specific type of long-term care services; rather, they are referred based on the people who deliver/provide the care—not the actual care given. The main differentiating factor between these two terms is the employment of (1) skilled versus nonskilled and (2) licensed versus unlicensed providers.
K. Generally, skilled care is available only for a short period of time after a hospitalization. Custodial care is for a much longer period of time. Sometimes, both levels of care are provided in the same facility (e.g., nursing home), and the patients (usually called *residents*) may transfer between levels of care within the facility without having to move from one room or unit into another.
L. A skilled and licensed care provider can provide custodial services; however, a nonskilled and unlicensed provider cannot provide skilled services. In rare situations, skilled services such as blood pressure monitoring, administering medications, or changing wound dressings may be given by a custodial care provider.

M. A long-term care treatment plan usually includes skilled and custodial services (care activities), goals, and expected outcomes. It addresses the following:
   1. Applied therapies
   2. Frequency of the therapies consistent with goals and expected outcomes
   3. Potential for patient's restoration and prognosis
   4. Time frame in which the physician/provider prescribing the treatment will review the plan and evaluate medical necessity and progress
   5. Maintenance, palliative relief, or measures to be implemented to prevent deterioration in the patient's status.
N. Medicare pays for skilled care. Custodial care is covered under Medicare if it is provided in a skilled care setting and under a skilled plan of care.
O. Medicare and other health insurance plans pay for the care of patients with certain acute medical needs where recovery is anticipated. Patients with chronic medical problems are usually covered under Medicaid.

Rehabilitation Levels of Care

A. Rehabilitation is the restoration of the handicapped individuals to the fullest physical, mental, social, vocational, and economic usefulness of which they are capable.
B. Rehabilitation is the process of providing, in a coordinated manner, those comprehensive services deemed appropriate to the needs of a person with a disability or complex medical illness, in a program designed to achieve objectives of improved health, welfare, and the realization of the person's maximal physical, social, psychological, functional, and vocational potential for useful and productive activity (Table 6-1).
C. Rehabilitation services are provided in many different settings, including the following:
   1. Acute care and rehabilitation hospitals
   2. Subacute facilities
   3. Intermediate rehabilitation facilities (IRFs)
   4. Long-term care facilities
   5. Comprehensive outpatient rehabilitation facilities (CORFs)
   6. Day rehabilitation services (DRSs)
   7. Home rehabilitation through home health agencies.
D. Regardless of setting, rehabilitation services are provided through an interdisciplinary rehabilitation team that revolves around the patient and family. The team helps set short- and long-term treatment goals for recovery and is made up of many skilled professionals (Box 6-11).
E. There are two fundamental requirements (criteria) for insurance coverage that must be met for inpatient hospital stays for rehabilitation care. The care/services must be:
   1. Reasonable and necessary (in terms of efficacy, duration, frequency, and amount) for the treatment of the patient's condition

(*text continues on page 148*)

TABLE 6-1 Summary of Rehabilitation Options and Criteria

Type of Rehab Services	Hours/Day Services Needed	Days/Week Services Needed	Approval Criteria	Funding Services	Target Turnaround Time
Acute care rehab	0.5–1.5	5–7	New or exacerbated disability	Billed as part of acute hospital stay	12 h
Outpatient rehab	0.5–2	3	Acute disability	Precertification	24 h
			At home, but can be transported	Medicare Part B cap $1,500/y	
			Ability to progress	Charges $75–$100/h	
Day rehab	3	5	Acute disability that does not prevent return home	Precertification except for Medicare	12 h
			Medically stable	Charges $400–$600/d	
			Participate in therapy 1 h 2× day		
			Ability to progress		
			Home support available		
Home health rehab	0.5–1	3	Homebound	Precertification	48 h
			Acute disability	Cap on total visits	
			Medically stable	Charges $75–$150/h	
			Ability to progress		
Inpatient rehab	3	5–7	Acute disability prevents return to home.	Precertification	24 h
			Medically stable	Coverage varies	
			Participate in therapy 1 h 2× day	Charges $50–$1,500/d	
			Ability to progress		
			Home support available		
Skilled nursing facility (SNF)	0.5–2	5–7	Acute disability	Precertification	48 h
			Medically stable	Coverage varies	
			Participate in therapy 1 h 2× day	Charges $120–$750/d	

Source: www.rrc.pmr.vcu.edu/misc/guide_to.htm (Virginia Commonwealth University, The Rehabilitation & Research Center).

BOX 6-11 Members of Rehabilitation Health Care Team

- Physicians such as a physiatrist—A physician who specializes in physical medicine and rehabilitation
- An internist or a specialist physician depending on the medical condition of the patient (e.g., a neurologist, in the case of a stroke patient)
- Rehabilitation nurses
- Physical therapists
- Occupational therapists
- Speech and language pathologists/therapists
- Dietitians
- Social workers
- Chaplains or clergy
- Psychologists, neuropsychologists, and psychiatrists
- Case managers
- Health educators

  2. Reasonable and necessary to furnish the care on an inpatient hospital basis, rather than in a less intensive facility such as an SNF or on an outpatient basis (Carr, 2005).

F. Determinations of whether inpatient rehabilitation hospital stays are reasonable and necessary are made through a preadmission screening process. These determinations are based on an assessment of each beneficiary's individual care needs. The screening involves a preliminary review of the patient's condition, medical record(s), and health history to determine if the patient is likely to benefit significantly from an intensive inpatient rehabilitation program.

G. For Medicare to pay for intensive inpatient rehabilitation center, a physician must certify that the patient needs the following:
  1. Intensive physical or occupational rehabilitation (at least 3 hours per day, 5 days per week)
  2. At least one additional type of therapy, such as speech therapy, occupational therapy, or prosthetics/orthotics
  3. Full-time access to a doctor with training in rehabilitation, including at least three visits per week
  4. Full-time access to a skilled rehabilitation nurse.

H. Rehabilitation may occur in specialized centers that:
  1. Are dedicated to the provision of such services
  2. Are staffed by the full gamut of rehabilitation professionals
  3. Include 24-hour physician coverage
  4. Develop an individualized program of intense rehabilitation that usually involves a minimum of 3 hours of therapy per day
  5. Include a team of professionals that meets at least once a week to evaluate the patient's progress and to amend the care plan.

I. The main goal of rehabilitation:
  1. A reduction in or reversal of impairment, disability, or handicap caused by disease, enabling individuals (patients) to achieve their fullest possible physical, mental, and social capability.

2. The range of goals varies according to the individual. Different goals and prognoses place patients into different levels of rehabilitation:
   a. Full activity after a severe illness
   b. Maximum achievable activity after a damaging illness
   c. As much independence as possible when continuing impairment is unavoidable.

J. The process of rehabilitation includes full patient and family assessment, goal setting, action planning and implementation, and evaluation/feedback.

K. Rehabilitation care and services are designed to meet each person's specific needs; thus, each program is different. Some general treatment components for rehabilitation programs include the following:
   1. Treating the basic disease and preventing complications
   2. Treating the disability and improving function
   3. Providing adaptive tools and altering the environment
   4. Teaching the patient and family and helping them adapt to lifestyle changes as caused by the disease and limitation in functioning.

L. The success of rehabilitation treatments depend on many variables, including the following:
   1. The cause, location, and severity of physical functioning
   2. The type and degree of any impairments and disabilities from the medical condition
   3. The overall health of the patient
   4. Family and community support
   5. The multidisciplinary health care team.

M. Rehabilitation services in a hospital/acute care setting (i.e., inpatient rehabilitation) are
   1. Considered to be reasonable and necessary for a patient who requires a more coordinated, intensive program of multiple services than is generally found outside of a hospital
   2. Appropriate for patients who have either one or more conditions requiring intensive and interdisciplinary rehabilitation services, or a medical complication/comorbidity in addition to their primary condition, so that the continuing availability of a physician is required to ensure safe and effective treatment
   3. Necessary if an individual requires and is able to tolerate an intensive level of rehabilitation; that is, at least 3 hours per day, 5 to 7 days per week, and of at least two different types of therapy and interdisciplinary services.

N. Rehabilitation programs offer a variety of services such as those shared in Box 6-12.

O. Any acutely hospitalized individual who has a new disability (or an exacerbation of an existing one) is often an appropriate candidate for acute rehabilitation services.

P. Individuals who meet the following criteria are appropriate for inpatient rehabilitation:
   1. Have an acute disability that prevents them from returning home with family care
   2. Have medical or surgical conditions that are sufficiently stable to allow participation in therapies

BOX 6-12 Rehabilitation Services

- Self-care skills—ADLs such as feeding, grooming, bathing, dressing, and toileting
- Mobility skills—Walking, transferring from bed to chair and vice versa, and self-propelling a wheelchair
- Communication skills—Speech, writing, and alternative methods of communication
- Cognitive skills—Memory, concentration, judgment, problem solving, and organizational skills
- Socialization skills—Interacting with others at home and within the community
- Vocational training—Work-related skills
- Pain management—Medicines and alternative methods of managing pain
- Psychological testing—Identifying problems and solutions with thinking, behavioral, and emotional issues
- Family support—Assistance with adapting to lifestyle changes, physical limitations, financial concerns, and discharge planning
- Education—Patient and family education and training about coping with illness (e.g., coping with stroke, amputation), medical care, and adaptive techniques

3. Have the ability to participate in at least 3 hour of therapy per day
4. Are able to make progress in acute care therapies
5. Have a social support system that will allow them to return home after reasonable improvement of function
6. Receive financial clearance from their insurer.

Q. Most health insurance plans will pay for acute care therapy-based rehabilitation.

R. The Centers for Medicare and Medicaid Services (CMS) has identified the specific evidence-based criteria to be used when evaluating potential candidates for placement in the inpatient rehabilitation setting (Table 6-2) (Carr, 2005).

TABLE 6-2 Rehabilitation Hospital Screening Criteria

Criteria	Explanation
1. Close medical supervision by a physician with specialized training or experience in rehabilitation	• A patient's condition must require the 24-h availability of a physician with special training or experience in the field of rehabilitation. The medical record should reflect frequent, direct, and medically necessary physician involvement in the patient's care, that is, at least every day for moderately stable patients to every 2 to 3 d for stable patients throughout the patient's stay.
2. Twenty-four-hour rehabilitation nursing	• The patient requires the 24-h availability of a registered nurse with specialized training or experience in rehabilitation. This degree of availability represents a higher level of care than is normally found in a skilled nursing facility (SNF) patient.

TABLE 6-2 Rehabilitation Hospital Screening Criteria, *continued*

Criteria	Explanation
3. Relatively intense level of rehabilitation services	• The general threshold of establishing the need for inpatient rehabilitation facility (IRF) services is that the patient must require and receive at least 3 h a day of physical and/or occupational therapy. In some cases, the 3 h a day requirement can be met by a combination of therapeutic services instead of, or in addition to, physical therapy and/or occupational therapy. Furnishing services no <5 d a week satisfies the requirement for "daily" services.
4. Multidisciplinary team approach to delivery of program	• A multidisciplinary team usually includes a physician, a rehabilitation nurse, a social worker, and/or a psychologist and those therapists involved in the patient's care, that is, speech–language pathologist and recreation therapist.

5. Coordinated program of care	• The patient's records must reflect evidence of a coordinated program, that is, documentation that periodic team conferences are held at least every 2 wk to:
	  ○ Assess the individual's progress or the problems impeding progress.
	  ○ Consider possible resolutions to such problems.
	  ○ Reassess the validity of the rehabilitation goals initially established.
	A team conference may be formal or informal. The decisions made during such conferences and any changes to the care plan and/or treatment goals and/or discharge planning must be recorded in the clinical record.

6. Significant practical improvement	• Hospitalization is covered only in those cases where a significant practical improvement can be expected in a reasonable period of time. • The expectation of improvement must be of practical value to the patient, measured against the patient's condition at the start of the rehabilitation program.
7. Realistic goals	• The most realistic rehabilitation goal for most beneficiaries is self-care or independence in the activities of daily living or sufficient improvement to allow the individual to live at home with assistance, rather than in an institution. The aim of treatment is to achieve the maximum level of function possible.

Reprinted from Carr, D. D. (2005). The case manager's role in optimizing acute rehabilitation services. *Lippincott's Case Management, 10*(4), 190–200, with permission.

Rehabilitation Services in Non–Inpatient Care Settings

A. Intermediate rehabilitation facilities (IRFs)
   1. IRFs are freestanding rehabilitation hospitals or rehabilitation unit(s) within acute care hospitals.
   2. IRFs provide an intensive rehabilitation program. Patients who are admitted to these facilities must be able to tolerate 3 hours of intense rehabilitation services per day, 5 to 7 days per week.
   3. IRFs are exempt from the Medicare Hospital PPS and are paid under the IRF PPS that went into effect in 2002. However, CMS collects patient assessment data only on Medicare Part A fee-for-service patients who are cared for in these facilities.
   4. In order to be paid under the IRF PPS structure, such facilities must submit specific data based on the IRF patient assessment instrument (PAI).
B. Comprehensive outpatient rehabilitation facilities (CORFs)
   1. CORFs are highly specialized outpatient facilities that provide services to individuals who require complex rehabilitative services.
   2. CORFs provide coordinated outpatient diagnostic, therapeutic, and restorative services, at a single fixed location. These services are geared toward rehabilitation of injured, disabled, or sick individuals.
   3. CORFs are designed to deliver physical therapy, occupational therapy, and speech–language pathology services. Other services available in these facilities may include the following:
      a. Prosthetic and orthotic devices, including testing, fitting, or proper training in the use of such devices
      b. Supplies, appliances, and equipment, including the purchase or rental of durable medical equipment (DME)
   4. CORFs tend to care for the mobile, more active patient.
   5. Individuals who meet the following criteria are appropriate for outpatient rehabilitation in a CORF facility:
      a. Having an acute disability or physical complaint (e.g., back pain)
      b. Having a medical or surgical condition that allows the individual to return home and be transported to and from therapy
      c. Ability to participate in therapy and to demonstrate progress toward agreed-upon goals
      d. Acceptance of fiscal responsibility by the insurer and/or patient.
   6. Individuals who are not homebound must receive this type of therapy after hospital discharge.
   7. Most insurers provide for outpatient therapy services; however, precertification is usually required and there are specific limits on the duration of services.
   8. Medicare Part B has a $1,500 per year cap on outpatient PT/OT services. Charges are typically $75 per hour to $150 per hour.
C. Day rehabilitation services (DRSs)
   1. Patients must be able to participate in at least a 3-hour rehabilitation program per day, 5 days per week, and use at least two different types of therapy.
   2. Interdisciplinary services are performed in a discrete location, often adjacent to an inpatient rehabilitation unit.

3. Transportation to and from the services is provided.
4. Some advantages of DRSs:
    a. Patients spend from 3 to 5 days per week in a facility that provides skilled nursing care and rehabilitation services.
    b. Patients may continue to live at home.
D. Skilled nursing facilities—Short-term subacute services
    1. Subacute rehabilitation care is comprehensive and cost-effective for patients who have been hospitalized for treatment of an injury or illness. This type of care is not limited to the elderly patient.
    2. The candidate for subacute care no longer requires the intensive procedures of an acute care hospital, but does require the diagnostic or invasive procedures of an inpatient health care facility.
    3. The patient's care still requires active physician direction, professional nursing care, significant ancillary services, an outcomes-focused interdisciplinary approach to care, and complex medical and/or rehabilitative care.
    4. Subacute rehabilitation care assists patients in regaining lost or diminished abilities and restoring independence and confidence by focusing on realistic, attainable goals.
    5. Subacute care usually requires that the patient is hospitalized for a short period of time and focuses on continuing the treatment plan initiated in the hospital/acute care setting while providing needed rehabilitation support to facilitate the patient's return to his or her prior living arrangement.
    6. Subacute care facilities or units provide rehabilitative care through an interdisciplinary team of professionals similar to inpatient and intensive rehabilitation services (Box 6-13).
    7. Subacute care facilities provide 4 or more hours of daily direct nursing care, plus 24-hour nursing supervision. Direct skilled nursing assessment is completed once per day.
    8. Care is led by a physician—internist, family practitioner, geriatric specialist, or physiatrist (a specialist in physical and rehabilitation medicine). Physicians are also available on call at all times to respond to emergency situations.
    9. Subacute care facilities see patients who have a variety of diagnoses requiring rehabilitation. Some of these are as follows:
        a. Orthopedic conditions such as hip and knee replacements, amputations, and multiple traumas

BOX
6-13   **Members of Subacute Rehabilitation Health Care Teams**

- Registered nurses
- Physical therapists
- Occupational therapists
- Speech pathologists
- Case managers
- Physicians
- Social workers
- Support staff such as physical therapy assistant and certified nurse's aide

   b. Neurological conditions, such as stroke, Parkinson disease and Guillain-Barré, brain injury, and spinal cord injury
   c. Other conditions such as postcardiac surgery, post–major abdominal surgery, infections requiring extended intravenous antibiotic treatment
   d. Complicated wounds and pressure ulcer/skin breakdown
10. Rehabilitation services in subacute care facilities focus on restoring function. Eligible patients are those who:
   a. Require skilled nursing services on a daily basis.
   b. Have a potential for improvement or ability to return to prior level of functioning in a reasonable amount of time.
   c. Have an acute disability.
   d. Have medical or surgical conditions that may not be sufficiently stable to allow full participation in therapies, but do not require acute inpatient hospitalization.
   e. Demonstrate the ability to participate in at least 1 hour of therapy per day.
11. Subacute care is not intended for chronic illnesses or disabilities. It is paid for by Medicare, following a qualifying hospitalization.
12. Subacute rehabilitation may take place in an SNF or a freestanding rehabilitation facility.
13. Subacute rehabilitation services can be divided into three broad categories (Box 6-14).

BOX 6-14   Subacute Rehabilitation Services

Short term/rehabilitative:
- Patients with significant medical and nursing needs and who are too ill to tolerate rigorous rehabilitation therapy in an acute care rehabilitation facility.
- Require 4.5 to 5.5 daily direct nursing care hours.
- High use of PT, OT, and SPT.
- Common medical problems include orthopedics (amputation, total hip or knee replacements) and neurology (stroke, brain or spinal injury).
- Length of stay/treatment ranges between 7 and 21 days.

Short-term complex medical:
- Patients who are postsurgical or medically stable but require intense medical and nursing management.
- Require 4.5 to 8.0 daily direct nursing care hours.
- High use of respiratory, laboratory, pharmacy, and medical supplies.
- Common medical problems include cardiology, oncology, pulmonary, renal disease, postsurgical, complex wounds, intravenous therapy, parenteral nutrition, and dialysis.
- Length of stay/treatment ranges between 7 and 21 days.

Long term/chronic:
- Patients who have experienced extended acute care stays and are medically stable but still have relatively high need for nursing and/or ancillary services.
- Require 4.5 to 8.0 daily direct nursing care hours.
- Common medical problems include head injury, coma, multiple trauma, and ventilator dependence.
- Length of stay/treatment is 25 days or longer.

14. Most insurers have subacute rehabilitation benefits, including non–managed care Medicaid.
    a. No limit on length of stay as long as progress occurs every 2 to 3 weeks.
    b. Non–managed care Medicare Part A (100 days coverage for each new disability as long as progress occurs every 2 to 3 weeks) and most private insurers.
    c. Subacute rehabilitation in an acute rehabilitation unit or acute hospital is only occasionally covered by insurers.
    d. Medicaid reimbursement for SNF-level care specifically directed at rehabilitation as opposed to medical needs is poor. Charges range from $120 to $400 per day (non–hospital-based SNF) to $450 to 750 per day (hospital or rehabilitation unit-based services).

E. Long-term acute care in specialty acute care hospitals
    1. Long-term acute care hospitals are facilities specializing in the treatment and rehabilitation of medically complicated, chronically ill, and critically ill patients.
    2. Areas of specialization may include pulmonary, ventilator dependency and weaning, cardiac, trauma, wound, and neurology.
    3. Average length of stay is 25 days or longer.
    4. Usually, the patient cannot tolerate more than 3 hours of therapy per day.
    5. Typically, patients are admitted to these facilities after illness such as stroke or severe infections.
    6. Care is directed by internal medicine and may include the following:
        a. Ventilator management, intravenous therapy, or other high-technology treatment available
        b. Daily physician assessments
        c. Complicated wound care
        d. Management of multisystem organ failure.
    7. Care provided in these facilities is usually covered by Medicare.

F. Long-term care—Skilled nursing facilities
    1. SNFs are considered cost-effective ways to enable patients with injuries, acute illnesses, or postoperative care needs to recover in an environment outside the acute care hospital setting.
    2. Individuals who require placement in SNFs are covered under Medicare Part A.
    3. Medicare coverage is only up to 100 days of skilled care during a benefit period and only if strict skilled criteria are met.
    4. SNFs are not intended for the care of patients with chronic illness or disabilities.
    5. All skilled services needed by patients must be "reasonable and necessary." Refer to the long-term care section above for more details.
        a. The individual must have potential for improvement or ability to return to prior level of function in a reasonable amount of time.
        b. Skilled service does not mean that the individual cannot care for himself or herself.
        c. Not intended to provide maintenance therapies to maintain function (e.g., restorative nursing).

G. Long-term care—Nursing homes
   1. Nursing homes primarily exist to serve a small portion of the elderly population—those with severe medical and/or disability problems that require 24-hour care.
   2. This population cannot stay in the home for many reasons, including the following:
      a. Financial resources are limited.
      b. Caregivers are unavailable.
      c. Personal choice.
      d. The intensity of the required home services is no longer possible.
      e. The elderly is no longer safe in a home environment.
      f. The elderly may require skilled care but has exhausted Medicare Part A benefits or is not eligible for Medicare Part A benefits.
   3. Long-term care in the nursing home setting may provide rehabilitation services (restorative nursing) to maintain function in the geriatric patient:
      a. Walking the patient on a daily basis
      b. Passive range-of-motion exercises
      c. Help with feeding activities.
   4. Functional characteristics may contribute to the decision to place a patient in a nursing home for long-term care. Examples may include:
      a. Difficulty with toileting and incontinence
      b. Memory or orientation problems
      c. Behavior problems
      d. Sensory and communication problems
      e. Speech therapy; does not include restorative speech programs.

Nonmedical Levels of Care

A. Assisted living facilities (ALFs)
   1. A type of living arrangement in which personal care services are provided as needed. These may include, but are not limited to, those listed in Box 6-15.
   2. ALFs are also called *residential care facilities* and tend to fill a gap between home care and nursing homes.

BOX
6-15   Services offered in Assisted Living Facilities

- Meals
- Housekeeping services
- Transportation services
- Assistance with activities of daily living
- 24-hour security and staff availability
- Emergency call systems
- Health care services such as visiting nurse
- Wellness and exercise programs
- Medications management
- Laundry services
- Social and recreational activities
- Food and grocery shopping

3. The physical environment of ALFs is set up with the geriatric/elderly patient in mind. They look more like apartment buildings with private rooms or suites. Some of the environmental characteristics include the following:
   a. Higher toilets
   b. Wheelchair accessibility
   c. Showers
   d. Electric outlets at hip level
   e. Communication devices
   f. Commodes.
4. Residents in ALFs can receive medication reminders and have access to health care professionals such as registered nurses, social workers, and nurse aides.
5. ALFs are not covered by Medicare.
6. Each state has its own licensing regulations or requirements for ALFs. Allowable services also vary among the states.
7. ALFs are known by various names in different states—*personal care, adult congregate living care, board and care, adult homes, adult living facilities, sheltered housing,* and *community-based retirement facilities.*

B. Group homes
1. Often, patients, known as *residents,* live in a facility with 4 to 10 other individuals.
2. Meals, recreation, and other housekeeping assistance are provided.
3. Residents must be able to ambulate to the bathroom and not require any skilled care.
4. Group homes are not covered by Medicare.
5. Used by state Medicaid systems to care for residents who have no other means of care or support.

C. Dementia care, adult day care, or 24-hour living units
1. Adult day care facilities (ADCFs) have been in use for more than 30 years. They are designed especially for the care of patients with Alzheimer disease or other types of dementia.
2. ADCFs may also be called *adult day centers, adult day health, adult day services, adult day residential care,* or *medical adult day care centers* (Box 6-16).

BOX
6-16   Functions and Services of Adult Day Care Facilities

- Offer an alternative to caregivers by providing a daytime care environment outside the home setting.
- Provide simple daily activities, supervision, and routine daily caregiving. They decrease stimulation and confusion.
- Maintain the individual's dignity and highest potential of functioning.
- Employ a family-centered approach to care and services and offer special training for caregivers and involved families.
- Focus on planned activities that fit the needs of elderly patients and help them to function as comfortably and independently as possible, for as long as possible.
- Aim to keep patients active and to teach them skills that will prevent them from needing to be in institutions such as nursing homes.

3. There are three types or models of ADCFs.
   a. The traditional model includes social services, activities, crafts, and individual attention from ADCF staff.
   b. The medical model includes, in addition to the services offered in the traditional model, skilled services by nurses, therapists, social workers, psychiatrists, and geriatricians.
   c. The Alzheimer model includes specialized services designed specifically for the care of the Alzheimer patient.
4. Some ADCFs may be eligible for Medicaid reimbursement or other public funds; however, most caregivers incur significant out-of-pocket payments for these services. Some are reimbursed under long-term insurance plans.

D. Green houses
1. Group homes, with a focus on elders' quality of life.
2. Focus on providing an environment that includes more "home" features and less of the clinical coldness of other care facilities.
3. Residents eat together like a family (communal dining).
4. Focus is not on care, rather on the dignity of the elder.
5. Built on a residential scale, not large scale like other facilities.
6. Residents are able to choose interior design of their own space.
7. Depending on their functional abilities, residents may help in the cooking of meals or daily routines, as if they were living in their own homes.
8. Caregivers have higher job satisfaction.
9. Less cost overall.

E. Aging in place
1. Occurs when a person chooses to remain in his or her living environment (home) and to remain as independent as possible, despite the physical or mental decline that may occur with chronic disabilities or the aging process.
2. This independence can be maintained by contracting with providers of any health services that are needed, including skilled care such as nursing care or skilled rehabilitative therapy services.
3. Independence may also be maintained by contracting with providers for other needs, such as the following:
   a. Assistance with ADLs
   b. Incontinence care
   c. Assistance with IADLs
   d. Assistance with personal and legal affairs.
4. Aging in place may face some barriers that are financial, community based, quality related, or individual related (Box 6-17).
5. Programs for aging in place:
   a. Federal—Older Americans Act of 1965
      i. Administration on Aging
      ii. Administers key programs to help vulnerable older Americans
      iii. Works closely with state, regional, and Areas of Aging agencies
   b. State and community programs
      i. Provide supportive in-home and community-based services
         a. Nutrition
         b. Transportation
         c. Senior center
         d. Homemaker services

6-17 Barriers to Aging in Place

Financial barriers:
- The individual may lack ability to pay for services.
- The individual may not want to pay for services.

Lack of community services:
- This may be an issue mainly in rural areas with no access to services.
- There may not be enough community services to meet needs.
- Frailness of the individual may require more assistance than possible or available from the community.

Quality of care concerns:
- Caregivers may not be properly trained.
- Caregivers may not be licensed or supervised adequately.
- Possible abuse and neglect.
- Lack of quality care.

Individual barriers:
- Owing to physical or psychological factors.
- Danger to self and/or others may exist.

    ii. Emphasis on elder rights programs
       a. Nursing Home Ombudsmen programs
       b. Legal and insurance counseling services
       c. Elder abuse prevention efforts
    iii. Contracts with public or private groups
       a. Referral, outreach, case management, escort, and transportation
       b. In-home services for homemakers, personal care, home repair, and rehabilitation
       c. Educational programs.

F. Custodial care
  1. A level of care that is available mainly for the purpose of performing ADLs and IADLs
  2. May be provided by persons without professional skills or training
  3. This level of care is intended to:
    a. Maintain and support the patient's existing level of health.
    b. Preserve health from further decline.
    c. May be provided in a long-term care (nursing home) setting.

Respite Care

A. Family members provide approximately 80% of the care needed by older relatives.
B. When caring for a loved one, it is easy for caregivers to overlook their own personal needs. They often juggle the demands of a family and career along with their responsibility to a sick or disabled family member or friend. Therefore, many caregivers often find themselves victims of stress and depression.
C. In order to maintain both their own and a loved one's quality of life, it is important for caregivers to take a rest.

D. A respite care program can offer temporary relief for a caregiver from the day-to-day demands of caring for an aging or disabled patient.

E. The idea of respite care emerged in the early 1970s when home care became a trend in the field of human services. It is typically defined as any type of "relief" care provided to families who care for a loved one having a chronic illness or disability.

F. Respite care may include temporary relief ranging from a few hours to a few weeks or periodic care up to a few months. This temporary relief may be provided on an emergency or regular basis.

G. Ideally, respite care should be preventive, rather than the result of a crisis. Planning ahead by seeking outside help will ensure that good care will be provided.

H. Respite care services are provided in many ways, depending on the needs of the family/caregiver. In general, there are three types of respite care services:
   1. Adult day programs
   2. In-home health aide or companion services
   3. Overnight care in a residential facility

I. Respite care services are part of an overall support system necessary for families or caregivers to provide care for a loved one at home.

J. One of the most important purposes of respite care is to give caregivers temporary relief from the stress they experience while providing care to an ill or disabled patient.

K. Respite care enables caregivers to take extended vacations or just a few hours off to spend time with friends or family or the opportunity to discuss a loved one's health status with a health care professional.

L. Most respite care programs are provided by health care organizations/ agencies such as hospitals, nursing homes, assisted living facilities, and private agencies. In some cases, families with an ill or disabled individual arrange for respite care with neighbors, family members, or friends.

M. Many caregivers are reluctant to rely on a respite care program. They may question the need for this type of service.

N. Respite care not only gives caregivers time to concentrate on themselves, but it provides an ill or disabled loved one with a change in their daily routine. It encourages the development of new relationships and friendships, boosts self-esteem and confidence, and inspires a move toward independence.

O. Case managers may engage in the following activities in relation to respite care:
   1. Educate family members and caregivers of patients about respite care, its goals/purpose, its availability, and how to access it.
   2. Encourage families and caregivers to take advantage of respite care programs.
   3. Arrange for respite care and coordinate its services.
   4. Counsel families and caregivers regarding their need for respite care.
   5. Support the actions of families and caregivers in obtaining respite care and assure them that this does not mean abandonment of their loved one.

Financial Aspects of Long-Term and Rehabilitation Care Settings

A. Prior to 1997, Medicare reimbursement for nursing homes was based on actual costs submitted on each patient. The Balanced Budget Act of 1996 forced Medicare to phase in a PPS of reimbursement that is currently fully implemented. Medicaid also reimburses for care based on the PPS.
   1. Reimbursement is determined based on intensity of care needed and the length of stay.
B. Nursing homes that only take Medicaid residents might offer longer term but less intensive levels of care. Nursing homes that do not accept Medicaid payment may make a resident move when Medicare coverage or the resident's own money runs out.
C. Medicare pays for 20 days of an SNF at full cost and the difference between $114 per day and the actual cost for another 80 days. These amounts are for 2015. Rates tend to change annually and one must refer to Medicare for current rates.
D. To qualify for Medicare nursing home coverage, a patient must stay in an acute care hospital setting for at least 3 full days and must have a skilled nursing care need that is ordered by a physician.
E. Medicaid covers skilled nursing care services when an individual spends down his/her liquid assets to $2,000.
F. Long-term care recipients of Medicaid come almost exclusively from the aged, blind, and disabled group of eligible beneficiaries, but very few of those are actually receiving Supplemental Security Income (SSI).
G. SSI is a welfare payment for certain disabled or handicapped individuals who are unable to work, have no assets, and have no extended family financial support.
H. Reimbursement in the rehabilitation care setting employs a PPS, similar to that of acute care/hospital-based care (i.e., the DRG system).
   1. This system includes a Patient Assessment Instrument (PAI) that captures a score that is used to place a patient in a case mix group (CMG) and to establish the reimbursement rate.
   2. In the CMG system, rehabilitation patients are classified into groups based on clinical/medical characteristics and expected resource consumption.
   3. Medicare Part A reimburses stays at an inpatient rehabilitation facility in the same way it reimburses acute care hospitals. Patients encounter an out-of-pocket cost.
      a. Medicare pays for the first 60 days of an IRF stay. After the 60th day in an IRF, and through the 90th day, patients pay a daily co-pay of $296. These amounts are for 2015. Rates tend to change annually and one must refer to Medicare for current rates.
      b. If IRF stay is more than 90 days during one episode of illness, the Medicare patient may use up to 60 additional "lifetime reserve" days of coverage. During those days, the patient is responsible for a daily coinsurance payment of $592. The 60 additional days are a patient's whole lifetime reserve, for both hospital and IRF stays combined. These amounts are for 2015. Rates tend to change annually and one must refer to Medicare for current rates.

I. SNFs also employ a PPS for reimbursement, similar to that of the acute care/hospital-based care (i.e., the DRG system); this system is called resource utilization groups (RUGs).
   1. The system classifies SNF patients into major hierarchies and specific RUGs based on information from the minimum data set (MDS). The classification is based on the type of services, therapies, and resource needs.
   2. The MDS includes data that reflects the patient's medical/clinical condition and resources/services required for care.
   3. Reimbursement is based on the assigned hierarchy and RUG.
J. Inquiries regarding finances are often difficult to initiate. In general, individuals are not comfortable providing information about their finances. This is especially true if the inquiries are over the telephone.
K. Economic issues can have a direct impact on the health of an elderly individual.
L. The Older Americans Resources and Services Multidimensional Functional Assessment Questionnaire (OARS) contains an assessment of financial resources case managers may use for the financial assessment of the elderly individual.
M. Case managers can arrange for this type of in-depth assessment of finances via the help of a social worker or, depending on the practice setting, may complete the assessment themselves.
N. Even without the complete assessment, the case manager should identify whether finances may be the root cause of other issues:
   1. Does the person fail to follow his or her special diet because of lack of funds?
   2. Does he or she ever alter the medication schedule to prolong the interval between refills to save money, or not take the medication at all?
   3. Does the patient miss his/her doctor's appointments for health maintenance or chronic illness management owing to insufficient funds?
   4. Does the patient's housing substandard or unsafe environment occur due to a lack of funding for a more suitable living situation?
O. Case managers may intervene in any of the above situations (or others) to limit the impact of financial issues on the health and well-being of all patients including older adults.
P. Case managers must understand the various care settings, eligibility criteria for admission into these settings, and the financial reimbursement methods associated with them so that they can best be able to assist their patients and ensure positive outcomes.

Case Management Roles in Long-Term and Acute Rehabilitation Care Settings

A. Case managers in the long-term and acute rehabilitation care settings balance the clinical and financial considerations of treatments.
B. Use of evidence-based criteria in the inpatient rehabilitation setting provides an excellent framework by which case managers are able to ensure that patients are admitted to the most appropriate level of care (Fig. 6-2).

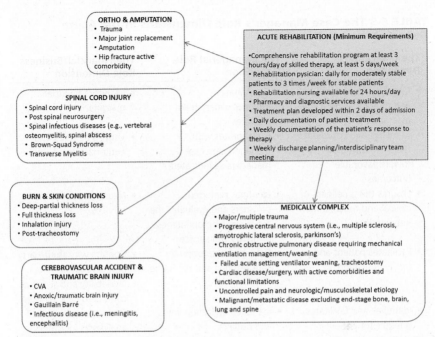

FIGURE 6-2 Acute rehabilitation criteria. (From Carr, D. D. 2005. The case manager's role in optimizing acute rehabilitation services. *Lippincott's Case Management*, *10*(4), 190–200.)

C. Registered nurse (RN) case managers in the long-term and rehabilitation care settings act as gatekeepers for health services, advocates for rehabilitation services and other treatment plans, and experts on case management issues.

D. Rehabilitation case managers are able to organize complex treatment plans and establish clear and attainable goals for the patient and family. They use creativity, adaptability, and flexibility to enhance resources, maximize health care benefits, and seek solutions to short- or long-term problems.

E. The case managers in the long-term and rehabilitation care settings must possess specialized knowledge related to the client population served; that is, they must act as clinical experts, insurance experts, and health care delivery systems and management experts.

F. The accomplishment of case management interventions depends largely on the case manager's ability to move effectively between the multidimensional aspects of their role. These dimensions are clinical, managerial, and financial/business as described by Carr (2005) and summarized in Table 6-3.

G. The case management process in the long-term or rehabilitation care setting begins with a referral from health care professionals in the acute care settings, including the acute care case managers. Case managers then initiate contact with the referring professionals and arrange for an onsite visit to assess the patient's condition and potential treatment needed.

TABLE 6-3 The Case Manager's Role Dimensions in the Acute Rehabilitation Setting

The Clinical Role Dimension	The Managerial Role Dimension	The Financial/Business Role Dimension
• Conducts the initial and ongoing clinical assessment	• Coordinates interdisciplinary team activities	• Monitors financial margins
• Manages and coordinates the treatment plan toward favorable outcomes	• Collaborates with managed care case managers as indicated	• Verifies benefits and authorization of services
• Ensures the timeliness of clinical and rehabilitation interventions	• Identifies preferred providers and evaluates the availability/appropriateness of goods and services	• Negotiates rates and services
• Facilitates patient and family education	• Determines appropriate care settings and discharge planning needs	• Confers with third-party payers regarding the availability and scope of continued care services
• Identifies and facilitates referrals for patient-related issues that require intervention	• Identifies utilization limits and outliers	• Conducts cost–benefit analysis as indicated
• Does early identification of potential problems that might adversely impact the plan of care	• Establishes and facilitates ongoing lines of communication with the team	• Maintains open lines of communication with third-party payers and facility business office
• Maintains open lines of communication with the team and the patient	• Ensures documentation supports the plan of care and treatment	• Acts as a liaison to the business office to facilitate services for the underinsured

Reprinted from Carr, D. D. (2005). The case manager's role in optimizing acute rehabilitation services. *Lippincott's Case Management, 10*(4), 190–200, with permission.

H. Whenever possible, the case manager may meet with members of the acute care multidisciplinary team and discuss the patient's condition and treatment plan before a decision is made to accept the patient into long-term or rehabilitation care setting.

I. As part of the patient assessment, the case manager:
  1. Completes a patient's history
  2. Gathers relevant data about hospital length of stay and treatment plan
  3. Meets with the patient and family to discuss the transfer to the rehabilitation or long-term care setting.

J. The role of the case manager in the rehabilitation or long-term care setting may include the following activities:
  1. Coordination of the flow of patients through the facility
  2. Collaboration with members of the multidisciplinary care team

3. Optimization of care outcomes, including safety, cost-effectiveness, and quality of life
4. Liaison between the referral sources, patient and family, managed care/insurance company, and community-based physicians
5. Negotiating services and resources and obtaining authorizations for such services
6. Advocating for patients and families.

 ## Resources for the Care of the Elderly

A. The American Association of Retired Persons (AARP) has information on virtually every aspect of successful aging and serves as a resource for case managers and patients.
B. The American Society on Aging has an extensive library of educational materials aimed at case managers and patients. In addition, it sponsors numerous conferences throughout the year for those working with older adults.
C. The Area Agency on Aging (AAA) offers a variety of programs, from information and referral to hands-on support programs. This is a number that should be in every case manager's telephone book. Both new and seasoned case managers should contact the AAA in their area and familiarize themselves with the services available.
D. Local public health departments often provide for in-home visits by public health nurses for health promotion activities. This is especially valuable for low-income elderly.
E. Service organizations such as the Salvation Army or St. Vincent DePaul Society often offer a variety of programs for the elderly population, such as:
1. Adult day health programs
2. Friendly visitor programs (on the phone or in person)
3. Equipment loan programs
4. Free or low-cost transportation.
F. Churches and religious groups often offer services to their members or the community at large.

The Geriatric and Older Adult Patient

A. According to the US Census Bureau, the number of people 65 years of age or older continues to rise. The Bureau's report published in 2014 using data from 2010 shows the following:
1. 40.3 million people are aged 65 years or older: 12 times the number in 1900.
2. The percentage of the population aged 65 and over increased from 4.1% in 1900 to 13.0% in 2010 and is projected to reach 20.9% by 2050.
3. Over 38% of those aged 65 and over had one or more disabilities, with the most common difficulties being walking, climbing stairs, and doing errands alone (US Census Bureau, 2014).
B. Medicare beneficiaries (65 years or older) in the United States suffer a number of chronic conditions and impairments; most commonly are high blood pressure (61%), high cholesterol (48%), ischemic heart disease (34%), arthritis (31%), diabetes (28%), heart failure (17%),

chronic kidney disease (15%), depression (27%), chronic obstructive pulmonary disease (12%), Alzheimer (13%), atrial fibrillation (9%), cancer (9%), osteoporosis (8%), stroke (5%), and asthma (4%) (CMS, 2012).

1. These conditions have a long duration, generally progress slowly, and must be managed on a continual basis.
2. Some of these chronic conditions can limit a person's independence and lower quality of life.
3. Almost two thirds of Medicare beneficiaries with 6 or more chronic conditions were hospitalized in 2010; of these, 16% had 3 or more hospitalizations; 27% had received more than 13 home care visits; and 49% were admitted to a postacute care facility (CMS, 2012).

C. Almost 70% of Medicare beneficiaries experience two or more chronic conditions, while 14% have six or more. Seventy eight percent of those between 75 and 84 years old experience two or more chronic conditions, and 83% of those 85 years or older have two or more conditions. The older the population is, the higher the percentage of those experiencing six or more chronic health conditions (CMS, 2012), raising concerns for care where case management services can make a difference.

D. Expertise in the case management of the older adult and geriatric patients is critical for case managers owing to the numbers of patients seen in this category and the diversity of health care delivery sites and services attending to this group of patients.

E. Numerous problems can occur in the geriatric and older adult populations and are characterized by the following:
1. Frequent occurrence
2. Underrecognition and undertreatment
3. Multiple causes
4. Impact on the individual's ability to function.

F. Case managers must be aware of the multitude of issues that may manifest themselves in a variety of ways in the elderly and older adult and act as precipitating cause of other problems.

G. Regardless of the case management setting, the case manager can ensure that the problems presented here are adequately assessed and appropriately addressed.

H. Altered mental status (AMS): An umbrella term linked to a variety of other descriptors of mental status, including confusion, delirium, obtundation, stupor, and coma.
1. A great deal of elder assessment depends on the assessment of a person's mental state. Changes in mental status can be very subtle and often go unrecognized.
2. There are several types and causes of cognitive decline. Dementia is one of the causes but not the only one and often is confused with delirium. Although both are types of AMS, *delirium* is a sudden change in mental functioning and/or acute confusion—*sudden* being the key word. *Dementia* is an *acquired* loss of intellectual functioning that occurs over a long period of time.
3. AMS can be the cause of many other problems identified by case managers (Box 6-18).

6-18 Health Care Effects of Altered Mental Status in the Elderly

- Nonadherence to treatment plans or medications or both
- Injuries such as falls and burns
- Nutritional deficits
- Agitation or aggressive behavior
- Depression
- Social isolation
- Fluid and electrolyte disturbances
- Infections
- Chemical withdrawal
- Chemical intoxicants

    4. A baseline assessment of mental status using standardized tools can help identify and track the progression of mental status. One popular tool is the Short Portable Mental Status Questionnaire for the Assessment of Organic Brain Disease in the elderly population; another is the Folstein Mini-Mental Status Examination.
       a. The choice of instrument depends on the case manager's practice setting.
       b. The case manager may not be the one who actually administers the test, but he or she should be aware of the availability of the various tools and recommend their use when appropriate.

I. Urinary incontinence.
    1. Although the urinary system is affected by changes in aging, incontinence should not be thought of as an inevitable part of aging.
    2. Assessment for incontinence or the risk of incontinence should be multifaceted and cover a number of factors (Box 6-19).
    3. Incontinence is often unreported and can have a significant impact on the life and functioning of the older adult.
    4. It is important for case managers to assess for and arrange interventions directed at resolving and/or improving the problem.

6-19 Focus of the Assessment for Incontinence in the Elderly

- Risk factors influencing elimination, such as prostate surgery.
- Social risk factors such as being able to read bathroom signs when out of the home.
- Signs and symptoms of actual dysfunction, such as leaking urine.
- Whether incontinence is acknowledged. Ask when the problem began, and what has been done about it.
- Fears about incontinence that include changing activities because of the need to go to the toilet.
- Behavioral signs, such as a urine odor or use of pads.
- Environmental factors that may contribute to incontinence, such as having to go upstairs to use the bathroom.
- Adverse drug responses.
- Delirium or hypoxia.
- Excessive fluid intake.
- Impaired mobility.
- Physiologic factors—history of prostatectomy, atrophic vaginitis, glycosuria.

6-20 Risk Factors for Falls in the Elderly

- Multiple risk factors are associated with falls in the elderly.
- Age-related changes such as:
  - Vision and hearing changes
  - Osteoporosis
  - Slowed reaction time
  - Altered gait
  - Postural hypotension
  - Nocturia.
- Medical problems.
- Psychosocial factors such as depression.
- Medications.
- Environmental factors.
- Any combination of the abovementioned items.
- Fear of falling and postfall anxiety syndrome are also well recognized as negative consequences of falls.

J. Safety issues.
    1. Falls: The case manager should assess for the presence of risk factors for falls as part of the comprehensive assessment of the elderly and older adult (Box 6-20).
        a. The case manager should assess for the possibility of falls and whether any of the assessment information collected puts the individual at greater risk such as previous falls both in the home and at other levels of the health care continuum.
        b. The fall assessment tool should include history of falls, confusion, impaired judgment, mobility status, cooperation, medications, physiological factors that may influence mobility or lack of mobility, and mobility aids, to mention a few.
        c. Some resources may be available to help the case manager with the assessment.
            i. The physical therapist can assess the individual's gait and balance.
            ii. A thorough home safety evaluation can identify environmental concerns.
            iii. A thorough history from the primary care physician that includes medications and health conditions can assist with identifying medical risk factors.
        d. The case manager should tailor the care interventions directed at preventing falls to the specific risk factors.
    2. Elder abuse and neglect: Often, victims of abuse and/or neglect unequivocally deny its occurrence. Box 6-21 describes the characteristics of elder abuse and neglect.
        a. In assessing elders for abuse and neglect and creating care plans of care, it is natural for the case manager to look to the family as a large part of the caregiver equation. It is critical that the case manager evaluate the potential for risk and intervene to reduce and/or eliminate the risk (Box 6-22).

6-21   Characteristics of Elder Abuse and Neglect

Victims' characteristics:
- Females are at a higher risk owing to the fact that they outlive men and because of gender issues.
- Persons 80 years and older suffer abuse and neglect two to three times more than the older population.
- Family members, especially children, are the most common perpetrators of elder abuse and neglect.
- Most elder abuse and neglect takes place at home, not in the nursing home.
- Advanced age.
- Greater dependency.
- Alcohol abuse.
- Intergenerational conflict.
- Isolation.
- Internalization of blame.
- Provocative behavior.
- Past history of being abused.

Abusers' characteristics:
- Alcohol and drug abuse
- Mental illness
- Caregiver inexperience
- History of abuse as a child
- Stress
- Economic dependence on elder

Families' characteristics:
- Caregiver reluctance.
- Overcrowding.
- Isolation.
- Marital conflict.
- History of past abuse.
- Caregiver spouse or companion caring for elder may have some dementia exhibited in abuse or neglect toward the other.

6-22   Case Management Interventions for Elder Abuse and Neglect

- Provide education to the caregiver about each aspect of the expected care.
- Discuss examples of situations in which the behavior of the elder patient causes frustration, anger, or feelings of helplessness in the caregiver. Help the caregiver identify appropriate responses to these feelings.
- Set realistic expectations, and frankly discuss the demands of caring for a dependent individual.
- Provide for direct observation of the home situation and the interaction between the elder family member and the caregivers. A home health nurse or a case manager may be able to identify subtle signs of trouble before it occurs.
- Assess the support system of the caregiver, and assist him or her in identification of support groups or respite from caregiver activities.
- Support and encourage the elderly person to continue to be as independent as his or her condition allows.
- Refer the caregiver to marital, substance abuse, or other specialized counseling services.
- Recommend different arrangements for the elderly person. Not every family can successfully provide care for the elder family member.

    b. Most states have specific reporting requirements for elder abuse and neglect. Most require reporting by the health care professionals who suspect the abuse. Case managers should be familiar with the state and federal agencies that receive reports of elder abuse and neglect—Area Agency on Aging (AOA), Adult Protective Services (APS), and National Domestic Hotline. They should also be aware of the reporting procedures and the organizational reporting policies.

    c. The case manager can recognize the possibility of elder abuse and neglect through signs such as the following:

      i. Direct reports by the elder of incidents

      ii. A rapid or unexplained decline in the physical condition of the elderly patient

      iii. Malnutrition

      iv. Suspicious injuries or conflicting reports of injury from the patient and the caregiver:

        a. Lacerations and bruises in multiple states of healing

        b. Multiple fractures in various states of healing

        c. Scald burns with demarcated immersion lines and no splash marks, involving the anterior or posterior half of extremity or to the buttocks or genitals

        d. Cigarette burns

        e. Rope burns or marks

        f. Refusal to go to the same emergency department for repeated injuries

        g. Evasiveness

    d. Although most health care professionals are trained to recognize abuse; it is still possible for them to miss the signs.

    e. Case managers may be the first to complete the picture and recognize abuse. This is especially true if the caregiver takes the patient to multiple providers and the case manager is the only constant of the health care team.

    f. Case managers will want to act as an advocate for the patient and take immediate steps to ensure the patient's safety.

K. Elder depression.

    1. Depression is underreported and undertreated in the elderly population. It is also widespread; at least 12% of Medicare beneficiaries suffer from depression; prevalence is higher in women than men; those who are dual eligible experience depression (27%) more than the nonduals (11%) (CMS, 2012).

    2. Risk factors for depression are family history, alcohol abuse, heart attack or stroke, anxiety disorders, mood disorders, chronic medical illnesses, and personality disorders.

    3. Common signs of depression are loss of interest in self-care or following medical advice, trouble sleeping or anxiety, little interest in outside activities, trouble concentrating or remembering things, unexplained aches and pains, change in appetite or weight loss, feeling hopeless about the future, feelings of helplessness, easily irritated or listless, or feeling one is a burden.

    4. Depression can be the root cause of many other observed problems in the elderly, such as:

    a. Nonadherence to treatment

    b. Social isolation

    c. Cognitive impairment

    d. Malnutrition

    e. Alcohol abuse.

  5. There are tools available to detect unrecognized depression in the geriatric individual. The Geriatric Depression Scale, Cornell Scale for Depression in Dementia (CSDD, detects depression in geriatric patients with dementia), and the Beck Depression Inventory are examples of these tools. In the PCMH, FQHC, and ACO settings, the PHQ-9 is most commonly used for depression screening and as an integral part of the care model and care planning.

  6. Even though the case manager may not be responsible for the administration of such tests, he or she should be aware of their existence, recommend them as appropriate, and incorporate the screening results in patient care planning, goals, and interventions.

  7. Appropriate referrals should be arranged if depression (actual or potential) is detected.

L. Constipation

  1. Constipation can be described as either functional (straining, hard stools) or rectal outlet delay (anal blockage or prolonged defecation). A number of risk health factors the elderly experiences as a natural aging process or due to chronic illnesses and associated care (Box 6-23).

  2. Interventions include diet, exercise, fluid intake, and laxative use, according to the individual situation.

M. Polypharmacy

  1. Older adults use more medications—prescription, over the counter (OTC), and supplements—than any other age group in the United States. Many take multiple medications at the same time.

    a. Experts report that two out of five Medicare beneficiaries report taking five or more prescription medications.

    b. Older patients tend to have more than one prescribing physician and use more than one pharmacy, making it more difficult to track all of their medications and identify potential problems (e.g., drug interactions, harmful doses, unnecessary medications with no health benefits).

6-23 Risk Factors for Constipation in the Elderly

- Recent abdominal surgery
- Limited physical activity
- Inadequate diet, with fiber less than 15 g per day
- Intake of medications known to contribute to constipation
- History of chronic constipation
- Laxative abuse history
- Other comorbidities known to cause constipation
- Endocrine or metabolic disorders
- Neurogenic disorders
- Smooth muscle or connective tissue disorders

    c. Older adults are at increased risk of serious adverse drug events, including falls, depression, confusion, hallucinations, and malnutrition, which are an important cause of illness, hospitalization and death among these patients.

    d. Drug-related complications have been attributed to the use of multiple medications (also called polypharmacy) and associated drug interactions, age-related changes, human error, and poor medical management (e.g., incorrect medication prescribed, inappropriate doses, lack of communication and monitoring).

2. The normal physiologic changes associated with aging cause the elderly individual to be more prone to medication-related problems.

3. The combination of several medications and the aging process can cause health issues in the elderly.

4. Medications adherence issues increase in proportion to the complexity of the regimen. Therefore, a thorough assessment of the individual's prescription and nonprescription medications is essential to the case management assessment of the elderly.

5. Case managers can enlist the aid of the physician or the pharmacist to review the medications used by the older person and can make recommendations for changes.

6. Majority of medication errors and adverse drug events can be attributed to lack of medication reconciliation. Each time a geriatric patient moves from one care setting to another, the case manager should make every effort to review medications with the care team.

7. Case managers should remember to consider medications in relation to other issues presenting in the patient's health condition or situation.

Identification of High-Risk Geriatric Patients

A. A brief history of early identification efforts.

1. In the early days of case management, cases were identified primarily through diagnostic criteria or through an event such as a workers' compensation injury. Most of the cases were identified after the diagnosis or event had already occurred.

2. With the advent of the managed Medicare programs, health maintenance organizations (HMOs) found themselves at financial risk for large populations of geriatric members. Once a geriatric member became ill, costs were greater and the illnesses were often more severe.

3. The added burden of comorbidities in this population made interventions by case managers more difficult.

4. There was an increasing demand for methods to identify geriatric patients before the onset of illness or a major decline in health status. Two reasons propelled the need for earlier identification:

    a. Once a geriatric member became ill, he or she consumed two to four times more resources than a healthy geriatric member. This problem increased costs of care.

    b. The more reactive style of case management that relied on a diagnosis or event did not fulfill the potential for case management impact in this population.

5. Early efforts at identification and prediction of risks were intuitive and based primarily on the case manager's or medical director's knowledge and experience. Questionnaires of varying lengths, some up to 12 pages, were mailed to geriatric health plan members, and trigger criteria were established to help identify geriatric patients who were, or could be, at high risk.

6. There were several pitfalls to the early use of questionnaires:
   a. Intuition has its limits. Some questions that a practitioner believes would be useful in predicting risk are not useful.
   b. Without a specific method of scoring the questionnaires, case managers were left to use their judgment regarding which geriatric members were at risk and should be contacted.
   c. Without a scoring methodology, case managers were still required to review each questionnaire. This did not yield any real efficiency or accuracy in the identification of high-risk geriatric patients.

B. Screening versus assessment.
   1. It is important to differentiate screening from assessment. Without a clear differentiation of these two concepts, case managers will spend time and resources where they are not necessary.
   2. When individuals are identified primarily because of a diagnosis or event, most of those individuals are ultimately deemed appropriate for case management.
   3. In the circumstance in which the overwhelming majority of the individuals who are referred to case managers actually need case management, assessment by the case manager is a logical first step.
   4. When the goal is to identify individuals who are at risk or in the very early stages of decline, different strategies are necessary.
   5. One method of addressing the issues of earlier identification and increasing the objectivity in follow-up was the development of screening tools that are valid and reliable in predicting risk.
   6. Use the example of a health fair, in which random blood glucose levels are obtained via finger stick. This is illustrative of several key principles of screening:
      a. The screening is aimed at a broad group of individuals to identify as many as possible and as early as possible.
      b. Individuals other than health care professionals can do the screening.
      c. The screening does not positively determine that the individual meets the criteria or diagnosis and requires further assessment by a health care professional.
   7. Screening accomplishes the following objectives:
      a. Identifying those geriatric patients who may be at risk before an adverse event without using case management resources
      b. Providing an objective method of determining which members require assessment by a case manager.
   8. Assessment also differs from screening in several other ways. Unlike screening:
      a. An assessment is reserved for those who have met some initial criteria not broadly applied.
      b. A qualified case manager should perform a comprehensive case management assessment.

      c. An assessment can determine whether the individual actually needs further follow-up.

  9. Goals of assessment include:

      a. Collection of data in order to identify problems or issues

      b. Determination of whether the problems or issues identified may be impacted by case management interventions

      c. Creation of an individualized plan of care.

C. Use of risk for readmission tools

  1. These tools are sued to predict risk for avoidable readmission to the hospital/acute care settings and implement specific interventions and strategies to prevent them and therefore reduce financial risk.

  2. The tools also are used to assess the reasons why a readmission occurred. Such information informs proactive intervention and necessary modifications to patient's plan of care including the postdischarge services.

D. SF (Short Form) 36—This document is a comprehensive short form with only 36 questions. Today, shorter versions of this questionnaire are also used.

  1. It yields an 8-scale health profile, as well as summary measures of health-related quality of life.

  2. SF-36 measures both physical and mental components of health:

      a. Physical component—Function, role, bodily pain, and general health

      b. Mental component—Mental health, emotional role, social function, and vitality.

  3. As documented in more than 4,000 publications, the SF-36 has proved useful in monitoring general and specific populations, comparing the burden of different diseases, differentiating the health benefits produced by different treatments, and screening individual patients. Most widely evaluated generic instrument that is used for the assessment of patient health outcome.

  4. The SF-36 is an excellent baseline measure, as is the SF-12 (a shorter version of the SF-36), which can be administered as part of the screening process to allow for comparison of outcomes after case management intervention.

  5. SF-12 is a shorter version of the SF-36. It is a single page scannable health survey that documents physical and mental health summary measures. It is useful to general and specific populations.

Comprehensive Geriatric Assessment

A. Geriatric patients benefit from a comprehensive geriatric assessment (Box 6-24), which is usually conducted by a team of geriatric experts from multiple disciplines and encompasses all aspects of the individual's health and functioning.

B. Geriatric assessment is recommended when there are multiple problems (recognized or unrecognized) and when the current plans are not addressing the identified problems or issues.

C. Caregivers should be a part of the geriatric assessment as they can help the case manager determine specific needs related to the patient and reflect the stresses experienced by caregivers of geriatric patients.

BOX
6-24 Elements of The Comprehensive Geriatric Assessment

- Physical
- Functional
- Psychosocial
- Mental and behavioral
- Financial
- Cognitive
- Nutritional
- Environmental
- Medications

Geriatric Assessment for Placement of the Geriatric Patient

A. Some assessments for the placement of a patient in a long-term facility are necessary. Often, these assessments are mandatory based on laws and regulations. Assessments are more necessary in the case of patients who are covered under state or federal health benefit programs. An example is functional ability assessment for placement of a patient in a skilled care facility (Box 6-25).

BOX
6-25 Functional Ability Assessment

- Activities of Daily Living (ADLs):
  - Assessment categories:
    - Bathing
    - Dressing
    - Toileting
    - Transferring
    - Continence
    - Feeding
  - Scoring: One point for every independent function:
    - A score of 6 indicates full function.
    - A score of 4 indicates moderate impairment.
    - A score of 2 indicates severe impairment.
- Instrumental Activities of Daily Living (IADLs):
  - Assessment categories focus on the following:
    - Use of the telephone
    - Getting to places beyond walking distance
    - Going shopping for groceries
    - Preparing own meals
    - Doing own housework
    - Doing own handyman work
    - Doing own laundry
    - Taking own medication
    - Managing own money
  - Scoring:
    - These items can be made gender specific by the interviewer.
    - The score range is 9 (poor) to 27 (good).
    - Scores are patient specific only.

6-26   Examples of Elderly Assessments for Placement in Postacute Care

Psychological health assessment that usually focuses on patient's mental, cognitive, and emotional state. An example is Folstein Mini-Mental State Examination with the following categories:
- Orientation to time, place, and date.
- Registration: Name three objects.
- Attention and calculation.
- Recall.
- Language: Repetition, commands, read, and repeat.
- Draw a clock.
- Assess level of consciousness.
- Scoring: Range is 0 (poor) to 30 (good); scores are patient specific.

Physical health assessment that includes the following:
- The defined diagnoses and symptom complexes
- Documentation of the number of days of hospitalization and disability to define the severity of health problems
- May use New York Heart Association Four Point Functional Disability Scale for clarification of degree of disability if the disorder is due to a cardiac problem
- A subjective assessment to determine the severity of congestive heart failure
- Scoring system with problem history of last 30 days

Nutritional assessment to identify the following:
- Amount of food eaten on a daily basis
- Kinds of foods consumed
- Problems eating certain kinds of food
- Likes and dislikes
- Ability to shop, cook, and prepare food
- Any dental or oral problems
- Awareness of any food preferences or only eating one type of food
- Obesity as signal of a nutritional concern

Oral health assessment that may include the following:
- Any gums, teeth, tongue, or dental pain issues
- Use of dentures and their condition

B. There are many aspects to the assessment of the elderly for placement in postacute and long-term care facilities or services other than functional ability. Examples are those in Box 6-26.

C. Pressure ulcers:
1. Because geriatric patients are always at risk for pressure ulcers due to decreased mobility or immobility, a case manager should be able to identify skin integrity issues. They may review findings of assessments completed by other professionals if they do not complete such assessment themselves; for example, use the "Braden Scale for Predicting Pressure Sore Risk" by nursing.
2. Geriatric patients have a risk of developing pressure ulcers due to immobility, friction while moving, decreased sensory perception, and poor circulation.

D. Visual acuity:
   1. Case managers should use the "Snellen Eye Chart" tool to screen for visual acuity.
   2. This will help determine the need for referral to an ophthalmologist if visual acuity is worse than 20/40 with glasses. This visual impairment can interfere with ADLs.

References

Agency for Healthcare Research and Quality (AHRQ). (2015). *Patient Centered Medical Home (PCMH)*. Rockville, MD: AHRQ. Retrieved from https://pcmh.ahrq.gov/page/tools-resources, on July 28, 2015.

Carr, D. D. (2005). The case manager's role in optimizing acute rehabilitation services. *Lippincott's Case Management, 10*(4), 190–200.

Case Management Society of America (CMSA). (2010). *CMSA standards of practice for case management*. Little Rock, AR: Author.

Centers for Medicare and Medicaid Services (CMS). (2012). *Chronic conditions among medicare beneficiaries, chartbook, 2012 edition*. Baltimore, MD: CMS.

Centers for Medicare and Medicaid Services (CMS). (June 5, 2014). *Rural Health Clinics (RHCs) and Federally Qualified Health Centers (FQHCs) billing guide*. Medicare Learning Network Matters, number SE1039. Retrieved from https://www.cms.gov/Outreach-and-Education/Medicare-Learning-Network-MLN/MLNMattersArticles/Downloads/SE1039.pdf

Centers for Medicare and Medicaid Services (CMS). (2015a). *Update to the Federally Qualified Health Centers (FQHC) Prospective Payment System (PPS)—Recurring file updates*. Medicare Learning Network Matters, October 9, 2015, number MM9348. Retrieved from https://www.cms.gov/Outreach-and-Education/Medicare-Learning-Network-MLN/MLNMattersArticles/Downloads/MM9348.pdf

Centers for Medicare and Medicaid Services (CMS). (2015b). *Accountable care organizations (ACOs, January 6, 2015)*. Retrieved from https://www.cms.gov/Medicare/Medicare-Fee-for-Service-Payment/ACO/index.html?redirect=/aco, on July 28, 2015.

U.S. Census Bureau. (2014). *65+ in the United States: 2010, P23-212*. Washington, DC: Government Printing Office.

US Department of Health and Human Services (USDHHS), Centers for Medicare and Medicaid Services. (2013). *Federally Qualified Heath Centers, Medicare Learning Network*. USDHHS ICN 006397.

US Department of Health and Human Services (USDHHS), Health Research and Services Administration (HRSA), Health Information Technology. (2015). *What are Federally Qualified Health Centers*. Retrieved from http://www.hrsa.gov/healthit/toolbox/ruralhealthittoolbox/introduction/qualified.html, on July 28, 2015.

Case Management in the Home Care Setting

Hussein M. Tahan

LEARNING OBJECTIVES

Upon completion of this chapter, the reader will be able to:

1. Discuss the different services available in the home health care setting.
2. Describe reimbursement and insurance issues in relation to the home health care setting.
3. Explain the importance of collaboration within the interdisciplinary health care team including durable medical equipment agencies and other support service representatives.
4. Explain the role of the case manager in the home health care setting.

IMPORTANT TERMS AND CONCEPTS

Advance Request
  Payment
Certified Home
  Healthcare Agency
  (CHHA)
Custodial Care
Home Care
Home Health Aide
Home Health Resource
  Groups (HHRGs)
Homebound

Intermittent or
  Part-Time Care
Long-Term Care
Low Utilization
  Payment
Nonskilled Services
Outcome and
  Assessment
  Information Set
  (OASIS)
Outlier Payment

Partial Episode
  Payment
Reasonable Care/
  Services
Significant Change in
  Condition Payment
Skilled Services

Introduction

A. Throughout history, medical care was provided in the home by family members, with some guidance from outpatient or home visiting professionals.

B. During the second half of the 20th century, medical practice shifted from this home-based model of care to the acute hospital-based care model. This allowed medical practice to expand its knowledge, widen its services, and improve individual outcomes and dramatically increase life expectancy.

C. As medical care costs have dramatically increased, they have brought about the necessity of controlling costs.

   1. In the private sector, health insurance companies sought to control costs through utilization review and management and establishment of health maintenance organizations (HMOs).

   2. In the public sector, the Centers for Medicare and Medicaid Services (CMS) have sought to control costs through the adoption of diagnosis-related groups (DRGs), all payer DRGs (APDRGs), and the inpatient prospective payment system (PPS). PPS ultimately expanded to various health care settings cross the continuum of care including home and long-term care.

   3. The development of DRGs and HMOs and the practice of utilization review have led to increased pressure on hospitals to control costs by limiting the number of days each patient spends in the hospital, that is, to reduce length of stay (LOS).

   4. The current pressure on hospitals has increased the need for home care services and, therefore, case management.

D. Hospitals have found that using interdisciplinary health care teams to collaboratively develop posthospital discharge and transition plans for their patients can confidently reduce length of stay without compromising patient safety and quality of care. These teams are best facilitated by case managers, as formal or informal leaders, to produce the most cost-effective care outcomes.

E. Home health care, when appropriate, serves two vital functions in reducing costs and limiting length of stay in institutional settings:

   1. First, home care serves as a less expensive extension to hospital-based care.

      a. The average home care visit cost is significantly less than the cost of a day in the hospital. The visit by a health care professional, such as a registered nurse, physical therapist, and/or social worker, can provide vital information to the physician (the provider responsible for care) that can confirm the plan of care or indicate the need for change in the plan.

      b. The assessment of a licensed health professional (e.g., case manager, registered nurse) in the home can provide reassurance to patients and their families (clients and their support systems) that the plan of care

NOTE: This chapter is a revised version of Chapter 5 in the second edition of *CMSA Core Curriculum for Case Management*. The contributor wishes to acknowledge the work of Elizabeth Alvarado and Edward Sutherland, as some of the timeless material was retained from the previous version.

or health regimen is appropriate and safe. The health professional can share the important information with the interdisciplinary health care team about conditions in the patient's home.

2. Second, home care serves as a less expensive and more satisfying alternative to other types of institutional care.

   a. The average cost of a home care visit is significantly less than the cost of a day in a skilled nursing care facility, and most, but by no means all, families would prefer to receive care in the patient's home setting.

   b. As an alternative to a hospital or skilled nursing facility, home health care shifts the burden of round-the-clock institutional care from the insurer (i.e., payer) and health care provider to the family. Therefore, across an effective continuum of care, one should expect to see increasing home care costs, not as a result of overutilization of home care services but as a result of shifting utilization away from more costly settings into home care.

F. Case management in the home health care setting is designed with similar goals in mind as those of case management in the acute care setting (Box 7-1). An overarching goal is ensuring the delivery of reliable, consistent, and cost-effective home care services to help the home care client achieve and maintain overall health and well-being, with reasonable degree of independence and self-care or self-management.

G. Patients who are eligible for home care services include those who were hospitalized in an acute care/hospital setting, those with chronic illnesses, or those with seriously complex medical conditions or injuries.

H. The demand for home care case management services has increased since the implementation of the federal home care PPS, the increase in managed care health insurance plans and capitation, the popularity of demand management programs, the growth of integrated care delivery systems, value-based purchasing, and the Patient Protection and Affordable Care Act of 2010, including CMS' Hospital Readmissions Reduction Program.

BOX
7-1   **Goals of Case Management in Home Care**

- Optimize the delivery of care across the continuum of health and human services
- Care for patients in less costly care settings
- Employ a proactive approach to patient care delivery by implementing strategies to keep patients out of costly acute care settings (e.g., avoidable hospital readmissions and access to emergency care)
- Monitor patients' conditions and prevent deterioration or avoidable disease progression
- Reduce patients' risks and need for acute care or emergency services
- Improve quality of care, continuity of care, and services
- Maintain patients' safety
- Improve patients' quality of life

Descriptions of Key Terms

A. Advance Request Payment—A home care services claim submitted at the completion of the initial assessment of the patient, upon admission into home care services, and at the completion of an initial Outcome and Assessment Information Set (OASIS) score. This claim includes a partial payment amount that does not exceed 60% of the specific Home Health Resource Group (HHRG)-designated reimbursement.

B. Certified Home Healthcare Agency (CHHA)—A company that meets all the eligibility criteria required by CMS before it is permitted to provide home care services for Medicare beneficiaries.

C. Custodial care—Care provided primarily to assist a patient in meeting the activities of daily living, but not requiring the services of a licensed professional, such as bathing and eating.

D. Home care—Health care services that are provided to patients while in their own homes. These services may include professional (i.e., skilled) and paraprofessional (i.e., supportive) services.

E. Home Health Resource Group (HHRG)—Groupings for prospective reimbursement under Medicare for home health agencies. Placement into an HHRG is based on the OASIS score. Reimbursement rates correspond to the level of home health services provided.

F. Homebound—Being confined to the home setting all (or almost all) the time. A patient who is considered homebound is only able to leave the home very infrequently and for short periods of time. Leaving the home requires a considerable or taxing effort with or without help. An example is a patient who experiences an unbearable and extreme effort to leave the home just for a clinic visit or to receive some sort of medical treatment.

G. Intermittent services—Care that is provided on a part-time basis; that is, for a portion of hours in a day and for few days of the week; for example, home care services provided by a nurse for 1 to 2 hours per day, 1 to 3 days per week.

H. Nonskilled services—Health care services that are provided by a paraprofessional or an unlicensed person. Examples of these services may include close observation, bathing, feeding, and transferring from bed to chair.

I. Outcome and Assessment Information Set (OASIS)—A uniform and standardized set of home care services–related outcomes data used by the CMS to examine the quality of home care services received by Medicare beneficiaries. The set includes clinical, financial, and administrative outcome indicators and is used by home health agencies for quality improvement.

J. Reasonable services—Services provided based on a patient's medical condition, acuity and severity of the disease, and the course of treatment meets what is described in national guidelines or standards.

K. Skilled services—Health care services that require delivery by a licensed professional such as a registered nurse, social worker, and physical, occupational, or speech therapists. Examples of these services may include wound care, vital signs assessment and monitoring, patient and family education, Foley catheter care, psychosocial counseling, physical rehabilitation, and intravenous medications administration.

Applicability to CMSA's Standards of Practice

A. The Case Management Society of America (CMSA) describes in its standards of practice for case management that case management extends across all health care settings across the continuum of care and patient populations. This also includes home care settings and care of patients while at home (CMSA, 2010).

B. The practice of case management in all care settings results in availability of case managers in these settings. Therefore, case managers in the home care settings may apply the CMSA standards in their practice, in addition to the organization-based policies, procedures, and guidelines.

C. Case managers in home care settings are often registered nurses. Sometimes, social workers function in the role of case manager, especially for patients with behavioral and mental health conditions. In these situations, nurses collaborate with social workers, especially during the initial assessment of the patient, which takes place during the first home visit.

D. Case managers who are nurses may assume responsibilities for both direct care provision and case management services.

E. Having awareness and knowledge of CMSA's standards of practice for case management allows case managers to gain more comfort in their roles and contributes to greater effectiveness. The standards may be used as a guide to identify expectations and assure appropriate focus of the role, especially in an environment of scarce case management resources.

The Role of the Hospital-Based Interdisciplinary Health Care Team

A. The primary care physician (attending physician of record), in cooperation with consulting physicians (i.e., specialty care providers), has responsibility for discharging a patient to home or transitioning to another care setting. All those involved in the patient's treatment plan, including the nursing staff, the case manager, the social worker, and the home care agency team, share in the responsibility and liability for providing appropriate posthospital discharge care.

B. Hospital-based interdisciplinary health care teams include physicians, nurses, social workers, care coordinators or case managers, physical therapists, occupational therapists, chaplains, nutritionists, and others.

C. Daily interdisciplinary patient care management rounds provide an effective forum to discuss the medical, financial, spiritual, functional, emotional, and psychosocial issues that impact the posthospital discharge/transition plan.

D. The role of the hospital-based case managers, whether they are called discharge planners or care coordinators, is to assess patient and family needs and available resources for posthospital discharge planning and to assist with linkage to the appropriate community-based providers who can provide services determined to be necessary by the interdisciplinary health care team.

E. Before considering home care services, the interdisciplinary health care team must know that the patient and family would appreciate and agree to a home care referral. The case manager can facilitate such discussion and follow-up on the referral with the patient, family, and a number of home care agencies depending on the type of health insurance plan the patient holds (i.e., payer).

1. Many people are reluctant to allow strangers into their homes, and some homes may be too small to accommodate patients, families, and home care professionals.
2. Other families may not be willing, or able, to participate in a plan of care, which includes home care.
3. Case managers educate their patients/families about the necessity and value of home care services to lessen the impact of present concerns.

F. The case manager, in collaboration with other members of the health care team, conducts an assessment of patient needs to identify type of home care services appropriate for the patient's condition (Box 7-2).

G. For a patient to be eligible for Medicare reimbursement of home care services, the patient must:
   1. Be homebound
   2. Require intermittent or part-time care
   3. Require skilled care/services
   4. Be under the supervision of a physician
   5. Receive services that are reasonable and necessary
   6. In addition, the agency must be a CHHA to provide the needed services.

H. In addition to the assessment of needs, the case manager must:
   1. Use the findings of the clinical evaluation of the patient to determine the type of services needed, such as skilled nursing, both at the professional and paraprofessional levels, rehabilitation therapies, and social work/services such as counseling.

BOX 7-2   Focus of the Assessment for Home Care Services

- Clinical/medical condition of the patient
- Reasons for home care services
- Plan of care for the postdischarge period
- Appropriateness of home care setting/level of care
- Financial status and health insurance benefits
- Evaluation of insurance benefits and restrictions placed by the patient's health plan on the:
  - Number of hours of home care to be provided per day
  - Number of home care visits to be provided per week
  - Total number of home care visits in an episode of care
  - Types of home care services and professionals needed
  - The vendors who have contracts with particular payers for provision of home health care services
  - Need for transportation upon discharge
  - Need for durable medical equipment and care supplies
  - Evaluate patient for adequacy of support system or backup resources in the home (e.g., an elderly patient living alone and not independent with activities of daily living may wish to go back home, but has no backup support system in the event of an emergency).
  - Assess patient's physical mobility (patient may be so anxious to go back home that he/she may not share inability to ambulate and transfer independently, or patient may have become deconditioned while in the hospital).

2. Decide on the needed services by applying knowledge of the operations of home care services, related rules and regulations, and policies and procedures.
3. Work closely with the interdisciplinary health care team on these assessments and in decision making about what is best for the patient and family.

I. Patients who are eligible for home care services and are known to benefit from these services may include:
   1. Those who may be recovering from a stroke, orthopedic or cardiac surgeries, or injuries or those learning to live with other neurological or cardiac disorders, diabetes, and other chronic health problems
   2. A number of high-risk populations require special attention, such as the frail elderly who live alone, those with limited cognitive or physical function, the severely mentally ill, the chemically dependent, the homeless, and people living with HIV/AIDS or other types of debilitating, chronic, and complex illnesses
      a. Individuals in these high-risk groups merit special attention in discharge planning because of specific vulnerabilities that may make them eligible for additional community support or that may preclude a safe home care posthospital discharge plan.

J. The case manager, on behalf of the health care team, works closely with health care professionals and support staff external to the hospital in coordinating the patient's discharge or transition plan and needed home care services. These may include the case manager of the managed care organization (i.e., payer), representatives from home care agencies such as the home care intake coordinator, staff from transportation agencies and laboratory services, and representatives of durable medical equipment.

 Home Health Care Visits

A. Home care professionals can be invaluable to patients and their families in making a home visit prior to scheduled admissions or prior to discharge from the hospital, especially in the case of emergency admissions, to anticipate minor changes in ordinary family routines. Such a visit could make all the difference in understanding the family preferences and the dynamics of the home environment.
   1. For example, the extension cord carelessly connecting a television set to the closest electrical outlet is known not to be safe, but for someone returning home from the hospital with decreased vision, balance, strength, or unsteady gait, it could become a deadly hazard.
   2. Home visits provide invaluable information about the way the family functions, the neighborhood supports, and the barriers to home care success and adherence to care regimen, including medication intake.

B. Information gathered during home care visits can be communicated to the hospital interdisciplinary health care teams during subsequent inpatient hospital stays and/or to ambulatory care providers (e.g., patient primary care provider) so that current or future discharge and transition of care plans can be structured in light of the specific reality of the individual patient in his or her own environment.

7-3 Types of Services Provided during a Home Care Visit

Professional services
- Skilled care in nature
- Care that requires the involvement of licensed professionals such as a registered nurse, social worker, or physical, occupational, and speech therapists
- Examples include the care provided by registered nurses, social workers, and therapists, such as respiratory, physical, and occupational.

Paraprofessional services
- Unskilled care in nature.
- Care that does not require the involvement of licensed professionals.
- Examples include the care provided by a home health aide, homemaker, housekeeper, or community health worker.

C. The number, type, length, and frequency of home care visits are determined based on the patient's medical/health condition and treatment regimen, capacity for self-care and self-management, intensity and complexity of the types of services required, health plan or insurance benefits, and applicable laws and regulations.

D. Home care visits may include the provision of professional and/or paraprofessional services (Box 7-3).

E. Medicare's Conditions of Participation stipulate that the initial home care evaluation visit be conducted by a registered nurse. This refers to the first home care visit to the patient's home after discharge from the acute care facility. The registered nurse in this evaluation and follow-up visits may engage in a number of important activities such as those listed in Box 7-4.

F. Home care case management is based on the individual's needs and goals. It is decided upon in consultation with other health care team members and the patient and family to ensure the care goals are achieved in the most efficient way possible.

7-4 Activities the Nurse Engages in during Home Care Visits

- Re-evaluate the patient's nursing and health care needs
- Initiate the plan of care and complete any necessary revisions
- Furnish those services requiring substantial and specialized nursing skills
- Initiate appropriate preventive and rehabilitative nursing procedures
- Review and assess for home safety
- Prepare the clinical and progress notes
- Coordinate the required services, especially those needed from other health care professionals and/or paraprofessionals
- Inform the physician and other personnel of changes in the patient's condition and needs
- Counsel the patient and family in meeting nursing and related needs
- Review medications
- Provide health instruction
- Supervise other personnel
- Evaluate patient's progress over time and examine whether the allocated number of home care visits is appropriate

G. Often, the home care case manager is a registered nurse. Responsibilities of the visiting nurse case manager include those shared in Box 7-4 in addition to the functions described in Box 7-5, if the visiting nurse and the case manager are the same person. Sometimes, the case manager is another member of the team and is not involved in direct care provision; rather, the case manager facilitates and manages the care virtually and with occasional home care visit(s) for patient's assessment and follow-up as warranted. In this case, the responsibilities are limited to those in Box 7-5, although there is always overlap in roles with the home care nurse.

H. The home care case manager assures that the health care team involved in the care of the home care patient includes the following:
1. Patient and patient's support system (e.g., family, friends, and caregivers)
2. Patient's physicians (primary and specialty care providers)
3. Other health professionals as indicated by the patient's condition and plan of care (e.g., physical therapists, pharmacist, holistic care specialist)
4. Other community-based providers (e.g., clergy or chaplain) and services (e.g., meals on wheels).

BOX 7-5   Functions of Home Care Case Managers

- Educate the patient, family, caregiver(s), and members of the health care team about treatment options, community resources, insurance benefits, self-management, and other concerns.
- Advocate for and assist the patient/family in obtaining the care they need—whether in the hospital or at home—and doing this in a timely way to ensure continuity of care and ongoing support for their needs.
- Ensure that a comprehensive care plan is in place and that it addresses all of the issues the patient and family are dealing with, not just the medical illness or condition.
- Establish and maintain regular contact with the patient and family and other members of the health care team and maintain communication among the parties.
- Serve as a liaison between the patient, the patient's physician, the home care agency and other health care providers, the health insurance plan/payer (e.g., Medicare, Medicaid, or a private company), and the employer (if applicable) to identify and obtain the services needed.
- Coordinate the necessary services and community resources that will help the patient return to the best physical function, health, and well-being possible.
- Focus home care activities on self-determination and work to safely move the individual to self-care whenever possible.
- Supervise any transition to another care setting in as timely, safe, and complete a manner as possible.
- Review the patient's health insurance plan and benefits and assure that the services provided are consistent with the plan's rules and procedures, for example, authorization for services and use of contracted providers if commercial insurance plan.
- Assist the patient and family in navigating the health care system.
- Oversee the quality data collection and submission to regulatory and other private agencies as necessary.
- Identify and engage in opportunities for performance improvement.

I. The home care nurse case manager determines the specific medical needs of the patient, ensures these are addressed in the home care plan, and coordinates their delivery. These may include skilled nursing care, a home health aide, a personal assistant, therapy, medication management, and medical supplies. The care plan must be comprehensive and include input from a variety of medical and health disciplines as well as incorporate the needs of the client's family.

Reimbursement for Home Health Care Services

A. Reimbursement for home health care services varies based on the health insurance plans the patients carry. Some follow the commercial or private insurance (e.g., managed care organizations) reimbursement methods; others apply the Medicare or Medicaid payment systems; while others are self-pay (Box 7-6).

B. Commercial insurance and managed care reimbursement is dependent on the contractual agreement between the provider and the payer/health insurance plan.
   1. Home care services are provided to enrollees in a commercial health insurance or managed care plan by an agency that is a contracted service provider.
   2. Authorization for home care services is usually expected prior to the delivery of these services.
   3. Patients' and family members' choice of provider is limited to those agencies that have a contractual agreement with the health insurance plan or managed care organization.

C. In 2000, reimbursement by CMS for home care services and visits provided to Medicare beneficiaries was changed to a PPS method.
   1. More visits no longer means higher reimbursement rates.
   2. Unlike the inpatient or hospital-based PPS, reimbursement for home care visits is determined based on a nursing assessment that is completed at the time a patient is admitted into home care services.
   3. Reimbursement is no longer based on the number and type of visits. Home care services are currently reimbursed based on an episode of care or 60 days.
   4. The dollar amount reimbursed is fixed regardless of the number of visits provided. It is determined based on the Outcome and Assessment Information Set (OASIS) score a patient receives.

BOX 7-6   Funding Sources for Home Health Care Case Management Services

- Private payers, such as employer-sponsored health insurance plans
- Medicaid, which includes options that allow for nonmedical services (e.g., the Medicaid Rehabilitation Option)
- Medicare and Supplemental Security Income (SSI) for disabled clients
- Social service providers (e.g., child welfare agencies)
- Private foundations and funds, such as United Way
- Private pay—fees may be billed directly to the individual who is using home care case management services

7-7 Circumstance of Special Medicare Payments for Home Care

1. If there is an interruption of service due to a patient's request for transfer from one home health agency to another before the conclusion of the 60 days of service. In this case, a partial episode payment is deemed appropriate.
2. If a patient is discharged from home care and then returns to the same agency within the 60-day period. In this case, a partial episode payment is considered appropriate—but only if the discharge from or return to service was not related to a significant change in the patient's condition.
3. If the patient experiences a change in condition that results in change in medical orders and course of treatment and ultimately leads to a change in the OASIS score or the hGHr assignment. In this case, a significant change in condition payment is deemed appropriate.
4. If a patient requires a minimal number of home care visits (e.g., five visits or fewer) during the 60-day period due to low acuity and resource utilization. In this case, a low-utilization payment is considered appropriate and the reimbursement is calculated based on the national standard per visit per discipline amount.
5. When unusual variations occur in the amount of medically necessary home health services. In this case, an outlier payment is considered appropriate.

---

     5. OASIS scores are determined based on three categories: clinical, financial, and service utilization.
     6. The OASIS score results in the assignment of the patient into one of 80 HHRGs. Each HHRG has a predetermined dollar amount attached to it.
  D. A CHHA may submit claims to Medicare for reimbursement on two occasions:
     1. An initial claim or a request for advance payment—completed upon admission of a patient into home care services and completion of the initial assessment of the patient (i.e., performing an initial OASIS assessment and score). The amount is limited to a maximum of 60% of the HHRG-designated rate.
     2. A final claim or request for payment—completed at the end of an episode of services and includes all line-item home care visit information or types of services rendered during the customary 60 days of service.
  E. Special payment rates by Medicare occur in five occasions including those described in Box 7-7.

Home Care Nursing Services

  A. When appropriate, home care services can extend the care of the hospital-based interdisciplinary health care team beyond the hospital boundaries and reduce length of stay or provide an alternative to institution-based custodial and skilled care.
  B. As an extension of hospital-based care, short-term home care services are reimbursable under Medicare benefits and many health plans offered by private insurance companies.
  C. Medicare and most health plans offered by private insurance companies may not provide long-term care or custodial care benefits; therefore, these services will not be reimbursed.

D. Medicaid, however, reimburses for long-term care and custodial care and therefore in some areas will reimburse for these same services at home.

E. To be reimbursable, short-term home care services must be medically necessary and for a limited period of time.
   1. Medicare requires that the condition of the patient presents a need for skilled services of a registered nurse, social worker, or therapist. In addition, services may include those provided by a registered nutritionist or a paraprofessional nursing aide.
      a. In some states such as New York, these aides are licensed as home health aides and follow a treatment plan performing tasks assigned by a registered nurse.
      b. Home health aides are trained to measure and report vital signs and assist patients with the activities of daily living to enable them to remain safely at home.

F. Long-term home care services may involve the same services as short-term home care; however, they also may involve transportation and use of a less-skilled paraprofessional personal care assistant.
   1. In some states such as New York, these assistants are licensed as home attendants.
   2. Personal care assistants are only permitted to assist with the activities of daily living that will enable the patient to remain safely at home.
   3. Over time, the CMS has permitted various demonstration projects in long-term home care, called "nursing homes without walls." Examples are the PACE program, which started in San Francisco and New York, and the Managed Long-Term Care Program.

G. The third type of home care services widely available in the United States is hospice care.
   1. Initially started by Dame Cicely Saunders when she opened St. Christopher's Hospital in London, the hospice movement spread to the United States as a volunteer nurse's program humanely caring for dying patients at home in the 1960s and 1970s. Hospice became a standard of care when the Congress adopted the Medicare reimbursement for home hospice services in 1983.
   2. Hospice care as determined by the Medicare regulations includes nursing, pastoral care, social work, and volunteer services.
   3. Hospice care also includes reimbursement for bereavement services, most often provided by social workers or volunteers, to the survivors (e.g., family members) for 13 months following the death of the patient.
   4. Hospice care allows inpatient care for symptom control or respite care relief for caregivers of the terminally ill individual. Inpatient care is at a length of stay determined by the hospice. Hospice care also covers services that are related to the terminal illness.

Home Care Rehabilitation Services

A. Rehabilitation therapy in the home is provided by a licensed physical therapist, occupational therapist, or speech therapist.

B. The goal of rehabilitation therapy is to maximize the patient's level of functioning to improve quality of life and avoid unnecessary readmission to the acute care/hospital setting.

C. Physical therapy includes therapeutic exercises, balance activities, and ambulation training that will help the patient regain functional mobility and motor skills.

D. Occupational therapists use motor, cognitive, perceptual, and sensory exercises and tasks to help improve the patient's ability to perform activities of daily living.

E. Speech/language therapists help patients improve their ability to produce and understand speech as well as help with communication skills. They also assist with swallowing disorders.

F. Professional therapists increase the value of home care services by providing therapy in the home where the patient lives. They can assess the patient, teach safety precautions and techniques, and provide exercise routines that work in the patient's home. Social workers may also be involved and provide the patient and/or family with counseling services especially for coping with major life changing events such as catastrophic illness or injury.

G. Case managers must be aware of these services and their purposes so that they can best incorporate them into the case management plans of care for their patients.

H. Case managers are effective in discussing the patient's need for these services with members of the interdisciplinary health care team and in incorporating such services into the patient's case management plan of care.

I. Case managers in the home care setting also follow up on the outcomes of these services for their specific patients and revise the home care plan of care accordingly to meet the patient's specific needs.

Durable Medical Equipment and Other Services

A. Many homes are not equipped to provide short-term or long-term patient care. Such situations warrant the use of durable medical equipment (DME) such as a hospital bed, wheelchair, glucose monitoring device, etc. Case managers facilitate the acquisition of equipment and monitoring devices, or other technologies as needed by the patients.

B. An important role for the hospital-based interdisciplinary health care team is to help the patient and family obtain the equipment and supplies they will need to ensure the success of home-based care.

C. DME, including hospital bed, walker, cane, portable oxygen, wheelchair, commode, tub chair, transfer bench, grab bars, stairs lifts, oxygen canisters, and concentrators, can be ordered and delivered to the patient's home prior to the patient's discharge from the hospital to ensure continuity of care and comfort when the patient arrives home.
   1. Sometimes, the DME is delivered to the patient while in the hospital (e.g., glucose monitoring device or wheelchair), at the time of discharge, in order for the case manager to ensure a safe transition to home.
   2. Sometimes, the DME is delivered to the patient's home (e.g., hospital bed) or installed in the patient's home (e.g., stairs lift) prior to discharge from acute care setting.

D. Supplies such as diapers, chucks, diabetic, wound and ostomy supplies, nebulizers, intravenous tubing, syringes, and even medications can be ordered prior to the patient's discharge for home delivery as a way to ensure continuity of care and comfort. This is especially true of newer medications, expensive medications, or less-often-used medications.

E. Case managers may alert patients and their families as well as the health care team that particular doses of pain medication or blood thinners, such as Lovenox, may not be available in all strengths at all pharmacies. In such situations, they negotiate the ordering of appropriate dosages or types of medications.

F. Case managers may educate patients and families and members of the health care teams about the variety of services provided in the varied patients' communities and provide them with lists of these services and contact information.

G. Case managers may not only teach patients about the choices available but also empower them to seek additional services and equipment as the patient's condition changes and new needs arise.

 ## Home Care Social Work Services

A. Although hospital social workers may be responsible for the completion of psychosocial assessments and the development of appropriate posthospital discharge plans, many times in the current health care environment, length of stay has shortened to the point that it is difficult to find time to educate patients and families about the range of social services available to them, let alone make appropriate referrals and have time to follow-up.

B. Social workers who come to the patient's home in the context of home care services usually are able to obtain additional important information about the patients' conditions including their home environment, social network, and caregivers. Such information is made available to them as they walk through the door as they are able to observe the condition of the home environment and the patient's living situation, and most of the time is not as apparent to the hospital-based colleagues.

C. Home visiting social workers can assist the patient in completing the patient's portion of the referral processes and follow-up. The fact that the patient is at home and has access to important documents and files facilitates this work.

D. Home visiting social workers also are able to assess why a particular referral may not have worked and assist the client in obtaining needed services through subsequent referrals.

E. Home care social workers can help families to identify strengths, overcome obstacles, and provide better care, which may result in improved outcomes for patients and their families.

F. As short-term home care services are about to be terminated, community-based social workers reassess patients and assist them, the interdisciplinary health care team, and family in developing the next plan of care. They may find it necessary to expand services or to adjust the type of services needed based on the patient's condition.

G. Plans of care may include transitioning the patient to long-term home care services, hospice services, or institutionalized care.

H. Adequate home care discharge or transition plans not only prevent the need for hospital readmissions or emergency services but also can optimize the patients' quality of life by helping them and their families to transition easily to new care plans.

The Role of the Hospital-Based Case Manager

A. The role of the hospital-based case manager varies from hospital to hospital depending on the ways the hospital, the case management program leaders, and the individual case managers have divided the work.

B. When the case manager or any member of the interdisciplinary team has identified a patient who would benefit from home care services, and the patient and family have agreed to a discharge plan that includes home care services, the patient/family must be educated about the agencies that offer the services recommended by the team so that they can identify the preferred agency. Next, the case manager facilitates the referral and the service brokerage process.

C. The Balanced Budget Act of 1996 requires that all patients be provided with written information about home health care, such as a list of agencies providing services in their area. The case manager may:
   1. Make the list available to patients
   2. Use the list to educate patients and their families about the role of the insurance company/health plan in authorizing and managing the home care services
   3. Inform patients of the procedures applied by managed care organizations in securing home care services, such as the use of preferred contracts and limits on the number of visits per calendar year.

D. When a home care agency has been selected and patient's permission for the release of medical information has been obtained, it is important for the case manager to consult with the indicated home care provider to confirm that the agency has a contract with the insurer (i.e., payer) and to discover whether the requested services are available through the agency.

E. In these times of growing shortages of professional nurses and therapists, case managers not only must check to see whether services are offered by the selected agency but also need to clarify that the agency has adequate personnel to deliver the needed services in a timely fashion and as the case management plan requires.
   1. Rehabilitation therapies following joint replacement, laboratory tests for Coumadin levels, and patient education about new medications or reinforcement of hospital-based diabetic education are three examples of services that must be delivered in a timely fashion.
   2. Serious complications in the patient's health condition may occur if home health care services are delayed. Complications in turn may warrant the patient's return to the hospital setting. Such return is considered avoidable readmission.

F. The case manager can facilitate the communication between the patient, family members, and the home health care agency. This communication is essential so that the patient and family know what is expected of them and the agency knows what the patient and family expects.

G. It is also important for the case manager to ask the agency and the insurer whether the patient is responsible for any costs associated with home care services and promptly relay the information to the patient and the family. It is also necessary to review with patients what home care is *not* about and go over their expectations.

   1. One type of cost is insurance policy deductible. If, for example, patients have Medicare benefits and have been hospitalized under the Medicare benefits, they will have already met their Medicare deductible.

   2. However, if a patient is hospitalized under the insurance policy of a spouse but the insurance company has refused to authorize home care services, then the astute case manager would make the patient aware of this and perhaps use the patient's Medicare benefit, if available.

   3. Many private insurance policies utilize per visit co-payments to discourage overuse of benefits. This strategy to reduce home care costs has been suggested but not approved for Medicare at this time.

H. The case manager should communicate with the community physician (e.g., primary care provider) responsible for the patient's follow-up and be sure that the community doctor is in agreement with the plan of care developed by the hospital-based interdisciplinary health care team, the patient, the family, and the home care agency.

I. The handoff of information is not only a courtesy but also provides continuity of care for the patient and provides the agency with ongoing physician orders for medical treatment that allows for a safe transition of care for the patient.

The Role of the Community-Based Case Manager

A. Community-based case management programs have evolved in response to changes in the health care delivery system and to mainly meet the needs of the disabled and noninstitutionalized elderly. Also recently, these programs have become more popular because of the following:

   1. Enactment of the Patient Protection and Affordable Care Act of 2010
   2. Value-based purchasing program
   3. Hospital Readmissions Reduction Program
   4. Reduction in reimbursement for hospital-based care.

B. Community-based case management is intended to improve the lives of high-risk patients through outreach, screening, and risk reduction programs.

C. The main purposes of community-based case management programs are care planning, continuity of care and services, and follow-up care.

D. Home care–based nurses and social workers work closely with community-based case managers who monitor the patient's medical and psychosocial progress, referrals, and interventions.

E. No one profession can be responsible to provide all the services a patient may need. Both social workers and nurses have different professional skills and talents. When working collaboratively, each brings a unique perspective within his/her discipline and then reaches across to improve patient care—when the focus is on the patient/client and not on professional self-image, the combination of the two worlds is dynamite.

Savings, Safety, and Satisfaction

A. Home care can provide savings to the health care system in two ways:
   1. By reducing the length of stay in the acute inpatient settings
   2. By reducing the length of stay in custodial or other institutional inpatient settings such as skilled nursing facilities.
B. As private and public insurance and institutional costs are controlled, it should never be forgotten that these reductions are possible not by eliminating costs but by shifting the burden of care from the health care system to the family.
C. Most families are ready, willing, and able to shoulder this burden, but case managers must never take their contribution for granted.
D. The most important issue of home care today is patient safety.
   1. When people have spent time in the acute care hospital setting, the inpatient acute rehabilitation unit, or the skilled nursing facility, they have been cared for by professional and paraprofessional staff around the clock. During such times, they develop, even after a short while, a type of dependency on the health care professional.
   2. No matter what pressures might exist to reduce patient stay and no matter how much patients may wish to return to the home setting, the only successful home care plan is a safe plan.
   3. Individuals who cannot ambulate, readily speak, or understand the speech of others, or are demented, cannot be safely left alone. If family members are not ready, willing, and able to stay with these individuals 24 hours a day, 7 days a week (or hire help), they cannot be safely discharged home.
E. Most patients are safer in their own homes surrounded by the loving care of their family and friends than in unfamiliar institutional settings.
F. If the patient, the family, the community physician, home care agency, and the interdisciplinary team have communicated effectively and developed a safe plan, there can be no more satisfying plan than home care.
G. Timely and expeditious transfer of a patient from the acute care/hospital to home care setting may reduce the risk of nosocomial illnesses— illnesses developed from a hospital-borne infection.
H. Home care encourages greater independence and promotes recovery by allowing patients to resume some parts of their ordinary life before they are completely healed. As a result, the patient and the family may feel more satisfied to be in their home environment while continuing to recover.
I. Home care also encourages loving care by family and friends rather than limiting care to visiting hours.
J. Home care can help reduce Medicare and Medicaid expenditures by caring for people in their homes and by reducing the number of far more costly days in skilled nursing facilities or hospitals.

Reference

Case Management Society of America (CMSA). (2010). *CMSA standards of practice for case management*. Little Rock, AR: Author.

CHAPTER 8

Case Management in the Palliative and Hospice Care Settings

Hussein M. Tahan

LEARNING OBJECTIVES

Upon completion of this chapter, the reader will be able to:

1. Understand the difference between palliative, hospice, and end-of-life care.

2. Recognize how case management practice applies to palliative, hospice, and end-of-life care issues.

3. Describe patient identification and criteria for palliative versus hospice care services.

4. Explain the main principles and scope of services for palliative and hospice care programs.

5. Describe the role of the case manager in the palliative, hospice, and end-of-life care settings.

IMPORTANT TERMS AND CONCEPTS

Advance Directives
Advance Care Planning
End-of-Life Care
Five Wishes Form
Futile Care
Good Death
Health Care Proxy
Hospice Care

Interdisciplinary
  Health Care Team
Palliative Care
Physician Orders for
  Life-Sustaining
  Treatment
Primary Palliative Care
  Level

Self-Determination
Specialty Palliative
  Care Level

Introduction

A. For more than 40 years, the venue for end-of-life care has been the hospice setting. Due to multiple barriers, hospice has been underutilized in the United States. However, since the enactment of the Patient Protection and Affordable Care Act in 2010, attention to end-of-life care issues and use of hospice and palliative care services have been increasing.

1. The majority of health care organizations have advanced the way these approaches to care are made available to the patients and support systems they serve.

2. For example, most acute care hospitals have established palliative care teams that are easily accessible for better patient care and ultimately quality of life.

B. Studies have consistently demonstrated that when patients are asked about their desires for end-of-life care, they indicate that they wish to die peacefully, with dignity and free of physical symptoms, and they do not want to die alone. They also share their preference to receive care that is person centered and in accordance with personal (especially spiritual) beliefs and in ways that honor the individual's life, culture, and value system and do not present a burden to the family, friends, and support system.

C. Over the past several years, demand for palliative and hospice care has grown tremendously. Palliative care and hospice care are provided across a variety of health care settings and professional disciplines. These areas of health care will continue to grow as the American population continues to age and seek desired alternatives to having their health care services met.

D. Since the advent of Education on Palliative and End-of-life Care (EPEC) and End-of-life Nursing Education Consortium (ELNEC), there has been an increasing understanding of the importance of symptom control (e.g., pain management and comfort care), advanced care planning, hospice care and patient's preferences, quality of life, and end-of-life care.

E. One long-standing barrier has been the lack of understanding by patients and health care providers, including physicians, about Medicare benefits for hospice and palliative care and misperception that palliative and end-of-life care are for individuals who are left with a limited number of days or weeks to live.

F. With the explosive growth of palliative care in hospitals and fledgling growth in the community, there has been further confusion with respect to the two levels of palliative care: primary and specialty care levels. Case managers must be aware of these levels and educate other health care team members and patients.

NOTE: This chapter is a revised version of Chapter 7 in the second edition of *CMSA Core Curriculum for Case Management*. The contributor wishes to acknowledge the work of Layla J. Correoso and Linda Santiago, as some of the timeless material was retained from the previous version.

G. The impact of increased cost to consumers and decreased insurance coverage for service delivery including Medicare capitation for end-stage illness has increased the need for palliative and hospice services in the community.
  1. Reimbursement capitation has led to the need for utilization of cost containment strategies to improve the efficiency and quality of services to those clients with end-stage illnesses.
  2. An example of such strategies is the coordination and management of service through palliative care and hospice programs.
H. The number of palliative care and hospice programs has grown in recent years in response to the growth in the population living with chronic, debilitating, and life-threatening illnesses. For example, in 2013, the number of hospice programs has grown to over 5,800 compared to 5,560 in 2012 (NHPCO, 2014).
I. Timely referrals to palliative care programs and hospice result in beneficial effects on patients' symptoms, reduced hospital costs, a greater likelihood of death at home rather than at an institutionalized facility, and a higher level of patient and family satisfaction than does conventional care.

 Descriptions of Key Terms

A. Advance directive—Legally executed document that explains the patient's health care–related wishes and decisions. It is drawn up while the patient is still competent and is used if the patient becomes incapacitated or incompetent.
B. Advance care planning—Involves multiple steps designed to help individuals learn about the health care options that are available for end-of-life care, determine which types of care best fit their personal wishes, and share their wishes with family, friends, and their physicians.
C. End-of-life care—Care provided by the health care team during the last few months of a person's life and when experiencing an end-stage illness that is life threatening or steadily progressing toward death. It is an integrated, patient-centered/family-centered and compassionate approach to care that is guided by a sense of respect for one's dignity and comfort. It also addresses the unique needs of patients and their families at a time when life-prolonging interventions are no longer considered appropriate or effective.
D. Futile care—The continued provision of medical care, treatments, and interventions to a patient where the prognosis is poor and when there is no reasonable hope of a cure or benefit.
E. Good death—Death that is free from avoidable distress and suffering for patients and their families and in accordance with the patient's and family's wishes. It is care that is considered reasonable and consistent with clinical, cultural, and ethical standards of care.
F. Health care proxy—A legal document that directs whom the health care provider/agency should contact for approval/consent of treatment decisions or options when the patient is no longer deemed competent to decide for himself or herself.
G. Hospice care—A model of quality and compassionate care at the end of life. It focuses on caring not curing and the belief that each person has the right to die pain free and with dignity.

H. Palliative care—A health care approach that seeks to provide the best possible quality of life for people with chronically progressive or life-threatening illnesses and in accordance with their particular values, beliefs, needs, and preferences.

I. Patient self-determination—Making treatment decisions, such as designating a health care proxy, establishing advance directives, deciding to refuse or discontinue care, and choosing to not be resuscitated or to withdraw nutritional support.

J. Primary palliative and hospice care level—Palliative and hospice care provided by the same health care team responsible for routine care of the patient's life-threatening or life-limiting illness.

K. Specialty palliative and hospice care level—Palliative and hospice care provided by a specialized health care team, with appropriately trained and credentialed professionals, such as physicians, nurses, social workers, chaplains, and others.

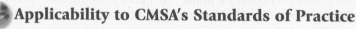

Applicability to CMSA's Standards of Practice

A. The Case Management Society of America (CMSA) describes in its standards of practice for case management that case management extends across all health care settings, including payer, provider, government, employer, community, and home environment, and various patient populations (CMSA, 2010). Effective palliative and hospice programs are those available in these various settings, thus, allowing case managers the opportunity to be actively involved in the care of this special population at the various stages of illness.

B. The number of adults who face a life-limiting or progressively worsening chronic disease(s) continues to rise. It is estimated that 90 million people in the United States live with at least one chronic illness, and 7 out of 10 die people from chronic disease (Wennberg, 2008). Some of these patients may benefit from palliative or hospice care, and case managers can assist in ensuring patient's access to such services.

C. Similar to case management practice and programs described in CMSA's standards, palliative care and hospice care are provided in a variety of care settings, such as the following:
   1. The patient's home
   2. Freestanding hospice centers
   3. Hospitals
   4. Skilled care facilities and nursing homes
   5. Long-term care facilities
   6. Ambulatory care clinics
   7. Residential facilities

D. Palliative and hospice care and services are beneficial to patients with any terminal illness or of any age, gender, religion, or race. The population served by palliative and hospice care is naturally a subset of that served by case managers. Therefore, case managers must be knowledgeable in identifying the patients who would benefit from these specialized services and facilitate timely access to them. They can apply the CMSA standards of practice for case management in this area of specialty practice.

E. The goal to maintain the best quality of life is important for every patient diagnosed with a life-limiting illness such as cancer. Research, however, shows that people with a terminal diagnosis often either do not receive palliative care or hospice or, if offered, it is too late in the course of the disease to make an impact on patient care outcomes including experience of care (Temel et al., 2010). Case managers in their roles almost in every health care setting are able to change this and enhance patient's timely access to palliative and hospice care.

F. Although the CMSA standard of practice pertaining to ethics applies to all aspects of case managers' practice and case management programs, it has specific and sensitive applicability when caring for patients with end-of-life issues and those with complex, chronic, and terminal illnesses.

1. Case managers must recognize that their primary obligation is to their patients. In this case, they must facilitate patients' access to timely palliative and hospice care and services. They also are obligated to educate patients and their families about such care options.

2. Case managers as patient/family advocates assure that the rights and wishes of patients and their families for certain care options, including palliative and hospice care, are respected.

3. Case managers respect patients' cultural values and beliefs, including their views on palliative and hospice care, while providing patient-centered care and services.

Palliative Care

A. Palliative care can be integral to end-of-life care in that it generally focuses on managing symptoms and providing comfort to patients and their families. While palliative care is common among people receiving end-of-life care, it is not necessarily restricted to people with terminal illnesses.

B. Palliative care is both a philosophy of care and an organized, highly structured care delivery system. The recent increase in popularity of palliative care has challenged the traditional assumption that more intensive and acute care is better for the management of patients with multiple chronic illnesses and that such means better care and enhances patient/family satisfaction.

C. Today, palliative care has demonstrated that it provides quality and safe care and improves outcomes (Box 8-1).

D. Palliative care can be delivered by an interdisciplinary health care team concurrently with medical life-prolonging measures or as the main focus of care. It may begin at the time a life-threatening, life-limiting, or debilitating illness or injury is diagnosed and continues through care or until after the patient's death—that is, into the family's bereavement period.

E. Palliative care is best defined as an interdisciplinary and system of care that aims to relieve suffering and improve quality of life for patients with advanced illness and their families. It is offered *simultaneously with all other appropriate medical treatment* (Meier, 2006) (Fig. 8-1).

1. It can be provided at any stage of progressively chronic illness even along with curative measures.

2. It may include hospice care even at the final stages of a chronic illness.

BOX 8-1 Benefits of Palliative Care Services

Palliative care is known to:
- Provide care consistent with patient's values and preferences.
- Lessen or relieve the pain chronically ill patients experience and other physical, emotional, and psychological suffering.
- Treat patients' symptoms effectively.
- Support patients' psychological and emotional needs.
- Provide patients and their families with support in making complex decisions.
- Improve overall patients' care and reduce its related cost.
- Facilitate smoother, timely, and safer transition from one setting to another more appropriate.
- Enhance patient and family satisfaction with and experience of care.
- Facilitate the coordination of services and safe and effective transition or discharge plans.
- Promote open and timely communication among health care team members and with patient and family.

From the Institute for Clinical Symptoms Improvement (ICSI). (2013). *A business case for providing palliative care services across the continuum of care.* Bloomington, MN: ICSI.

F. Palliative care involves addressing the physical, intellectual, emotional, social, and spiritual needs of patients and their families. It facilitates the patient's autonomy, self-determination, access to critical information, and right to choice of care and treatment options.

G. Palliative care programs aim to improve or optimize the quality of life for patients with advanced illness in collaboration with their families and caregivers. This is achieved by anticipating, preventing, and treating suffering.

H. The delivery of palliative care may occur in the setting of the administration of life-prolonging therapy (e.g., acute care/hospital stay) or in a setting where the sole aim is amelioration of suffering (e.g., patient's home or a hospice facility).

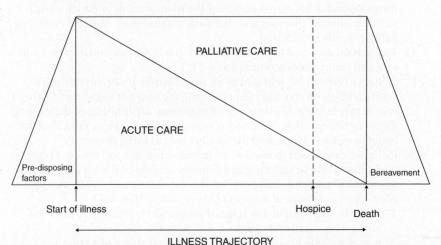

FIGURE 8-1. Palliative and hospice care across the continuum of health and illness.

I. Palliative care may require end-of-life care and services. The delivery of such services necessitates the involvement of health care professionals who possess specialized skills, knowledge, and competencies in caring for the terminally ill at the end stage of illness or when nearing death.

J. Medicare's hospice benefit also covers palliative care for beneficiaries with terminal illness.

Hospice Care

A. Hospice care is a service delivery system that provides comprehensive and compassionate care for patients suffering from a terminal illness and who have a limited life expectancy—generally 6 months or less if the disease follows its usual course.

   1. The hospice population includes a subset of palliative care patients who have entered the end-of-life stage of their illness.

   2. The care is patient centered and extends to the care of the family unit as well. Family is often defined by the patient.

   3. Care requires comprehensive biomedical, psychosocial, and spiritual support, especially during the final stage of illness.

   4. Hospice care supports family members coping with the complex consequences of illness as death nears, as well as post death during the bereavement phase.

B. The hospice benefit is designed to cover the needs of a patient with respect to physician services, medications, durable medical equipment, nursing services, home health aid, social services, and spiritual care. Essentially, costs are related to the services required to care for the terminal diagnosis for which a patient is on hospice care.

   1. For terminally ill Medicare beneficiaries who do not want to pursue curative treatment, Medicare offers a comprehensive hospice benefit covering an array of services, including nursing care, counseling, palliative medications, and up to 5 days of respite care to assist family caregivers.

   2. Medicare patients who elect the hospice benefit have little to no cost-sharing liabilities for most hospice services.

   3. In order to qualify for hospice coverage under Medicare, a physician must confirm that the patient is expected to die within 6 months if the illness runs a normal course. If the Medicare patient lives longer than 6 months, hospice coverage may continue if the physician and the hospice team recertify the eligibility criteria.

C. Home is considered the patient's residence and is not necessarily limited to a "typical" home setting. Home could also be a nursing home, jail or prison, hospice residence, or assisted living facility.

D. The National Hospice and Palliative Care Organization (NHPCO) has estimated that about 1.6 million patients received hospice care or services in 2013. It also estimated that about 1.1 million patients died in 2013 while under hospice care (NHPCO, 2014). The number of those who received hospice care in 2013 is small considering the estimated 90 million people in the United States who are living with one or more complex and chronic illness.

E. The National Hospice and Palliative Care Organization also reported that 84% of those who received hospice care in 2013 were 65 years of age or older (about 41% being 85 years or older). It also estimated that 1% of hospice care recipients were pediatric and young adults—25 years of age or younger (NHPCO, 2014).

F. Hospice statistics continue to demonstrate that one of the barriers to receiving good hospice care is late referrals.
1. Patients are often not referred until the last few days or weeks of life as opposed to earlier when they would be able to benefit more fully from the end-of-life care and services that are offered to them and their family (e.g., palliative care).
2. The reasons for late referrals are multifactorial and may include but are not limited to those shared in Box 8-2.

G. With the improvement in the level of education of case management staff, including case managers, about the barriers to hospice care, it is hoped that better communication, collaboration, and coordination of care will move patients upstream early for palliative and hospice care referrals.

H. The barrier most commonly encountered by health care providers, including case managers, is timely identification of patients with chronic illnesses who have entered into the end-stage phase of the disease trajectory.
1. Patients with cancer are more easily identifiable.
2. Patients with end-stage illnesses other than cancer are not easily recognized.

I. The National Hospice and Palliative Care Organization has guidelines that are used to select patients that are appropriate for hospice care. (These are available at www.nhpco.org.)

J. Recent educational efforts have tried to simplify for health care providers the identification of appropriate patients for hospice or palliative care. As a rule of thumb, health care providers have been encouraged to ask themselves "Would you be surprised if this patient died within the next 6 months to a year?" If you would not be surprised, then the patient could be receiving palliative care measures or hospice benefits.

BOX 8-2   Reasons for Late Patient Referrals to Hospice Care

- Physicians' and/or other providers' overly optimistic views of their patients' prognoses.
- Reluctance of physicians to provide bad news to patients and their families/caregivers.
- Physicians and/or other providers do not discuss hospice as an option for care at the end of life.
- Misperception that hospice care is only necessary within few days of a patient's imminent death.
- Lack of knowledge or expertise in hospice care.
- Hospice (and palliative) care not viewed as a legitimate medical specialty by some providers.
- Lack of availability of hospice care team or experts in this area of practice.
- Patient and/or family disagreeing or uncomfortable yet with hospice care.
- Lack of or limited resources.

BOX 8-3   Karnofsky Performance Status Scale Use for Hospice and Palliative Care

Definitions Rating (%) Criteria
The Karnofsky Performance Scale Index allows patients to be classified as to their functional impairment. This can be used to compare effectiveness of different therapies and to assess the prognosis in individual patients. The lower the Karnofsky score, the worse the survival for most serious illnesses.

Able to carry on normal activity and work; no special care needed
100   Normal, no complaints; no evidence of disease
90   Able to carry on normal activity or do active work; minimal signs or symptoms of disease
80   Normal activity with effort; some signs or symptoms of disease

Unable to work; able to live at home and care for most personal needs; varying amount of assistance needed
70   Cares for self; unable to carry on normal activity or do active work
60   Requires occasional assistance, but is able to care for most personal needs
50   Requires considerable assistance and frequent medical care

Unable to care for self; requires equivalent of institutional or hospital care; disease may be progressing rapidly
40   Disabled; requires special care and assistance
30   Severely disabled; hospital admission is indicated although death is not imminent
20   Very sick; hospital admission necessary; active supportive treatment necessary
10   Moribund; fatal processes progressing rapidly
0   Dead

Adapted from Doyle, D., Hanks, G., Cherny, N., & Calman, K. (Eds.) (1993). *Oxford textbook of palliative medicine* (p. 109). Oxford, UK: Oxford University Press, with permission.

K. For more detailed information about identification of patients to benefit from hospice and palliative care, refer to Boxes 8-3 and 8-4. Once the patient has been identified, plans for case management of this patient can be developed.
L. Many studies suggest that medical care for patients with serious and advanced illnesses is characterized by the undertreatment of symptoms (e.g., pain, labored breathing, anxiety, insomnia), conflicts about decision making regarding care options, inadequate support for patients/ families, and inadequate utilization of resources.
M. Deficits in care provider's support for palliative and hospice care services include palliation of symptoms, rehabilitation, combination of life-prolonging treatments (when possible and appropriate), support for families, and advanced care planning.
N. Several studies have demonstrated that the personal and practical care needs of patients who are seriously ill and their families are not adequately addressed by routine office visits or hospital and nursing home stays and that this failure results in substantial burdens—medical, psychological, and financial—on patients and their caregivers (Meier, 2006; Temel et al., 2010).

(*text continues on page 205*)

BOX 8-4 Common Indicators of End-Stage Disease

The patient may exhibit one or more of the following core and disease-specific indicators.

Core Indicators
- Physical and functional decline
- Weight loss
- Multiple comorbidities
- Serum albumin <2.5 g/dL
- Dependence in most ADLs
- Karnofsky score ≤50%
- Desire/will to die

Amyotrophic Lateral Sclerosis
Unable to walk, needs assistance with ADLs
Barely intelligible speech
Difficulty swallowing
Nutritional status down
Declines feeding tube
Significant dyspnea, on O_2 at rest
Declines assisted ventilation
Medical complications—pneumonia, upper respiratory infection, sepsis

Cerebrovascular Accident and Coma
Level of consciousness down; coma
Persistent vegetative state
Dysphagia age >70
Paralysis poststroke dementia
Nutritional status down (despite feeding tube if present)
Medical complications up
Family wants palliative care

Debility Unspecified
Multiple comorbidities with no primary diagnosis
Emphasis on core indicators

Dementia
Unable to walk without assistance
Urinary and fecal incontinence
Speech limited to ≤6 words/day
Unable to dress without assistance
Unable to sit up or hold head up
Complications—aspiration pneumonia, urinary tract infection, sepsis, decubitus ulcers
Difficulty swallowing/eating
Nutritional status down
Weight loss

Failure to Thrive
Body Mass Index ≤22 kg/m²
Declining enteral/parenteral support
Not responding to nutritional support
Karnofsky score ≤40%

8-4   Common Indicators of End-Stage Disease

Heart Disease/Congestive Heart Failure
NYHA class IV
Ejection fraction $\leq$20%
Discomfort with physical activity
Symptomatic despite maximal medical management with diuretics and vasodilators
Arrhythmias resistant to treatment
History of cardiac arrest
Cardiogenic embolic CVA

Liver Disease
No liver transplant
PT >5 s above control
Ascites despite maximum diuretics
Peritonitis
Hepatorenal syndrome
Encephalopathy with asterixis, somnolence, coma
Recurrent variceal bleeding

Pulmonary Disease/Chronic Obstructive Pulmonary Disease
Dyspnea at rest
FEV1 < 30% after bronchodilators
Recurrent pulmonary infections
Cor pulmonale/right heart failure
pO_2 $\leq$55 mm Hg; O_2 sat $\leq$88% (on O_2)
Weight loss >10% in past 6 mo
Resting tachycardia >100/min
pCO_2 >55

Renal Disease
Creatinine clear <10 mL/min (<15 mL/min in diabetics)
No dialysis, no renal transplant
Signs of uremia (confusion, nausea, pruritus, restlessness, pericarditis)
Intractable fluid overload
Oliguria < 40 mL/24 h
Hyperkalemia > 7.0 mEq/L

Note. Visiting Nurse Services of New York (VNSNY). *End stage disease indicators for non-cancer diagnoses: Common indicators of end-stage disease.* Published with permission.

O. Communication is an essential core skill for palliative care. Clear communication leads to the successful assessment and management of pain and other associated symptoms. This starts with the identification of each individual patient's/family's needs (Box 8-5).

P. Hospice care can be provided in four general venues as described below (NHPCO, 2014). Case managers are beneficial in these venues of care provision.

1. Routine or intermittent home-based hospice care at the place where the patient resides. This option is most common today.

2. Continuous home-based hospice care at the place where the patient resides. Licensed health professionals such as nurses provide such care. Sometimes, this option is offered briefly during periods of crises and patient returns to intermittent home-based care or transferred to a hospice facility.

Sample Patient and Family Needs during Hospice or Palliative Care Period

BOX 8-5

- Pain management
- Symptom control (i.e., labored breathing, anxiety, and insomnia) including other routine medical care (e.g., medications, speech, and physical therapy)
- Treatment decision making
- Financial burdens
- Psychological and emotional support
- Caregiver burdens
- Grief and bereavement counseling to surviving family
- Spiritual support, especially in aspects of dying
- Patient-centered care
- Funeral preparation and care of the family post patient's death
- Patient and family instruction about care provision and expectations

3. General inpatient (or hospital) hospice care offered in an inpatient facility especially for pain management and control or for other acute complex symptoms management.
4. Inpatient respite care where the patient receives hospice care on a temporary or short-term basis while providing respite for the patient's family.

 ## Guiding Principles and Goals of Palliative and Hospice Care Programs

A. End-of-life care encompasses all health care provided to someone in the days or years before death, whether the cause of death is sudden or a result of a terminal illness that runs a much longer course.
B. There are general principles that guide palliative and hospice care programs; most common are those in Box 8-6.

 General Guiding Principles for Palliative and Hospice Care

BOX 8-6

- Provision of information to patient and family (or health care professionals) to support care decisions.
- Treating the patient's and family's values, beliefs (cultural and social), and preferences with respect.
- Addressing the total needs of the patient and family—symptom control, especially pain and suffering; psychosocial distress; spiritual issues; social, practical, financial, and legal ramifications of the patient's condition; patient/family education; and bereavement services.
- Care and services are delivered by an interdisciplinary health care team and coordinated by a designated health care professional such as a case manager. Members of the core team are competent and knowledgeable in palliative and hospice care and practices.
- Care and services are administered across all settings of the continuum of care.
- Access to palliative and hospice care is available across care settings and patient populations regardless of ethnicity, race, age, ability to pay, and so on.
- Palliative and hospice care professionals, including case managers, act as advocates for patients and their families.

> ### BOX 8-7   General Goals of Palliative and Hospice Care Programs
>
> - Addressing and controlling pain and other symptoms
> - Promoting advance care planning, especially incorporating the principles of palliative and hospice care in the case management plan and by all members of the health care team, regardless of the care setting
> - Providing patients and their families with the needed information that may be crucial for decision making, especially regarding treatment and care options
> - Advocacy, coordination and facilitation of care activities, especially as patients transition from one level of care/setting into another or from one health care provider to another
> - Preparing both the patient and the family for dignified death when it is anticipated
> - Providing bereavement support to the family after the patient's death
> - Providing palliative and hospice care that is patient and family centered

C. The general goals of palliative and hospice care programs are several (Box 8-7). They focus on enhancing the patient's quality of life and quality of death.

D. Patients with cancer diagnoses continue to be the number one condition of those who receive hospice care. NHPCO reports that 36.5% of hospice admissions were cancer patients (NHPCO, 2014). Box 8-8 lists the diagnoses of patients who tend to receive palliative or hospice care.

E. The Patient Protection and Affordable Care Act of 2010 addresses some aspects of end-of-life care, which has advanced the focus of health care professionals on the use of palliative and hospice care as an option for their terminally ill patients or those with complex chronic and potentially life-limiting illnesses.

F. Although palliative care for the chronically ill is not a universally reimbursable expense, it is a service that hospitals are providing to select patient populations. Hospital executives and other health care professionals deem this service valuable and sustainable because of the overall cost savings in health care expense they are able to achieve.

> ### BOX 8-8   Common Diagnoses of Patients Under Palliative or Hospice Care
>
> - Cancer
> - Dementia
> - Heart disease
> - Progressive pulmonary or lung disease
> - End-stage renal/kidney disease
> - Stroke or coma
> - Liver disease
> - Progressive neurological conditions such as amyotrophic lateral sclerosis (ALS) and Alzheimer disease
> - HIV/AIDS

G. Medicare covers a comprehensive set of health care services that beneficiaries are eligible to receive up until their death. Many of these Medicare-covered services may be used for either curative or palliative (symptom relief) purposes or both.

1. These services include care in hospitals and several other settings, home health care, physician services, diagnostic tests, and prescription drug coverage through a separate Medicare benefit.
2. Medicare beneficiaries with a terminal illness are eligible for the Medicare hospice benefit that includes additional services—not otherwise covered under traditional Medicare—such as bereavement services.

 ## Scope of Palliative and Hospice Care and Services

A. A primary principle in palliative and hospice care is that services are provided seamlessly across all care settings and phases of illness.
1. Palliative care is provided at any stage of a patient's illness.
2. Hospice services are provided to patients who are entering the terminal stages of their illness as a result of a life-threatening or debilitating illness or injury.
3. The patient population receiving palliative and hospice care encompasses individuals of all ages and those with a broad range of diagnostic categories that reduce their life expectancy.

B. Palliative and hospice care is provided in all care settings including those listed below. Length of stay and applicable criteria vary across these various settings; case managers must be aware especially when engaged in developing care plans, discharge, and transition of care plans.
1. Inpatient
    a. Acute care hospitals
    b. Acute and subacute rehabilitation facilities
    c. Dedicated hospice and/or palliative care units within a facility
    d. Freestanding hospice and palliative care facilities
2. Outpatient clinics
3. Chronic care facilities
4. Nursing homes or other skilled nursing facilities
5. Assisted living facilities
6. Boarding care and residential care facilities
7. Home

C. Palliative and hospice care and services are provided at two levels—primary and specialty.
1. The primary level is care provided to the patient by the same interdisciplinary health care team who is responsible for routine care of the terminal illness.
2. The specialty level is care provided by a specialized palliative and hospice care team of "core" health care professionals who are trained and credentialed in such specialties.

D. Health care team members who may be involved in the care of a patient receiving palliative or hospice care may include those listed in Box 8-9.

BOX 8-9   Members of Palliative or Hospice Interdisciplinary Health Care Teams

- Physicians: the patient's primary care provider and the palliative and hospice care specialist
- Nurses
- Hospice aides
- Social workers
- Case managers
- Home health aides
- Therapists: respiratory, physical, occupational, speech
- Chaplains, clergy, or other spiritual counselors
- Psychiatrists, psychologists, or bereavement counselors
- Pharmacists
- Nutritionists
- Trained volunteers
- Administrators

 ## Advance Directives and Health Care Proxies

A. The patient Self-Determination Act has set the tone for health care providers to ensure patients' and families' education about the need for the designation of a health care proxy and the completion of an advance directive. It is necessary for patients to choose a person, or an advocate, to speak on their behalf in the event that they become unresponsive or incompetent. This designation is a necessity whether a person is healthy or has an advanced disease state.

B. An advance directive (AD) is a set of written instructions that, when completed, outlines what types of treatment the patient would or would not desire when faced with a terminal illness.

1. Examples of ADs include a living will, health care proxy, a health care power of attorney, advanced directive to physicians, or a medical directive.

2. These documents are recognized in situations where the patient has been diagnosed to have a terminal illness or condition where treatments would only artificially prolong the process of dying or the patient is in a permanent, unconscious condition.

3. The legal acceptance of these documents varies from state to state. Case managers should become familiar with their individual state's legislation with respect to these items.

4. NHPCO has an excellent website resource for ADs (www.nhpco.org).

C. A health care proxy (HCP) is a person, an advocate, who has been selected by the patient to speak for the patient in the event that he or she is unable to speak for himself or herself.

1. The HCP can be anyone that the patient trusts. It does not necessarily have to be a family member.

2. The HCP should have a sense of what the person would desire since they will be providing substituted judgment for the patient.

    3. The patient should have discussions with the HCP about wishes and desires for care. This dialogue is crucial for the HCP to be able to adequately represent the person's wishes.

    4. Details that should be covered with an HCP include but are not limited to:

      a. Resuscitation

      b. Feeding tubes and nutritional support

      c. Dialysis

      d. Mechanical respirator/ventilator support

      e. Transfusions of blood and blood products

      f. Antibiotics

D. In developing an AD and selecting an HCP, patients and families should be aware of the importance of these documents and the role they play in decision making regarding health care options.

E. Copies of ADs should be given to the HCP and the primary care physician. Should the dynamics of a family change and a new AD needs to be created, this can be done at any time as long as the process and the documents conform to state regulations.

F. ADs can be drafted, but not completed, by a lawyer. A lawyer is not necessary to legitimize an AD. Proper witnessing and signatures are required but do not entail the use of a notary. However, an AD can be certified as a legal document when signed in front of a notary and notarized. Additionally, an AD can be considered a legal document, without notarization, if witnessed and signed by two individuals who bear no financial or other interests as a result of the AD.

G. Case managers may find it difficult to explain to patients the need for ADs and HCPs. Regardless, they should be addressing this need while discussing palliative, hospice, or routine care with patients and their families.

    1. In communicating this to a family and patient, it is best to use simplified concepts that patients/families may comprehend.

    2. Equating the AD to a road map of life and the HCP as the designated driver may assist families and patients in better understanding the concepts.

H. When traumatic events do occur and the HCP and AD are needed and followed, these documents can be empowering and comforting to the family because they feel confident that they are following their loved one's wishes.

I. When having end-of-life conversations with their physicians and/or other health care professionals, patients end up experiencing less costly care, especially during the last weeks of their lives. They also experience better quality of life and less drastic care measures.

J. One may prepare an AD at any time, even if does not suffer from a serious illness or disease at the time. To be valid, an AD must be dated and signed in the presence of two witnesses. Both witnesses must also sign. The witnesses may not be:

    1. Related to the person executing an AD by blood or marriage

    2. Entitled to inherit money or property from this person

    3. People to whom the person executing the AD owe money

    4. The person's attending doctor or the doctor's employee

    5. An employee of a health facility where the person is a patient

BOX 8-10	The Wishes Included in the "Five Wishes Form"

1. Naming a health care agent, which should match the name(s) of the agent(s) listed in the Durable Power of Attorney
2. Description of the health care matters, treatments interested in receiving, and those prefer not to receive
3. Comfort
4. Preference as to be treated by others
5. Things wanting loved ones to know

K. In addition to an AD, one may also complete the Physician Orders for Life-Sustaining Treatment (POLST) form. The POLST is an 8 ½ × 11 type document, green in color, two-sided form that acts as a summary for health care and emergency personnel of the person's wishes regarding life-sustaining measures and treatments. This document is intended for individuals with an advanced life-limiting illness.
   1. One may obtain the POLST form from the primary care provider.
   2. This document has replaced the EMS-No CPR form used in the past (Emergency Medical Services—No Cardiopulmonary Resuscitation).
   3. The POLST form covers the patient's wishes for resuscitation, medical interventions, antibiotics, and artificial feedings.
   4. This form is portable, which means it can be taken from health care to long-term care settings without the need to complete another form. The POLST form specifically translates one's wishes into actual physician orders.
L. In addition to the AD and POLST form, one may also complete the "Five Wishes Form." This form offers an alternative to what is typically thought of as an AD. Once completed and notarized, it constitutes a legal document. This form (Box 8-10):
   1. Sets forth the types of medical treatments one wishes to have and those one does not want.
   2. Goes further to clarify the comfort measures one desires to have implemented at the end of life.
   3. Covers how one prefers to be treated and what one wants loved ones to know about his/her preferences.
   4. Acceptable in the majority of the states. Case managers must be familiar whether the Five Wishes form is acceptable in the jurisdiction where they work so that they are better able to advise patients, support systems, and fellow health care professionals about its use.

Case Management Services in Palliative and Hospice Care Programs

A. Using case management strategies in palliative and hospice care, case managers engage in functions and activities such as those described in Box 8-11.
B. Palliative care acts as a bridge for the hospice referral and services. The case manager can play a major role in ensuring that timely and appropriate referrals are made and in clarifying misconceptions.

BOX

8-11 Common Activities of Case Managers in Palliative and Hospice Care

- Assessment
- Treatment planning
- Treatment decision making
- Collaboration with other disciplines and care providers
- Implementation of the case management plan of care
- Evaluation of care outcomes and care experience
- Ensuring that the patient's/family's needs are met
- Provision of bereavement services for the family
- Patient and family health education and instruction
- Managing the practical burdens of illness
- Conferencing with the patient and family and health care team to facilitate communication and decision making regarding the plan of care
- Coordinating respite care
- Transitions of care

C. Hospice service coverage includes physician and nursing care, durable medical equipment, medications for pain and other symptom management, home health aide or a certified nursing assistant services, social work, physical therapy, occupational therapy, short hospitalization stay, crisis care, and respite services as they relate to the terminal illness. The case manager oversees these services and ensures patients' access to these services.

D. Palliative and hospice care include end-of-life care that is focused on symptom management, pain management and control, and assisting patients and families in providing care at home while assisting with advanced care planning.

E. Once an initial assessment for palliative and/or hospice care is made by the coordinator of care (COC), the initial plan of care is set and agreed upon by the core team. The interdisciplinary team meets at least every 2 weeks (14 days) and collaborates regarding each individual patient's plan of care, evaluates the effectiveness of the plan, and revises the plan as indicated. The patient and family are actively involved in the care planning process.

F. The COC is the case manager (most of the time an RN) responsible for overseeing and facilitating the care of each patient.

G. Ensuring reimbursement is a primary role for the case manager in hospice and palliative care programs. Utilization management practices, principles and concepts, and roles and responsibilities of case managers are similar to those applied in other care settings.
   1. Hospice services provided under Medicare are a capitated service. Once the Medicare benefit is signed over to hospice, the hospice receives (national average) $126 daily for management of the patient's certified terminal illness.

H. In addition to the goals of palliative and hospice care described above, the goals/outcomes of case management are:
   1. Efficient utilization of services, decreased emergent care, and emergency department utilization
   2. Improved patient outcomes and quality of life (especially in end-of-life issues)
   3. Increased knowledge and confidence for care provision regarding end-stage diagnosis and symptom management

4. Increased consistency of care delivery
5. Increased patient/family satisfaction
6. Honoring patient/family wishes regarding whether care is to be at home or inpatient placement

I. The COC plays a significant role as a case manager in hospice to help facilitate the patient's care through advanced care planning and bereavement psychosocial support services. The COC as a case manager facilitates communication and care provision with the patient, family, physician, and interdisciplinary team to achieve outcomes/goals mutually set in a collaborative fashion.

J. The expected patient/case management program outcomes using palliative care and hospice services include:
1. Efficient utilization of services
2. Cost-effectiveness through the coordination and management of health care services
3. Improved patient outcomes such as satisfaction with care, quality of life, and symptom management
4. Resolution of identified issues while maintaining the patient at home with support of the caregiver

K. The achievement of these goals results in decreased use of emergent or acute care, better symptom control, provision of quality and cost-efficient care, and interdisciplinary team concept and approach to care while meeting the terminally ill patient's/family's wishes to care for their loved ones in their own home or facility.

L. Palliative and hospice services and the role of the case manager in the provision of these services are crucial in helping patients/caregivers navigate the difficult terrain of end-of-life issues.

References

Case Management Society of America (CMSA). (2010). *CMSA standards of practice for case management*. Little Rock, AR: Author.

Institute for Clinical Symptoms Improvement (ICSI). (2013). *A business case for providing palliative care services across the continuum of care*. Bloomington, MN: ICSI.

Meier, D. (2006). *The case for palliative care*. Retrieved from website: www.capc.org, on July 26, 2006.

National Hospice and Palliative Care Organization (NHPCO). (2014). *Facts and figures: Hospice care in America*. Alexandria, VA: NHPCO.

Temel, J. S., Greer, J. A., Muzikansky, A., Gallagher, E. R., Admane, S., & Jackson, V. A. (2010). Early palliative care for patients with metastatic non-small-cell lung cancer. *New England Journal of Medicine, 363*(8), 733.

Wennberg J. E. (2008). *Tracking the care of patients with severe chronic illness*. Lebanon, NH: The Dartmouth Institute for Health Policy and Clinical Practice, The Dartmouth Atlas of Health Care.

CHAPTER 9

Case Management in the Remote and Rural Care Settings

Marietta P. Stanton

LEARNING OBJECTIVES

Upon completion of this chapter, the reader will be able to:

1. Describe the major components of rural case management.
2. Differentiate the definitions of "rural" for health care purposes.
3. Discuss the characteristics of rural individuals or population and the implications for case management both in urban and rural areas.
4. Identify essential skills for the case manager working in a rural care setting.
5. Describe a model for rural case management that addresses access issues for health care.
6. Explain the similarities and differences between rural case management programs and those in other care settings.

IMPORTANT TERMS AND CONCEPTS

Federal Office of
  Rural Health Policy
  (ORHP)
Health Professional
  Shortage Areas
  (HPSA)
Metropolitan Statistical
  Areas (MSA)

Medically Underserved
  Area (MUA)
Medically Underserved
  Population (MUP)
Micropolitan Statistical
  Area
Rural
Rural Areas

Rural Area Commuting
  Area (RUCA)
Urbanized Areas
Urbanized Clusters

Introduction

A. The issues faced by health care providers and patients in rural areas are different than those in urban areas. A unique set of factors creates disparities in health care services and resources not typically found in urban areas (Bushy, 2000). The following are a summary of facts from Health and Human Services (USDHHS, 2013):
   1. Economic factors, cultural and social differences, educational shortcomings, lack of recognition by legislators, and the sheer isolation of living in remote rural areas impede rural Americans in their struggle to lead a normal, safe, and healthy life.
   2. During the implementation of the Patient Protection and Affordable Care Act (PPACA) of 2010, some interesting facts demonstrated how case management in the rural environment requires different approaches. For instance:
      a. Nearly one in five uninsured Americans lives in a rural area.
      b. A greater proportion of rural residents lack health insurance in comparison to urban residents.
      c. Due to lower income levels, a large segment of the rural population is eligible for subsidized insurance coverage through the Health Insurance Marketplaces or Exchanges (Marketplaces).
B. The Health Insurance Marketplaces are expected to increase competition in the insurance market not only in urban but also in rural areas—especially in the 29 mostly rural states, where a single insurer currently dominates more than half the health insurance market (USDHHS, 2013; Joo, 2014).
C. In states that are expanding Medicaid benefits and reach, rural residents are more likely to be eligible for affordable coverage under this coverage expansion.
D. This is especially important in rural areas, where research has shown that one in five farmers faces medical debt, and families, on average, pay nearly half of their health care costs out of pocket (USDHHS, 2013).
E. Only about 10% of physicians practice in rural America despite the fact that nearly one fourth of the population lives in these areas. This is complicated by the existing shortages in primary care providers.
F. Rural residents are less likely to have employer-provided health care coverage or prescription drug coverage, and the rural poor are less likely to be covered by Medicaid benefits than their urban counterparts.
G. Although only one third of all motor vehicle accidents occur in rural areas, two thirds of the deaths attributed to these accidents occur on rural roads.
H. Rural residents are nearly twice as likely to die from unintentional injuries, other than motor vehicle accidents, than are urban residents. Rural residents are also at a significantly higher risk of death by gunshot than urban residents.
I. Rural residents tend to be poorer. On the average, per capita income is $7,417 lower than in urban areas, and rural Americans are more likely to live below the poverty level. The disparity in income is even greater for minorities living in rural areas. Nearly 24% of rural children live in poverty.

J. People who live in rural America rely more heavily on the Federal Food Stamp Program.

K. There are 2,157 Health Professional Shortage Areas (HPSAs) in rural and frontier areas of all states and US territories compared to 910 in urban areas.

L. Abuse of alcohol and use of smokeless tobacco are significant problems among rural youth. The rate of driving while under the influence of alcohol (DUI) arrests is significantly greater in nonurban counties. Forty percent of rural 12th graders reported using alcohol while driving compared to 25% of their urban counterparts. Rural eighth graders are twice as likely to smoke cigarettes (26.1% vs. 12.7% in large metro areas).

M. Anywhere from 57% to 90% of first responders in rural areas are community volunteers.

N. There are 60 dentists per 100,000 individuals in urban areas versus 40 per 100,000 in rural areas.

O. Cerebrovascular disease is reportedly 1.45 higher in nonmetropolitan statistical areas (non-MSAs) than in MSAs.

P. Hypertension is also higher in rural than urban areas (101.3 per 1,000 individuals in MSAs and 128.8 per 1,000 individuals in non-MSAs).

Q. Twenty percent of nonmetropolitan counties lack mental health services versus 5% of metropolitan counties.

R. The suicide rate among rural men is significantly higher than in urban areas, particularly among adult men and children. The suicide rate among rural women is escalating rapidly and is approaching that of men.

S. Medicare payments to rural hospitals and physicians are dramatically less than those to their urban counterparts for equivalent services. This correlates closely with the fact that more than 470 rural hospitals have closed in the past 25 years.

T. Medicare patients with acute myocardial infarction (AMI) who were treated in rural hospitals were less likely than those treated in urban hospitals to receive recommended treatments and had significantly higher adjusted 30-day post AMI death rates from all causes than those in urban hospitals.

U. Rural residents have greater transportation difficulties reaching health care providers, often traveling great distances to reach a doctor or hospital (Morgan & Fahs, 2007).

V. Death and serious injury accidents account for 60% of total rural accidents versus only 48% of urban.

   1. One reason for this increased rate of morbidity and mortality is that in rural areas, prolonged delays can occur between a crash, the call for EMS, and the arrival of an EMS provider.

   2. Many of these delays are related to increased travel distances in rural areas and personnel distribution across the response area.

   3. National average response time, from motor vehicle accident to EMS arrival, in rural areas is about 18 or 8 minutes greater than in urban areas.

W. The federal government uses two definitions for "rural," along with many variants that are important for the case manager to know. These designations and descriptions may result in different funding and reimbursement opportunities or may provide benefits not available to urban areas.

X. Case managers and program leaders, especially those who practice in rural and remote areas, must be knowledgeable in the issues and concerns rural area residents and health care seekers face. Such awareness assists in designing effective case management programs, roles, and strategies, which ultimately enhance the health of the rural communities (Davis et al., 2014).

Descriptions of Key Terms

A. Health Professional Shortage Areas (HPSAs)—Areas designated by the Health Resources and Services Administration (USDHHS, HRSA, 2015) as having shortages of primary care, dental care, or mental health providers. They may be geographic (e.g., a county or service area), population (e.g., low income or Medicaid eligible), or facilities (e.g., Federally Qualified Health Centers or state or federal prisons).

B. Index of Medical Underservice (IMU)—A score that is used to determine whether a geographic area can be designated as underserved or well served. The index involves four variables: ratio of primary medical care physicians per 1,000 population, infant mortality rate, percentage of the population with incomes below the poverty level, and percentage of the population age 65 or over. The value of each of these variables for the service area is converted to a weighted value, according to established criteria. The four values are summed to obtain the area's IMU score (HRSA, 2015).

C. Metropolitan Statistical Areas (MSA)—A geographical region with a relatively high population density at its core and close economic ties throughout the area. Such regions neither are legally incorporated as a city or town would be nor are they legal administrative divisions like counties and states. Such designation is made by the Office of Management and Budget (OMB) for use by Federal statistical agencies in collecting, tabulating, and publishing Federal statistics. An MSA is core urban area with 50,000 or more population size.

D. Medically Underserved Area (MUA)—A designation of a geographic area that is given based on the Index of Medical Underservice (IMU) score. The IMU scale ranges from 0 to 100, where 0 represents completely underserved and 100 represents best served. Under the established criteria, each service area found to have an IMU of 62.0 or less qualifies for designation as an MUA (HRSA, 2015).

E. Medically Underserved Population (MUP)—A designation that involves application of the Index of Medical Underservice (IMU) to data on an underserved population group within an area of residence to obtain a score for the population group. Population groups where MUP determination is considered are usually those with economic barriers such as low-income or Medicaid-eligible populations or experiencing cultural and/or linguistic access barriers to primary medical care services. The MUP process involves assembling the same data elements and carrying out the same computational steps as stated for MUAs (HRSA, 2015).

F. Micropolitan Statistical Area—A geographic region that contains an urban core population of at least 10,000, but less than 50,000 (US Census Bureau, 2015).

G. Rural—Characteristics of country life. Encompasses all populations, housing, and territories not included in designated "urban" areas.

H. Rural Areas—(See rural) Nonurban areas characteristic of low population density, small settlements, and tend to focus more on agriculture as life resources.

I. Rural–Urban Commuting Area (RUCA)—Is a census tract–based classification scheme completed using the standard Bureau of Census' urbanized area and urban cluster definitions (population density and urbanization) in combination with work commuting information. The classification contains two levels. Whole numbers (1 to 10) delineate metropolitan, micropolitan, small town, and rural commuting areas based on the size and direction of the primary (largest) commuting flows. 1 indicates most urban flow, while 10 indicates most rural flow (USDA, 2015).

J. Urbanized Area—Is a location characterized by high human population density and vast human-built features in comparison to the areas surrounding it. Urban areas may be cities or towns. The geographical territory is identified according to criteria and must encompass at least 2,500 people, at least 1,500 of which reside outside institutional group quarters (US Census Bureau, 2010).

K. Urban Clusters—Based on the Census Bureau's geographical designations, an urban cluster represents densely developed territory and encompasses residential, commercial, and other nonresidential urban land uses. To be designated as an UC, the area must have at least 2,500 and less than 50,000 people, compared to urbanized areas (UAs), which require to have 50,000 or more residents (US Census Bureau, 2010).

Applicability to CMSA's Standards of Practice

A. The Case Management Society of America (CMSA) describes in its standards of practice for case management (CMSA, 2010) that case management practice extends across all health care settings and by providers of various professional disciplines. This without a doubt applies to the provision of case management services in rural areas.

B. Rural case management programs are designed similarly to those in urban and metropolitan areas. They include same aims/goals, roles, functions, strategies, and approaches as those of general practice or care settings. Case managers share similar responsibilities; however, the population served and the health care concerns addressed vary because the health care disparity issues, resources, and services available in rural regions are different than urban areas (Stanton & Packa, 2001).

C. Rural case managers may use the CMSA standards as a guide for the implementation of their roles. All of the standards are relevant to the practice of rural case managers including the legal and ethical considerations.

D. Case managers in the rural care settings must demonstrate awareness and competence in the CMSA standards of practice. They also must inform their employers and other professionals they collaborate with when dealing with clients/support systems about the existence of these standards and their value and need to adhere to them (Mullahy, 2014; Pyrillis, 2015).

E. This chapter introduces case managers to the differentiating factors and principles of rural case management practice, characteristics of the rural client population, and role of the case manager in such care settings. It also explains how collaboration may occur between case managers in the rural and other care settings, especially the urban-based health care organizations and providers.

 ## Understanding Designation of Areas Within United States

A. The US Census Bureau (2015) defines various areas within the United States as either urban areas or urban clusters. These are basically delineation of geographical areas based on population density and other factors such as residential, commercial, or nonresidential.
   1. Urbanized areas (UAs) are those of 50,000 or more people.
   2. Urban clusters (UCs) are those areas of at least 2,500 and less than 50,000 people.
B. The Census Bureau describes "rural" as an area that encompasses all population, housing, and territory not included within an urban area. Whatever is not urban is considered rural.
   1. The Census Bureau recognizes that "densely settled communities outside the boundaries of large incorporated municipalities are just as 'urban' as the densely settled population inside those boundaries."
   2. The Census Bureau definition does not always follow city or county boundaries and so it is difficult sometimes to determine whether a particular area is considered urban or rural.
   3. Under this definition, about 21% of the US population in 2000 was considered rural, but over 95% of the land area was classified as rural. In the 2010 Census, 59.5 million people, 19.3% of the population, was rural, while over 95% of the land area is still classified as rural.
C. According to the White House Office of Management and Budget (OMB, 2013), a metropolitan area contains a core urban area of 50,000 or more in population size. A micropolitan area is an area that contains an urban core of at least 10,000 (but less than 50,000) in population size as micropolitan. Rural area, on the other hand, is any county that is not part of a metropolitan statistical area (MSA). Micropolitan counties are considered nonmetropolitan or rural along with all counties that are not classified as either metropolitan or micropolitan.
   1. Under this definition, about 17% of the population in 2000 was considered nonmetropolitan, while 74% of the land area was contained in nonmetropolitan counties.
   2. After the 2010 Census, the nonmetropolitan population was 46.2 million people, about 15% of the total population. For more information on metropolitan and rural areas, refer to the US Census Bureau statistical area classifications page available at http://www.census.gov/population/metro/. Designations tend to be reviewed every 10 years.
D. There are measurement challenges with both the Census Bureau and OMB definitions. Some policy experts note that the census definition classifies quite a bit of suburban area as rural. The OMB definition includes rural areas in metropolitan counties including, for example,

the Grand Canyon, which is located in a metropolitan county. Consequently, one could argue that the Census Bureau standard includes an overcount of rural population, whereas the OMB standard represents an undercount of the rural population. Case managers must be aware of these issues especially if the rural case management programs are funded and the funding is impacted by the designation.

1. The Office of Rural Health Policy (ORHP) accepts all nonmetropolitan counties as rural and uses an additional method of determining "rurality" called the Rural–Urban Commuting Area (RUCA) codes. Like the MSAs, these are based on census data, which are used to assign a code to each census tract.

2. Tracts inside metropolitan counties with the codes 4 to 10 are considered rural. While use of the RUCA codes has allowed identification of rural census tracts in metropolitan counties among the more than 70,000 tracts in the United States, there are some that are extremely large and where use of RUCA codes alone fails to account for distance to services and sparse population.

3. In response to these concerns, ORHP has designated 132 large area census tracts with RUCA codes 2 or 3 as rural. These tracts are at least 400 square miles in area with a population density of no more than 35 people.

4. Following the 2010 Census, the ORHP definition included approximately 57 million people, about 18% of the population and 84% of the area of the United States. RUCA codes represent the current version of the Goldsmith Modification.

E. The United States Department of Agriculture (USDA, 2015) defines urban (100 persons per square mile), frontier (6 or few persons per square mile), and rural (7 to 99 persons per square mile).

F. The United States Department of Agriculture (USDA, 2015) Economic Research Service (ERS), Rural Economy and Population, defines rural in terms of the economic and social factors. An area's economic and social characteristics have significant effects on its development and need for various types of public programs.

G. To provide policy-relevant information about diverse county conditions to policymakers, public officials, and researchers, ERS has developed a set of county-level typology codes that captures differences in economic and social characteristics.

1. The 2004 County Typology Codes classify all US counties according to six nonoverlapping categories of economic dependence and overlapping categories of policy-relevant themes. The economic types include farming, mining, manufacturing, services, federal/state government, and unspecialized counties.

2. The policy types include housing stress, low education, low employment, persistent poverty, population loss, nonmetro recreation, and retirement destination. In addition, a code identifying counties with persistent child poverty is available.

H. Health professional shortage areas (HPSA) describe the distribution and density of health professionals in a given area. These designations assist in understanding the access patients have to health care providers, services, and resources. Usually, they are designated on the basis of counties within each state, and these can exist in all three of the following categories:

1. A Primary Health Care HPSA acknowledges the physician shortage in a service area. The physician shortage is calculated based physicians availability in the specialties of pediatrics, obstetrics, gynecology, general internal medicine, and family practice only.
2. A Dental Health Care HPSA acknowledges the shortage of dentists in a service area. The dental shortage is calculated from general dentists only; however, age and auxiliary assistance are also considered as important factors.
3. A Mental Health Care HPSA acknowledges the shortage of psychiatrists and core mental health professionals in a service area. The psychiatric shortage is calculated from ratios of population to mental health care providers.

I. To better understand health professions shortages in various geographical area designations, it is important for the case manager to be familiar with the four types described below and to apply each HPSA category. This is especially important for case managers involved in health policy and access to care and services.

1. Geographic HPSA: A geographic HPSA is a term used to refer to a region that is determined to be a sound rational service area (RSA). It can be a portion of a city or a county, or it can be an entire county. It is based on primary care hours for the general population.
2. Low-Income Population HPSA: A low-income population HPSA is used to describe a region that is determined to be a sound rational service area focusing on only that population living below the 200% federal poverty level. The shortage of primary care physicians is based on the time spent serving this population.
3. Specialty Population HPSA: A specialty population HPSA denotes a region that is determined to be a sound rational service area focusing on only that population that may fall into one of the following populations: Medicaid populations below the 100% federal poverty level, ethnicity, homeless, and migrant farm workers.
4. Facility HPSA: A facility HPSA is a term used to refer to one of the following facilities: state and federal prisons, correctional facilities, community health centers, rural health clinics, and Federally Qualified Health Centers (FQHC).

J. Medicare Bonus—When an area is designated as a geographic HPSA, all physicians working in the HPSA are eligible for an additional 10% Medicare payment. From primary care physicians and specialists to optometrists, chiropractors, podiatrists, and medical teleconsultants, they are all eligible for the incentive payment for practicing in the geographic HPSA.

1. Although the HPSA project is based on the study of primary care, all disciplines benefit.
2. As of January 2011, all primary care physicians and surgeons working in a geographic HPSA have become eligible for a 20% Medicare bonus payment.

K. Loan Forgiveness—The goal of the National Health Services Corps (NHSC, 2015) is to expand access to health care services and improve the overall health of individuals living in medically underserved areas across the United States.

1. Through the active recruitment of primary care, dental, and mental health providers, the NHSC is able to place these physicians within the service areas with the highest needs.

2. In exchange for 3 years of service in a site approved by the NHSC, education loan relief is made available for medical service providers. These placements are based on Health Professional Shortage Area designations.

L. Visa Waiver—This program excuses foreign nationals from meeting some of the usual requirements for obtaining permanent residence in the United States. Such program enhances the provision of health care services in remote and rural areas where health care resources and services are short.

1. A J-1 visa, also called an "exchange visitor visa," is a visa used by foreign nationals who come to the United States for the purpose of teaching, training, studying, research, and so on. Foreign nationals are required to physically return to their home country or the country of last residence for at least 2 years before they are eligible to apply for any other nonimmigrant visa or lawful permanent residence.

2. In exchange for working in an underserved area, a visa waiver will remove the requirement for the foreign physician to return home for 2 years.

3. The use of the H-1B petition allows an employer to temporarily employ a foreigner in the United States on a nonimmigrant basis in various specialty occupations. The H-1B petition authorizes the employee to work for a limited period of time for the specific employer, in the specific position outlined in the petition.

M. Veterans Health Administration (VHA, 2015), Office of Rural Health (ORH)—The VHA plays an active role in rural health care. The mission of the VHA ORH is to improve access and quality of care for enrolled rural and highly rural veterans by developing evidence-based policies and innovative practices to support the unique needs of enrolled veterans residing in geographically remote areas. Rural designation of VHA medical centers is one way of determining where health care resources may require special attention.

N. Rural designation of VHA's health care facilities may use three schemes as follows:

1. Facility URH Classification: The Veterans Administration Medical Center (VAMC) classification system, which applies a 3-category scheme. The system designates each facility as urban (U), rural (R), or highly rural (H) based on census block population density, making up the URH classification (Kaboli & Glasgow, 2011).

   a. Urban refers to any facility located in a US Census urbanized area.
   b. Rural denotes any facility not defined as urban.
   c. Highly rural is any facility defined as rural but located in counties with average population density of less than 7 civilians per square mile.

2. Patient URH Classification: This system examines the geocoded (geographic code) location of the home of each patient discharged

from a given VHA facility. Patients are classified as urban, rural, or highly rural using the same criteria as the facility URH classification system (Kaboli & Glasgow, 2011).

3. Patient RUCA Classification: This system examines the Rural–Urban Commuting Area (RUCA) classification, which is also based partially on census tracts, but takes into consideration patient location in relationship to larger urban areas (Kaboli & Glasgow, 2011).

Rural Culture Health Care Considerations

A. Awareness of rural health emerged in the 1980s when health care workers began to notice disparate status of health care utilization in rural regions (RR).

B. During the 1980s, rural hospitals began to close due to low census, increased regulation and financial failure, and persistent shortages of health care professionals.

C. The 1990s witnessed anxiety and concerns about how cost containment and managed care would impact rural health. Lawmakers did not know about the implications of managed care (Coughlin, Long, & Graves, 2008).

D. There were numerous concerns about rural and remote health care delivery and resources: some of which still exist today (Box 9-1).

E. There continues to be some concerns about the state of contemporary rural health care. These are described in Box 9-2. Case management is the perfect force to mitigate the negative issues and barriers to health care delivery in rural areas (Meyer & Morrisey, 2007).

F. Rural Populations—According to the 2010 Census, 78% of the rural population is white or non-Hispanic compared to 46% of the nation as

---

BOX 9-1   Past Concerns of Rural Health

- Rural obscurity abating in professional schools, in health care literature, and health care texts and other publications.
- Emergence of frontier versus rural delineations based on population density.
- Rural health care intertwined with characteristics of rural locale so there is variation in the composition of the rural populations in different areas.
- Rural residents exhibit self-reliance, hardiness, resourcefulness, and creativity in meeting challenges.
- Wald and Breckenridge pioneers in developing a framework for rural health that is relevant today.
- Post–World War II, the Hill-Burton Act resulting in the proliferation of small community hospitals.
- Access to health care professional is poor for hospitals in RRs.
- Imprecise definitions for what constitutes rural has had many resource and policy implications for rural health care and rural populations.
- Incomplete and conflicting health utilization data.
- Inadequacy of infrastructures to support rural health care.
- Fewer people living in remote areas.
- Failure of managed care in rural areas.
- Poor recruitment, retention, and education of health professionals.

BOX 9-2 Issues for Contemporary Rural Health Care

- Technology links need to increase for rural residents and providers.
- Quality assurance and measurement of outcomes addressing rural situations is still lacking.
- Partnership models of rural health care delivery are limited; collaborations between various levels of care, providers, and facilities must be pursued.
- Ethical issues especially related to allocation of scarce resources must be continuously monitored.
- Evidence-based health care programs that targets rural areas are a must: currently lacking or limited.

a whole. Although whites represent the largest group in rural America, they only account for 2% of the increase in the rural population.

1. In 2000, African Americans comprised 8.2% of the rural population and ranked as the largest percent of racial or ethnic minorities. In 2010, there was a modest increase of 2.9% in this population.
2. The majority of African Americans live in rural or small towns; nearly 9 out of 10 African Americans reside in the south in the "Black Belt" region, which extends from Louisiana, Mississippi, Alabama, Georgia, South Carolina, North Carolina, and the delta region of Arkansas, Louisiana, and Mississippi.
3. Hispanics are the largest group in rural and small towns representing 9.3% of the population. Although they have moved into a number of rural areas throughout the country, the largest concentration resides in Arizona, New Mexico, Texas, and California with a proximately one quarter of these residing in rural Texas.
4. Native Americans represent about 1.5% of the residents in rural and small towns but about half of the Native Americans live in small towns near the reservations or on the trust lands in the southwest, Midwest plains, and Alaska.
5. Asian and Pacific Islanders comprise less than 3% of the rural population but in the past decade have experienced double-digit growth. Their numbers increase consistently over time.

G. Of the 7.8 million veterans, approximately 3 million (38%) live in rural areas. As the challenges of providing care to these veterans are better understood, it becomes increasingly important to identify those facilities that require the most resources to meet the needs of veterans they serve (Mohamed, Neale, & Rosenheck, 2009).

1. Currently, there are just over 3.4 million rural veterans enrolled in the VA system. This represents 41% of the total enrolled veteran population. Nearly 43% (2.27 million) of veteran patients and 15% (914,000) of veterans with at least a service-connected disability are from rural and highly rural areas.
2. From October 1, 2009, to December 31, 2010, approximately 416,132 rural veterans were impacted by Office of Rural Health (ORH) projects. Over the last few years, ORH has supported the opening of 51 community-based outpatient clinics and 41 outreach clinics in rural and highly rural areas.

BOX 9-3   Special Issues of Rural Homeless

- Rural homeless tend to stay with relatives, in church facilities, and camps, sheds, or abandoned farms.
- Many are homeless because of farm evictions, transient homeless, family dissolution, and marital conflicts.
- More working near poor white Americans, more women with children, more intact two person families.
- Lead less visible lives; may live in campers in public lot tents or campers in relatives' yards or remote spots.
- Usually homeless for a shorter time compared to urban counterparts, more transient.
- Incidence of substance abuse is lower in rural homeless than urban.
- Lack subculture of urban homeless.
- Depend more on faith community.
- Health problems include higher incidence of TB, HIV, hepatitis, diabetes, and chronic mental illness than regular population.
- Illiteracy.

3. From Fiscal Year 2010 to Fiscal Year 2011, 1st quarter, approximately 57,191 unique patients were seen at ORH-funded rural community-based outpatient clinics. The number of rural health outpatient mental health visits increased from 3.4 million in Fiscal Year 2009 to 3.9 million in Fiscal Year 2010.

H. Rural Homeless—7% to 14% of the nation's homeless live in rural areas. The majority are families with children, runaways, single adult men, the elderly, and the mentally ill (National Alliance to End Homelessness, 2010).

   1. Characteristics of the rural homeless as described in Box 9-3 are of special importance for the rural or remote area case manager and the design of case management programs for this population.

   2. Important for case managers to partner with others on the prevention of rural homelessness and to offer financial counseling, promote community awareness, address the common problems this population suffers, and engage in outreach programs to this vulnerable populations to mitigate the situation (Austin, McClelland, & Gursansky, 2006; Mobley et al., 2014; Olivia, 2008; Sadowski, Devlin, & Hussain, 2012; Shah et al., 2010).

I. More rural health care providers are required to care for the rural population and address existing concerns of health disparities (Derrett et al., 2014). Additionally, more programs are needed to prepare health providers in rural health and rural case management including use of telehealth and telemedicine technology and remote monitoring (Davis et al., 2014). Other needs necessary to improve health care for the rural Americans (*News Briefs*, 2008; O'Neill & Klepack, 2007) are listed in Box 9-4.

Rural Case Management Programs and Services

A. Rural case management programs are similar in structure and processes to those in other geographical regions. They address similar goals and objectives and, however, face challenges unique to rural health care settings and delivery systems.

BOX 9-4

Ways to Enhance Health Care and Case Management Services for Rural Populations

- Educate health care students to function independently and to be able to tailor services to unique communities.
- Offer rural health care providers training and experience in case management and managing transitions from urban medical centers to rural primary care providers and other agencies.
- Prepare nurses and other health care providers in expanded roles to then be able to manage primary care issues in rural and remote settings.
- Prepare health care professionals in interdisciplinary collaboration and partnerships especially across care setting and urban area designations.
- Recruit rural minorities for health professions, including case management.
- Recruit rural health care providers from rural communities for special training in urban setting/academic medical centers in the hopes they will return to those rural and remote communities.
- Prepare rural case managers in evidence-based practice and use of clinical practice guidelines.
- Develop strong networks of providers to render comprehensive and primary care.
- Increase access to educational programs in the rural area to enhance recruitment of natives to the health care workforce.
- Create partnerships between schools, faith-based, and community organizations.
- Implement use of telemedicine and other innovative technology for rural regions, especially in partnership with other urban-based health care facilities.

B. Some of the theoretical foundations for rural case management outreach programs are similar to general outreach approaches. Case managers must be knowledgeable in a number of specific health care knowledge and practice areas (Box 9-5) and use such knowledge and skills to maximize their outreach efforts and case management successes.

C. It is important to conduct a community health assessment when designing and implementing a rural case management program. The assessment informs the goals and objectives the program must address and the needed resources and services. The community health assessment process may include a systematic collection and utilization of data to identify, prioritize, and resolve a community's related concerns.

D. The assessment relies heavily on network and partnering theory.

BOX 9-5

Important Knowledge and Practice Areas for Effective Rural Case Management

- Health Beliefs Model (HBM)
- Theory of Hardiness
- Collaborative Practice Models, especially across various area designations
- Case Management Theories, Concepts, and Principles
- Cultural Competence, Sensitivity, and Health Literacy
- Characteristic of successful Models of Rural Case Management
- Phenomena of "Ruralness": Occupational, Ecological, and Sociocultural Dimensions of Rural Health Care
- Telehealth/Telemedicine/Telemonitoring

E. Providers weigh in on partnering with community leaders and other health care professional to plan the types of rural community interventions.

F. The process of serving as a rural health care provider organization or program depends on key community stakeholders, informants, and use of available primary and secondary data.

G. Seeking funding from government and nongovernment agencies or charitable organizations is important to support the conduct of the assessment and the development of a program plan.

H. Rural case management programs and case managers apply specific care delivery strategies, interventions, and approaches to assure effective health care delivery that ultimately impacts the health of the communities they serve (Box 9-6).

I. The rural patient population may be considered vulnerable or disadvantaged for many reasons, for example, issues of health disparity. To reduce the concerns of vulnerability, case managers must apply their specialized knowledge of how to care for such populations and be skilled in engaging these individuals in their own health care including decision making about care options, self-management, and adherence to health regimens.

J. Plan the case management services to meet the needs of special and at-risk individuals, not just the general population.

K. Address the needs of persons with special needs (e.g., behavioral health, homelessness) while considering the social and human services.

BOX 9-6   Strategies and Interventions of Rural Case Management Programs

- Identifying special at-risk populations such as individuals who are vulnerable and disadvantaged physically, socially, cognitively, economically, or psychologically
- Identifying real and potential occupational and lifestyle risks
- Implementing predictive modeling and population health risk stratification process
- Tracking population trends
- Implementing health promoting interventions and lifestyle behavior changes
- Defining a theory to guide and refine research and practice
- Identifying educational needs of clients and providers living in that community
- Understanding of definitions that have shaped and will shape rural policy
- Identifying health professional shortage areas (HPSAs)
- Implementing appropriate services in the community
- Coordinating care that satisfies the targeted population(s)
- Delineating and measuring care outcomes (individual, population., program, and organizational levels)
- Developing partnerships within the community and promote health care services
- Developing evidence to enhance best practices
- Use of interdisciplinary practice models and approaches (across settings, communities, and providers)
- Eliminating or mitigating disenfranchisement of groups that are separated from the mainstream of society
- Determining vulnerability—disadvantaged physically, socially, or psychologically
- Examination of issues of higher incidence such as obesity, diabetes, higher mortality from cancer, and how they affect health care outcomes
- Identifying area health condition ranking compared to other states (e.g., perinatal health, incidence of chronic illness, infant mortality, cost of health care per capita)

L. Establish contingencies for medical indigence and serious inabilities to pay for health care services if underinsured or completely uninsured.

M. Investigate multiple epidemiological factors that promote vulnerability and negative health outcomes with special application to rural health and remote communities.

N. Develop an understanding to how poverty is linked to health risk, vulnerability, and negative health outcomes.

O. Remember that poor communities have higher incidence of minorities, single mothers, unemployment, and low wages. Often, most vulnerable poor are the very young or elderly.

P. Understand the poverty threshold and poverty guidelines for the rural area on concern; poverty reports are updated annually by the federal government.

Q. Implement counterbalancing measures such as support networks to mitigate negative consequences of poverty; use faith-based programs or other cultural and charitable contingencies.

R. It is important to use formal evaluation methodologies when studying the impact of the rural case management program on the health of the population. Use both formative and summative approaches.

S. Outcomes management evaluation designs of general case management programs apply similarly in the rural case management specialty.

T. Value-based purchasing program measures also apply similarly.

U. Quality improvement methods and tools also apply for improving the care delivery systems and associated outcomes of rural case management programs.

V. Stanton and Packa (2001) described an effective model for rural community case management practice. This model is patient centered and incorporates special characteristics of the rural population and its unique health care needs. The model includes the following seven features:

1. Center care delivery on the patient/client and support system and maintain a holistic approach.

2. Consider the individual, groups of people, and community health care factors and needs.

3. Focus on the role of the case manager, use of specific case management tools and technologies, and application of the case management process (e.g., assessment, planning, intervention, evaluation, and interaction).

4. Incorporate the three levels of prevention into the case management services: primary, secondary, and tertiary.

5. Address the rural community factors in care delivery design. These may include diversity, isolation, independence, health and work beliefs, lack of anonymity, and insider and outsider views.

6. Measure outcomes in an effort to evaluate the impact of the rural case management program on individual and community health. Outcome categories/classification may include clinical, financial, functional well-being, satisfaction with care, human services/humanistic, and quality.

7. Address stakeholders' interests and concerns in the design and purpose of the model, delivery of services, and health care goals. Stakeholders may include customers, payers, health care providers, regulators, vendors/sellers of goods, and volunteers/community leaders.

Behavioral Health Care in Rural Areas

A. Behavioral health care in rural areas consists of mental health, substance abuse, and other issues similar to those that apply in urban areas (Fig. 9-1).
   1. Five to twenty percent of those in rural areas with physical problems also suffer from behavioral problems.
   2. Rural residents may experience high incidence of depression, alcohol abuse, domestic violence, and child neglect.
   3. Forty percent of rural behavioral health personnel are hospital based compared to 20% in the United States.
   4. These characteristics make the provision of case management services to this vulnerable population more necessary and complex.
B. The array and quality of behavioral health care services and resources in rural areas are tied to stability of small acute care or critical access hospitals and their partnerships or collaborations with other organizations, especially in urban areas such as academic medical centers.

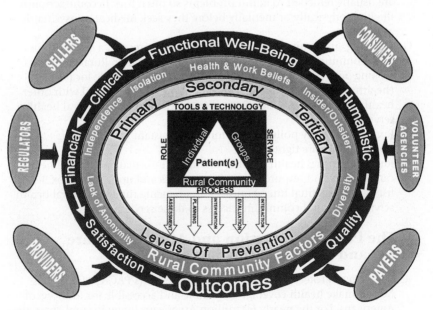

FIGURE 9-1. Rural community case management model. This model encompasses components of case management services and steps in the case management process. The model also addresses the characteristics of rural residents, outcomes for rural case management practice, and influences on the case management system. Reprinted from Stanton, M. P., & Packa, D. (2001). Nursing case management: A rural practice model. *Lippincott's Case Management, 6*(3), 97. Reprinted with permission.

C. Lack of health care personnel is another issue in rural health that contributes to the lack of enough behavioral health services and resources.
   1. Social workers, counselors, physicians, case managers, and advance practice registered nurses (APRNs) with backgrounds in psychiatry are lacking.
   2. Rural area–based registered nurses may assume multiple roles and lack of savvy about reimbursement, utilization management, and quality and outcomes management.
   3. There is a need for rural case managers to handle a wide variety of issues beside coordination of behavioral health care and resources. This usually contributes to role confusion and overload.
D. Rural social structures stigmatize powerless rural minorities with mental health issues and ostracize those who seek mental health assistance. Therefore, many do not seek help and tend to hide behavioral problems. They rather tolerate risky health behaviors.
E. Unlike urban counterparts, first-tier neighbors are major support for rural residents with health or behavioral health needs. Second-tier support consists of faith-based agencies sand congregations, community advocates, firefighters, volunteers, and emergency medical services. Third tier includes formal health services, however, altered based on persistent poverty.
F. Self-Reliance versus Dependency: Rural residents do not like to depend on others for help. They pride themselves in their self-reliance. They are usually reluctant to admit problems so often they become seriously ill either physically or mentally before they seek medical or psychiatric attention.
G. Ensuring anonymity and confidentiality: This presents a challenge in rural communities where everyone knows each other. Rural residents seeking behavioral health services look to find accessible locations (health care providers and agencies) but must be colocated with other health services or facilities that will mask the use of behavioral health services.
H. Rural community political structures are resistant to "outsiders." Communities are tightly knit.
I. Rural behavioral health requires linking of informal and formal health care services and resources to increase access and utilization. Box 9-7 lists some potential interventions for enhancing rural behavioral health services and rural community access to these services.

The Patient Protection and Affordable Care Act and Rural Case Management

A. The Patient Protection and Affordable Care Act (PPACA) of 2010 has helped make health coverage affordable and accessible for millions of Americans. For the nearly 60 million Americans living in rural areas, the law has addressed:
   1. Inequities in the availability of health care services
   2. Increasing access to quality and affordable health coverage
   3. Investment in prevention and wellness programs
   4. Increasing individuals' and families' control over their health care

9-7 Rural Behavioral Health Interventions

- Avoid duplication of services.
- Avoid turf disputes.
- Educate other health care professionals about rural catchment areas.
- Develop directories of formal and informal regional health services and resources.
- Develop web pages for rural communities with hyperlinks to other Web sites to enhance ease of access to resources and health information.
- Develop associations of and partnerships among telehealth, telemedicine, telenursing, and telecase management providers.
- Ensure having contingency plans for community emergencies.
- Use a case management partnership model to coordinate behavioral health services.
- Develop meaningful discharge plans. Have clients and their support systems actively participate in the development of their discharge plans including identification of services needed and contingency plans for crisis situations.
- Provide dedicated hotlines for farmers to address farms-related stresses and other behavioral health problems.
- Designate responsible persons for coordination of services and resources especially where access is limited.
- Coordinate and confirm follow-up services after patient's discharge from acute care or post other episodes of care.
- Educate the community; target informal networks—health information better accepted by women especially in faith-based communities and organization; rural women tend to be more motivated to learn about health and emotional and behavioral health.
- Seek to partner with rural business owners; they may be amenable to participating in health care initiatives.

B. Rural Americans experience higher rates of chronic diseases, disabilities, and mortality rates. The PPACA has offered important reforms to improve the health of these rural communities.

C. Key facts regarding rural coverage in the Health Insurance Marketplace of special value for rural case managers and case management programs are:

1. Beginning in 2014, it was estimated that there were 7.8 million uninsured rural Americans under age 65 who would enroll.
2. Due to lower income levels, a large segment of the rural population is eligible for subsidized insurance coverage through the Health Insurance Marketplaces (Marketplaces).
3. The Health Insurance Marketplaces are expected to increase competition in the insurance market in rural areas, especially in the 29, mostly rural states, where a single insurer carrier has traditionally dominated more than half the health insurance market.
4. In states that have been expanding the Medicaid benefits, rural residents are more likely to be eligible for affordable coverage under this expansion.
5. By increasing competition, the Health Insurance Marketplaces help lower health care costs. This is especially important in rural areas, where studies show that one in five farmers face medical debt and families pay on average nearly half of their health care costs out of pocket.

D. Uninsured individuals living in rural areas are able with the PPACA to use the Health Insurance Marketplaces to compare options of qualified health plans based on price, benefits, quality, and other factors with a clear picture of premiums and cost-sharing amounts. This opportunity helps rural individuals to choose the qualified health insurance plan that best fits their needs (USDHHS, 2013).
   1. Each insurance plan offered through the Marketplaces covers essential health benefits, including prescription drugs, inpatient and emergency services, pediatric care, and behavioral health treatment.
   2. The 30 million rural Americans with private insurance now have access to expanded preventive services with no cost sharing. These services include well-child visits, blood pressure and cholesterol screenings, Pap tests and mammograms for women, and flu shots for children and adults.
   3. More than 11 million elderly and disabled rural Americans who receive health coverage from Medicare also now have access to many preventive services with no cost sharing, including annual wellness visits with personalized prevention plans, diabetes and colorectal cancer screening, bone mass measurement, and mammograms.
   4. It is estimated that nearly 600,000 young rural Americans between ages 19 and 26 now have coverage under their parent's employer-sponsored or individually purchased health plan.
   5. Lifetime limits can no longer be included in private insurance policies, and annual limits cannot be less than $2,000,000. Annual limits have been prohibited as of 2014.
   6. Children, under age 19, cannot be denied coverage, because of a pre-existing condition. This protection also was extended to adults in 2014 (USDHHS, 2013).
E. Where Rural Americans Can Go for Consumer Assistance:
   1. A total of $5.5 million in Navigator funding went to organizations that focus on rural issues and also receive grants through the Federal Office of Rural Health Policy (ORHP), which focuses on rural health.
   2. The ORHP has made almost $1.3 million available to support 52 rural community and health care organizations to provide outreach and assistance to the uninsured in rural areas.
   3. Through $1.25 million in funding provided by the Centers for Medicare & Medicaid Services, a network of Cooperative Extension Service educators in 12 states will help uninsured and underinsured consumers make informed decisions about participating in the Marketplaces (USDHHS, 2013).
F. The Department of Health and Human Services operates a 24/7 call center to assist consumers in more than 150 languages. Consumers also have access to an online, live chat available at www.health.gov, which connects them to a customer service representative able to answer a range of questions. These resources for consumer assistance may be especially useful in rural areas where there is less broadband access and lower population density (USDHHS, 2013).
G. The Federal Office of Rural Health Policy frequently holds webinars to make rural health care stakeholders aware of new opportunities for coverage through the PPACA. These sessions provide a forum for rural

health care providers and organizations to share best practices, ask questions, and learn more about resources for consumer outreach and education. For more information on these webinars, you may contact ORHP-ACAQuestions@hrsa.gov.

H. Best Practice Models for Rural Case Management: Three clinics collaborated in care provision. Care integration was supported by two fundamental changes to organize and deliver care to patients:

1. Empanelment with a designated group of patients being cared for by a health care provider.

2. An interdisciplinary team able to address rural health issues. New funding and organizational initiatives of the PPACA may help to further improve care integration, although additional solutions may be necessary to address particular needs of rural communities.

I. Assertive community treatment would seem ideally suited to areas lacking services because of its self-contained interdisciplinary health care treatment team approach. However, rural programs have been forced to make several adaptations to the assertive community treatment model, including smaller teams, less comprehensive staff, and less intensive services.

1. There is no published evidence that these adaptations are able to produce the same results as full-fidelity teams.

2. Evidence suggests that intensive case management programs are effective only in community settings where there is an ample supply of treatment and support services.

3. Some believe that intensive case management may be an alternative to assertive community treatment in rural settings because intensive case management emphasizes individual caseloads, fewer staff, less intensive contacts, and brokered services.

4. To build the evidence base for the effectiveness of these models, much more attention needs to be focused on evaluating the current wave of assertive community treatment and intensive case management dissemination in rural areas.

J. A quality improvement project developed a rural community-based nursing case management program to decrease preventable readmissions to the hospital and emergency department by providing telephonic case management and, if needed, onsite assessment and treatment by a clinical nurse specialist (CNS) with prescriptive authority. It also used advanced practice nurses in transitional care.

1. This transitional care follow-up by the hospital can prevent readmissions, resulting in cost avoidance.

2. The coordination of community resources during patient's transition from hospital to home is a job best suited for CNSs, because they are educated to work within organizations/systems.

3. The money saved with this project more than justified the cost of hiring a CNS to lead it.

4. Guidelines for this intervention need to be developed. Replicating the cost-avoidance transitional care model can help other facilities limit that loss.

K. A telehealth program was used to follow up with congestive heart failure (CHF) patients. Results showed five broad themes of effectiveness:

(*text continues on page 241*)

TABLE 9-1 Rural Case Management Projects and Research

Journal Citation	Abstract	Clinical	Data-Based
Joo, J. Y. (2014). Community-based case management, hospital utilization, and patient-focused outcomes in Medicare beneficiaries. *Western Journal of Nursing Research, 36*(6), 825	There is limited research about the impact of community-based case management (CBCM) services and its outcomes with longitudinal analysis. The purpose of this study was to evaluate the effectiveness of a CBCM intervention on patient outcomes in Medicare beneficiaries with chronic illness in a CBCM service in the rural Midwest. A descriptive, repeated measures design was used, and a secondary analysis of a data set containing longitudinal CBCM data, originally collected from 2002 to 2007, was conducted. Two years of case management (CM) interventions, three health service utilization outcomes, and three patient-focused outcomes were examined. The study findings showed that a CBCM had significant effect on reducing patients' number of hospitalizations and increasing patients' symptom control and quality of life. The impact of CM on length of stay and emergency department visits was indeterminate. Findings suggest that CBCM can be used as an effective intervention program for Medicare beneficiaries.		√
Davis, M. M., Currey, J. M., Howk, S., DeSordi, M. R., Boise, L., Fagnan, L. J., & Vuckovic, N. (2014). A qualitative study of rural primary care clinician views on remote monitoring technologies. *The Journal of Rural Health, 30*(1), 69–78	Remote monitoring technologies (RMTs) may improve the quality of care, reduce access barriers, and help control medical costs. Despite the role of primary care clinicians as potential key users of RMTs, few studies explore their views. This study explores rural primary care clinician interest and the resources necessary to incorporate RMTs into routine practice. Researchers conducted 15 in-depth interviews with rural primary care clinician members of the Oregon Rural Practice-Based Research Network (ORPRN) from November 2011 to April 2012. The multidisciplinary team used thematic analysis to identify emergent themes and a cross-case comparative analysis to explore variation by participant and practice characteristics.		√

continued

Clinicians expressed interest in RMTs most relevant to their clinical practice, such as supporting chronic disease management, noting benefits to patients of all ages. They expressed concern about the quantity of data, patient motivation to utilize equipment, and potential changes to the patient–clinician encounter.

Direct data transfer into the clinic's electronic health record (EHR), availability in multiple formats, and review by ancillary staff could facilitate implementation. Although participants acknowledged the potential system-level benefits of using RMTs, adoption would be difficult without payment reform.

Adoption of RMTs by rural primary care clinicians may be influenced by equipment purpose and functionality, implementation resources, and payment. Clinician and staff engagement will be critical to actualize RMT use in routine primary care.

To explore the perceived barriers, resources, and training needs of rural primary care providers in relation to implementing the American Medical Association Expert Committee recommendations for assessment, treatment, and prevention of childhood obesity.

In-depth interviews were conducted with 13 rural primary care providers in Oregon. Transcribed interviews were thematically coded.

Barriers to addressing childhood obesity fell into 5 categories: barriers related to the practice (time constraints, lack of reimbursement, few opportunities to detect obesity), the clinician (limited knowledge), the family/patient (family lifestyle and lack of parent motivation to change, low family income and lack of health insurance, sensitivity of the issue), the community (lack of pediatric subspecialists and multidisciplinary/tertiary care services, few community resources), and the broader sociocultural environment (sociocultural influences, high prevalence of childhood obesity). There were very few clinic and community resources to assist clinicians in addressing weight issues. Clinicians had received little previous training relevant to childhood obesity, and they expressed an interest in several topics.

Findholt, N. E., Davis, M. M., & Michael, Y. L. (2013). Perceived barriers, resources, and training needs of rural primary care providers relevant to the management of childhood obesity. *The Journal of Rural Health, 29*(s1), s17–s24

TABLE 9-1 Rural Case Management Projects and Research, *continued*

	Rural primary care providers face extensive barriers in relation to implementing recommended practices for assessment, treatment, and prevention of childhood obesity. Particularly problematic is the lack of local and regional resources. Employing nurses to provide case management and behavior counseling, group visits, and telehealth and other technological communications are strategies that could improve the management of childhood obesity in rural primary care settings.
Shah, M. N., Caprio, T. V., Swanson, P., Rajasekaran, K., Ellison, J. H., Smith, K., ..., Katz, P. (2010). A novel emergency medical services–based program to identify and assist older adults in a rural community. *Journal of the American Geriatrics Society, 58*(11), 2205–2211	Rural-dwelling older adults experience unique challenges related to accessing medical and social services. This article describes the development, implementation, and experience of a novel, community-based program to identify rural-dwelling older adults with unmet medical and social needs that leveraged the existing emergency medical services (EMS) system. The program specifically included geriatrics training for EMS providers; screening of older adult EMS patients for falls, depression, and medication management strategies by EMS providers; communication of EMS findings to community-based case managers; in-home evaluation by case managers; and referral to community resources for medical and social interventions. Measures used to evaluate the program included patient needs identified by EMS or the in-home assessment, referrals provided to patients, and patient satisfaction. EMS screened 1,231 of 1,444 visits to older patients (85%). Of those receiving specific screens, 45% had fall-related, 69% medication management–related, and 20% depression-related needs identified. One hundred and seventy-one eligible EMS patients who could be contacted accepted the in-home assessment. Of the 153 individuals completing the assessment, 91% had identified needs and received referrals or interventions. This project demonstrated that screening by EMS during emergency care for common geriatric syndromes and linkage to case managers is feasible in this rural community, although many will refuse the services. Further patient evaluations by case managers, with subsequent interventions by existing service providers as required, can facilitate the needed linkages between vulnerable rural-dwelling older adults and needed community-based social and medical services.

continued

Eack, S. M., Greeno, C. G., Christian-Michaels, S., Dennis, A., & Anderson, C. M. (2009). Case managers' perspectives on what they need to do their job. *Psychiatric Rehabilitation Journal, 32*(4), 309

The purpose of this brief report is to identify the perceived training needs of case managers working on community support teams in a community mental health center serving a semirural/suburban area. Semistructured interviews were conducted with 18 case managers and 3 supervisors to inquire about areas of training need in case management. Interviews were coded and analyzed for common themes regarding training needs and methods of training improvement. Identified training needs called for a hands-on, back-to-basics approach that included education on the symptoms of severe mental illness, comorbid substance use problems, and methods of engaging consumers. A mentoring model was proposed as a potential vehicle for disseminating knowledge in these domains. Case managers identify significant training needs that would address their basic understanding of severe mental illness. Programs targeting these needs may result in improved outcomes for case managers and the individuals with psychiatric disabilities they serve.

McGovern, R. J., Lee, M. M. Johnson, J. C., &Morton, B. (2008). ElderLynk: A community outreach model for the integrated treatment of mental health problems in the rural elderly. *Ageing International, 32*(1), 43–53

In 2000, a rural consortium of health care education and service providers established a geriatric mental health outreach program (ElderLynk) for the underserved elderly (aged 65 and older) in 10 rural counties in Northeast Missouri. ElderLynk evaluated the efficacy of an integrated community-based treatment model through the creation and evaluation of a clinical database. Ten rural counties in Northeast Missouri were chosen because they were designated as mental health shortage areas (MHSAs) and because their elderly population approximates the projected level of elderly in the United States in 2020. All patients were managed by a geriatric nurse with treatment planning and oversight provided by a community-based interdisciplinary team, which included a psychiatrist, geriatrician, psychologist, and social worker. Using the Geriatric Depression Scale (GDS); the Government Performance and Results Act (GPRA) data to assess life satisfaction, independence/ autonomy, psychosocial functioning, and overall health; the instrumental activities of daily living (IADL); the mini-mental status examination (MMSE); and patterns of service usage (number of hours of case management and number of counseling sessions), ElderLynk patients improved significantly in overall psychological functioning, level of depression, and reported life satisfaction despite significant declines in mental status, daily function, and overall health.

TABLE 9-1 Rural Case Management Projects and Research, *continued*

Oliva, N. L. (2008). *The impact of RN case management on inpatient and ED utilization in a chronically ill, older adult, community-dwelling population.* (Doctoral dissertation). Retrieved from: ProQuest Dissertations and Theses. Accession Order No. AAT 3339201.

This study examines the characteristics and impacts of RN case management on patients' inpatient and emergency department (ED) admissions in a 65+ Medicare-enrolled community-dwelling, chronically ill population. Data are from a multiyear randomized controlled trial (RCT) of Medicare Coordinated Care Demonstration (MCCD) program participants in the Carle Clinic health care system. This study is a secondary analysis of case management data on 1,551 treatment group patients from 2002 through 2005. All patients had at least one of five qualifying chronic health conditions: atrial fibrillation, congestive heart failure, coronary artery disease, chronic obstructive pulmonary disease/asthma, or diabetes mellitus. Patient characteristics were analyzed to determine association with increased admission risk. The timing and time allocated to RN case management interventions for all participants were analyzed to document case management activities in each of 21 standardized nursing care categories. The association of case management activity type, timing and time with all-cause ED, and inpatient admission and readmissions was analyzed to determine which case management activities reduce or increase ED admission or inpatient admission/readmission risk.

Analysis revealed that age, gender, race, urban or rural status, and number of diagnoses were not significantly associated with risk of all-cause inpatient readmission. Of 14 RN case managers, 6 were associated with significant reductions in all-cause readmission risk, and one was associated with increased readmission risk. The Identify Needs: Medicare activity, which can include identifying the need for inpatient or outpatient Medicare-covered health services, was associated with a decrease in inpatient readmission log odds. All monitor case management activities and patient-specific travel were significantly associated with increased ED admission hazard. A final multivariate model identified CHF (OR 2.7, $p = .01$), as well as Assessment (OR 1.06, $p = 0.03$) and Identify Needs (OR .663, $p = .06$) activities as the strongest predictors of inpatient readmission risk.

Patients with 1 inpatient admission vs. patients with 2+ admissions received significantly greater amounts of case management time in the categories of Assessment, Identify Needs: Medicare, and Identify

Needs: Non-Medicare in most 0- to 180-day intervals after an index admission. These results indicate that RN case management intervention type, timing, and time (amount) were associated with reduced readmission risk in the study population.

continued

Meyer, P. S., & Morrissey, J. P. (2007). A comparison of assertive community treatment and intensive case management for patients in rural areas. *Psychiatric Services,* 58(1), 121–127

Objective: This article reviews the evidence for the effectiveness of community-based services for rural areas, specifically assertive community treatment and intensive case management. Service delivery to persons with severe mental illness in rural areas is challenged by low population densities, limited services, and shortages of professionals. Methods: A comprehensive literature search identified six studies of rural assertive community treatment, only two of which were controlled studies, and four rural intensive case management studies, only one of which was a controlled study. Assertive community treatment would seem ideally suited to areas lacking services because of its self-contained multidisciplinary treatment team approach. However, rural programs have been forced to make several adaptations to the assertive community treatment model, including smaller teams, less comprehensive staff, and less intensive services. There is no published evidence that these adaptations are able to produce the same results as full-fidelity teams. Some believe that intensive case management may be an alternative to assertive community treatment in rural settings because intensive case management emphasizes individual caseloads, fewer staff, less intensive contacts, and brokered services. Conclusions: The evidence suggests that intensive case management programs are effective only in community settings where there is an ample supply of treatment and support services. To build the evidence base for the effectiveness of these models, much more attention needs to be focused on evaluating the current wave of assertive community treatment and intensive case management dissemination in rural areas.

TABLE 9-1 Rural Case Management Projects and Research, *continued*

Kopelman, T., Huber, D. L., Kopelman, R., Sarrazin, M. V., & Hall, J. A. (2006). Client satisfaction with rural substance abuse case management services. *Care Management Journals*, 7(4), 179–190	Although many substance abuse organizations offer case management services, little is known about clients' satisfaction as consumers of case management services. The purpose of this study was to evaluate consumer preferences regarding the delivery of case management services in a rural substance abuse treatment program. For this study, 120 clients (30 in each of four research conditions) were interviewed about their experiences in the Iowa Case Management Project (ICMP), a field-based clinical trial evaluating a strengths-based model of case management for rural clients in drug abuse treatment. A mixed-method approach evaluated clients' responses from a semistructured interview. Most clients preferred meeting with their case manager in their own home. Clients also stated that they preferred specific characteristics of case management services, namely, convenience, privacy, comfort, and accessibility. Finally, clients wanted more time with their case managers over time. Although clients in drug treatment are not often considered as consumers, we found that client satisfaction with case management services could be studied and that clients appreciated being asked about their experiences. By targeting perceived and actual barriers to meeting with case managers (e.g., availability of transportation), service utilization by clients may be increased along with overall satisfaction.

improved knowledge, improved self-care behaviors, improved health outcomes, cost reduction, and patient satisfaction.

1. Telehealth technologies have proven effective in the management of CHF patients by detecting changes in health status earlier, decreasing the rates of hospital readmission and emergency department visits, decreasing costs, and improving self-care behaviors and quality of care.
2. Evidence from clinical trials supports the use of telehealth in disease management in general as well as future development of strategies for management of CHF in rural populations.

L. As good health is necessary to learning and educational achievement, and because rural residents frequently face difficulties accessing health care services, the availability of and access to quality health service affects the health of rural children and their families.

1. Schools are leading institutions in rural communities and hold promise to act as the point of service for child and family health.
2. APRNs and school nurses are key providers of health care in rural schools, thus decision-making frameworks are important to promote access to care, decrease service fragmentation, decrease costs, promote better collaboration and resource utilization, as well as reconcile clinical interventions with desired outcomes relevant to the community context.

M. Refer to Table 9-1 for a list of projects that demonstrate the use of case management in a rural environment.

References

Austin, C. D., McClelland, R. W., & Gursansky, D. (2006). Linking case management and community development. *Care Management Journals*, 7(4), 162–168.

Bushy, A. (2000). *Orientation to nursing in the rural community.* Thousand Oaks, CA: Sage Publications, Inc.

Case Management Society of America. (2010). *Standards of practice for case management.* Little Rock, AR: Author.

Coughlin, T. A., Long, S. K., & Graves, J. A. (2008). Does managed care improve access to care for Medicaid beneficiaries with disabilities: A national study. *Inquiry, 45*(4), 395–407.

Davis, M. M., Currey, J. M., Howk, S., DeSordi, M. R., Boise, L., Fagnan, L. J., & Vuckovic, N. (2014). A qualitative study of rural primary care clinician views on remote monitoring technologies. *The Journal of Rural Health, 30*(1), 69–78.

Depression; reports by D. Lombardi and co-researchers describe recent advances in depression. (2011). *Obesity, fitness & wellness week, 1539.*

Derrett, S., Gunter, K. E., Nocon, R. S., Quinn, M. T., Coleman, K., Daniel, D. M., … Chin, M. H. (2014). How 3 rural safety net clinics integrate care for patients: A qualitative case study. *Medical Care, 52*(11), S39–S47.

Eack, S. M., Greeno, C. G., Christian-Michaels, S., Dennis, A., & Anderson, C. M. (2009). Case managers' perspectives on what they need to do their job. *Psychiatric Rehabilitation Journal, 32*(4), 309.

Findholt, N. E., Davis, M. M., & Michael, Y. L. (2013). Perceived barriers, resources, and training needs of rural primary care providers relevant to the management of childhood obesity. *The Journal of Rural Health, 29*(s1), s17–s24.

Joo, J. Y. (2014). Community-based case management, hospital utilization, and patient-focused outcomes in Medicare beneficiaries. *Western Journal of Nursing Research, 36*(6), 825.

Kaboli, P. and Glasgow, J. (Winter 2011). VAMC facility rurality: Comparison of three classification approaches. Veterans Rural Health Resource Center-Central Region, Issue Brief #4. Office of Rural Health, VHA Office of Rural Health.

Kopelman, T., Huber, D. L., Kopelman, R., Sarrazin, M. V., & Hall, J. A. (2006). Client satisfaction with rural substance abuse case management services. *Care Management Journals, 7*(4), 179–190.

McGovern, R. J., Lee, M. M. Johnson, J. C., &Morton, B. (2008). ElderLynk: A community outreach model for the integrated treatment of mental health problems in the rural elderly. *Ageing International, 32*(1), 43–53.

Meyer, P. S., & Morrissey, J. P. (2007). A comparison of assertive community treatment and intensive case management for patients in rural areas. *Psychiatric Services, 58*(1), 121–127.

Mobley, S. C., Thomas, S. D., Sutherland, D. E., Hudgins, J., Ange, B. L., & Johnson, M. H. (2014). Maternal health literacy progression among rural perinatal women. *Maternal and Child Health Journal, 18*(8), 1881–1892.

Mohamed, S., Neale, M., & Rosenheck, R. A. (2009). VA intensive mental health case management in urban and rural areas: Veteran characteristics and service delivery. *Psychiatric Services, 60*(7), 914–921.

Morgan, L., & Fahs, P. (2007). *Conversations in the disciplines-sustaining rural populations.* Binghamton, NY: Global Academic Publishing.

Mullahy, C. (2014). *The case manager's handbook* (5th ed.). Burlington, MA: Jones & Bartlett.

National Alliance to End Homelessness. (January 17, 2010). Fact sheet: Rural homelessness. Washington, DC. Retrieved from http://www.endhomelessness.org/library/entry/fact-sheet-rural-homelessness

News briefs. (2008). *Psychiatric Services, 59*(9), 1072.

Olivia, N. L. (2008). *The impact of RN case management on inpatient and ED utilization in a chronically ill, older adult, community-dwelling population* (Doctoral dissertation). Retrieved from: ProQuest Dissertations and Theses. Accession Order No. AAT 3339201.

O'Neill, L., & Klepack, W. (2007). Electronic medical records for a rural family practice: A case study in systems development. *Journal of Medical Systems, 31*(1), 25–33.

Pyrillis, R. (2015). Small, Rural + Smart. *Hospitals & Health Networks, 89*(1), 22–27.

Sadowski, D., Devlin, M., & Hussain, A. (2012). Diabetes self-management activities for Latinos living in non-metropolitan rural communities: A snapshot of an underserved rural state. *Journal of Immigrant and Minority Health, 14*(6), 990–998.

Shah, M. N., Caprio, T. V., Swanson, P., Rajasekaran, K., Ellison, J. H., Smith, K., & Katz, P. (2010). A novel emergency medical services–based program to identify and assist older adults in a rural community. *Journal of the American Geriatrics Society, 58*(11), 2205–2211.

Stanton, M. P., & Packa, D. (2001). Nursing case management: A rural practice model. *Lippincott's Case Management, 6*(3), 96–103.

U.S. Census Bureau. (2010). 2010 census urban and rural classification and urban area criteria. Retrieved from http://www.census.gov/geo/reference/ua/urban-rural-2010.html

U.S. Census Bureau. (2015). *Geography: Urban and rural classification.* Retrieved from https://www.census.gov/geo/reference/urban-rural.html

U.S. Department of Agriculture (USDA), Economic Research Service. (2015). *County typology codes.* Retrieved from http://www.ers.usda.gov/data-products/county-typology-codes.aspx

U.S. Department of Health and Human Services (USDHHS). (September 20, 2013). *The affordable care act: What it means for rural America* [Fact sheet]. Retrieved from http://www.hhs.gov/healthcare/facts/factsheets/2013/09/rural09202013.html

U.S. Department of Health and Human Services (USDHHS), Health Resources and Services Administration (HRSA). (2015). *Shortage designation: Health professional shortage areas & medically underserved areas/populations.* Retrieved from http://www.hrsa.gov/shortage/

U.S. Department of Health and Human Services (USDHHS), National Health Service Corps (NHSC). (2015). *Students to service program.* Retrieved from https://nhsc.hrsa.gov/loan-repayment/studentstoserviceprogram/programoverview%20-%20s2s%20left%20nav/index.html

U.S. Department of Veterans Affairs, Veterans Health Administration (VHA), Office of Rural Health. (2015). *About the VHA office of rural health.* Retrieved from http://www.ruralhealth. va.gov/about/index.asp

U.S. Office of Management and Budget (OMB). (February 28, 2013). *Revised delineations of metropolitan statistical areas, micropolitan statistical areas, and combined statistical areas, and guidance on uses of the delineations of these areas* (OMB Bulletin No. 13-01). Retrieved from https://www.whitehouse.gov/sites/default/files/omb/bulletins/2013/b-13-01.pdf

CHAPTER 10

Transitional Care and Case Management

Cheri Lattimer

LEARNING OBJECTIVES

Upon completion of this chapter, the reader will be able to:

1. Define transitions of care.

2. Identify four key barriers and gaps related to transitions of care.

3. Describe three transition of care models and their impact on reducing avoidable hospital readmissions.

4. Relate the key case management competencies necessary for the effective management of transitions of care throughout the continuum of health and human services and by the interprofessional health care team.

5. Determine the impact of the Patient Protection and Affordable Care Act on transitions of care and case management practice.

6. Review key aspects of financial alignment related to chronic care management and the coordination of transitions of care activities.

IMPORTANT TERMS AND CONCEPTS

Accountable Care
  Organizations (ACOs)
Care Coordination
Care Plan
Chronic Care
  Management
Discharge Plan
Follow-Up Care

Handoff
Handover
Health Literacy
Interprofessional Care
  Planning
National Transitions
  of Care Coalition
  (NTOCC)

Patient-Centered Care
Patient-Centered Medical
  Home (PCMH)
Patient Protection and
  Affordable Care Act
  (PPACA)
Transitions of Care
Transitional Plan

Introduction

A. Transition of care involves the movement of a patient from one health care practitioner or setting to another as the patient's condition and care needs change.
   1. Transitions occur at multiple care settings, that is, emergency room to inpatient admission, critical care unit to a hospital ward, hospital discharge to home or a skilled nursing facility, primary care referral to a specialist provider, and facility to facility (Coleman & Boult, 2003).
   2. According to the National Transitions of Care Coalition (NTOCC), each transition can involve multiple gaps and barriers such as those listed in Box 10-1 (NTOCC, 2010).
   3. Transitions also present risks for suboptimal care or unsafe practices or patient experiences. Therefore, they are opportunities for case managers' interventions to ultimately assure quality and safe care and outcomes.
B. The focus on improving transitions of care has been the work of several researchers starting in the early 1990s such as:
   1. Dr. Eric Coleman's Care Transition Intervention
   2. Dr. Mary Naylor's Transitional Care
   3. Dr. Chad Boult's Work in Guided Care
C. The passage of the Patient Protection and Affordable Care Act (PPACA) of 2010 brought a much higher visibility to the issues of transitions of care and elevated the recognition of case management and its contribution to outcomes. PPACA highlighted the need for case management interventions to bring about the improvement in care coordination and transitions within the continuum of care.
D. One of the challenges for case managers is recognition of their roles within the interdisciplinary health care teams and appropriate attribution for their case management participation, especially as documented in the patient's electronic medical record reflective of their key care interventions (Box 10-2).

 Applicability to CMSA's Standards of Practice

A. The Case Management Society of America (CMSA) describes in its standards of practice for case management (CMSA, 2010) that case management practice extends across all health care settings, including payer, provider, government, employer, community, and home

BOX
10-1   Gaps and Barriers in Transitions of Care

- Miscommunication among providers, patient, and family caregiver
- Unreconciled medication lists and poor medications management
- Lack of patient and family caregiver engagement and health education
- Inadequate transfer and exchange of information across settings and providers
- Lack of follow-up care and visits
- Inadequate patient and family caregiver tools and resources
- Minimal performance measures focused on transitions of care

BOX 10-2   Examples of Case Manager's Interventions and Care Contributions

- Assessment of needs
- Identification of patient's priority areas of focus and care goals
- Care planning
- Health literacy assessment
- Cultural competency and provision of patient-centered care
- Engagement and health education of the patient and family caregiver
- Medication management
- Patient and family caregiver advocacy
- Monitoring and evaluation of the patient's response to care and progress toward achieving care goals

environment. The standards also recognize that it is natural for patients to transition among these care settings based on their care needs.

B. Professional case managers are essential to improving transitions of care and the patients' experiences during transitions. They provide interventions for care coordination across the continuum of care and bring value in improving clinical and financial outcomes.
   1. Case managers have the opportunity to take a key role within the interprofessional health care team to achieve patient-centered and directed care, enhanced patient safety, and clinical and humanistic outcomes.
   2. Case managers who accept these responsibilities take leadership roles as change agents devoted to reengineering the currently fragmented health care delivery process to ultimately maximize quality, cost, and safety outcomes for all stakeholders: patients, their families, health care providers, payers, and employers.

C. The case manager works at the top of his/her license addressing professional case management practice, which requires knowledge of and proficiency in the following practice standards described by CMSA (CMSA, 2010):
   1. Client assessment
   2. Problem/opportunity identification
   3. Care planning
   4. Monitoring
   5. Facilitation, coordination, and collaboration
   6. Advocacy
   7. Cultural competency
   8. Outcomes

Descriptions of Key Terms

A. Accountable Care Organization (ACO)—The ACO concept is evolving, but it is generally considered that an ACO is as a set of health care providers, including primary care physicians, specialists, and hospitals, working together collaboratively and accepting collective accountability for the cost and quality of care delivered to a population of patients (Accountable Care Facts, 2015).

B. Accreditation—Accreditation is an evaluative, rigorous, transparent, and comprehensive process in which a health care organization undergoes an examination of its systems, processes, and performance by an impartial external organization to ensure that it is conducting business in a manner that meets predetermined criteria and is consistent with the standards set forth by the accrediting organization (URAC, 2015a). Criteria may include standards of care and operations, quality, safety, outcomes management, and performance improvement.

C. Care Coordination—The deliberate organization of patient care activities between two or more participants (including the patient) involved in a patient's care provision, to facilitate the appropriate delivery of health care services.

1. Organizing care involves marshaling personnel and resources needed to carry out all required patient care activities and is often managed by the exchange of information among participants responsible for different aspects of care (Agency for Healthcare Research and Quality [AHRQ], 2014).

2. Care coordination delivers health benefits to those with multiple needs while improving their experience of the care system and driving down overall health care (and societal) costs.

3. Care coordination is a mechanism to assess the effectiveness of the care plan and make adjustments in order to avoid the need to deliver care in more expensive environments such as acute care facilities (Craig, Eby, & Whitington, 2011).

4. Care coordination aims at improving the transfer of patient care information and establishing accountability by clearly delineating who is responsible for which aspect of patient care delivery and communication across the care continuum. There is substantial evidence that enhanced access and improved care coordination result in improved health outcomes and patient satisfaction and decreased total costs of care for a defined population (Patient Centered Primary Care Collaborative, 2011).

D. Care Plan—A written individual plan of care, developed from an evidenced assessment with the patient, family caregiver, and interdisciplinary health care team. The care plan should detail the patient's health, behavioral, social and health system needs, and personal preferences.

E. Certification—Is a process by which an agency or association grants recognition to an individual who has met certain predetermined qualifications specified by that agency or association and usually relevant to the specialty.

F. Care Team—A collaborative care team for a given patient consisting of the various health care professionals—physicians, advanced practice nurses, pharmacists, clinical nurses, social workers, case managers, and other allied health care professionals.

G. Discharge Planning—Conducted to plan for when a patient leaves a care setting or health care encounter. The health care professional(s) and the patient participate in discharge planning activities that aim to identify the most appropriate setting the patient may access and the necessary services and resources required (Centers for Medicare and Medicaid, 2014a).

H. Handover—Sometimes also referred to as handoff. It is the communication between two parties that ensures consistent patient care and requires both the sender and receiver to understand the information and have the ability to clarify any questions or concerns. Although handovers have been practiced by nurses during shift changes for many years, the term/concept is now being used to enhance communication during transitions of care and among various health care providers and patients/families.

I. Health Literacy—Defined as the degree to which individuals have the capacity to obtain, process, and understand basic health information needed to make appropriate health decisions and services needed to prevent or treat illness (Health Resources and Services Administration, 2015). Low health literacy is more prevalent among older adults, minority populations, those who have low socioeconomic status, and medically underserved populations. Patients with low health literacy may have difficulty being engaged in own health care and may experience certain challenges (Box 10-3).

J. Interprofessional Practice (IPP)—A collaborative practice that occurs when various health care providers work with people from within their own profession, with people outside their profession, and with patients and their families (Canadian Interprofessional Health Collaborative, 2009) for the purpose of meeting patient care goals and needs.

   1. Interprofessional practice enhances the provision of comprehensive health and human services to patients/families by multiple caregivers who work collaboratively to deliver quality care within and across care settings.

   2. The Interprofessional Education Collaborative (IPEC) Expert Panel identified four main competencies for interprofessional collaborative practice (2011) (Box 10-4) that are relevant to case managers, especially in their roles on interdisciplinary care teams.

K. Patient-Centered Care—The Institute of Medicine (IOM) defines patient-centered care as providing care that is respectful of and responsive to individual patient preferences, needs, and values and ensuring that patient values guide all clinical decisions (2001).

L. Patient-Centered Medical Home (PCMH)—A care delivery model whereby patient treatment is coordinated through the primary care physician to ensure the patient receives the necessary care when needed and where needed, in a manner the patient can understand. PCMH takes responsibility for coordinating the patient's health care plan and needed resources across care settings and services over time in consultation and collaboration with the patient and family caregiver. The interdisciplinary

BOX
10-3   **Consequences of Health Literacy Concerns**

- Locating providers and services
- Filling out complex health forms
- Sharing their medical and medications history with providers
- Seeking preventive health care services
- Knowing the connection between risky lifestyle behaviors and health
- Managing chronic health conditions
- Understanding directions on medications
- Being engaged in own care and self-management activities

10-4 Interprofessional Collaborative Practice (IPEC) Competencies

1. *Values and ethics for interprofessional practice*
   - Work with individuals of other professions/disciplines to maintain a climate of mutual respect and shared values.
2. *Roles and responsibilities*
   - Use the knowledge of one's own role and those of other professions and disciplines to appropriately assess and address the health care needs of the patients, families, and populations served.
3. *Interprofessional communication*
   - Communicate with patients, families caregivers, communities, and other health professionals in a responsive and responsible manner that supports a team approach to the maintenance of health and the treatment of disease.
4. *Teams and teamwork*
   - Apply relationship-building values and the principles of team dynamics to perform effectively in different team roles to plan and deliver patient-/population-centered care that is safe, timely, efficient, effective, and equitable.

health care team in the PCMH setting has a number of responsibilities toward patient care such as those summarized in Box 10-5 (American College of Physicians, 2007).

M. Transitions of Care—Refers to the movement patients make between health care practitioners and settings as their condition and care needs change during the course of a chronic or acute illness or an episode of care. For example, in the course of an exacerbation of a chronic illness, a patient may receive care from a primary care physician or specialist in an outpatient setting and then transition to a hospital physician and nursing team during an inpatient admission before moving on to

10-5 Care Team Responsibilities in a Patient-Centered Medical Home Setting

- Help a patient choose specialist care providers and obtain medical tests when necessary. The team informs specialists of any necessary accommodations for the patient's needs.
- Help a patient access other needed providers or health services including those not readily available in the patient's community (e.g., in a medically underserved area).
- Track referrals and test results, share such information with patients/families, and ensure that patients receive appropriate follow-up care and help in understanding results and treatment recommendations.
- Ensure smooth transitions by assisting patients and families as the patient moves from one care setting to another, such as from hospital to home.
- Have systems in place that help prevent medical errors or unsafe events when multiple clinicians, hospitals, or other providers are caring for the same patient, such as medication reconciliation and shared medical records.
- Have systems in place to help patients with health insurance eligibility, coverage, and appeals or to refer patients to sources that can be of assistance. In each of these, the team works with the patient and, when appropriate, the family caregiver to identify and meet patient needs.

yet another care team at a skilled nursing facility. Finally, the patient may return home where he/she receives care from a visiting nurse. Each of these shifts from care providers and settings is defined as a care transition (Care Transitions Intervention Program, 2015).

NTOCC Care Transitions Bundle: Seven Essential Intervention Categories

A. The National Transitions of Care Coalition (NTOCC) was founded in 2006. It consists of a group of professional organizations, associations, and individuals who have joined together to address actual and potential problems concerning transitions of care: the movement of patients from one practice setting or provider to another. NTOCC believes that during these transitions, poor communication and coordination between professionals, patients, and caregivers can lead to serious and even life-threatening situations. In addition, these inefficiencies may result in wasted resources and frustrate health care consumers (NTOCC, 2015).
   1. NTOCC's Board of Directors collaborates with over 30 industry-leading professional associations, medical specialty societies, standards bodies, regulators, and government organizations, which make up the Advisors Council to guide and develop NTOCC tools and resources.
   2. Over 450 organizations participate in the review, test, critique, and implementation of NTOCC's tools and materials, which aim to improve transitions of care.
   3. NTOCC has created a variety of white papers and statements defining transition of care issues; tools to help health care professionals, patients, and caregivers establish safer transitions; and resources for practitioners and policymakers to improve transitions throughout the health care system. Most of these resources are available free of charge at NTOCC's Web site www.ntocc.org (NTOCC, 2015).
B. One of the key tools or materials NTOCC developed based on available evidence and expert opinions is the *Transitions Bundle*, which consists of *"seven essential intervention categories"* for improving transitions of care (NTOCC, 2011). The bundle provides examples of essential care transition intervention strategies that health care professionals interested in implementing improvements in care transition can consider for use (Box 10-6).
C. The concepts of the *Care Transitions Bundle* apply to all care transition exchanges across providers and care settings. They are categorized into

BOX 10-6) Care Transitions Bundle: Seven Essential Intervention Categories

- Medications management
- Transition planning
- Patient and family caregiver engagement and health education
- Information transfer
- Follow-up care
- Health provider engagement
- Shared accountability across providers and organizations

main topics containing concrete practices and descriptive language. Descriptions of each of the elements and examples are provided below to aid health care professionals in easily adopting these strategies.

D. *Bundle Element 1: Medication Management*
1. Ensures the safe use of medications by patients and their families based on the patient's plan of care.
2. Assessment of the patient's medication regimen including medication review, identification of problem medications, use of polypharmacy, adherence, persistence, and medication schedule (e.g., timing).
3. Patient and family caregiver education and counseling and teach-back reinforcement.
4. Careful and thorough conduct of medication reconciliation and management. This process should be a partnership role between the physician, pharmacist, case manager, the patient and family caregiver (as appropriate). Shared accountability can enhance a comprehensive medication review and list that should be shared with the patient and their family caregiver.

E. *Bundle Element 2: Transition Planning*
1. A formal process to facilitate the safe transition of a patient from the one level of care to another including home or from one practitioner to another. Transition planning is clearly defined in order to facilitate and coordinate a patient's transition plan.
2. Responsibility for transition planning includes a case manager who conducts a comprehensive assessment of the patient's needs, barriers, and strengths and coordination of the transition plan, inclusive of the patient and caregiver, with an interdisciplinary care team.
3. Collaboration across providers and settings in the safe execution of the transition plan with special focus on coordination with the team to assume care for the patient and family caregiver post transition.

F. *Bundle Element 3: Patient and Family Caregiver Engagement/Education*
1. Focus on patient and family caregiver active engagement in the plan of care and related decisions. This includes health education based on an assessment of the patient's health literacy and engagement in own care.
2. To enhance the active participation of the patient in health care, including informed decision making.
3. A patient must be knowledgeable about his or her condition and plan of care.
4. The case manager enhances communication at transition points and ensures that all care team members take the patient preferences into consideration.
5. The case manager assesses and understands patient health literacy, cultural norms, and motivation in order to work with the care team and in order to improve patient adherence and outcomes.

G. *Bundle Element 4: Information Transfer*
1. Sharing important care information with the patient, family caregiver, and care team members in a timely and effective manner is imperative.
2. Timely bidirectional communication that supports feedback and feedforward of information by utilizing specific communication models and tools (e.g., personal health record, transition transfer tool, transition summary). Transfer of patient information is preferred within 24 to 48 hours.

3. Case managers play an important role in assuring that all health care providers involved in a patient's care are well aware of the plan of care, transition plan, and patient's progress toward achieving care goals. Also keeping the patient and family caregiver apprised at all times.

H. *Bundle Element 5: Follow-Up Care*

1. Ensures each patient has access to key health care providers and services in a timely manner following an episode of care.
2. This may require staff to make follow-up care appointments prior to patient's discharge from an episode of care such as a hospital admission.
3. The case manager ensures telephonic or face-to-face reenforcement of the transition plan takes place and problem solving with the patient and family caregiver occurs within 24 to 48 hours after transition.

I. *Bundle Element 6: Health Care Provider Engagement*

1. Improve the flow of information between the hospital and community-based providers (e.g., outpatient physicians) and access to timely information on hospital admissions and emergency room visits.
2. Give the patient and family caregiver a written discharge summary or transition plan and health instructions that they can understand and feel confident about their responsibilities toward the plan at the time of discharge. Provide similar information to health care providers to assume responsibility for the patient post transition.
3. Assure that the patient and/or family caregiver can perform self-care activities as described in the posttransition plan of care.
4. When possible, clearly identify the patient's personal physician (primary care provider) and coordinate the transfer of patient information. This is important to secure follow-up care, enhance continuity, and assure safety.

J. *Bundle Element 7: Shared Accountability across Providers and Organizations*

1. Accountability for care enhanced across the continuum of health and human services including various care settings and providers involved in a patient's care.
2. Enhancing the transition of care process through accountability for care of the patients by both the health care provider or organization transitioning and the one receiving the patient.
3. No single entity is wholly responsible for the success of the transition process. This requires shared responsibility as a functional, collaborative care team, ensuring clear and timely communication of the patient's care plan and ensuring that a health care provider is responsible for the care of the patient at all times.
4. Improving the patient care experience and outcomes (i.e., quality, safety, and cost) depends on accountability of the health care team across the continuum and not just those involved in a specific care setting independent of the rest.

Legislative and Regulatory Considerations Pertaining to Transitions of Care

A. In March 2010, the Patient Protection and Affordable Care Act was signed into law. This legislation is also referred to as PPACA, ACA, and ObamaCare. For the rest of this chapter, the term Affordable Care Act (ACA) is used.

B. The ACA focuses on increased access to health care services, reducing costs via payment reductions and special attention to wellness and prevention. It seeks to reward value-based care and quality, safe care delivery.

C. The implementation of the ACA brought about increased attention to the skill and proficiency of case managers and case management programs. Within the ACA, Section 2717 Care Management, four areas were highlighted, which focus on improving the quality of care (NCQA, n.d.).

1. "Improve health outcomes through the implementation of activities such as quality reporting, effective Case Management, Care Coordination, chronic Disease Management, and medication and care compliance initiatives, including through the use of the medical homes model."

2. "Implement activities to prevent hospital readmissions through a comprehensive program for hospital discharge that includes patient-centered education and counseling, comprehensive discharge planning, and postdischarge reinforcement by an appropriate health care professional."

3. "Implement activities to improve patient safety and reduce medical errors through the appropriate use of best clinical practices, evidence-based medicine, and health information technology under the plan or coverage."

4. "Implement wellness and health promotion activities."

D. The Affordable Care Act brought a significant focus on improved transitions of care and care coordination, especially in relation to hospital readmissions, which are still a concern today.

1. Jencks, Williams, and Coleman (2009) in their analysis of Medicare claims data from 2003 to 2004 showed that of the 11,855,702 Medicare beneficiaries discharged from the hospital:

   a. 19.6% (nearly 1/5) were rehospitalized within 30 days of discharge.

   b. 34% were rehospitalized within 90 days of discharge.

   c. 50.2% of those rehospitalized within 30 days following a medical discharge, there was no claim for a physician office visit.

2. This study began the wheels turning to reduce avoidable hospital readmissions and improved care coordination across the continuum of care.

E. Provisions within the ACA required multiple changes for the health care delivery system, including those described in Table 10-1 (Kaiser Family Foundation, 2013).

F. The restructuring and changes within the health care system also required new payment or reimbursement models.

1. Financial incentives focused on value-based payments, bundling of health care payments, and financial alignment for value rather than volume and fee-for-service arrangements.

2. New care coordination, transition of care, and chronic care management billing codes were implemented supporting case/care management services in the primary care and specialist office practices. These codes are discussed later in the chapter.

TABLE 10-1 Examples of Changes in Health Care Delivery as a Result of the ACA

Approach to Expanding Access to Coverage	Individual Mandate	Employer Mandate
Expansion of public programs	Premium and cost-sharing subsidies to individuals	Premium subsidies to employers
Health insurance exchanges (HIE)	Benefit design—changes to private insurances	State roles
Cost containment	Improving quality/health system performance	Prevention and wellness
Long-term care		

G. Case managers, care managers, care coordinators, and transition of care specialists have become more popular as a result of renewed interest in care/case management, care coordination, and transitions of care programs in the various settings across the continuum of care.

 Transition of Care Models and Delivery Systems

A. Improving transitions of care is not only an important component of ensuring the high delivery of quality of care, but enhances patient safety and reduces the cost of care. Several new and emerging models of care are demonstrating that effective and coordinated care transitions lead to improved communication, reduced medication errors, better patient engagement, and cost savings.

B. *The Care Transitions Intervention (CTI)*
   1. Developed by Eric Coleman, MD, MPH, CTI is a program that provides specific tools to patients with complex care needs and allows them to work with a transitions coach to learn transition-specific self-management skills.
   2. Evidence has shown that participants in CTI are significantly less likely to be readmitted to the hospital and the benefits are sustained for 5 months after the end of the 1-month intervention. Rather than simply managing posthospital care in a reactive manner, imparting self-management skills pays dividends long after the program ends.
   3. Anticipated net cost savings for a typical transition coach panel of 350 chronically ill adults with an initial hospitalization over 12 months is conservatively estimated at $365,000. Patients who received this program were also more likely to achieve self-identified personal goals around symptom management and functional recovery (Coleman, Parry, Chalmers, & Min, 2006).

C. *The Transitional Care Model (TCM)*
   1. Developed at the University of Pennsylvania and spearheaded by Mary Naylor, PhD, RN.
   2. TCM establishes an interdisciplinary team, led by a master's prepared transitional care nurse to treat chronically ill, high-risk older patients before, during, and after discharge from the hospital.

3. Significant reductions in total health care costs (e.g., hospital, home health, physician visits) after accounting for the additional costs of the intervention have been demonstrated in a number of multisite, NIH-funded randomized clinical trials.

D. *The Guided Care Model*
1. Developed at Johns Hopkins University, the Guided Care model is driven by a highly skilled Guided Care nurse (GCN) who coordinates care for chronically ill patients.
2. After 1 year into a randomized controlled trial, Guided Care patients experienced (on average) 24% fewer days in hospital, 37% fewer skilled nursing facility days, 15% fewer emergency department visits, and 29% fewer home health care episodes, as well as 9% more specialist visits (GuidedCare.com, 2015).

E. *Project Reengineered Discharge (RED)*
1. Project RED is a research group at Boston University Medical Center that develops and tests strategies to improve the hospital discharge process in a way that promotes patient safety and reduces rehospitalization rates.
2. The Project RED intervention is founded on 12 discrete, mutually reinforcing components and has been proven to reduce rehospitalizations and yields high rates of patient satisfaction.
3. Virtual patient advocates are currently being tested in conjunction with the Project RED intervention.

F. *The Bridge Model*
1. Rush University Medical Center's Enhanced Discharge Planning Program is now referred to as the Bridge Model. It is designed to aid in patient transitions from hospital to home.
2. Transitional care is delivered by a Masters-level social worker providing telephonic follow-up and short-term care coordination for recently discharged adults. The social worker conducts a biopsychosocial assessment through a review of medical records, discharge plans, and participation in predischarge interdisciplinary rounds and collaborates with the patient following discharge to identify gaps in care and intervene to resolve identified needs.
3. This model provides a resource for each patient as well as an opportunity for the social worker to provide early intervention should difficulties arise.
4. A randomized control trial showed a decreased readmission rate at 30, 60, 90, and 120 days post discharge. Participants were more likely to make and keep follow-up appointments, had a better understanding of medication management, experienced reduced caregiver burden, and had lower mortality rates (Rush University Medical Center, 2015).

G. *Project BOOST*
1. The Project BOOST is a national mentored implementation program led by the Society of Hospital Medicine (SHM). It focuses on improvement of patient care during transition from hospital to home.
2. Project BOOST is a yearlong initiative during which hospitals receive expert mentoring and peer support to aid in the improvement of patient care transitions from hospital to home.

3. BOOST provides a suite of evidence-based clinical interventions that may be adapted and integrated into unique hospital environments. In a study of 11 hospitals that implemented one or more Project BOOST tools, hospitals reduced 30-day readmissions by an average of 13.6 percent (Society of Hospital Medicine, 2014).

H. *Accountable Care Organization (ACO)*
1. The ACO is one way in which CMS is working to ensure better health care, better health, and lower growth in expenditures through continuous improvement.
2. The Medicare Shared Savings Program provides incentives for ACOs that meet standards for quality performance and reduce cost while putting patients first.
3. Established by the ACA, CMS published final rules for the Shared Savings Program on November 2, 2011. Working in concert with the Shared Savings Program, the Innovation Center is testing an alternative ACO, the Pioneer ACO Model (Centers for Medicare and Medicaid, 2015a).

I. *Comprehensive Primary Care (CPC) Initiatives*
1. The CPC initiative is a 4-year multipayer initiative designed to strengthen primary care. Since its October 2012 launch, CMS has collaborated with commercial and state health insurance plans in seven US regions to offer population-based care management fees and shared savings opportunities to participating primary care practices to support the provision of a core set of five comprehensive primary care functions. These five functions are:
   a. Risk-stratified care management
   b. Access and continuity
   c. Planned care for chronic conditions and preventive care
   d. Patient and caregiver engagement
   e. Coordination of care across the medical neighborhood
2. The initiative is testing whether provision of these functions at each practice site, which is supported by multipayer payment reform, the continuous use of data to guide improvement, and meaningful use of health information technology, can achieve improved care, better health for populations, and lower costs and can inform future Medicare and Medicaid policy (Centers for Medicare and Medicaid, 2015c).

J. *Patient-Centered Medical Home (PCMH)*
1. The medical home model holds promise as a way to improve health care in America by transforming how primary care is organized and delivered.
2. Building on the work of a large and growing community, the Agency for Healthcare Research and Quality (AHRQ) defines a medical home not simply as a place but as a model of the organization of primary care that delivers the core functions of primary health care.
3. The medical home encompasses the following five functions and attributes.
   a. Comprehensive care
   b. Patient centered
   c. Coordinated care
   d. Accessible services
   e. Quality and safety

4. A 2013 study reported in the American Journal of Managed Care found a clinic-level population-based PCMH redesign can decrease downstream utilization and reduce total health care costs in a subpopulation of patients with common chronic illnesses (Liss et al., 2013).

 ## Transitions of Care and Implications for Case Management Practice

A. Improving transitions of care requires the skills of professional case managers and their knowledge of and experience with care coordination. Successful transitions mean having the case manager as an integral part of the interdisciplinary clinical team from the beginning of care.

B. Enhancing transitions of care requires a focus on patient-centered care and supporting meaningful communication among care team members and with the patient/family caregiver.

C. Case managers through their focus on patient engagement and education can assist the provider, patient, and family caregiver to reach a collaboration of care planning and self-management and improve the patient's health care experience.

D. Case managers work in every aspect of the health care continuum, which provides a framework for improved communication and warm handoffs (or handovers) of patient information to assist in reducing miscommunications and improve patient follow-up. Case managers bring in other members of the interdisciplinary or interprofessional health care team to reduce fragmentation of care issues.

E. In the complex and hurried world of health care, the professional case manager links patients with appropriate providers and resources across the continuum of care services.

F. Case managers may apply NTOCC's Care Transitions Bundle in their work settings and when caring for patients and their families or collaborating with other members of the health care team internal and external to their settings.

G. Refer to Chapter 13 for more details on transitional planning and transitions of care and their applicability in case management practice.

Roles and Functions Associated with Transitions of Care

A. The National Transitions of Care Coalition highlights seven key principles associated with improving transitions, described previously in NTOCC Care Transitions Bundle: Seven Essential Intervention Categories

B. The case manager plays a key role in care transition by conducting a thorough case management assessment ensuring that the medical, behavioral, psychosocial, emotional, financial, and health system needs of the patient have been clearly documented.

1. The assessment drives the care plan including problem identification, a reconciled medication list, and both clinical and nonclinical goals developed with the patient.

2. Ensuring that the patient and family caregiver have an understanding of the clinical and nonclinical issues incorporated in the care plan and that the plan encourages greater engagement with the patient and family caregiver as well as communication.

C. Effective communication and greater engagement with each patient and family caregiver are important functions of the case manager. The case manager ensures that information provided to the patient takes into account his/her health literacy status and that the information is actionable, meaning that the patient is able to take productive steps to accomplish the action plan.

D. The case manager helps enhance the patient and family caregiver engagement in own care and demonstrate better self-management skills by carefully attending to existing health literacy issues identified based on an assessment and through applying specific health literacy strategies that improve patient's understanding of health condition and ultimately adherence to health care regimen (Box 10-7).

E. Use of the teach-back method is an excellent way of assessing the level of understanding that the patient and family caregiver have achieved about their medical and health condition, medication list, follow-up care, and safety.

1. The case manager is an excellent coach to ensure that patients feel comfortable in asking questions of the clinical care team and that they know which questions to ask.

BOX
10-7
Strategies for Clear Communication with Patients/Families and Improving Health Literacy

- Identification of literacy limitations
- Use of straightforward and simple language using short sentences and defining technical terms
- Supplementing instruction with appropriate materials (e.g., videos, models, pictures)
- Asking the patient to explain instructions (e.g., teach-back method) or to demonstrate the procedure
- Asking questions that require an explanatory response and begin with how and what, rather than posing closed-ended questions that require yes or no response
- Organizing information by emphasizing the most important point(s) and repeating key information
- Reflecting the age, cultural, ethnic, and racial diversity of the patient in instructions and examples
- For limited English–proficiency (LEP) patients, providing information in the primary, preferred written language
- Improving the physical care environment through use of universal symbols
- Offering assistance with completing forms
- Maintaining eye contact during in-person interactions
- Listening carefully and using patient's own words
- Demonstrating how care activities (e.g., Insulin injections) are expected to be done
- Inviting patients to ask question and to be active participants

From the Agency for Healthcare Research and Quality (AHRQ). (August 2015). AHRQ health literacy universal precautions toolkit. Accessed on October 6, 2015 from http://www.ahrq.gov/professionals/quality-patient-safety/quality-resources/tools/literacy-toolkit/index.html

F. Improving communication between providers, patients, and families or caregivers can be improved by using bidirectional communication especially during transitions of care. According to the NTOCC, it is imperative that there is accountability for both the sender and receiver of patient-related information.

    1. The care transition-based interactions between the accountable providers of care occur in a care coordination hub context with a primary aim of ensuring effective and safe transitions of care between settings and/or providers. See Figure 10-1 and Table 10-2 for clarification (NTOCC, 2008).

G. Ensuring that critical patient information is transferred and coordinated in a timely and effective manner with all members of the interdisciplinary health care team is an important intervention at the point of transition.

    1. Often, the communication role is part of the case manager's practice whether in an acute care setting, health plan, or outpatient services.

    2. Successful communication requires excellent listening, written, and verbal communication skills.

H. Ensuring that patients and family caregivers have an updated medication list after each transition means that the interdisciplinary health care team must work together to ensure coordinated medication reconciliation and communication with the patient and family caregiver. An emerging model is the interdisciplinary partnership between the pharmacist and case manager collaborating to ensure there is a complete assessment and transfer of information.

I. After a patient is transitioned from the hospital to home, a follow-up call or home visit is another intervention associated with improving transition of care for hospitalized patients. Studies have shown that follow-up intervention is an excellent time to review discharge instructions, identify concerns, clarify miscommunication, and provide problem resolution with the patient and family caregiver.

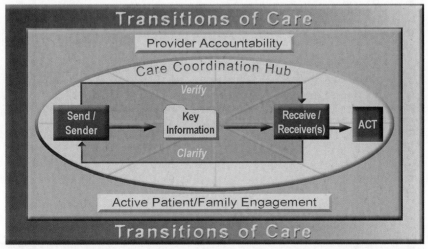

FIGURE 10-1. Conceptual model for transitions of care. (From National Transitions of Care Coalition (NTOCC). (2008). Transitions of care measures. Retrieved from http://www.ntocc.org/Portals/0/PDF/Resources/TransitionsOfCare_Measures.pdf, on October 6, 2015.)

TABLE 10-2 Clarifying the Transitions of Care Interaction between the Sender and Receiver

	Who	What	To Whom	When	Verify/Clarify	Act Upon	How is This Documented
SENDER	Accountable provider on sender team	• Tests • Consultations • Medication reconciliation • Transition summary • Assessments • Patient education • My medicine list • Other	Accountable provider and patient	Send the information timely for appropriate intervention with patient	Sender • Verifies information that is received by the intended recipients • Clarifies information for recipient	Sender • Documents transaction • Sender will resend information if not received by intended recipient.	Sender documents data source. • Paper medical record • Electronic health record (HER), electronic medical record (EMR) • Checklist
RECEIVER	Accountable provider on receiver team	• Tests • Consultations • Medication reconciliation • Transition summary • Assessments • Patient education • My medicine list • Other	Accountable provider and patient	Received the information timely for appropriate intervention with patient	Receiver • Acknowledges having document • Asks questions for clarification of information received	Receiver • Uses the information and takes actions as indicated • Ensures continuity of plan of care/ services	Receiver documents data source. • Paper medical record • EHR, EMR • Checklist

From National Transitions of Care Coalition (NTOCC). (2008). Transitions of care measures. Retrieved on October 6, 2015 from http://www.ntocc.org/Portals/0/PDF/Resources/TransitionsOfCare_Measures.pdf

Reimbursement Issues

A. The focus on improved transitions of care and care coordination within the ACA prompted the development of new International Classification of Diseases—Clinical Manual (ICD-CM), Ninth Revision (ICD-9) payment codes. The new codes recognized the importance of the transitional care and provide reimbursement to primary care and specialty providers. These codes have carried over to the Tenth Revision.

B. In January 2013, transitional care codes were implemented. Transitional Care Management Services rendered within 30 days of discharge from acute care setting can be billed using the following Current Procedural Terminology (CPT) codes:

1. 99495 required the following elements:
   a. Communication (direct contact, telephone, electronic) with the patient and/or caregiver within 2 business days of discharge
   b. Medical decision making of at least moderate complexity during the service period
   c. Face-to-face visit, within 14 calendar days of discharge (Santa Clara County Medical Association/Monterey County Medical Society, 2013)

2. 99496 recognized a more intense level of service:
   a. Communication (direct contact, telephone, electronic) with the patient and/or caregiver within 2 business days of discharge
   b. Medical decision making of at least high complexity during the service period
   c. Face-to-face visit within 7 calendar days of discharge (Santa Clara County Medical Association/Monterey County Medical Society, 2013)

C. These CPT codes provided a scope of practice for nurses and social workers rendering case management services under a physician's supervision and collaboration, inclusive of the reimbursable care activities described in Box 10-8.

D. In January 2015, CPT code recognizing outpatient chronic care management (CCM) became effective.

1. The mechanism for financial reimbursement applies for primary care and specialty providers for care management of chronically ill

---

BOX

 10-8   **Reimbursable Case Management Activities under the Transitional Care Management Service Codes**

- Communicate with the patient or family caregiver (by phone, e-mail, or in person).
- Communicate with a home health agency or other community service that the patient needs.
- Educate the patient and/or caregiver to support self-management and activities of daily living.
- Provide assessment and support for treatment adherence and medication management.
- Identify available community and health resources.
- Facilitate access to services needed by the patient and/or caregivers.

patients, 24 hours a day, 7 days a week (Centers for Medicare and Medicaid, 2014b, 2015b).

2. Conditions for use of the CCM code (Reimbursement Code 99490) are listed in Box 10-9.

Certification and Accreditation in Transitions of Care

A. The new models of care addressing better care coordination and transitions brought about the need for both individuals and organizations to demonstrate meeting national standards for certification and accreditation.

B. There are numerous case management–related certifications. Some are specific to transitions of care, and others are related to the general practice of case management assuming that transitions of care is one of the aspects these certifications address (refer to Chapter 17 for more information).

C. Individual certification in transitions of care may be attained through the following organizations:

1. American Board of Quality Assurance and Utilization Review Physicians (ABQAURP)
   a. ABQAURP requires each candidate to complete the health care quality and management (HCQM) core certification after which he/she may sit for one or more subspecialty certification.
   b. The transitions of care subspecialty certification demonstrates that the health care professional possesses the background, knowledge, and tools required to critically evaluate issues associated with transitions of care, to identify evidence-based practice of care, and to make recommendations providing better health, care, and cost (ABQAURP, 2015).

2. The Commission for Case Management Certification (CCMC)
   a. Offers the Certified Case Manager (CCM) credential, which demonstrates a case manager's knowledge, expertise, skill, and ability to practice competently.
   b. The CCM underscores the case manager's ability to work effectively on today's multidisciplinary team environment.

   c. The CCM is a certification in general practice of case management of which transitions of care is an aspect.

   d. The credential is available to individuals who meet the rigorous qualification criteria and pass the written examination (CCMC, 2015).

  3. Medical–Surgical Nursing Certification Board (MSNCB)

   a. Offers the Certified in Care Coordination and Transition Management (CCCTM) credential, which recognizes that the highest standards of care coordination nursing practice have been achieved.

   b. CCCTM certification requires successfully completing the certification examination, which validates proficiency in care coordination and transition management nursing (MSNCB, 2015).

 D. Organizational accreditation and/or program certification may be attained through the following organizations:

  1. National Committee on Quality Assurance (NCQA)

   a. The Accountable Care Organization (ACO) accreditation standards and guidelines incorporate whole-person care coordination throughout the health care system.

   b. The ACO accreditation helps health care organizations demonstrate their ability to improve quality, reduce costs, and coordinate patient care.

   c. The ACO accreditation verifies availability of and patients' access to care, patient rights and responsibilities, primary care, care management and coordination capabilities, practice patterns and performance reporting, and program operations (NCQA, 2015).

  2. URAC

   a. Accountable Care Accreditation is a model focusing on total population health and care coordination for improving the health of a defined segment or entire population. By validating the key components of population health (e.g., population needs assessment, risk stratification), improved quality of care may be provided to all consumers.

   b. URAC's Accountable Care Accreditation program works through an approach building on a framework of clinical integration and focuses on the following five areas:

    i. Patient centeredness and engagement

    ii. Health information technology

    iii. Population-based risk management

    iv. Quality management

    v. Case management (URAC, 2015b)

References

Accountable Care Facts. (2015). *What is an accountable care organization.* Retrieved from http://www.accountablecarefacts.org/topten/what-is-an-accountable-care-organization-aco-1, on September 29, 2015.

Agency for Healthcare Research and Quality (AHRQ). (2014). *What is care coordination?* Retrieved from http://www.ahrq.gov/professionals/prevention-chronic-care/improve/coordination/atlas2014/chapter2.html, on September 29, 2015.

American Board of Quality Assurance and Utilization Review Physicians. (2015). *Sub-specialty certifications.* Retrieved from http://www.abqaurp.org/ABQMain/Certification/Sub-Specialty_Certifications/ABQMain/Sub-Specialty.aspx?hkey=45e64f2f-5093-4bdd-bad3-786b71f2760e, on October 4, 2015.

American College of Physicians. (2007). *Joint principles of the patient centered medical home.* Retrieved from https://www.acponline.org/running_practice/delivery_and_payment_models/pcmh/demonstrations/jointprinc_05_17.pdf, on September 29, 2015.

Canadian Interprofessional Health Collaborative (CIHC). (2009). *What is collaborative practice?* Accessed on October 6, 2015; Available at http://www.cihc.ca/files/CIHC_Factsheets_CP_Feb09.pdf

Care Transitions Intervention Program. (2015). *What is transitional care?* Retrieved from http://caretransitions.org/#transitionalcare, on September 29, 2015.

Case Management Society of America. (2010). *CMSA Standards of practice for case management, revised 2010.* Retrieved from http://www.cmsa.org/portals/0/pdf/memberonly/StandardsOfPractice.pdf, on September 29, 2015.

Centers for Medicare and Medicaid. (2014a). *Discharge planning.* Retrieved from https://www.cms.gov/Outreach-and-Education/Medicare-Learning-Network-MLN/MLNProducts/Downloads/Discharge-Planning-Booklet-ICN908184.pdf, on September 29, 2015.

Centers for Medicare and Medicaid. (2014b). *Proposed policy and payment changes to the Medicare Physician Fee Schedule for Calendar Year 2015.* Retrieved from https://www.cms.gov/Newsroom/MediaReleaseDatabase/Fact-sheets/2014-Fact-sheets-items/2014-07-03-1.html, on September 30, 2015.

Centers for Medicare and Medicaid. (2015a). *Pioneer ACO fact sheet.* Retrieved from http://innovation.cms.gov/initiatives/Pioneer-ACO-Model/PioneerACO-FactSheet.html, on September 30, 2015.

Centers for Medicare and Medicaid. (2015b). *Chronic care management services.* Retrieved from https://www.cms.gov/Outreach-and-Education/Medicare-Learning-Network-MLN/MLNProducts/Downloads/ChronicCareManagement.pdf, on October 4, 2015.

Centers for Medicare and Medicaid. (2015c). *Comprehensive primary care initiative.* Retrieved from http://innovation.cms.gov/initiatives/comprehensive-primary-care-initiative/, on September 30, 2015.

Coleman, E. A., & Boult, C. (2003). Improving the quality of transitional care for persons with complex care needs. *Journal of the American Geriatrics Society, 51*(4), 556–557.

Coleman, E. A., Parry, C., Chalmers, S., & Min, S. J. (2006). The Care Transitions Intervention: Results of a randomized controlled trial. *Archives of Internal Medicine, 166*(17), 1822–1828. Retrieved from http://caretransitions.org/our-publications, on September 29, 2015.

Commission for Case Management Certification. (2015). Board certified case manager. Retrieved from http://ccmcertification.org/case-managers/board-certified-case-manager, on October 2, 2015.

Craig, C., Eby, D., & Whittington, J. (2011). *Care coordination model: Better care at lower cost for people with multiple health and social needs.* IHI Innovation Series white paper. Cambridge, MA: Institute for Healthcare Improvement. Retrieved from http://www.ihi.org/resources/Pages/IHIWhitePapers/IHICareCoordinationModelWhitePaper.aspx, on September 29, 2015.

Health Resources Services Administration (HRSA). (2015). Effective communication tools for healthcare professionals: Addressing health literacy, cultural competency, and limited English proficiency (LEP). Retrieved from https://www.train.org/DesktopModules/eLearning/CourseDetails/CourseDetailsForm.aspx?tabid=62&CourseID=1010508, on September 29, 2015.

GuidedCare.com. (2015). Program history and results. Retrieved from http://www.guidedcare.org/program-history-results.asp, on September 29, 2015.

Institute of Medicine (IOM). (2001). *Crossing the quality chasm. Crossing the quality chasm: A new health system for the 21st century.* Washington, DC: National Academy Press.

Interprofessional Education Collaborative (IPEC) Expert Panel. (2011). *Core competencies for interprofessional collaborative practice: Report of an expert panel.* Washington, DC: Interprofessional Education Collaborative.

Jencks, S. F., Williams, M. V., & Coleman, E. A. (2009). Rehospitalization among patients in the medicare fee-for-service program. *New England Journal of Medicine, 360*, 1418–1428. doi: 10.1056/NEJMsa0803563. Retrieved from http://www.nejm.org/doi/full/10.1056/NEJMsa0803563, on September 29, 2015.

Kaiser Family Foundation (KFF). (2013). *Summary of the affordable care act.* Retrieved from http://kff.org/health-reform/fact-sheet/summary-of-the-affordable-care-act, on September 29, 2015.

Liss, D. T., Fishman, P. A., Rutter, C. M., Grembowski, D., Ross, T. R., Johnson, E. A., & Reid, R. J. (2013). Outcomes among chronically ill adults in a medical home prototype. *American Journal of Managed Care, 19*(10), e348–e358. Retrieved from http://www.ncbi.nlm.nih.gov/pmc/articles/PMC4074014/, on October 2, 2015.

Medical Surgical Nursing Certification Board (MSNCB). About MSNCB. Retrieved from https://www.msncb.org/about, on October 4, 2015.

National Committee on Quality Assurance (NCQA). (n.d.). *Implementation of section 2717: Ensuring the quality of care.* Retrieved from http://www.ncqa.org/Portals/0/Public%20Policy/Implementation%20of%20Section%202717-%20Ensuring%20the%20Quality%20of%20Care.pdf, on September 29, 2015.

National Committee on Quality Assurance (NCQA). (2015). *Accountable care organization accreditation.* Retrieved from http://www.ncqa.org/Programs/Accreditation/Accountable CareOrganizationACO.aspx, on October 4, 2015.

National Transitions of Care Coalition (NTOCC). (2008). *Transitions of care measures.* Retrieved on October 6, 2015 from http://www.ntocc.org/Portals/0/PDF/Resources/TransitionsOfCare_ Measures.pdf

National Transitions of Care Coalition (NTOCC). (2010). *NTOCC improving transitions of care. Findings and considerations of the "Visions of the National Transitions of Care".* Retrieved from http://www.ntocc.org/Portals/0/PDF/Resources/NTOCCIssueBriefs.pdf, on September 29, 2015.

National Transitions of Care Coalition (NTOCC). (2011). *Care transition bundle, seven essential intervention categories.* Retrieved from http://www.ntocc.org/Portals/0/PDF/Compendium/ SevenEssentialElements_NTOCClogo.pdf, on September 29, 2015.

National Transitions of Care Coalition (NTOCC). (2015). *About us.* Retrieved on October 6, 2015. Available at http://www.ntocc.org/AboutUs.aspx.

Patient Centered Primary Care Collaborative. (2011). *Core value, community connections: Care coordination in the medical home.* Retrieved from https://www.pcpcc.org/sites/default/files/ media/carecoordination_pcpcc.pdf, on September 29, 2015.

Rush University Medical Center. (2015). *Bridge model.* Retrieved from https://www.rush.edu/ services-treatments/geriatric-services-older-adult-care/enhanced-discharge-planning-pro-gram-rush, on September 29, 2015.

Santa Clara County Medical Association/Monterey County Medical Society. (2013). *CPT— Transitional Care Management Services (99495-99496).* Retrieved from http://www.sccma-mcms.org/Portals/19/assets/docs/TCM-CPT.pdf, on October 4, 2015.

Society of Hospital Medicine. (2014). *Project BOOST 2014 Fact Sheet.* Retrieved from http:// www.hospitalmedicine.org/Web/Quality_Innovation/Implementation_Toolkits/Project_ BOOST/Web/Quality___Innovation/Implementation_Toolkit/Boost/First_Steps/Fact_ Sheet.aspx, on October 4, 2015.

URAC. (2015a). *What is accreditation.* Retrieved from https://www.urac.org/accreditation-and-measurement/accreditation-and-measurement, on September 29, 2015.

URAC. (2015b). *Accountable care accreditation.* Retrieved from https://www.urac.org/ accreditation-and-measurement/accreditation-programs/all-programs/accountable-care-accreditation/, on October 4, 2015.

Roles, Functions, and Essential Practice Considerations for Case Managers

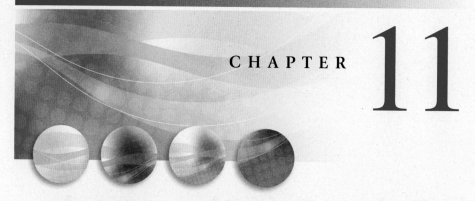

CHAPTER 11

The Roles, Functions, and Activities of Case Management

Hussein M. Tahan

LEARNING OBJECTIVES

Upon completion of this chapter, the reader will be able to:

1. Differentiate among a role, a function, and an activity and how each applies to the case manager.

2. Understand how the practice of the case manager has changed and expanded over time in the United States.

3. Identify how and why clients/patients and other health care providers have embraced and accepted case management services.

4. Explain why the case manager's role continues to change and be dynamic in practice.

5. List five various functions case managers perform across the different practice settings across the continuum of health and human services.

IMPORTANT TERMS AND CONCEPTS

Activity	Context	Role
Care Management	Domain	Task
Care Manager	Function	Transition of Care
Case Management	Job Description	
Case Manager	Practice Setting	

Introduction

A. Roles and functions of case managers are defined by professional organizations/societies (e.g., Case Management Society of America [CMSA], American Nurses Association [ANA], Commission for Case Manager Certification [CCMC], American Case Management Association [ACMA], and National Association of Social Workers [NASW]), based on scientific evidence, literature published by organizations that have implemented case management programs, and educational materials used in training and education of case managers.

B. Roles and functions of case managers are usually written in an organization in the form of job descriptions. However, the research literature that addresses what case managers do tends to report a taxonomy (or a list) of activities and tasks of case management based on which job descriptions can be delineated.

C. The role of the case manager has been implemented in every setting of the health care continuum (preacute, acute, postacute, rehabilitative, and end of life) and is assumed by a variety of professionals from different health disciplines, such as nurses, social workers, rehabilitation counselors, disability specialists, workers' compensation specialists, pharmacists, and others.

D. The role of the case manager has also been implemented in health care provider organizations for the care of special populations such as clients with multiple chronic illnesses, congenital anomalies, developmentally and mentally disabled, and other vulnerable age groups. Case managers care for these client populations in various settings.

E. There is no standard job description for case managers today in the United States. However, the literature shares common or core aspects of case management practice: clinical/patient care, managerial/ leadership, financial/business, quality and safety, and information management.

 Descriptions of Key Terms

A. According to the *Merriam-Webster Dictionary* (Merriam-Webster, 2015), key case manager role-related terms are defined as follows:
   1. Domain—A sphere of knowledge, influence, or activity. In case management, it refers to an area or category of practice and/or knowledge.
   2. Function—Any of a group of related tasks contributing to a larger action; also indicates an official position. In case management, it is the activities a case manager performs in his or her job.
   3. Role—A function or part performed especially in a particular operation or process; the proper function of a person or thing. In case management, it refers to the case manager's job title or position.
   4. Setting—The scene or locale of any action or event; the time, place, and circumstances in which something occurs or develops. In case management, it refers to the type of agency/organization a case manager works in and what population he or she serves.

B. Tahan and Campagna (2010) defined the terms *activity, function, knowledge,* and *role* as described below and used these conceptualizations to guide their research on roles and functions of case managers.
1. Activity—A concrete and discrete action, task, or behavior that is derived from a function and performed by the person in the role to meet the goals of the role; for example, "list the medications a patient takes while at home."
2. Function—A grouping or composite of specific activities within the role. These activities are interrelated and share a common goal, for example, "coordination of care activities."
3. Role—A general, conceptual, and abstract term that refers to a set of behaviors and expected results that is associated with one's position in a social structure. This includes theoretical descriptions that guide one's expected behaviors. A proxy usually used for the role is the individual's title, for example, the "case manager."
4. Knowledge—A grouping of specific facts, information, skills, and abilities necessary for effective execution of one's role and related expected behaviors, for example, knowledge of "health care reimbursement methods."
C. Other case management–related terms are as follows:
1. Case manager—A health care professional who works with the patient and family as well as the health care team in the coordination of care activities and treatment or case management plan of care. He or she may be engaged in many activities such as patient and family education, counseling, outcomes monitoring, utilization management, and others. The case manager may be a registered nurse, a social worker, a physical therapist, a vocational rehabilitation counselor, or some other licensed health care professional.
2. Context—The environment or work structure in which a case manager functions, for example, managed care organization or payer-based case manager, hospital, or acute care.
3. Job description—A document that describes roles and responsibilities, which when appropriately executed produces intended results. It also describes general tasks, responsibilities, and functions; identifies the individual/position to whom the case manager reports; and specifies the required qualifications for the job such as educational background, years of experience, and certification.

Applicability to CMSA'S Standards of Practice

A. The Case Management Society of America (CMSA) describes the roles, functions, and activities of case managers in its standards of practice for case management (CMSA, 2010). The standards emphasize the importance of differentiating among the terms "role," "function," and "activity," before describing what case managers do.
B. The standards of practice advocate for having a clear and contextual understanding of the roles and responsibilities of case managers, which start with delineation what a "role," "function," and "activity" mean. The standards define these terms based on the scientific work of Tahan, Huber, and Downey (2006). These definitions continue to apply in today's case management practice.

C. The case manager, according to the CMSA standards of practice (CMSA, 2010), performs the primary functions of assessment, planning, facilitation, advocacy, monitoring and evaluation which are achieved through collaboration with the client and other health care professionals involved in the client's care.

D. Key responsibilities of case managers have been identified by nationally recognized professional societies and certifying bodies, usually through case management roles and functions research and evidence. The CMSA standards of practice broadly define the major functions involved in the case management process necessary to achieve desired outcomes.

E. The CMSA standards of practice also clearly caution that successful outcomes cannot be achieved without case managers exhibiting specialized skills and knowledge throughout the case management process and while caring for clients and their support systems. The skills and knowledge base of a case manager may be applied to individual clients, or to groups of clients, such as in disease management or population health models (CMSA, 2010).

F. The CMSA standards of practice highlight key knowledge areas and a set of skills case managers must possess for effective role performance. These are, but should not be limited to those, presented in Box 11-1.

G. The CMSA standards of practice for case management identify a specific set of essential roles and functions of case managers, which can be applied to various care settings across the continuum of health and human services and regardless of professional discipline or background of the case manager. These include, but are not limited to, those presented in Box 11-2.

H. This chapter describes the roles and functions of case managers in greater depth in an effort to expand on those CMSA highlights in its standards of practice and to offer a greater understanding of the complex roles and responsibilities entrusted in case managers.

BOX 11-1   Essential Knowledge Areas and Skills for Case Managers

Knowledge areas
- Funding sources
- Health care services
- Human behavior dynamics
- Health care delivery and financing systems
- Clinical standards and outcomes

Skills
- Positive relationship building
- Effective written and verbal communication
- Negotiation
- Ability to effect change
- Ongoing evaluation and critical analysis
- Ability to plan and organize effectively

From Case Management Society of America (CMSA). (2010). *Standards of practice for case management*. Little Rock, AR: CMSA.

11-2 Roles and Functions of Case Managers

- Conducting a comprehensive assessment of the client's health and psychosocial needs, including health literacy status and deficits.
- Development of case management plans of care collaboratively with the client and family or caregiver.
- Planning with the client, family and caregiver, the primary care physician or provider, other health care providers, the payer, and the community, to maximize health care responses, quality, and cost-effective outcomes.
- Facilitating communication and coordination among members of the health care team, involving the client in the decision-making process in order to minimize fragmentation in the services and maximize efficiency and cost-effectiveness.
- Educating the client, the family or caregiver, and members of the health care delivery team about treatment options, community resources, insurance benefits, psychosocial concerns, and case management services, so that timely and informed decisions can be made.
- Empowering the client to problem-solve by exploring options of care, when available, and alternative plans, when necessary, to achieve desired outcomes.
- Encouraging the appropriate use of health care services and striving to improve quality of care and maintain cost-effectiveness on a case-by-case basis.
- Assisting the client in the safe transitioning of care to the next most appropriate level.
- Striving to promote client self-advocacy, self-determination, and right to choice including refusal of care.
- Advocating for both the client and the payer to facilitate positive outcomes for the client, the health care team, and the payer. However, if a conflict arises, the needs of the client must be the priority.

From Case Management Society of America (CMSA). (2010). *Standards of practice for case management.* Little Rock, AR: CMSA.

 Background

A. Over the past several decades, the field of case management has evolved to meet the changing nature of the health, social, political, and medical care systems. Although the process of case management remains the same, the roles, functions, and venues continue to change and evolve.
   1. The process of case management permeates every aspect of the health and medical care systems, and now, this process is beginning to be used in other industries as well (e.g., legal and business).
   2. This chapter focuses on how the roles and functions of a case manager are executed via the case management process.

B. In 1982, when the U.S. Congress passed the Tax Equity and Fiscal Responsibility Act (TEFRA), it pushed third-party payers to integrate case management services across all lines of health, social, financial, and medical services to control costs and manage limited resources.

C. The case management community established several professional case management associations and organizations that were focused on advancing the practice of case management and its value in the United States. For example:
   1. Case Management Society of America (CMSA)—established in 1990.

2. National Association of Professional Geriatric Care Managers (NAPGCM)—established in 1985.
3. Commission for Case Manager Certification (CCMC)—established in 1992 and offers certification in case management.
4. The American Case Management Association (ACMA) has offered certification in hospital-based case management practice since 2005.

D. In the 1980s, the difference between *case* and *care* management was established.
1. *Case management* is a term used to refer to the management of acute and rehabilitative health care services. Services are delivered under a medical model, primarily by nurses.
2. *Care management* is a term used to refer to the management of long-term health care, legal, and financial services by professionals serving social welfare, aging, and nonprofit care delivery systems. Services are delivered under a psychosocial model.
3. In the mid-1980s, case and care management entrepreneurs emerged and started independent for-profit companies or private practices that focused on selling case management services as a niche product for the care of a specific population (e.g., the disabled, the work-related severely injured, and most recently the chronically ill).

E. By the 1990s, other health care–related professionals (e.g., physical, occupational, and speech therapists; gerontologists, etc.) began to offer case and care management services on a fee-for-service basis in different practice venues.

F. In 1997, the Foundation for Rehabilitation Education Research (FRER) and NAPGCM cosponsored a case/care management summit to discuss the future of case and care management in the United States.
1. The summit was held in Chicago in October, 1997. Sixteen professional associations/organizations attended to discuss their vested interest in case/care management and its future in the United States. Participants included the following:
   a. American Association of Occupational Health Nurses
   b. American Nurses Credentialing Center
   c. American Society on Aging
   d. Case Management Society of America
   e. Certification of Disability Management Specialist Commission
   f. Commission for Case Manager Certification
   g. Commission on Rehabilitation Counselor Certification
   h. Foundation for Rehabilitation Education and Research
   i. Health Insurance Association of America
   j. Institute of Case Management
   k. National Academy of Certified Care Managers
   l. National Association of Case Management
   m. National Association of Professional Geriatric Care Managers
   n. National Association of Social Workers
   o. National Guardianship Association
   p. National Guardianship Foundation
2. The goal of the 1997 Case and Care Management Summit was to "foster cost-efficient, collaborative professional interactions that effectively integrate the medical, psychological, and social elements of each client/provider relationship in a manner that includes the

essential activities of case management in order to provide timely, appropriate and beneficial service delivery to the client. These activities include, but are not limited to, assessment, planning, coordination, implementation, monitoring, education, evaluation, and advocacy. Such integration would encompass, but not be limited to, clients and their families, health care providers, community agencies, legal and financial resources, third-party payers and employers" (Bodie-Gross & Holt, 1998, p. 4).

3. The 1998 summit also recommended that a second summit be organized to:

  a. Examine and establish minimum standards for qualified case management practitioners and how case managers demonstrate ongoing competency (includes reviewing the different levels of education required for existing credentials and determining the need to standardize the entry level criteria).

  b. Document successful case management outcomes in order to demonstrate the value of the case manager credential.

  c. Develop educational materials to answer basic questions and inform consumers about the qualifications of various providers as well as the types of services care and case managers offer their clients.

  d. Use market research to identify the information needs of specific stakeholders.

  e. Review organizational codes of ethics in order to establish a common code of conduct that all care and case managers could endorse (in addition to their existing codes). Overall code would include, at a minimum, individual scope of practice, requirements for professional disclosure, clarity on conflicts in interests, cultural competency of practitioners, and client confidentiality.

  f. Identify minimum requirements for a qualified practice, develop a mechanism to standardize existing credentials, conduct periodic review of professional development criteria, and determine the need for advanced credentials for care and case managers.

4. The Second Case and Care Management Summit (1999) was held in Chicago to discuss the topics outlined in the 1998 Summit I Discussion Paper. Participants remained the same, except that the Institute on Case Management did not attend. At the conclusion of this summit, the Coalition for Consumer-Centered Care and Case Management was established. The Coalition was dissolved in 2001 due to a lack of funding.

G. In 1999, Michaels and Cohen (2005) redefined care and case management as follows:

1. *Care* management establishes a system of care for a particular condition, across the continuum of care to ensure seamless transition to the right services, right providers, and at the right time and encourages patients and their family/caregiver to manage their own health. Such care is facilitated by a case manager.

2. *Case* management is a way of managing unique and high-risk situations often associated with costly acute care and hospital stay. Typically, those who require case management are individuals whose self-care capacity is diminished at a time when their health condition is most complex or even life threatening. Such care is facilitated by a case manager.

H. In the early 2000s, care coordination as a term began to become popular and organizations started to use it somewhat interchangeably with case management, although it is different. Experts argue that care coordination is one important function under the broader umbrella of case management. The National Quality Forum (NQF) in 2006 introduced a definition and framework for care coordination.
   1. NQF defined care coordination as a "function that helps ensure that the patient's needs and preferences for health services and information sharing across people, functions, and sites are met over time" (NQF, 2006).
   2. NQF in its framework identified five key domains: Healthcare "Home"; Proactive Plan of Care and Follow-up; Communication; Information Systems; and Transitions or Handoffs (NQF, 2006).
   3. The definition and framework have been used extensively since then and seem to remain widely adopted as established in 2006.
I. The Patient Protection and Affordable Care Act of 2010 has increased the popularity of case management and the continued need to focus on transitions of care to ultimately enhance patient safety, quality of care, and the experience of care. The Act also has emphasized the impact of value-based purchasing on reimbursement with the shift from volume to value, placing the provider of health care services at financial risk. Case management is a desirable strategy for controlling such financial risk.

Case Management Roles

A. Since the 1980s, the case manager's role has evolved, transforming itself from being an evaluator of health care services (quality, cost, and safety) to a procurer and negotiator of health, medical, social, legal, and financial services. The role of a case manager has become more sophisticated and active in the care of an individual. Case managers are required to professionally and legally provide state-of-the-art, quality, safety, cost-effective, and ethical services.
B. The changes that have catapulted case managers into the forefront of the health and medical care delivery systems include the following:
   1. Increased complexity of coordinating and financing health/medical care services.
   2. Almost 50 million Americans are uninsured or do not have appropriate health insurance plans and need a case manager to help them navigate and procure needed health/medical care services with limited financial resources.
   3. Due to the economy, many health, medical, and social care agencies and institutions are reducing their list of services because they are deemed to be unprofitable or a "losing asset."
   4. Many social service agencies have reduced or eliminated services and subsidies (e.g., sliding scales) due to a lack of government funding and grants.
   5. Nonprofit and federally/state-funded social service agencies and organizations are closing down due to a lack of overall funding. This situation is referred to as the "dissolution of the U.S. social service infrastructure."
   6. The Patient Protection and Affordable Care Act of 2010 has resulted in a decrease in the number of uninsured Americans by over 15 million

individuals. The health insurance plan these individuals have today may not be enough to cover all their health care needs. Case managers are needed to work closely with these newly insured to address their multiple complex needs and assure they receive timely, quality, affordable, and safe care and resources.

C. Most important case management roles as identified by Tahan (2005) and Powell and Tahan (2010) include those described below and listed in Box 11-3. However, case managers may assume other roles as determined by their organizations and employers or the care setting they operate in.

1. Educator—Given the complexities of our health, medical, and long-term care systems, case managers are able to:
   a. Assess the educational needs of their clients/patients and their family members or caregivers and educate them in the areas identified, which may include medications, treatments, healthy lifestyles, and illness risk reduction strategies.
   b. Educate health/medical/social service clinicians about the services they offer and how to obtain these needed services. Case managers also educate clinicians about health insurance benefits, reimbursement, and other appropriate aspects of care delivery.

2. Coordinator—Case managers are coordinators of complex service patterns. Through multidisciplinary collaboration efforts, they are able to:
   a. Organize service providers so that they meet the needs of their clients/patients and their families
   b. Facilitate the delivery of care, such as the completion of tests and procedures, transition planning, and teaching activities

3. Communicator—Case managers are effective communicators. They articulate, and clearly communicate, the needs of their clients/patients to family members, health/medical clinicians, and other service providers so that clients can reach their highest level of functioning.

4. Collaborator—Case managers are able to collaborate with numerous health, medical, and social service providers about the needs of their

BOX 11-3 Diversity of the Roles Assumed by Case Managers

- Educator
- Coordinator
- Communicator
- Collaborator
- Clinician
- Utilization manager
- Transitional planner
- Leader
- Negotiator
- Quality manager
- Advocate
- Researcher
- Risk manager

clients/patients. Some health care professionals with whom case managers collaborate are internal to the organization where they work such as physicians, pharmacists, and physical therapists; others are external to the organization such as representatives from durable medical equipment agencies, employers of injured workers, and providers of transportation services.

5. Clinician—Case managers are expert clinicians as well. They possess a level of expertise in a particular specialty such as cardiac, oncology, or disability care. Some of them, however, are general practitioners. They use their knowledge to identify the client's problems and develop an effective plan of care.

6. Utilization manager—Case managers ensure cost-effective care delivery and use of services as well as reimbursement. They focus on the continuum of care and the transition of patients from one level of care to another. In addition, they conduct specific reviews for the purpose of securing certification/authorization of care from the managed care/insurance company.

7. Transition planner—Case managers facilitate the movement of patients from one level of care to another across the continuum of health and human services and care and settings. They also identify and broker the services and resources (e.g., durable medical equipment, home care) a patient needs post an episode of care/illness (e.g., acute care hospital stay). They accomplish this by examining the patient's condition, necessary treatment options, and where the relevant services are available and by developing a plan of care that includes a discharge or transition plan, for example, a plan that addresses the transition of a patient from most to least acute care settings.

8. Leader—Case managers assume leadership responsibilities in their role especially in the areas of allocation and utilization of resources, gatekeeping of services, reimbursement review and revenue management, changing the care delivery systems, and performance review and management.

9. Quality manager—Case managers are responsible for ensuring patient safety and improving the quality of the care provided. They identify variances or delays in care (system-, practitioner-, and patient-/family-related variances) and institute action. They also participate in activities of a quality improvement team and function as team leaders, facilitators, or members. In addition, they evaluate the effectiveness of case management services through monitoring organizational and client-oriented outcomes.

10. Negotiator—Case managers assume an important role in negotiating the plan of care and services. They are skilled in coordinating the scheduling of tests and procedures and the communication of results. They also are effective in negotiating with managed care organizations the services required for patients, length of hospital stay, community-based services, and reimbursement for care provided.

11. Advocate—Case managers ensure that the needs of patients and their families are met and place their interests above all others. In addition, they educate patients about their treatment options and facilitate the making of informed decisions.

12. Researcher—Case managers evaluate case management services and outcomes via research and recommend the utilization of research outcomes in their practice and changes in standards of care, policies, procedures, and treatment protocols; that is, they ensure evidence-based practice.

13. Risk manager—Case managers identify areas of risk in the care environment and processes while they review patient care and services and recommend, if not execute, an action plan. They are first to identify significant events that warrant immediate attention and resolution. They also ensure that the organization and other professionals adhere to regulatory and accreditation standards at all times.

Case Management Functions and Activities

A. In 1998 when the Case and Care Management Summit I Paper was distributed, for the first time, it was publicly stated that the function of a case manager was dependent upon his or her job title (role) and practice or work setting (venue).

B. Often, a case manager's role does not correlate with or reflect his or her job function, so it is important to know where the case manager works and whom he or she serves.

C. Regardless of work setting or clinical specialty, case managers perform the essential activities of case management (assessment, planning, goal setting, coordinating, managing, monitoring, advocating, communicating, and evaluating), but these activities are greatly influenced or directed by a case manager's venue of practice setting.

D. Case management functions are also influenced by the expectations a client/patient, family member, health/medical/social service provider, or employer has of the role. Case managers must always weigh the functions of their job against what is realistic to expect in a given situation or case.

E. Every 5 years, the CCMC conducts a formal role and function study to identify those changes that have taken place in the case management practice, field, or industry. The most recent study was concluded in 2014, and the results were published by Tahan, Watson, and Sminkey (2015, 2016). This study identified the six essential activity domains of the case manager's practice based on the opinion of almost 7,700 practicing case managers. The domains are listed below, and the details for each domain are described in Box 11-4.
   1. Delivering Case Management Services
   2. Managing Utilization of Health Care Services
   3. Accessing Financial and Community Resources
   4. Evaluating and Measuring Quality and Outcomes
   5. Delivering Rehabilitation Services
   6. Adhering to Ethical, Legal, and Practice Standards

F. Another study sponsored by the CCMC (Tahan & Huber, 2006) reported the use of more than 75 case management activities by case managers working in a variety of settings and specialties throughout the United States. The researchers identified these activities based on a qualitative analysis of more than 1,000 case manager job descriptions obtained

(*text continues on page 281*)

BOX 11-4   **CCMC's Six Essential Activity Domains of Case Management**

1. Delivering Case Management Services Domain:
   a. Identifying clients who meet eligibility for case management services
   b. Assessing client's understanding, readiness, and willingness to engage in case management services
   c. Communicating the client's needs to other health care providers including the physician and stakeholders
   d. Identifying barriers that affect clients' engagement in their care
   e. Assessing client's health condition, needs, and situation, developing the case management plan accordingly, and focusing the assessment on client's physical, social, emotional, psychological, financial/economic, cognitive, and vocational condition
   f. Facilitating and coordinating care activities and services and collaborating with others involved while being accountable for keeping communication open among care providers
   g. Reviewing and modifying the delivery of health care services as needed while incorporating both the behavioral and nonbehavioral health issues and concerns
   h. Assessing the client's health history, language needs, health literacy, readiness for change, and involvement in healthy lifestyle behavior
   i. Assessing the respite care needs of the client's caregiver
   j. Counseling client on health condition, care interventions, care choices, and facilitating client's empowerment
   k. Communicating case management assessment findings to providers, payers, employers, family, and other key stakeholders
   l. Collaborating with the client and other stakeholders in establishing comprehensive goals, objectives, and expected outcomes of care
   m. Organizing resources and integrating the delivery of health care services
   n. Identifying multicultural, spiritual, and religious factors that may impact client's health status and care provision and incorporating these in the plan of care
   o. Documenting client's progress, assessment findings, communication with other providers and outcomes of care, case closure and termination of case management services, and changes in the plan of care
   p. Educating clients about health condition, case management plan, self-management, and adherence to health regimen
   q. Communicating termination of service notification to stakeholders
   r. Bringing the case manager–client relationship to closure
2. Managing Utilization of Health Care Services Domain:
   a. Reviewing the client's insurance coverage, determining medical necessity, negotiating rates to maximize the funding available for an individual's health care needs, and appealing service denials such as admission to an acute care setting
   b. Performing utilization management activities such as obtaining authorizations for care and services, notification of services based on payer's requirements, and appealing service denials
   c. Collaborating with physician advisor in the management of service denials and other care management activities
   d. Identifying clients who would benefit from alternate levels of care such as subacute, skilled nursing, and home care
   e. Advocating the provision of care in the least restrictive care setting

continued

   f. Evaluating the cost-effectiveness of treatments and conducting cost–benefit analysis of services

   g. Mitigating identified delays and variances in care and assuring care progression

   h. Educating health care team members about appropriate utilization of resources and related regulatory standards

   i. Ongoing communication with payers and insurance companies

   j. Reviewing the completeness of the care providers' documentation in the client's record

   k. Identifying cases at high risk for complications and those that would benefit from additional types of services (e.g., disease management, physical therapy, durable medical equipment, vocational services, diagnostic testing, counseling, and assistive technology)

3. Accessing Financial and Community Resources Domain:

   a. Incorporating client's health insurance benefits in the development of the case management plan of care

   b. Identifying the need and eligibility for private and public sector funding for services and educating clients of availability of such funds

   c. Coordinating language interpreter services

   d. Coordinating client's social service needs such as transportation, housing, and food/meals

   e. Referring clients to formal and informal community support services and resources

   f. Research community resources applicable to the client's situation such as alternate treatment programs and meals on wheels

   g. Reviewing information about a client's social and financial resources, family dynamics, cultural issues, and resources and integrating specific interventions related to issues identified into case management practice

   h. Evaluating the ability and availability of the designated caregiver to deliver the needed services

4. Evaluating and Measuring Quality and Outcomes Domain:

   a. Collection of both client- and organizational-specific outcomes data

   b. Analysis and reporting of care outcomes (e.g., clinical, physical/vocational functioning, financial, variance, quality of life, patient satisfaction, and productivity)

   c. Monitoring care interventions and client's progress in achieving goals, objectives, and expected/desired outcomes of the case management plan of care

   d. Evaluating the quality of care interventions and services and the effectiveness of the case management plan of care including transitional plan

   e. Ensuring client's access to timely and necessary services including referrals to other specialty care providers

   f. Using evidence-based practice guidelines in the development of the case management plan

   g. Coordinating referrals of potential quality of care and risk management issues or client's complaints and grievances to appropriate parties for follow-up

   h. Preparing reports in compliance with regulatory requirements

5. Delivering Rehabilitation Services Domain:

   a. Collaborating with other health care providers to clarify restrictions and limitations related to client's physical or vocational functioning

BOX
11-4

CCMC's Six Essential Activity Domains of Case Management
continued

   b. Identifying the need for modifications in the client's home environment to eliminate accessibility barriers

   c. Identifying the need for specialized services (e.g., rehabilitative services) to facilitate achievement of an optimal level of wellness, functioning, and productivity

   d. Arranging for rehabilitation assessment and services

   e. Coordinating client's job analysis for job modifications and accommodation; recommending job modifications and accommodations to employers

   f. Facilitating the achievement of optimal wellness, functioning, or productivity such as return to work and return to school

   g. Coordinating specialized rehabilitative services or use of assistive devices such as teletypewriter, telecommunication technology for the deaf, and mobility devices

6. Adhering to Ethical, Legal, and Practice Standards Domain:

   a. Protecting client's privacy and confidentiality

   b. Adhering to ethical standards that govern case management practice such as serving as an advocate for an individual's health care needs

   c. Adhering to ethical and legal standards that govern professional licensure and certification

   d. Complying with legal, regulatory, and accreditation requirements pertinent to case management practice such as informed consent, Health Insurance Portability and Accountability Act, and Americans with Disabilities Act

   e. Documenting case management activities with accuracy and in a timely manner reflecting state, federal, and payer-based requirements

   f. Facilitating completion of legal documents such as advance directives, health care proxy, and guardianship

   g. Educating clients about their rights and appealing service denials

From Tahan, H. A., Watson, A. C., & Sminkey, P. V. (2016). Informing the Content and Composition of the CCM® Certification Examination: A National Study from the Commission for Case Manager Certification-Part II. *Lippincott's Case Management*, accepted for publication.

from different health care organizations during the time of application for the Certified Case Manager (CCM) examination/credential. The activities the researchers found to be included most in the case managers' job description are listed in Box 11-5—not in any order of priority or frequency. These activities are still common today, however, with increased focus on care coordination and transitions of care activities, including handoff communication.

G. The care settings case managers work in usually determine how many and what type of the functions/activities described above are required and necessary to succeed in a specific case management role.

H. The case manager's roles, responsibilities, and functions are impacted by the type of health care organization, purpose of the role, the specific practice setting, and the patient population served.

I. Case managers are found to function in variety of settings such as those listed in Box 11-6.

BOX
11-5

Case Manager's Activities Based on Review of a Sample of Job Descriptions

- Evaluating case management outcomes
- Monitoring patient care and progress
- Assuming the role of patient advocate
- Assessing patient's progress
- Writing summary reports
- Engaging in quality assurance activities
- Determining patient needs and resources, including insurance/financial
- Acting as liaison between payers and health care team
- Determining medical necessity of admissions and services
- Assessing patient's level of impairment
- Identifying patients using a high level of services
- Preventing overutilization/underutilization of resources
- Analyzing data
- Communicating with health care team
- Collecting medical history information
- Acting as a professional role model
- Collaborating in the development of treatment plan/care plan
- Identifying gaps in treatment plan/care plan
- Communicating with patients and their family/caregivers
- Avoiding the use of high-cost services
- Developing quality assessment methods
- Determining patient compliance with the treatment plan
- Ensuring care is provided in the most appropriate setting
- Meeting time management and quality assurance standards
- Completing necessary documentation
- Monitoring the appropriateness of test procedures and care settings
- Communicating with payers
- Completing admission reviews
- Analyzing medical files for effectiveness of case management
- Reviewing active cases with employers
- Attending or holding case conferences
- Maintaining confidentiality
- Educating patients in health promotion
- Implementing cost management strategies
- Engaging in discharge planning activities
- Identifying community resources
- Analyzing utilization patterns and denied cases
- Processing appeal requests
- Developing and documenting policies and procedures
- Establishing new client files
- Implementing treatment plans
- Maintaining URAC accreditation standards
- Reporting inappropriate utilization of resources
- Identifying gaps in general treatment
- Monitoring medical progress
- Scheduling medical evaluations
- Collecting data on utilization patterns and denied cases
- Meeting billing requirements
- Coordinating transfers to appropriate facilities, home care, or alternative settings
- Fostering professional development of personnel
- Traveling to patients' homes, job sites, or other health care facilities
- Collecting general data

| BOX 11-5 | Case Manager's Activities Based on Review of a Sample of Job Descriptions *continued* |

- Ascertaining the reasons for high service use
- Obtaining approval for contacts
- Educating and training other staff
- Training case managers on computer systems
- Initiating vocational service referrals
- Coaching case managers on time management
- Training case managers on philosophy, systems, and departmental guidelines
- Assessing staff competencies
- Reviewing files for claims adjusters
- Supervising staff
- Facilitating return to work (RTW)
- Monitoring physical care and therapy
- Completing clerical functions
- Obtaining claims records
- Planning for resolution of audit issues
- Completing quality audits
- Engaging in budget activities
- Overseeing consultant work for thoroughness
- Completing referral activities to other services
- Assessing need for follow-up
- Coordinating discharge planning activities and services
- Developing short- and long-term care goals
- Performing job site evaluations
- Initiating discharge planning
- Engaging in marketing activities
- Planning medical rehabilitation processes
- Coordinating patient care

 ## Case Management Knowledge for Practice and Qualifications

A. In addition to the case manager's essential activities, the role and functions study completed by CCMC in 2014 also identified five main knowledge domains for effective case management practice (Tahan, Watson, & Sminkey 2015, 2016). The domains are listed below, and the details for each domain are described in Box 11-7.
   1. Care Delivery and Reimbursement Methods
   2. Psychosocial Concepts and Support Systems
   3. Rehabilitation Concepts and Strategies
   4. Quality and Outcomes Evaluation and Measurement
   5. Ethical, Legal, and Practice Standards
B. Tahan and Huber (2006), in their job description analysis study, also reported on the qualifications considered by employers in hiring case managers. These qualifications were identified based on the qualitative analysis of more than 1,000 job descriptions of case managers working in variety of health care practice settings. These qualifications are described in Box 11-8—not in any order of priority or frequency. They continue to be relevant today; however, there has been an increased interest in case managers with advanced degrees and certification.

BOX 11-6 · Various Case Manager's Practice Settings

- Acute and medical case management
- Traditional group or individual medical insurance plans
- Health insurance companies and managed care organizations (e.g., HMOs, PPOs, EPOs, etc.)
- Long-term care health insurance plans
- Hospital-based or acute care settings
- Home health care companies
- Government-based benefit programs (e.g., Medicaid, Medicare, etc.)
- Long-term care facility (e.g., skilled nursing facility, assisted living, acute and subacute rehabilitation, etc.)
- Community-based organizations
- Hospice and palliative care
- Social service agencies
- Not-for-profit and religious organizations
- Agencies on aging
- Workers' compensation companies
- Disability management companies
- Independent case management companies
- Life care planning
- Law firms
- Day care centers
- Nontraditional sites of care such as retail stores (e.g., CVS, Target and Walgreens Pharmacy)
- Health outreach, wellness, and prevention agencies

BOX 11-7 · CCMC's Five Knowledge Area Domains of Case Management

1. Care Delivery and Reimbursement Methods Domain:
   a. Processes of case management practice and tools
   b. Continuum of care, continuum of health and human services, care settings and levels of care, and alternative levels of care
   c. Goals and objectives of case management practice
   d. Health care delivery systems and models of care
   e. Financial resources, public and private benefit programs, and cost containment principles
   f. Health care providers and interdisciplinary care teams and roles and functions of various members including case managers
   g. Management of acute and chronic illnesses and medication reconciliation and management
   h. Transitions of care
   i. Reimbursement methods, utilization review, and management
   j. Factors that impact client's acuity and severity levels
   k. Adherence to care regimen
2. Psychosocial Concepts and Support Systems Domain:
   a. Client's self-care management and behavioral change theories and stages
   b. Behavioral health concepts
   c. Community resources, support programs, and resources for the uninsured
   d. Wellness and illness prevention; health coaching; client activation, empowerment, and engagement; and health literacy assessment

BOX 11-7   CCMC's Five Knowledge Area Domains of Case Management *continued*

   e. Multicultural, spiritual, and religious factors impacting health condition and care options and family dynamics

   f. Psychosocial aspects of chronic illness and disability

   g. End-of-life issues

   h. Crisis intervention strategies and abuse and neglect

   i. Conflict resolution and interviewing techniques

3. Rehabilitation Concepts and Strategies Domain:

   a. Rehabilitation post an injury, acute health condition, and hospitalization

   b. Functional capacity evaluation

   c. Assistive devices

   d. Vocational aspects of chronic illness and disability and vocational rehabilitation

4. Quality and Outcomes Evaluation and Measurement Domain:

   a. Accreditation standards and requirements

   b. Sources and types of quality indicators/measures

   c. Quality and performance improvement concepts

   d. Data analytics, interpretation, and reporting

   e. Program evaluation and research methods

   f. Case load calculation

   g. Cost–benefit analysis

5. Ethical, Legal, and Practice Standards Domain:

   a. Ethics related to care delivery and professional practice

   b. Clinical pathways and practice guidelines

   c. Privacy and confidentiality

   d. Risk management

   e. Standards of practice

   f. Legal and regulatory requirements

   g. Health care– and disability-related legislation

   h. Affordable Care Act and meaningful use

   i. Case recording and documentation

   j. Use of tools such as clinical pathways and evidence-based guidelines

   k. Self-care and well-being as a professional

From Tahan, H. A., Watson, A. C., & Sminkey, P. V. (2016). Informing the Content and Composition of the CCM® Certification Examination: A National Study from the Commission for Case Manager Certification-Part II. *Lippincott's Case Management,* accepted for publication.

C. To be successful in their roles, case managers must possess specific skills that allow them to carry out their roles, functions, and activities and apply their knowledge into practice. Box 11-9 contains a list of important and common skills case managers must possess (Powell & Tahan, 2010; Tahan, 2005).

D. In its standards of practice for case management, CMSA notes that case managers should maintain competence in their area(s) of practice by having one of the following:

   1. Current, active, and unrestricted licensure or certification in a health or human services discipline that allows the professional in the role of case manager to conduct an assessment independently as permitted within the scope of practice of the discipline.

   2. In the case of a health professional in a state that does not require licensure or certification, the individual must have a baccalaureate or

BOX 11-8   Qualifications for Case Manager's Role based on Job Descriptions Research

Education, Certification, and Licensure
• Education—Bachelor or Master's degree
• Professional licensure such as registered nurse, social worker, and rehabilitation counselor
• Licensure and specialty certification, such as Case Management Certification

Experience
• Clinical experience in a specific specialty
• Utilization management experience
• Supervisory/managerial experience
• Long-term care experience
• Past experience in case management

Skills
• Independent decision making
• Teamwork
• Computer literacy such as skills in word processing, spreadsheets, and presentation software
• Customer service
• Critical thinking and creativity
• Initiative
• Multitasking abilities
• Flexibility
• Negotiation
• Mentoring
• Communication

Knowledge
• Knowledge or experience in Workers' Compensation
• Knowledge or experience in disability management
• Knowledge of medical technology and vocabulary
• Knowledge of medical management
• Knowledge of age-related differences in care needs
• Knowledge of Americans with Disabilities Act/Law
• Knowledge of specialized services, including referrals to other providers or services
• Knowledge of cost analysis, cost–benefit analysis, and cost-effectiveness analysis methods
• Knowledge of labor laws and benefits
• Knowledge of reimbursement and benefit systems—prospective payment systems, managed care, etc.
• Knowledge in data analysis and management

graduate degree in social work or another health or human services field that promotes the physical, psychosocial, and/or vocational well-being of the persons being served (CMSA, 2010).

a. CMSA explains in the standards that the educational degree, in the case of states that do not require licensure, must be from an institution that is fully accredited by a nationally recognized educational accreditation organization, and the individual must have completed a supervised field experience in case management, health, or behavioral health as part of the degree requirements (CMSA, 2010).

BOX
11-9   **Common Skills for Case Managers According to Powell and Tahan (2010)**

Clinical and patient care
a. Direct and indirect care provision
b. Expertise in a clinical area/specialty
c. Patient and family/caregiver teaching, health instruction, and health literacy assessment
d. Transitional planning
e. Coordination, facilitation, and expedition of care activities
f. Holistic and pastoral care
g. Crisis intervention and counseling
h. Development and implementation of case management plans of care

Managerial and leadership
a. Problem solving and conflict resolution
b. Critical thinking, clinical reasoning, and clinical judgment
c. Project management
d. Conducting meetings
e. Goals setting
f. Management of change
g. Management of ethical and legal issues
h. Time management and priority setting
i. Delegation
j. Negotiation
k. Cultural competence
l. Consensus building
m. Integration
n. Advocacy

Business and financial
a. Resource allocation
b. Utilization review and management
c. Certification/authorizations of services
d. Financial analysis/cost–benefit (and cost-effectiveness) analysis
e. Financial reimbursement methods and procedures
f. Claims and denials management
g. Gatekeeping
h. Health benefits and entitlements

Information management and communication
a. Customer relations
b. Cultural sensitivity
c. Writing reports
d. Information sharing
e. Communication: interprofessional, interdisciplinary, and with client/family/caregiver
f. Documentation and case recordings
g. Dealing with challenging people
h. Active listening
i. Collaboration
j. Motivational interviewing

Quality and safety
a. Variance and delay management
b. Outcomes management
c. Quality and performance improvement
d. Data collection, analysis, and reporting (e.g., core measures)

continued

BOX
11-9
Common Skills for Case Managers According to Powell and Tahan (2010) *continued*

e. Value-based purchasing
f. Access to appropriate care and services
g. Effective handoff communication among providers

Professional
a. Research and evidence-based practice
b. Specialty certification
c. Writing for publication
d. Consulting
e. Networking
f. Membership in professional organizations and regional or national taskforces

E. Other qualifications CMSA articulates in its standards relate to ongoing education, maintenance of work setting-related competencies and current knowledge, and seeking the support and consultation of other health care professionals.
1. Possession of the education, experience, and expertise required for the case manager's area(s) of practice
2. Adherence to national and/or local laws and regulations that apply to the jurisdictions(s) and discipline(s) in which the case manager practices
3. Maintenance of competence through relevant and ongoing continuing education, study, and consultation
4. Practicing within the case manager's area(s) of expertise and making timely and appropriate referrals to, and seeking consultation with, other health care professionals and peers when needed (CMSA, 2010)

Case Management Knowledge and Skills According to the American Nurses Credentialing Center

A. The American Nurses Credentialing Center (ANCC) offers a certification in case management practice and conducts roles and functions studies on regular basis to inform the focus of the certification. These studies allow ANCC to identify the knowledge and skill areas required of case managers.
B. The ANCC certification in case management is offered only to registered professional nurses, unlike the one offered by CCMC, which is interdisciplinary.
C. The most recent ANCC study was completed in 2013, which resulted in the findings summarized in Box 11-10. The main domains of knowledge and practice of case management that the certification examination covers are those listed below (ANCC, 2013).
1. Fundamentals of case management practice
2. Resource management
3. Quality management
4. Legal and ethics
5. Education and health promotion

BOX
11-10
ANCC's Identified Knowledge and Skills of Case Management Practice

Knowledge of Case Management Practice
 a. Nursing case management concepts (e.g., functions, principles, roles)
 b. Standards of practice for case management and scope of services
 c. Tools (e.g., assessment, evaluation, screening), clinical guidelines, and pathways
 d. Biopsychosocial health and characteristics of illness
 e. Evidence-based practice
 f. Utilization of management concepts (e.g., authorizations, benefits, contract management, denials and appeals)
 g. Discharge planning, community and support resources, medical supplies, and durable medical equipment
 h. Payor and reimbursement methodology (e.g., government, private, disability, workers' compensation)
 i. Benefit and payment options for support services (e.g., insured, uninsured, charity)
 j. Scope of services for providers (e.g., primary care, specialty providers, and ancillary services)
 k. Outcome evaluation tools, quality indicators (e.g., core measures), data management, predictive modeling, benchmarking principles, and quality and performance improvement processes and concepts
 l. Accreditation and licensure
 m. Governmental regulations and policies that affect health care delivery
 n. Legal responsibilities (e.g., abandonment, abuse and neglect, malpractice, guardianship)
 o. Risk management concepts
 p. Nursing code of ethics and professional code of conduct for case managers
 q. Patient's bill of rights, advanced directives and living wills, informed consent, interpretation services, and cultural perspectives
 r. Change theories and concepts (e.g., motivational interviewing, behavioral change)
 s. Disease management, wellness promotion, and disease prevention

Skills Required of Case Managers:
 a. Conducting screenings and assessments and identifying and managing risk factors and barriers
 b. Developing a client-focused plan of care using evidence-based practice, verifying if interventions are consistent with the client's needs and goals, and linking the client to available resources
 c. Implementing a client-focused plan of care using evidence-based practice, modifying the plan and services based on the evaluation of outcomes, and referring clients for interventions (e.g., health maintenance, symptom management, wellness promotion)
 d. Communicating the plan, interventions, and outcomes to stakeholders
 e. Collaborating with stakeholders and problem solving and conflict resolution with stakeholders
 f. Determining level of care using utilization review criteria
 g. Negotiating benefits for clients and facilitating resolution of denials and appeals
 h. Planning for transition of care and collaborating with multiple providers to facilitate access to care
 i. Negotiating for support services (e.g., medical supplies, durable medical equipment, pharmaceuticals)
 j. Identifying potential risks and liabilities (e.g., client, facility, financial, safety), conflicts of interests, and ethical concerns and facilitating resolution

continued

BOX 11-10   **ANCC's Identified Knowledge and Skills of Case Management Practice** *continued*

k. Collecting data (e.g., variance tracking, benchmarking) and synthesizing data to improve services (e.g., client, program)
l. Conducting a cost–benefit analysis
m. Documenting the case management process
n. Advocating for the client throughout the continuum of care
o. Assessing client's readiness for change
p. Selecting educational materials for specific learner needs, providing client-focused instruction, and evaluating educational outcomes
q. Conducting population screenings and identifying at-risk individuals

From American Nurses Credentialing Center. (2013). *Nursing case management board certification: Test content outline.* Silver Springs, MD: ANCC.

 Conclusion

A. The case management industry will continue to expand and evolve in response to the dynamic health care environment so that it can meet the challenges of tomorrow: elderly population with multiple ands complex chronic illnesses, focus on value instead of volume of care, and provider accountability for care and outcomes (quality, safety, and cost) across the continuum of care.

B. Case management services will continue to be integrated into exciting new models and sites of care especially those nontraditional in nature, thus challenging how we will educate and train future case managers.

C. The above descriptions of the roles, functions, activities, knowledge, and skills of case managers and case management practice are a guide for designing job descriptions for the case managers of today and the future. These lists should be taken into consideration carefully and applied in a way specific to the practice setting of case management. They are not to be applied in totality in any setting; rather, health care and case management executives should incorporate in the case manager's job description what is considered applicable to their organization, the specialty or service, and the practice setting.

References

American Nurses Credentialing Center. (2013). *Nursing case management board certification: Test content outline.* Silver Springs, MD: ANCC.

Bodie-Gross, E., & Holt, E. (1998). Care and Case Management Summit, October 19–20, 1997. *The White Paper,* Chicago, IL. Sponsored by the National Association of Professional Geriatric Case Managers, Tucson, AZ and the Foundation for Rehabilitation, Education and Research, Rolling Meadows, IL. FRER, IL.

Case Management Society of America (CMSA). (2010). *Standards of practice for case management.* Little Rock, AR: CMSA.

Merriam-Webster, Incorporated. (2015). *Dictionary.* Retrieved from http://www.merriam-webster.com/dictionary, on July 12, 2015. Merriam-Webster-Incorporated.

Michaels, C., & Cohen, E. (2005). Two strategies for managing care: Care management and case management. In E. Cohen & T. Cesta (Eds.), *Nursing case management: From essentials to advanced practice applications* (4th ed., pp. 33–37). St Louis, MO: Elsevier Mosby.

National Quality Forum (NQF). (2006). *NQF-endorsed definition and framework for measuring and reporting care coordination*. Washington, DC: NQF.

Powell, S. K., & Tahan, H. A. (2010). *Case management: A practical guide for education and practice* (3rd ed.). Philadelphia, PA: Lippincott Williams & Wilkins.

Tahan, H. (2005). The role of the nurse case manager. In E. Cohen & T. Cesta (Eds.), *Nursing case management: From essentials to advanced practice applications* (4th ed., pp. 277–295). St Louis, MO: Elsevier Mosby.

Tahan, H., & Campagna, V. (2010). Case Management Roles and Functions across Various Settings and Professional Disciplines. *Professional Case Management, 15*(5), 245–277.

Tahan, H., & Huber, D. (2006). The CCMC's national study of case manager job descriptions: An understanding of the activities, role relationships, knowledge, skills, and abilities. *Lippincott's Case Management, 11*(3), 127–144.

Tahan, H., Huber, D., & Downey, W. (2006). Case managers' roles and functions: Commission for Case Manager Certification's 2004 research, Part I. *Lippincott's Case Management, 11*(1), 4–22.

Tahan, H. A., Watson, A. C., & Sminkey, P. V. (2015). What Case Managers Should Know about Their Roles and Functions: A National Study from the Commission for Case Manager Certification-Part I. *Professional Case Management, 20*(6), 271–296.

Tahan, H. A., Watson, A. C., & Sminkey, P. V. (2016). Informing the Content and Composition of the CCM® Certification Examination: A National Study from the Commission for Case Manager Certification-Part II. *Professional Case Management, 21*(1), 3–24.

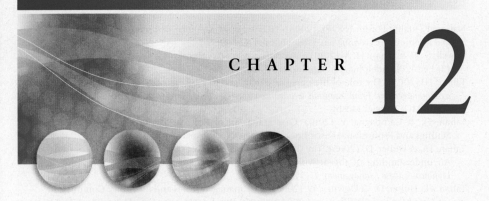

CHAPTER 12

The Case Management Process

Hussein M. Tahan

LEARNING OBJECTIVES

Upon completion of this chapter, the reader will be able to:

1. List the seven steps of the case management process.
2. Describe the process of patient identification and selection for case management services.
3. Discuss the difference between the case selection and the assessment/problem identification steps/phases.
4. Explain the steps in the development and coordination of the case management plan and care activities.
5. Discuss the importance of the "evaluation and follow-up" step of the case management process and how it relates to the achievement of outcomes.
6. Explain the roles and benefits of continuous monitoring, reassessment, and re-evaluation activities and how they are related to the evaluation and follow-up step.

IMPORTANT TERMS AND CONCEPTS

Advocacy
Assessment
Client Identification
Client Selection
Collaboration
Continuum of Care

Continuum of Health
  and Human Services
Coordination
Core Measures
Evaluation
Implementation

Intervention
Monitoring
Outcomes
Planning
Problem Identification
Transitions of Care

Introduction

A. Case management is an interdisciplinary practice that focuses on the coordination of the care activities and interventions and the allocation of resources required by a client/patient during an acute or nonacute episode of illness or encounter with a health care provider.

B. A case manager manages, facilitates, coordinates, and evaluates the necessary care activities, interventions, and treatments, applying an approach to care delivery that is called the *case management process*.

C. The case manager also manages communication among the varied care providers and other essential parties (or stakeholders) internal and external to the health care organization.

D. The case manager communicates with the client, family, and/or caregiver on an ongoing basis to assure active engagement in decision making about care options and that care meets the client's interests, goals, and preferences.

E. The case management process focuses on the identification of clients/patients who would benefit from case management services and the activities of assessment, problem identification, care planning, care delivery, advocacy, monitoring, and evaluation of the care provided, specifically for its relevance to the needs of the patient/family and for the health care team's ability to meet the desired outcomes and established goals.

F. Each client/patient is unique, and the case management process takes into consideration the individual needs of the patient, family, and caregiver. This is not only limited to the patients' medical condition and treatment; rather, it includes their financial and psychosocial state as well as their culture, values, and belief system.

G. Each case manager has her or his own unique style of case management based on one's own experience, education, skills, knowledge, ability, competence, creativity, clinical specialization (e.g., critical care, organ transplantation, rehabilitation, home care), professional discipline (e.g., nursing, social work, rehabilitation counselors, workers' compensation specialists), professional networks, and advanced credentials (e.g., certification in case management or clinical specialty).

H. The case management process is a set of steps applied by case managers in their approach to patient care management. It is similar to the nursing process or problem-solving approaches (and other processes used by other disciplines such as social work and medicine).

  1. The nursing process is applied to the care of patients in a particular setting by all nurses in that setting.

  2. The case management process is used by case managers only in settings where case management is the care delivery system in use; today, case management is practiced in virtually every setting across the continuum.

  3. The process of case management is much broader than the nursing process.

    a. The nursing process assesses the patient for changes in the physical, medical, psychosocial, cultural, and safety needs; plans how to meet these needs; implements these plans; and evaluates the results of these plans.

b. The case management process entails—in addition to the activities assumed in the nursing process—collecting assessment data and services used (e.g., home care), including those before the onset of the current illness; assessing the environmental, financial (e.g., availability of health insurance plan and coverage), and support systems present to meet the identified needs; planning future care; and evaluating the impact of case management care delivery on both patient- and organization-based outcomes.

I. The case management process has been applied in the care of a select group of clients/patients based on certain criteria determined by the health care organization or provider and dependent on the care setting. These criteria are the necessary factors that indicate the patient's need for case management services.

1. In some organizations or programs, such as health insurance plans/ payer based, disease management, population health, patient-centered medical home, and accountable care organizations, predictive modeling and risk stratification approaches using service utilization history among other factors to identify patients who would benefit most from case management services.

2. In some organizations, the case managers screen all patients for case management services, identify their needs, and implement the case management process accordingly.

3. In other organizations, case managers work with a client/patient based on a referral from other health care providers.

4. In some care settings, such as patient-centered medical home or acute rehabilitation, all clients/patients may be followed by case managers.

J. Some activities of the case management process may vary significantly based on the case management setting (preventive, preacute, acute, postacute or payer-based/managed care, ambulatory, hospital, community, home, skilled facilities, and so on) and the population served (pediatric, geriatric, behavioral health, well individuals, and so on).

1. Activities that may vary based on the above variables are case selection/identification, implementation of the case management plan of care, utilization management, transitional planning, and the necessary evaluation and follow-up postcare encounter.

2. Other activities of the case management process may apply similarly to case management practice in many of the care settings. These activities are assessment/problem identification; development and coordination of the case management plan; and continuous monitoring, reassessing, and re-evaluation.

K. Through the case management process, case managers eliminate fragmentation and/or duplication in care delivery. They also maintain open and timely communication with all parties involved in care in an effort to ensure continuity, safety, quality, timely, and cost-effective outcomes.

L. The case management plan designed by the case manager in collaboration with the client/patient, family, and other health care providers identifies client's immediate, short-term, and ongoing needs, as well as where and how these care needs can be met.

1. The plan sets goals and time frames for achieved goals that are appropriate to the individual and his or her family/caregiver and are agreed to by the patient or family and health care treatment team.

2. The case manager ensures that funding (e.g., health insurance plan benefits) or community resources, or both, are available to support the implementation of the case management plan.

Descriptions of Key Terms

A. Advocacy—"The act of recommending, pleading the cause of another, to speak or write in favor of" (CMSA, 2010, p. 24). Case managers demonstrate advocacy when they are acting on behalf of those who are not able to speak for or represent themselves and when defending others and acting in their best interest.

B. Advocate—A person or group involved in activities of advocacy is called an advocate.

C. Assessment—The collection of "in-depth information about a client's situation and functioning to identify individual needs and in order to develop a comprehensive case management plan that will address those needs. In addition to direct client contact, information should be gathered from other relevant sources (patient/client, professional caregivers, nonprofessional caregivers, employers, health records, educational/military records, etc.)" (CCMC, 2015, p. 7). CMSA describes assessment as a "systematic process of data collection and analysis involving multiple elements and sources" (CMSA, 2010, p. 24).

D. Collaboration—Working together with the client/family, other health care providers and agents who are both internal and external to the health care organization for the purpose of achieving consensus on the client's care goals, case management plan and to maximize the achievement of desired care outcomes.

E. Continuum of a concept involving an integrated system of care that guides and tracks clients/patients over time through a comprehensive array of health services across all levels of intensity of care. It reflects care provided over time in various settings, programs or services and spanning the illness-wellness continuum with varying degrees of complexity, acuity and intensity depending on the care setting. It refers to the different settings and types of health care services an individual may access for the purpose of wellness, prevention or treatment of a disease. Case managers use the continuum of care while engaged in the case management process to match the ongoing needs of their clients with the appropriate level and type of health, medical, financial, legal, and psychosocial care for services within a setting or across multiple settings or providers.

F. Coordination—"Organizing, securing, integrating, modifying, and documenting the resources necessary to accomplish the goals set forth in the case management plan" (CCMC, 2015, p. 7).

G. Discharge planning—The process of assessing the patient's needs of care after discharge from a health care facility or a care encounter and ensuring that the necessary services are in place before discharge. This process ensures a patient's timely, appropriate, and safe discharge to the next level of care or setting, including appropriate use of resources necessary for ongoing care.

H. Evaluation—"Determining and documenting the case management plan's effectiveness in reaching desired outcomes and goals. This might lead to a modification or change in the case management plan in its entirety or in any of its component parts" (CCMC, 2015, p. 8).

This activity is repeated at appropriate intervals and is adjusted or changed as necessary based on the plan and the client's condition.

I. Facilitation—An activity assumed by the case manager to promote communication among the client/family and the health care team members including the insurer. Facilitation also focuses on collaboration among all parties to achieve the case management goals and to ensure informed decisions by the client and that the necessary interventions are happening as intended.

J. Implementation—"Executing and documenting specific case management activities and/or interventions that will lead to accomplishing the goals set forth in the case management plan" (CCMC, 2015, p. 7). Implementation of the case management plan also means linking the patient's assessed needs with private and community services, filling the gaps in care and services, avoiding duplication of services, and obtaining agreement on the plan of care from the patient and his or her support systems. The main goal in these activities is maximizing the safety and total well-being of the patient.

K. Intervention—Planned strategies and activities that are employed to modify or manage a maladaptive behavior or state of being (e.g., health condition) and facilitate improvement, resolution, growth, or change. Intervention is also analogous to the medical term *treatment*. Intervention may include activities such as advocacy, medications management, health instructions, physical therapy, or speech–language therapy.

L. Monitoring—Reviewing and "gathering sufficient information from all relevant sources and its documentation regarding the case management plan, and its activities and/or services to enable the case manager to determine the plan's effectiveness" (CCMC, 2015, p. 7).

M. Outcomes—The measurable results of a process or action such as adherence to health regimen. Used to assess the effectiveness of case management interventions to determine their impact and consequences as they relate to the client (e.g., clinical, financial, variance, quality/ quality of life, client satisfaction) (CCMC, 2015).

N. Planning—"Determining and documenting specific [case management] objectives, goals, and actions designed to meet the client's needs as identified through the assessment process… [usually] action-oriented and time specific" (CCMC, 2015, p. 7).

O. Problem identification—Use of objective data gathered through careful assessment and examination of a client's situation to articulate concerns and areas of interest that require special attention. This process allows the case manager to decide on the focus of case management services and implementation of necessary interventions reflecting practice patterns and trends wherein client outcomes can be positively influenced.

Applicability to CMSA's Standards of Practice

A. The Case Management Society of America (CMSA) describes the roles, functions, and activities of case managers in its standards of practice for case management (CMSA, 2010). The standards emphasize the importance of differentiating between the terms "role," "function," and "activity," before describing what case managers do.

B. The case management process is carried out within the ethical and legal realm of a case manager's scope of practice, using critical thinking and evidence-based knowledge. The overarching themes in the case management process include the tasks described below.

12-1 **Key Steps in the Case Management Process**

1. Client identification and selection: Focuses on identifying clients who would benefit from case management services. This step may include obtaining consent for case management services, if appropriate.
2. Assessment and problem/opportunity identification: Begins after the completion of the case selection and intake into case management and occurs intermittently, as needed, throughout the case.
3. Development of the case management plan: Establishes goals of the intervention and prioritizes the needs of the client, support system, and/or family caregiver, as well as determines the type of services and resources that are available in order to address the established goals or desired outcomes.
4. Implementation and coordination of care activities: Puts the case management plan into action.
5. Evaluation of the case management plan and follow-up: Involves the evaluation of the client's status and goals and the associated outcomes.
6. Termination of the case management process: Brings closure to the care and/or episode of illness. The process focuses on discontinuing case management when the client transitions to the highest level of function, the best possible outcome has been attained, or the needs/desires of the client change.

C. Case management is neither linear nor a one-way exercise. For example, the assessment responsibilities will occur at all points in the process, and functions such as facilitation, coordination, and collaboration will occur throughout the client's health care encounter.
D. Primary steps in the case management process according to Powell and Tahan (2008) include those described in Box 12-1.

 Steps of the Case Management Process

A. The case management process is a systematic approach to patient care delivery and management.
   1. The process identifies what the case manager should do, how much, and at what time intervals or frequency during the patient's course of treatment.
   2. The case manager works closely with the various members of the interdisciplinary health care team in implementing the case management process and interventions.
   3. The process consists of seven steps that are executed as necessary and as indicated by the patient's condition or the demands of the health care delivery system.
   4. The main steps do not always occur in a linear or specific chronological manner. Case managers may go back and forth executing the steps or actions within steps as necessitated by the client's condition and care needs.
B. Step 1: Client identification/selection—Focuses on identifying clients who would benefit from case management services.
   1. In some health care organizations, it is considered the first step in the case management process. In others, it is viewed as being unnecessary due to the fact that case managers may follow all types of patients regardless of acuity levels, intensity of services and resources required, or needs.

2. In organizations where selection is necessary, the case manager identifies the clients who will most benefit from case management services based on certain criteria specific to the organization and the services available in the setting where the client is receiving care.
3. According to the Case Management Society of America (CMSA), identification of clients for case management services is accomplished through the use of methods and tools that include, but are not limited to, those in Box 12-2 (CMSA, 2010, p. 15).
4. Health care organizations often have a policy, procedure, or guideline explaining the process for client selection for case management. Such process may be designed based on the following:
   a. Health risk screening
   b. Evidence-based criteria
   c. Risk stratification through data management
   d. Referrals from other health care providers such as physicians and clinical nurses
5. Client identification/selection may be applied in the evaluation of individuals who are referred by other health care providers to the case manager for the purpose of providing case management services.
   a. The case manager decides whether to accept the individual based on the established set of criteria developed by the health care organization where she or he works.
   b. The criteria applied enable the case manager to determine whether the patient needs case management services and the type of services that will be needed.
6. Criteria for case management services are not limited to a single condition or diagnosis. For example, sentinel or significant/reportable quality and safety events may be considered by some organizations as automatic situations that necessitate full case management services and follow-up by case managers.

BOX
12-2   **General Screening Criteria for Client Selection for Case Management Services***

- Age
- Poor pain control
- Low functional status or cognitive deficits
- Previous home health and durable medical equipment usage
- History of mental illness or substance use, suicide risk, or crisis intervention
- Chronic, catastrophic, or terminal illness
- Social issues such as a history of abuse, neglect, no known social support, or lives alone
- Repeated emergency department visits
- Repeated admissions
- Need for admission or transition to a postacute facility
- Poor nutritional status
- Financial issues

* The criteria represent examples only and not a comprehensive list.
From Case Management Society of America (CMSA). (2010). *Standards of practice for case management*. Little Rock, AR: Author.

7. Through client identification and selection, the case manager is able to systematically review all patients' situations and select those individuals who absolutely need case management services and would benefit from them the most. This activity is essential for streamlining the case managers' workloads and to allow them to spend their time and efforts where they are needed the most.

8. During the client identification/selection step, case managers determine the necessity for case management services using a rapid and brief assessment or a special screening tool. Not all patients need a case manager. Case management services may *not* always be necessary for certain clients (Box 12-3).

9. Selection criteria can be generic and applicable across care settings and levels of care or specific to a population or setting. Regardless, they must be based on issues that may affect length of stay or service, quality, safety, and cost of care. Their use by case managers should be based on the condition and anticipated needs of the patient.

10. Selection criteria must be prospectively identified by an organization and communicated to all staff in a case management policy or procedure format.

11. Avoid exclusively using length-of-stay and claims data as selection criteria. These criteria are late indicators of case management needs. By the time the patient has exceeded the established length of stay and maximum dollar expenditure for the diagnosis, much case management intervention could have already taken place.

12. The selection criteria are to be used with caution or in conjunction with other factors. For example, in the acute care/hospital setting, selection criteria for case management services may include, but are not limited to, those listed in Box 12-4.

C. Step 2: Assessment and problem identification—This step of the process begins after the completion of the case selection and client's intake into case management.

BOX 12-3 Provision of Case Management Services

Examples of When Case Management Services Are Unnecessary
- The client meets intensity of services and severity of illness criteria of the level of care the client has accessed. This means appropriate for the level and may not require a case manager's intervention.
- No major discharge barriers are identified.
- If readmission to the hospital or service is not a concern (i.e., planned readmission such as client receiving chemotherapy treatment).
- No financial, payer, or psychosocial barriers present.
- Excellent self-management skills in engagement in own care with appropriate family caregiver or support system.

Examples of When Case Management Services Are Necessary
- Multiple and complex medical issues or comorbidities
- Needs for complex and costly services/resources
- Complex postdischarge or postcare encounter needs
- Complex psychosocial and socioeconomic issues
- Risks for untoward events including legal/ethical concerns
- Compromised financial situations or absence of health insurance
- Poor self-management and engagement and suboptimal psychosocial support system.

BOX 12-4 Example of Case Management Selection Criteria in Acute Care Setting

- Lives alone or with someone with a disability
- Age over 65 years
- Payer source, for example, managed care–type insurance/health plans
- Readmission or readmissions within 15 and up to 30 days of hospital discharge
- Multiple physician involvement including specialists
- Overdose (unintentional/intentional)
- Chemical dependency (alcohol and drugs)
- Eating disorder (e.g., bulimia, anorexia nervosa, failure to thrive)
- Chronic mental illness
- Alzheimer/dementia
- Noncompliance
- Uncooperative, manipulative, or aggressive behavior
- Coexisting behavioral and physical conditions
- Miscellaneous conditions (Munchausen syndrome)
- Socioeconomic indicators
- Suspected child or elder abuse and neglect
- Victim of violent crime
- Homelessness
- Poor living environment
- No known social or family support system
- Admission from an extended care facility (ECF) or sheltered living arrangement
- Need for transitional care in an ECF or sheltered living arrangement
- Out-of-state or out-of-country residence, undocumented immigrants
- Residence in rural community with limited or nonexistent services
- Limited or no financial resources
- Absence of or inadequate health insurance
- Single or first-time parent
- Dependent in activities of daily living and inability to shop for groceries, drive, or cook for self
- Repeated admissions to acute care
- Frequent visits to the emergency room (ER), family physician, or clinic
- Disruptive or obstructive family member or significant other
- Poor self-management and engagement state

1. A thorough assessment must be done at this point in order to determine the needs of the clients/patients and their families, particularly as they relate to the case management plan, treatment, and transitional/discharge plan.
2. An inaccurate or poor assessment can lead to an unsafe case management and discharge/transition plans.
3. Sources of assessment data are:
   a. Patient and family/caregiver
   b. Family physician or primary care provider
   c. Office and hospital medical records, including old and current emergency department records
   d. Ancillary staff
   e. Employers
   f. Medications
   g. Claims and other administrative paperwork

    h. Other external agencies such as extended/skilled care facilities and home care services
4. The assessment must be comprehensive and address the following:
    a. Patient's health demographics and history
    b. Appropriateness for admission to the level of care or setting the patient is in
    c. Current health and medical status, including the chief complaint that prompted the patient to seek medical care
    d. Nutritional status
    e. Adjustment to illness
    f. Health education needs
    g. Medication assessment
    h. Financial assessment including health insurance, status of certification, or authorization for care and services
    i. Functional assessment and environmental factors
        i. Home environment assessment
        ii. Activities of daily living (ADLs) and instrumental ADLs (IADLs) assessment
    j. Psychosocial assessment, including family and support systems
    k. Cultural, spiritual, and religious characteristics
5. Based on the assessment data and findings, case managers, in conjunction with the patient and family/caregiver and in collaboration with other health care providers, are able to:
    a. Identify the actual and potential problems to be addressed
    b. Set the goals of the treatment
    c. Identify the necessary interventions and strategies that will need to be incorporated in the case management plan of care in order to achieve the goals
    d. Determine the resources needed for addressing these problems
    e. Assure patient and family interests, beliefs, and preferences are incorporated into the process and findings
6. In its standards of practice for case management, CMSA explains that case managers assess and reassess their clients on an ongoing basis. It also emphasizes the need for case managers to complete these health and psychosocial assessments, while taking into account the cultural and linguistic needs of the clients and their families. CMSA also indicates that case managers may demonstrate such expectation through documentation using assessment tools, which consist of elements pertinent to the practice or care setting. Box 12-5 shares examples of these elements (CMSA, 2010).
D. Step 3: Development of the case management plan—The case management plan is necessary to establish goals of the treatment, prioritize the patient's needs (i.e., actual and potential problems), and determine the types of services and resources required to meet the established goals/desired outcomes.
    1. The case management plan is interdisciplinary in nature and requires input from those involved in the care including the client (patient) and the client's family and caregivers.
    2. A well-developed case management plan helps decrease the risk for incomplete interventions or inappropriate care. It also provides a seamless approach to care that supports the standards of accreditation and regulatory agencies.

BOX 12-5   Examples of Assessment Elements Important to Include in Case Managers' Documentation

- Physical/functional
- Medical and surgical history including past course(s) of treatment
- Psychosocial behavioral
- Mental health
- Cognitive
- Client strengths and abilities
- Environmental and residential
- Family, caregiver, or support system dynamics
- Spiritual
- Cultural
- Financial
- Health insurance status and available benefits
- History of substance use
- History of abuse, violence, or trauma
- Vocational and/or educational
- Recreational/leisure pursuits
- Caregiver(s) capability and availability
- Learning and technology capabilities
- Self-care, self-management and engagement capability
- Health literacy
- Health status expectations and goals
- Transitional or discharge plan
- Advance care planning
- Legal and ethical
- Transportation capability and constraints
- Health literacy and illiteracy
- Readiness to change
- Resource utilization
- Cost management activities
- Current diagnosis(es) or complaints
- Goals of care (short and long term)
- Provider options

From Case Management Society of America (CMSA). (2010). *Standards of practice for case management*. Little Rock, AR: CMSA.

3. Case managers may answer the following questions to ensure the appropriateness of the case management plan:
   a. What are the patient's and family's problems that need to be addressed in this episode of care? Are the patient and family in agreement with these problems? What are the client's interests, desires, preferences, needs, and goals?
   b. What are the treatment goals and desired outcomes the health care team must accomplish and the patient/family are interested in?
   c. What are the necessary interventions (both diagnostic and therapeutic) that would address these problems and goals?
   d. What time frame(s) should be established for meeting the goals and outcomes?
   e. What are the barriers to meeting the goals and the desired outcomes?
4. The case management plan is used by all health disciplines and providers when caring for the client and family. The case manager,

along with the client and family, facilitates the development of the plan and the revision of plan as she or he engages in ongoing assessment and reassessment of the client's condition, goals of treatments, and progress toward achieving desired outcomes.

5. The CMSA standards of practice for case management note the importance of identifying the problems and opportunities before the development of the case management plan. Therefore, it is necessary for case managers to articulate the client's problems or opportunities that would benefit from case management interventions (CMSA, 2010).

6. The CMSA standards of practice require case managers to document they have established agreement among the key stakeholders (e.g., the client, family or caregiver, and the other involved health care providers and other organizations or vendors) about the problems and opportunities identified and the goals of the interventions. Examples of opportunities case managers may identify when working with a client/family or caregiver are available in Box 12-6.

7. One important aspect of the case management plan development is planning the care based on the problems identified during the client's comprehensive assessment. In this regard, CMSA explains in its standards of practice for case management (CMSA, 2010) that case managers should identify immediate, short-term, long-term, and ongoing needs, as well as develop appropriate and necessary case management strategies, interventions, and goals to address these needs.

8. Case managers' documentation of the planning and development of the case management plan should reflect those elements or activities described in Box 12-7.

BOX 12-6

Examples of Opportunities Case Managers May Identify to Address in the Case Management Plan

- Lack of established, evidence-based plan of care with specific goals
- Overutilization or underutilization of services
- Use of multiple providers/agencies
- Use of inappropriate services or level of care
- Poor self-management and engagement skills, and nonadherence
- Nonadherence to plan of care (e.g., medication adherence)
- Lack of education or understanding of the disease process, current health condition(s), and medication list
- Medical, psychosocial, and mental health and/or functional limitations
- Lack of a support system (e.g., family caregiver) or presence of a support system under stress
- Financial barriers to adherence of the plan of care
- Determination of patterns of care or behavior that may be associated with increased severity of condition
- Compromised client safety
- Inappropriate discharge or delay from other levels of care
- High cost injuries or illnesses
- Complications related to medical, psychosocial, or functional issues
- Frequent transitions between settings

From Case Management Society of America (CMSA). (2010). *Standards of practice for case management*. Little Rock, AR: CMSA.

BOX 12-7

Elements of Case Manager's Documentation that Pertain to the Case Management Plan

- Relevant, comprehensive information and data using interviews, research, and other methods needed to develop the case management plan of care
- Recognition of the client's diagnosis, prognosis, care needs, preferences, preferred role in decision-making, and outcomes of the goals articulated in the case management plan of care
- Validation that the case management plan of care is consistent with evidence-based practice, when such guidelines are available and applicable
- Establishment of measurable goals and indicators within specified time frames, for example, access to care, cost-effectiveness of care, quality of care, and safety
- Client's or client's caregiver/support system participation in the written case management plan of care
- Agreement with plan, including agreement with any changes, eliminations, or additions
- Facilitation of problem solving and conflict resolution
- Evidence of supplying the client/family with information and resources necessary to make informed decisions
- Awareness of maximization of client outcomes by all available resources and services
- Adherence to payer expectations, especially with respect to how often to contact and re-evaluate the client

From Case Management Society of America (CMSA). (2010). *Standards of practice for case management*. Little Rock, AR: CMSA.

E. Step 4: Implementation and coordination of care activities—In this step, the case manager puts the case management plan into action.

F. Step 4 also encompasses all the interventions indicated in the plan that are meant to meet the treatment goals and resolve the patient's problems or presenting chief complaint.

   1. Implementation and coordination requires case managers to reassess the patient's condition on an ongoing basis looking for:

      a. Resolution of the identified problems

      b. Status of the treatment goals, case management interventions, and the transitional plan

      c. Whether new needs have arisen that require modification in the plan

   2. In this step, case managers continue to obtain certifications/authorizations for care and services from managed care organizations as needed. They engage in concurrent reviews as well as follow-up on any outstanding issues with the insurer/payer or members of the health care team.

   3. Case managers facilitate and coordinate the work of the health care team and advocate for the client in an effort to promote cost-effective, safe, and efficient care. This may include:

      a. The required tests and procedures

      b. Patient and family health education and instruction

      c. Discharge/transitional planning

      d. Brokerage of services such as specialty consultations, physical therapy, and home care services

      e. Completion of all required paperwork such as those needed for the placement of patients in skilled nursing, rehabilitation facilities, or home with visiting nurse services

4. For effective implementation and coordination of the case management plan, case managers work closely with:

      a. Health care providers internal to the organizations that employ them, such as physicians, social workers, and physical therapists

      b. Key health care providers and agents external to the organizations, including staff from transportation agencies, durable medical equipment vendors, home care agencies, charitable organizations, and skilled nursing facilities

5. Case managers also address the family's needs to help members of the patient's family cope with illness and sometimes hospitalization. These may include:

      a. The need for hope and the need for information about their family member's condition (seen by the patient's family as the most important of all the needs identified)

      b. Communicating accurate information to the family to enable them to make informed decisions, thereby assisting them to gain understanding and a feeling of control over a difficult situation

6. For effective implementation of the case management plan and for ensuring that it is patient and family centered, case managers may answer the following questions:

      a. Does the patient/family have any new needs that must be incorporated into the case management plan?

      b. Are the patient, family, and health care team in agreement with the plan?

      c. What is the appropriate time frame for implementing the treatments and interventions? Is this time frame appropriate for resolving the identified problems?

      d. Does the transitional/discharge plan meet the patient's condition and needs?

      e. Have all the necessary authorizations for treatment and services been obtained?

      f. Have the barriers to meeting the plan been addressed or resolved?

7. The case manager during the implementation of the case management plan facilitates, coordinates, communicates, and collaborates with the client and other stakeholders in order to achieve goals and maximize positive client outcomes (Box 12-8).

8. CMSA addresses the case manager's responsibility toward plan implementation in its standards of practice for case management and recognizes the importance of the case manager's professional role and practice setting in relation to that of other providers and organizations caring for the client and working toward achieving desired goals (CMSA, 2010).

G. Step 5: Evaluation of the case management plan and follow up—This step involves the evaluation of the patient care activities and treatments, and their associated outcomes, including client's progression toward achieving agreed-upon and set goals.

> ### BOX 12-8 Focus of the Case Manager's Implementation of the Client's Plan of Care
>
> - Development and maintenance of proactive, client-centered relationships and communication with the client and other necessary stakeholders to maximize the achievement of desired outcomes.
> - Evidence of transitions of care, including:
>   - A transfer to the most appropriate health care provider/setting.
>   - The transfer is appropriate, timely, and complete.
>   - Documentation of collaboration and communication with other health care professionals, especially during each transition to another level of care within or outside of the client's current setting.
> - Adherence to client privacy and confidentiality during collaboration.
> - Use of mediation and negotiation to improve communication and relationships when necessary.
> - Use of problem-solving skills and techniques to reconcile potentially differing points of view and reach consensus.
> - Collaboration with other stakeholders to optimize client outcomes. This may include working with:
>   - Community, local, and state resources
>   - Primary care physician and other primary or specialty providers
>   - Other members of the health care team
>   - The payer
>   - Other relevant health care stakeholders
> - Evidence of collaborative efforts to maximize adherence within the case manager's practice setting to regulatory and accreditation standards.
> - Advocating for the client, client's support system and caregiver to assure the plan of care is client-centered and serves the client's best interest.
>
> From Case Management Society of America (CMSA). (2010). *Standards of practice for case management.* Little Rock, AR: CMSA.

H. Case managers complete this evaluation by examining the patient's condition and the status of the goals and desired outcomes. During these activities, case managers may answer the following questions:
   1. Are the activities and outcomes on target?
   2. Is care progressing according to the case management plan's milestones?
   3. Are treatments occurring as per the established timeline?
   4. Is the patient ready for discharge or transition to another level of care?
   5. Is the patient being cared for in the appropriate level of care or setting?
   6. Are there any issues with reimbursement? Have all required authorizations been obtained?
   7. Does the case management plan meet the needs and interests of the patient and family?
   8. Are there any legal or ethical risks present?
   9. What modifications in the case management plan are necessary and when?
   10. What is the status of the client's self management and engagement skills? How optimal is the presence and involvement of the client's support system or family caregiver in client's care?
I. Case managers continuously monitor and reassess the client to measure response to the plan of care. Such activities are necessary for ensuring

timely care delivery and patient-focused modifications of the plan. These also include special focus on the following (CMSA, 2010):

1. Client's condition, responses to interventions, and progress toward recovery
2. Verification that the plan of care continues to be appropriate, understood, accepted by client and support system, and documented
3. Awareness of circumstances necessitating revisions to the plan of care, such as changes in the client's condition, lack of response to the care plan, preference changes, transitions across settings, and barriers to care and services
4. Collaboration with the client, providers, and other pertinent stakeholders regarding any revisions to the plan of care
5. Ongoing collaboration with the client, family and caregiver, providers, and other pertinent stakeholders, so that the client's response to interventions is reviewed and incorporated into the plan of care and documented in the medical record

J. Case managers also ensure that the discharge/transition plan is safe and that the patient and family are satisfied with care and the postdischarge services and resources.

K. During the evaluation and follow-up step, case managers are able to measure outcomes of care, identify any variances or delays in the care, and address them immediately as indicated. These activities enhance client's health, safety, adaptation to illness, and self-management abilities. They also ensure that care is efficient, safe, of high quality, cost-effective, and of optimal experience (Box 12-9).

L. Step 6: Termination of the case management process—This step brings closure to the care, services, and the episode of illness. It focuses on discontinuing the case management services and the transition of the patient back to a community-based level of care including the patient's home.

1. Case managers determine the need for terminating the case management services based on the patient's and family's condition or

---

BOX 12-9   Focus of the Evaluation and Follow-Up Step of the Case Management Process

- Evaluation of the extent to which the goals documented in the plan of care have been achieved
- Demonstration of the efficacy, quality, and cost-effectiveness of the case manager's interventions in achieving the goals documented in the plan of care
- Measurement and reporting of the impact of the case management plan of care
- Utilization of adherence guidelines, standardized tools, and proven processes, which can be used to measure individuals' preference for and understanding of:
  - The proposed plans for their care
  - Their willingness to change
  - Their support to maintain health behavioral change
- Utilization of evidence-based guidelines in appropriate client populations
- Evaluation of client satisfaction with case management
- Evaluation of the client, support system and caregiver's involvement in client's care.

From Case Management Society of America (CMSA). (2010). *Standards of practice for case management*. Little Rock, AR: CMSA.

choice, the health care team, the payer/insurer, and the status of the case management plan and related goals.

2. Situations that may require termination of case management services may include, but are not limited to, the following:
   a. Achievement of targeted goals and outcomes.
   b. Required change in health care setting or level of care.
   c. Loss of or change in the benefits (i.e., client no longer meets program or benefit eligibility requirements, reaching maximum benefits).
   d. Client/family wishes (e.g., client refuses further services).
   e. Case manager is no longer able to provide case management services.
   f. Patient and family met maximum benefit from case management services.
   g. Client and/or family exhibits nonadherent behaviors to the case management plan of care.
   h. Client's death (CMSA, 2010).

3. When terminating the case management process and/or services, case managers must provide ample notice and explanation to the patient, family, and health care team members. Such decisions should be discussed with all involved in the care and must be made based on the situations shared above.

4. The case manager should appropriately terminate case management services based upon established case closure guidelines. These guidelines may differ in various case management practice settings and health care organizations.

5. In its standards of practice for case management, CMSA emphasizes the need for case managers to (CMSA, 2010):
   a. Have evidence of agreement of termination of case management services by the client, family or caregiver, payer, case manager, and/or other appropriate parties before actual termination
   b. Provide a reasonable notice to the client/family and other appropriate parties of the termination of case management services that is based upon the facts and circumstances of each individual case
   c. Document that both verbal and written notice of termination of case management services has been given to the client and to treating and direct service providers
   d. Communicate, with permission from client/family and in accordance with laws, regulations, and ethical standards, client information to transition providers to maximize positive outcomes and continuity to care

M. Step 7: Follow-up postdischarge or transition from the health care encounter—This step highlights the importance of following up with the client/family and caregiver postdischarge from an episode of care or transition to another level of care or provider. This is important primarily to assure client's safety and quality of care.

N. If the client had been discharged to the home setting, the case manager in this step may follow up with the client/family or caregiver to:
   1. Ensure the client is safe
   2. Assess the client's (or caregiver's) level of comfort and knowledge in self-management
   3. Examine client's adherence to care regimen

4. Answer any questions the client/family and caregiver has
5. Ascertain the quality of the client's experience of care and identify opportunities for improvement
6. Identify opportunities for intervention to avoid unnecessary readmission to acute care setting or return to emergency department
7. Assure that follow-up appointment with primary care provider (or other providers) is set and client has no concerns about that
8. Confirm that postdischarge services arranged for prior to discharge or transition are in place as planned

O. If the client had been transitioned to another level of care or provider, the case manager in this step may follow up with the health care team at the other level of care to:
1. Ensure continuity of the client's plan of care and that all materials about the client's care pretransition have been received by the team (e.g., care summary, medications list)
2. Answer any questions the team may have about the plan of care
3. Ascertain the quality and safety of the handoff communication (transition of care communication) and identify opportunities for improvement
4. Identify opportunities for intervention to avoid unnecessary readmission to acute care setting or return to emergency department
5. Assure that tests or procedures planned to occur posttransition are happening as planned
6. Clarify any misunderstanding

P. Follow-up postdischarge or transition has gained increased importance recently, especially because of the Patient Protection and Affordable Care Act of 2010, value-based purchasing, and Hospital Readmission Reduction Programs. These have moved quality of care from volume to value and emphasized the need to ensure client's safety during transitions. Case managers play an essential role in this regard.

Special Actions Occurring Throughout the Case Management Process

A. Throughout the case management process, case managers engage in other necessary activities. These activities are applicable to almost all of the steps of the case management process. They are advocacy, continuous monitoring, reassessment, and re-evaluation.
1. Advocacy focuses on being patient and family or caregiver centered in the case management activities, that is, meeting the patient and family needs, interests, preferences, and wishes and ensuring that care activities and decisions on treatment options focus on what is in the best interest of the patient and family.
2. Continuous monitoring where the case manager uses a method of checking, regulating, rechecking, and documenting the quality of care, services, and products delivered to the patient to determine whether the goals of the case management plan are being achieved or whether the goals remain appropriate and realistic while assuring the patient is safe at all times.
3. Reassessment is similar to continuous monitoring and focuses on frequently examining the patient's and family's condition and the

status of the case management plan of care, looking for data that allow the case manager to decide whether the case management plan is on target or if it requires any modifications.

4. Re-evaluation is an activity case managers engage in especially after they have instituted action, such as examining whether their attempts to expedite the reporting of test results or to counteract the effects of a delay in care have been successful and, if not, to determine the next necessary steps.

5. The frequency of these activities depends on the care setting or level of care where case management services are provided. For example, case management services in a hospital setting may require more frequent follow-up (e.g., hourly, daily, or every shift) than for an individual in a private home (e.g., few times a week), clinic (e.g., quarterly), or extended care facility (e.g., weekly).

B. Reassessment, ongoing monitoring, and re-evaluation of the client/ family and plan of care may be necessary if certain situations occur such as those presented in Box 12-10.

C. Case managers may decide to repeat the case management process at any time during the episode of care, or they may revisit any of the six steps:

1. Engaging in activities such as continuous monitoring, reassessment, and re-evaluation requires the case managers to go through every step of the case management process or those that are most relevant to the concern at hand. This is important to assess whether a goal has been met or an outcome needs to be revisited.

2. Repeating the process is one way of ensuring that care activities are being completed as predetermined, the transitional/discharge plan is safe, and care is of utmost quality, efficient, and cost-effective.

D. Throughout the case management process, case managers also:

1. Document their observations, decisions, actions/interventions, and outcomes in the patients' records

2. Keep a record of their assessment, monitoring, and evaluation findings

3. Keep a record of the modifications they make to the case management plan, including the rationale for the change

4. Document their interactions with the patient/family, the insurer/ payer, and other health care providers/agents internal and external to their organization

---

BOX
12-10

Sample Reasons for Reassessment and Re-evaluation of Client's Situation and Care

- Change in the client's medical or health condition
- Change in the client's social stability and network
- Quality of care issue
- Delays in care ultimately impacting care progression
- Risk management issue
- Concern regarding the transitional/discharge plan or postdischarge services
- Change in the client's functional, mobility, or cognitive capacity
- Evolving health educational needs
- Issues in the availability of community resources/services
- Reimbursement concerns or denials for services issued by the payer
- Issues in client's self-management and engagement skills and concerns about availability and involvement of client's support system or family caregiver.

References

Case Management Society of America (CMSA). (2010). *Standards of practice for case management*. Little Rock, AR: Author.

Commission for Case Manager Certification (CCMC). (2015). *CCM certification guide*. Rolling Meadows, IL: Author.

Powell, S., & Tahan, H. (2008). *CMSA Core Curriculum for Case Management* (2nd ed.). Philadelphia, PA: Lippincott Williams & Wilkins.

CHAPTER 13

Transitional Planning and Transitions of Care

Jackie Birmingham

LEARNING OBJECTIVES

Upon completion of this section, the reader will be able to:

1. Define transitional planning as it relates to continuity of care.
2. List two federal Conditions of Participation that influence transitional care from acute care hospitals.
3. List other selected federal rules that have significance in transition planning.
4. Discuss factors that impact case management in cross-setting measures.
5. Describe specific topics related to selected levels of care to which inpatients are referred.
6. Describe Value-Based Purchasing and impact on transition management and readmissions.
7. List additional qualifications and experience needed to be a case manager who manages the transition of care as stated in discharge planning Conditions of Participation.

IMPORTANT TERMS AND CONCEPTS

Americans with Disabilities Act
Assessment Domains
Discharge Planning
Discharge Status Codes

Efficiency Score
Health Information Privacy and Accountability Act
Hospital Value-Based Purchasing

Improving Medicare Post-Acute Care Transformation Act
Key elements of care coordination
Levels of Care

Notice of Hospital Discharge	Preadmission Screening and Resident Review	Surveyor guidelines
Olmstead Decision		Transfer MS-DRG
Overlap of functions	Privacy	Transitional Planning
	Readmission	Utilization Review

Introduction

A. The importance of transition planning is high on the need-to-know index for case managers regardless of experience level (e.g., novice, expert) or hierarchical position (e.g., frontline staff, management).
   1. Transition planning is an example of demonstrating trust in other case managers across the care continuum.
   2. Sending a patient to another care setting involves a handover of responsibility. The sending case manager presumes that the receiving case manager possesses the knowledge, experience, and adherence to case management practice standards in order to assume responsibility for the patient and his/her identified goals and concerns.
   3. This handover requires the receiving case manager to perform case management activities in accordance with practice standards to ensure the patient's case management needs are identified and addressed in an ongoing and progressive manner.
B. Transition management is not a new topic for case managers.
   1. The article, One Patient, Numerous Healthcare Providers, and Multiple Care Settings: Addressing the Concerns of Care Transition Through Case Management, sets the stage for attention to the influence of case managers on patients as they move through the health care settings (Tahan, 2007).
      a. In the 8 to 9 years since this definitive article was written, much has changed for case managers, not in the essential process or practice but in the health care industry as a whole.
      b. One of the most significant change resulted from the Patient Protection and Affordable Care Act of 2010 with goals that have impact on payment for health care services based on quality and outcomes versus quantity of services provided (CMS-ACA, 2011).
      c. The outcome of the success is based on the appropriate transition of patients, from acute care to self-care and all the steps in between.
C. The hallmark of patient-centered transition of care is based on a case manager's ability to work with a team of professionals on both sides of the continuum.
   1. All participants in the transitions of care must also work with the patient and family and determine what is the next best appropriate level of care in time and place, keeping in mind that the patient's preferences met as far as is reasonably possible.
   2. Nobody said it would be easy; however, it makes a huge difference for patients across the care continuum both your institution and the facilities and vendors that accept your transitioned patients.

Descriptions of Key Terms

A. Conditions of Participation—The Centers for Medicare and Medicaid Services (CMS) develops Conditions of Participation (CoPs) that health care organizations must meet to participate in the Medicare and Medicaid programs. These standards are used to improve quality and protect the health and safety of beneficiaries. The CMS also ensures that the standards of accrediting organizations recognized by the CMS, such as The Joint Commission (TJC) or the American Osteopathic Association (AOA), through a process called *deeming*, meet or exceed Medicare standards as stated in the CoPs. The standards apply to anyone receiving services, regardless of payment source.
   1. Discharge planning—CoPs are associated directly with the hospital's responsibility for discharge planning.
   2. Patients' rights—CoPs are associated with assuring that patients' rights to freedom of choice and other issues are followed.
   3. Medical records—CoPs are associated with the patient's inpatient medical record and the need to ensure that the closed record contains information related to the course of the hospital stay and plans for follow-up care.
B. Continuity of care—The coordination of care received by a patient over time and across multiple health care providers and settings. This is usually of most concern during patient's transition from one provider or level of care to another.
C. Discharge—The formal release, or signing out by a physician, of a patient from an episode of care. The episode of care can be in the form of hospital inpatient status, observation status, emergency room stay, or a clinic visit. A discharge can also be applied to an inpatient skilled nursing facility, acute and subacute rehabilitation facility, or a home health episode of care.
   1. Discharge status—Disposition of the patient at discharge indicating to what level of care a patient has been transferred or discharged. Discharge status, particularly from acute care, has significance in how a hospital is paid and in how health care organizations track care. Disposition status also may refer to the patient's state at the time of concluding care and services, which may be either alive or expired.
   2. Leaving Against Medical Advice (LAMA) or Against Medical Advice (AMA)—A term used to describe a patient who is discharged from the hospital against the advice of his or her attending physician. The person signing out is usually asked to sign a form stating his or her awareness that the discharge is against medical advice.
   3. Patient elopement—A term used to describe a situation in which a patient leaves without the knowledge of the hospital staff. The patient is then determined to be "missing."
D. Discharge planning—The process of assessing the patient's needs of care after discharge from a health care facility and ensuring that the necessary services are in place before discharge. This process ensures a patient's timely, appropriate, and safe discharge to the next level of care or setting, including appropriate use of resources necessary for ongoing care.

E. Functional status—The assessment of an individual's ability to manage his or her own care needs.
1. Activities of daily living (ADLs)—Activities that are considered an everyday part of normal life. These include dressing, bathing, toileting, transferring (e.g., moving from and into a chair), and eating. The functional levels of ADLs are used to measure the degree of impairment and can affect eligibility for certain types of insurance benefits.
2. Instrumental activities of daily living (IADLs)—Regularly necessary home management activities, including meal preparation, housework, grocery shopping, and other similar activities.
3. Executive function—An integrated set of cognitive abilities that allow an individual to process available information in planning, prioritizing, sequencing, self-monitoring, self-correcting, inhibiting, initiating, controlling, or altering behavior. It includes evaluation of such parameters as "capacity" and "competency." Evaluating a patient's executive function is a multidisciplinary process involving physicians, nurses, social workers, and other health care professionals and can, in some situations, involve the court system.
F. Handoff—The exchange of a patient's care between incoming and outgoing caregivers; any transfer of role and responsibility from one person to another or one setting to another. Successful handoffs overcome barriers such as physical setting, social setting, language and communication barriers, and time and convenience.
G. Level of care—Different kinds and locations of care provided to patients, based on a scale of intensity or amount of care/services provided.
1. Acute level of care—The most intense level of care related to necessity for medical (physician) services.
2. Subacute level of care—The level of care that combines a high need for nursing, therapy, and physician services. Intermediate between acute and chronic, this level of care can be provided in acute care facilities or other facilities as determined by licensing in each state.
3. Transitional care unit (TCU)—A unit of care, usually in a hospital, that is dedicated to supporting a patient's transition of care from acute to a lesser level of care. The level of care is similar to subacute.
4. Skilled nursing facility (SNF)—A facility offering 24-hour skilled nursing care along with rehabilitation services, such as physical, speech, and occupational therapy; assistance with personal care activities, such as eating, walking, toileting, and bathing; coordinated management of patient care; social services; and activities. Some nursing facilities offer specialized care programs for Alzheimer disease or other illnesses or short-term respite care for frail or disabled persons when a family member requires a break from providing care in the home. Payment for a stay in an SNF varies depending on the payer criteria, whether the patient was an inpatient in a hospital for 3 consecutive days, and the reason for admission.
5. Home health care services—Care provided to individuals and families in their place of residence for the purpose of promoting, maintaining, or restoring health, or for minimizing the effects of disability and illness, including terminal illness. Patients must meet the definition of homebound status and require intermittent professional services,

including nursing, physical therapy, occupational, and speech–language services, or social work services. Eligibility criteria for insurance coverage for home care services vary between payer groups.

6. Hospice—A program that provides special care for people who are near the end of life and for their families, either at home, in freestanding facilities, or within hospitals.

H. Prospective payment system (PPS)—A method of reimbursement used by the CMS that bases Medicare payments on a predetermined, fixed amount. The payment amount derived for a particular episode of care is based on a classification system of a specific level of care and an episode of care, for example, *diagnosis-related groups* (DRGs) classification for inpatient hospital services, *resource utilization groups* (RUGs) classification for nursing facilities, and *home health resource groups* (HHRGs) classification for home health agencies.

1. Diagnosis-related groups (DRGs)—The system used to pay for acute inpatient care that is based primarily on the patient's principal diagnosis.

2. Resource utilization groups (RUGs)—The system used to pay for care provided in a nursing facility that is based on the amount, intensity, and type of "resources used," including nursing care and therapies.

3. Home health resource groups (HHRGs)—The system used to pay home health agencies for services based on the resources used and the duration of the services.

I. Readmission—The admission of a patient back into the hospital, for the same disease or condition as the previous admission. Some payers review both admissions if they occur within a specified number of days, for example, 72 hours or 15 or 30 days. Readmission is the focus of a great deal of attention by health professionals and regulators especially with the advent of the Patient Protection and Affordable Care Act of 2010 and the proliferation of the Value-Based Purchasing Program and Hospital Readmissions Reduction Program.

J. Referral—The process of sending a patient from one practitioner to another for health care services; in the case of transitional planning, usually for services related to the current episode of care (e.g., rehabilitation consultation).

K. Transfer—The planned action of sending a patient from one place of care to another. It can be to the same level of care (acute to acute) or to a lower level of care (acute to postacute), or vice versa. The planning of the transfer involves notification of the next level of care and the transfer of necessary medical information.

L. Transfer/qualified DRG—A situation in which a patient's care is coded as being within a predetermined list of DRGs, the patient is discharged to either a skilled nursing facility or home health agency for services related to the reason for hospitalization, and the patient is transferred before the national geometric length of stay for that DRG. Because the patient is determined to be leaving prior to the number of days in that DRG, and because the patient is receiving continuing care for which Medicare is paying, the hospital is paid only for the days of care provided and not the full DRG.

M. Transitional planning—The process that case managers apply to ensure that appropriate resources and services are provided to patients and that these services are provided in the most appropriate setting or level of care, as delineated in the standards and guidelines of regulatory and accreditation agencies. It focuses on moving a patient from the most complex to less complex care settings (Commission for Case Manager Certification [CCMC], 2005).

N. Transitional care—Transitional care includes all the services required to facilitate the coordination and continuity of health care as the patient moves between one health care service provider to another (Case Management Society of America [CMSA], 2010).

O. Transitions of care—Transitions of care is the movement of patients from one health care practitioner or setting to another as their condition and care needs change. This phrase is sometimes known as care transitions (CMSA, 2010).

 ## Applicability to CMSA's Standards of Practice

A. In its Standards of Practice for Case Management, the Case Management Society of America (CMSA) describes that case management practice extends across all health care settings, including payer, provider, government, employer, community, and home environment (CMSA, 2010).

B. CMSA explains that case management practice varies in degrees of complexity and comprehensiveness based on four factors:
   1. The context of the care setting (e.g., wellness and prevention, acute, subacute, rehabilitative, or end of life)
   2. The health conditions and needs of the patient population(s) served including those of the patients' families
   3. The reimbursement method applied for services rendered (payment), such as managed care, workers' compensation, Medicare, or Medicaid
   4. The health care professional discipline assuming the role of the case manager such as registered nurse, social worker, or rehabilitation counselor

C. Transitional and discharge planning standards are also addressed in the CMSA's Case Management Standards of Practice. In this regard, the standards discuss the roles and responsibilities of the case manager in care planning, including identifying needs and developing short- and long-term goals, planning with the patient and family and obtaining their consent to the transitional plan, working with other professionals internal and external to the organization to meet the patient's and family's needs, brokering of services and procurement of health care resources as needed by the patient, and working in concert within payer demands and expectations.

D. This chapter describes transition planning across the continuum of health care and human services and focuses on the role of the case manager in these settings and the case management services provided. Because of the contemporary focus on transitions from acute care settings, content frequently mentions this care setting.

E. This chapter addresses case management practice that requires knowledge of and proficiency in the following practice standards: client assessment, problem/opportunity identification, planning, facilitation/coordination/collaboration, legal, ethics, advocacy, resource management, and stewardship.

Transitional Planning as it Relates to Continuity of Care

A. From the first introduction of the Standards of Practice (Case Management Society of America, 1995), to the revisions in 2002 (Case Management Society of America, 2002), and most recently in 2010 (CMSA, 2010), the term "transition of care" has been increasingly used and now can be found in one form or another in all of the Standards of Practice.

B. The Standards of Practice for Case Management: a Foundation for Care Coordination Across the Entire Care Continuum (McLaughlin Davis, 2014) provides a crosswalk between CMSA Standards, the Centers for Medicare and Medicaid (CMS) Condition of Participation, and the Joint Commission Standards. Each references the transition process and emphasizes the importance of transitioning patients through multiple levels of care in a timely manner with goals of satisfactory outcomes and financial efficiency.

C. Clarification about the essential definition of care coordination, as it relates to transition management, was addressed in the book, *Closing the Quality Gap: A Critical Analysis of Quality Improvement Strategies* (Shojania, McDonald, Wachter, & Owens, 2007).

   1. The chapter, Definitions of Care Coordination and Related Terms (Shojania et al., 2007), shows the importance of care coordination, including transitions of care, and its relationship to quality improvement.

   2. In this chapter, the editors list five key elements compromising care coordination.

      a. Numerous participants are typically involved in care coordination.

      b. Coordination is necessary when participants are dependent upon each other to carry out disparate activities in a patient's care.

      c. In order to carry out these activities in a coordinated way, each participant needs adequate knowledge about their own and others' roles and available resources.

      d. In order to manage all required patient care activities, participants rely on exchange of information.

      e. Integration of care activities has the goal of facilitating appropriate delivery of health care services.

D. Transition of care and discharge planning. Although the term used in this chapter, and in seminars, publications, and innovative projects, is frequently referred to as transition planning, the concept arises out of the practice and process referred to as discharge planning.

   1. In the September 27, 2014 Interpretive Guidelines (CMS SOM-A, 2014) in the section on Discharge Planning, §482.43 Condition of Participation for Discharge Planning, CMS cited the distinction between these two terms, particularly in the use of either term, transition planning or discharge planning to denote facilitating care across the continuum:

      a. Much of the interpretive guidance for these CoPs have been informed by newer research on care transitions, understood broadly. At the same time, the term discharge planning is used both in Section 1861(ee) of the Social Security Act as well as in §482.43. In this guidance, therefore, we continue to use the term discharge planning.

2. The term discharge planning in the CMS COPs is centered on the practice as carried out in hospitals, as opposed to the practice of continuity of care for other non–hospital health care provider settings.

    a. In contrast to the CMSA Standards of Practice that applies across the continuum, §482.43 of the Conditions of Participation for hospitals is targeted to patients in hospitals.

    b. The amendment was passed in 1988 and the standards have been in effect since then, relatively unchanged. However, the process of transition planning has been adapted into COPs for other levels of care. For example, the COPs for home health agencies include the requirement of a policy for discharge of a patient from services (CMS-COP HHA, 2015).

    c. Regardless of setting type, know the Conditions of Participation, which all include information on how to transition/discharge patients to the next level of care.

E. The role of a department manager in transition of care has distinct characteristics in addition to the functions of any person at the manager level (Box 13-1).

1. If you are a department manager that carries out transition of care functions, along with a myriad of other functions, review articles focused on managing transition of care from the managerial perspective.

F. It is necessary for the caser manager to differentiate the use of the terms transitional planning and discharge planning especially because of the subtle differences that exist between these two terms.

1. Transitional care planning is a general term that is used to describe the focused planning for patients who are moving through the health care system.

2. Discharge planning is a term generally applied to the process in which patients in an acute care setting are assessed for continuing care needs required after discharge from an acute setting.

3. Discharge planning is a specialty process within transitional planning.

BOX 13-1 Seven Domains of the Role of Transitions of Care Department Manager

- Staffing and human resources
- Compliance and accreditation
- Discharge planning responsibilities
- Utilization review responsibilities
- Internal department relationships
- External relationships
- Revenue cycle accountability

G. Discharge planning is mandated by federal regulations. The process involves identifying patients who are at risk for adverse outcomes after discharge without specific interventions (Box 13-2).

H. Transitional planning has been mandated by federal agencies in the form of legislation, by accreditation agencies in the form of accreditation or professional performance standards, and by professional organizations and societies in the form of policies or practice guidelines.

I. Currently, there are specific case management standards and guidelines available that explain the roles and responsibilities of case managers in both transitional and discharge planning. These standards are advocated for by case management professional organizations such as the Commission for Case Manager Certification (CCMC), the CMSA and others that promote case management practice such as the American Nurses Association (ANA) and the National Association of Social Workers (NASW).

J. Transitional or discharge planning is one of the core knowledge areas usually covered in case management certification examinations. This topic addresses specific knowledge that pertains to case management practice, including the continuum of care, levels of care and services, care planning and goal setting, community services and resources, rehabilitation services and support programs, assistive technologies and durable medical equipment, continuity of care, and benefit programs.

BOX 13-2 Characteristics of Discharge Planning

- All patients are required to have a discharge plan, but not all patients need the detailed interventions required by regulations.
- Determining whether the patient's ongoing needs are related to the reason for admission to an acute care setting, or if the ongoing needs are related to a chronic health condition or nonacute health problem, is involved. Reimbursement for postacute services depends on the origin of the need (acute vs. chronic).
- Assessment of the patient's postacute care needs is based on the patient's predicted functional status and the capacity for self-care and management.
- Level of care determinations is based on the patient's assessed functional needs at or near the time of discharge. Functional assessment is a more reliable predictor of level of care than is the patient's principal diagnosis.
- The focus of discharge planning is moving the patient from the complex–acute care health system to the next appropriate level of care, which is usually less complex. Patients may need to move through two or three levels before they are in the least complex setting.
- The least complex setting can be described as the level of care where the patient is stabilized from a functional point of view and has reached his or her maximum capacity for self-care.
- Although case managers participate in discharge planning activities, it is the physician who determines the patient's readiness for discharge and appropriateness of the next level of care based on the patient's health condition and needs.

Federal Conditions of Participation that Influence Transitional Care From Acute Care Hospitals

A. The CM job description includes a variety of functions assigned to a department known by a variety of names (e.g., Case Management Department, Care Coordination Department, Care Continuity Department).

B. There are two basic regulations that influence CM job descriptions.
   1. Those two basic regulations are utilization review (UR) and discharge planning (DP) (eCFR, 2015).
   2. Some departments separate staff to perform the UR and DP functions; others combine the functions into a single position. Some facilities maintain two separate departments.
   3. Regardless of the department configuration of the department, the two functions most closely related to transition management are UR and DP (Birmingham, Case Management: Two regulations with coexisting functions, 2007).

C. Utilization review. This section describes the overlap of utilization review and discharge planning as it affects case managers whose responsibilities include transition management.
   1. Utilization review is an amendment to the Social Security Act that occurred in 1972.
      a. The original rule stated that hospitals must review their own patient population for the following:
         i. Appropriateness of admission
         ii. Continued stay
         iii. Professional services used
      b. The terms medical necessity, reasonable, and necessary came into discussions about whether to admit, or not, a patient and, after admission, when and to what level to discharge.
   2. In 1995, the UR process added the requirement that the hospital contract with a Professional Standards Review Organization (PSRO) for outside review.
      a. A PSRO was charged with determining whether services were medically necessary, provided in accordance with federal standards and rendered in the appropriate setting (Neumann, 2012; Sprague, 2002).
      b. The PSRO came to be known as the Quality Improvement Organizations (QIO) to more reflect its work on improving quality of care for Medicare beneficiaries.
   3. In 2014, the CMS split two main QIO functions previously combined in one organization, which resulted in the two functions being managed by two separate entities contracting for each function, Beneficiary and Family-Centered Care (BFCC) and Quality Innovation Network (QIN). In the new structure, case review and quality improvement functions are performed by different contractors.
      a. BFCC manages all beneficiary complaints, quality-of-care reviews, and appeals to ensure consistency in the review process while taking into consideration local factors important to beneficiaries and their families. For additional information, see the section on the Important Message from Medicare.

      b. QIN works regionally with providers and the community on multiple, data-driven quality initiatives to improve patient safety, reduce harm, and improve clinical care at their local and regional levels (HSAP, 2014).

   4. Why talk about UR in a chapter on Transitions of Care? As mentioned, there is a significant overlap in functions of UR and DP.

      a. UR monitors admission with the patient's physician, monitors continued stay based on accepted criteria sets (e.g., InterQual, Milliman), and, by so doing, has a baseline for length of stay and can trigger more action in the discharge planning process when discharge is anticipated.

      b. Both rules working in synergy result in a viable discharge plan as soon as the patient no longer meets medical necessity for continued stay.

      c. These parallel functions mean that the patient will get the right care, at the right level at the right time.

D. Discharge planning—The four-stage process in transition planning as outlined by the CMS in the hospital COPs applies across the continuum. The stages are site neutral—regardless of where you work with patients, these steps can guide you in planning for the patient's next phase of care.

   1. The DP CoPs (and Section 1861(ee) of the Act on which the CoPs is based) provides for a four-stage discharge planning process:

      a. Screening all inpatients to determine which ones are at risk of adverse health consequences postdischarge if they lack discharge planning

      b. Evaluation of the postdischarge needs of inpatients identified in the first stage, or of inpatients who request an evaluation, or whose physician requests one

      c. Development of a discharge plan if indicated by the evaluation or at the request of the patient's physician

      d. Initiation of the implementation of the discharge plan prior to the discharge of an inpatient (CMS SOM-A, 2014)

   2. Although listed in numbered phases, it is important to understand that the process is dynamic and not always linear. The following scenarios demonstrate this point:

      a. On admission screening, a patient may appear to be appropriate for discharge to home with only family/caregiver support. However, as the hospitalization progresses, the patient's condition may worsen (e.g., unplanned surgery, medical complication) and so transition needs should be reevaluated.

      b. A patient is referred to a skilled nursing facility (SNF), but none meeting his needs are available on his expected date of discharge and he remains in the hospital a few more days getting the physical therapy for which he was referred. His evaluation for discharge level of care will be repeated. He may be able to go home with home physical therapy.

         i. In the event that the patient is medically ready for discharge but no bed is available at the SNF, the CM works with the physician to assure that certification for continued stay and need for hospitalization because an appropriate SNF bed is unavailable.

      ii. A physician may certify or recertify need for continued hospitalization if the physician finds that the patient could receive proper treatment in an SNF, but no bed is available in a participating SNF.

     iii. If this is the basis for the physician's certification or recertification, the required statement must so indicate; and the physician is expected to continue efforts to place the patient in a participating SNF as soon as a bed becomes available (LII Cornell, 2015).

     iv. Because in this case the patient may reach outlier status, CMs actively work on a patient's discharge plan and must document all activities regarding the continued facility search.

     v. UR committee collaboration is essential in this situation.

3. The constant movement of planning for transition is one of the greatest challenges facing case managers. The process is not complete until the patient moves to the subsequent appropriate and available level of care.

Other Selected Federal Rules that have Significance in Transition Planning

A. The Health Improvement Protection and Accountability Act of 1996 (HIPAA).

1. Title II of HIPAA changed the exchange of information between health care providers as no other law has.

    a. The intent of Title II in the Law is to protect the privacy of health information of individuals.

    b. The explanation of what can be exchanged for the purpose of coordinating care is best understood, when the fact that care transitions is considered by HIPAA as a treatment. Transition planning, aka discharge planning, is clearly a treatment.

2. Transition management is focused on the use of medical privacy of health information and the sharing or exchange of protected health information (PHI) when the information is exchanged electronically. The Health Information Technology for Economic and Clinical Health Act (HITECH) covers the requirements of PHI, but for purposes of this chapter, the focus will be on what type of information can be shared, not how it is shared.

3. Frequently, questions arise regarding the consent to share information for transition/discharge planning.

    a. HIPAA does not require patients to sign consent forms before doctors, hospitals, or ambulances may share information for treatment purposes (MLN-HIPAA, 2014).

    b. However, because transition management is regarded as a treatment, the CM may reinforce that the patient signed the consent for treatment and services upon admission to the hospital.

    c. When a patient is admitted through the emergency department, there is a higher risk for not having obtained a signature authorizing consent to treatment. The CM ensures a consent form has been signed. Regardless of the signature status, the patient (and family) must be kept aware of the transition planning process.

4. Please note that HIPAA is a federal law. Many states maintain separate legislation and regulation. State-specific regulations regarding PHI sharing, especially pertaining to behavioral health issues, are frequently more restrictive. Know the laws and regulations governing PHI within your particular jurisdiction.

B. Preadmission Screening and Resident Review (PASRR).

1. PASRR is a federal requirement to help ensure that individuals are not inappropriately placed in nursing homes for long-term care. It requires that
   a. All applicants to a Medicaid-certified nursing facility be evaluated for mental illness and/or intellectual disability
   b. All applicants be offered the most appropriate setting for their needs (e.g., community, SNF, acute hospital)
   c. All applicants receive the services they need in those settings (PASRR, 2015)

2. PASRR programs are managed on a state-by-state process, meaning that each state has its own rules for how the federal mandate is run.
   a. Most states require that all applicants for nursing home care have a level I PASRR screen by hospital staff to determine if there is evidence of a mental illness (MI) or developmental disability (DD) that requires further evaluation.
   b. If the patient demonstrates any of the state's criteria for MI/DD, the patient may require further evaluation by a specialized, approved health care professional who must conduct what is known as a level II evaluation.

3. The process of completing the PASRR requirement for patients being considered for nursing home placement can take several days; therefore, persons doing transition management should start the PASRR level I as soon as that level of care is being considered. If you are unsure about anything to do with PASRR, there is a PASRR technical organization, which provides free, up-to-date assistance (PTAC-PASRR, 2015).

C. Olmstead v. L.C.

1. On June 22, 1999, the Supreme Court of the United States held that unjustified segregation of persons with disabilities constitutes discrimination in violation of title II of the Americans with Disabilities Act (ADA).

2. The Court held that public entities must provide community-based services to persons with disabilities when the following exist:
   a. Such services are appropriate.
   b. The affected persons do not oppose community-based treatment.
   c. Community-based services can be reasonably accommodated, taking into account the resources available to the public entity and the needs of others who are receiving disability services from the entity (ADA-Olmstead, 2015).

3. A case manager participating in transition management for person with disabilities must assure that the individual with disabilities is discharged to the least restrictive environment, regardless of their previous level of care.
   a. For example, a disabled individual is admitted to the hospital from an SNF. His subsequent medical condition and necessary

treatment make transition to the community an appropriate
level of care. The case manager must assess and consider different
options as part of transition planning.

D. The Americans with Disabilities Act. The ADA is mentioned in the CoPs
for DP (CMS SOM-A, 2014). Case managers must assess individuals
qualified as disabled for special needs as part of the transition planning
(OCR-ADA 504, 2015).

E. Notice of Hospital Discharge (Important Message [IM]).

   1. Part of the CMS Beneficiary Notice Initiatives it serves in the
   beneficiary protection process, one of the notices is the Notice of
   Hospital Discharge, also known as The Important Message from
   Medicare (IM).

   2. This notice resulted in much discussion regarding who can/should
   deliver the initial copy and the follow-up copy, how is it recorded,
   and how to meet 100% compliance requirement for short stay
   patients.

   3. The IM is intended not only to notify patients of their right to
   participate in their discharge planning but also that they have a right
   to appeal the discharge and ask for review by a CMS contracted,
   outside agency, now known as the BFCC-QIO (CMS-IM, 2015).

   4. As previously mentioned, the CMS undertook a restructuring of the
   QIO functions into two separate entities, placing the responsibility of
   being the outside reviewer for patients who appeal a discharge to the
   BFCC.

      a. This first phase of the restructuring allows two Beneficiary and
      Family-Centered Care (BFCC) QIO contractors to support the
      program's case review and monitoring activities apart from the
      traditional quality improvement activities of the QIOs.

         i. The two BFCC QIO contractors are Livanta LLC in Annapolis
         Junction, Maryland, and KePRO in Seven Hills, Ohio.

         ii. Both organizations are responsible for ensuring consistency
         in the review process with consideration of local factors
         important to beneficiaries (CMS-BFCC, 2014).

      b. There are concerns regarding the geographic distance of agencies
      receiving appeals as well as the requirement that QIOs invest in
      education of providers.

      c. Case management professionals must monitor changes in CMS
      regulations to be knowledgeable and helpful to beneficiaries and
      providers.

      d. Communication skills are important to developing strong working
      relationships with the BFCC responsible for service coverage in
      your region regardless of geographic proximity.

F. Jimmo v. Sebelius.

   1. In this landmark case, the courts clarified critical points with regard
   to Medicare policy pertaining to patient status improvement as a
   condition continued eligibility for services in postacute services.

      a. A beneficiary's lack of restoration potential cannot, in itself,
      serve as the basis for denying coverage, without regard to an
      individualized assessment of the beneficiary's medical condition
      and the reasonableness and necessity of the treatment, care, or
      services in question.

b. Conversely, coverage in this context would not be available in a situation where the beneficiary's care needs can be addressed safely and effectively through the use of nonskilled personnel (CMS, 2014).

2. Specifically, in accordance with the settlement agreement, the manual revisions clarify that coverage of skilled nursing and skilled therapy services in the skilled nursing facility (SNF), home health (HH), and outpatient therapy (OPT) settings "…does not turn on the presence or absence of a beneficiary's potential for improvement, but rather on the beneficiary's need for skilled care" (CMS-Jimmo, 2014).

3. Skilled care may be necessary to improve a patient's current condition, to maintain the patient's current condition, or to prevent or slow further deterioration of the patient's condition" (CMS-Jimmo, 2014).

4. This means that assessing a patient for skilled care needs should not solely focus on the potential for improvement, but should include the need for skilled care. Skilled services may be needed to prevent further deterioration of the condition or to maintain the patient's current status.

5. Case managers are responsible for understanding the Jimmo ruling.

G. Discharge Status and Condition Codes and Hospital Transfer Policies.

1. In transition planning, the final plan documentation has significant impact on the revenue cycle of a hospital. Coders rely upon medical record documentation to ensure the proper code selection for claim submission.

2. Proper coding is also helpful for the postacute provider revenue cycle. What is used in the acute facility claim, tracks to the postacute care claim (e.g., SNF, HH). Eligibility criteria and reimbursement are also affected.

H. Hospital Transfer MS-DRG Payment Policy.

1. Case managers should be informed as to Transfer DRG and associated payment rules as they pertain to coding.

a. If a patient is discharged before the geometric mean length of stay (GMLOS) and is referred to postacute care for the condition for which the patient was inpatient, the destination and the reason for selection of that provider must be documented.

i. The GMLOS is a statistical term calculated by multiplying all of the lengths of stay and taking the nth root of that number (where n = number of patients).

ii. The advantage of the GMLOS is that it minimizes the outlier impact. When the number of patients is relatively low, one patient with an uncharacteristically long or short LOS significantly impacts the ALOS. However, that same patient's impact on the GMLOS is less noticeable (Case Management Innovations, 2015).

b. If the patient is referred to home health, capturing the start of care date is important because if it occurs more than 3 days after discharge, it is not considered a transfer. As a result, the hospital can bill for the entire DRG rather than the transfer formula.

    c. This is a financial concept; however, case manager documentation regarding the status of the referral is critical to claims processing.

    d. The list of MS-DRGs included in the transfer policy is updated annually and is found in Table 5 of the hospital inpatient prospective payment system (CMS-Table 5, 2014).

    e. Your institution's Chief Financial Officer should be consulted to better understand the impact of these issues on your day-to-day activities.

    f. Auditors carefully monitor for evidence of keeping a patient in the acute setting in order to reach the LOS so the full MS-DRG will be paid, which is reviewed carefully by auditors, basically for the fact that the patient is staying beyond the medically necessary stay, and this action will be considered as fraudulent.

2. The official list of discharge disposition codes can be found in a Special Edition of Medicare Learning Network. In this MLN publication, there is also clarification of coding for patients whose DRGs fall into the Transfer Rule for payment (MLN—Dispo Codes, 2014).

Factors that Impact Case Management in Cross-Setting Measures

A. The Improving Medicare Post-Acute Care Transformation Act of 2014 (IMPACT) and Cross-Setting Measures

1. The IMPACT Act of 2014 is the result of years of study about how patients move across settings and what factors about the patient are important across settings (CMS IMPACT Act, 2014).

    a. The idea of a Uniform Needs Assessment Instrument was first mentioned in a Report to Congress on June 30, 1992, and in a report titled "Uniform Patient Assessment for Post-Acute Care" in 2006 (Kramer, 2006).

    b. The goal of this act is to establish assessment domains, which will follow the patient across all levels of care, identify outcomes, and potentially devise a predictive model based on the patient's functional stats and medical status for hospital case managers to use to determine the next best level of care.

    c. A decision support tool, a clue about what might happen to a patient at the next level of care with certain assessment categories that drive the decision for referrals.

2. IMPACT is directed toward postacute care, and thus, the domains of attention are directed at what the patient needs after discharge, rather than what utilization review assessment categories reviews for admission and continued stay to a hospital.

3. One of the most challenging aspects of a case manager's work is looking forward, more or less trying to predict what a patient will need after discharge and what the best level of care is.

    a. The importance of taking time to assess–predict and counsel cannot be overstated. So much depends on your skill and knowledge of assessment domains.

    b. The data collection of these domains will be phased in over the next few years allowing the CMS to collect enough data on outcomes to validate a useful assessment tool.

13-3   IMPACT 2014 Domains

- Skin integrity and changes in skin integrity
- Functional status and changes in function
- Cognitive function and changes in cognitive function
- Medication reconciliation
- Incidence of major falls
- Transfer of health information and care preferences when an individual transitions
- Resource use measures, including total estimated Medicare spending per beneficiary
- Discharge to community
- All-condition risk-adjusted potentially preventable hospital readmissions rates

Source: CMS IMPACT Act, 2014 September 18). *IMPACT Act 2014.* Retrieved from IMPACT Act of 2014 & Cross Setting Measures: http://www.cms.gov/Medicare/Quality-Initiatives-Patient-Assessment-Instruments/Post-Acute-Care-Quality-Initiatives/IMPACT-Act-of-2014-and-Cross-Setting-Measures.html, on March 27, 2015.

4. IMPACT includes the list of domain measures to be standardized across settings are in the following table, and the subsequent table lists other categories for which patients should be assessed (Box 13-3). Assess the patient for these domains to begin making a difference in postacute level of care selection and improved patient outcomes.
5. In addition to these domains, a case manager's comprehensive assessment of patients ready for transition to another level of care (across settings) should include a number of domains or factors including those listed in Box 13-4.

13-4   Additional Assessment Domains

- Language literacy and health literacy
- Culturally sensitive care practices
- Functional status (activities of daily living and instrumental activities of daily living)
- Capacity and competency
- Potential for mandatory reporting of abuse, neglect, exploitation
- Financial resources including insurance or private resources
- A patient's right to refuse discharge planning
- Family or responsible person readiness, willingness, and ability to provide care needed
- Family and responsible party disagreement on the transition plan
- Patient choice (among available and appropriate providers)
- Patient preferences that conflict with team plan for transition because of anticipated risks
- The right of appeal of a discharge plan
- Homelessness; lack of safe environment in the community

© 2015 Birmingham. Reprinted with permission.

Selected Levels of Care to Which Inpatients are Referred

A. There are multiple levels of care (LOC) to which a patient may transition. These transitions take place across the entire continuum, not simply from hospital to another location. The movement of patients across the continuum takes place with increasing rapidity and complexity; there are many contributing factors such as patient choice, available options, network structure, availability, and financial incentives. The patient's medical and social needs trump financial incentives, but financial incentives are a reality due to network structure and other preferential arrangements.

B. Case managers influence patient outcomes by knowing basic information about each level of care. This section provides the level of care information to be used when selecting and advocating for the patient's transition. Please cross-reference this section with other chapters, which present similar content from different perspectives. Please dig deeper for more specifics on each level of care, work setting and state-specific regulations, organizational policy, and evidence-based criteria.

C. The discussion presented herein includes a definition of the various levels and admission criteria. There may also be mention of the assessment tool used primarily for that care level. It's important to understand what subsequent levels of care use for assessments. This provides insight as to requirements for transitioning patients to those care settings. This information is also intended to aid you in describing various care settings to your patients. The information in this section is found in the Social Security Act §1861, Part E—Miscellaneous Provisions (HHS-SSA, 2015). The information on average length of stay is found in the Healthcare Cost and Utilization Project (HCUP) (AHRQ). For payer-specific information, kindly refer to the appropriate primary source.

D. Levels of Care.
   1. Short-Term Care Hospital
      a. This is the hospital setting, which provides short-term acute care services. Recently, the CMS has referred to this type of facility as short-term care hospital (STCH) to distinguish the expected length of stay as short term as compared to a long-term care hospital (LTCH). In 2012, the average length of stay for patients in an STCH was 4 to 5 days (all payers included).
      b. A hospital is defined in the Social Security Act as an organization primarily engaged in providing, by or under the supervision of physicians, to inpatients (A) diagnostic services and therapeutic services for medical diagnosis, treatment, and care of injured, disabled, or sick persons or (B) rehabilitation services for the rehabilitation of injured, disabled, or sick persons
      c. Pediatric children's hospitals (e.g., Texas Children's, Boston Floating), cancer hospitals (e.g., Dana Farber Cancer Institute, MD Anderson), and behavioral/psychiatric hospitals (e.g., McLean's) are considered STCH. Although they are considered hospitals, they often have different rules pertaining to access and payment.

2. Critical Access Hospital
   a. A Critical Access Hospital (CAH) is a hospital, which is certified under a specific set of Medicare Conditions of Participation (CoPs). A distinguishing characteristic of CAH is being located in a rural area at least 35 miles drive away from any other hospital or CAH. Additional requirements include no more than 25 inpatient beds, annual average length of stay of no more than 96 hours for acute inpatient care, and offering 24-hour, 7-day-a-week emergency care (Health Resources and Services Administration [HRSA], 2015).
   b. The limited size and short stay length encourage a focus on providing care for common conditions and outpatient care and accessing larger facilities for the treatment of more complex conditions.
   c. A CAH also provides a service commonly referred to as a swing bed. These beds are used for the provision of extended care services that would otherwise be provided at a skilled nursing facility (SNF) level of care (HRSA, 2016; Rural Assistance Center, 2015).
   d. Because CAH is considered an acute care hospital, there is no specific assessment tool, but they use the same criteria sets to review for appropriateness of admission on continued stay.
3. Long-Term Acute Care Hospital (LTACH)
   a. Long-term care hospitals (LTCH or LTACH) are certified as acute care hospitals, but LTCH facilities focus on patients who require an average LOS of more than 25 days. Many of these patients are transferred to LTCH from an intensive or critical care unit because these facilities specialize in the care of patients with more than one serious condition and who may improve over a longer period of time with intensive care and services. These patients may eventually return home.
   b. LTCHs typically provide services including comprehensive rehabilitation, respiratory therapy, head trauma treatment, and pain management.
   c. A patient may be transferred directly from an STCH or admitted to an LTCH within 60 days of being discharged from an STCH hospital stay (CMS-LTCH, 2014). If the patient has had either an STCH stay or a qualified SNF stay within the last 60 days, he/she is covered by the CMS for LTCH stay.
   d. Emergency room case managers are critical in determining the treatment history of a patient before recommending the level of care to which the patient should be admitted. Understanding level of care qualifications is essential to ensuring the admission covered by Medicare.
   e. For beneficiaries enrolled in managed Medicare programs, the case manager should also be mindful of the specific rules for direct admission to an LTCH. The collaboration between payer and hospital case managers is essential to ensure coverage and effective advocacy on the patient's behalf.
   f. LTCH is considered a hospital. Assessment tools vary according to facility and there is not a mandated tool. However evidence-based criteria are utilized to evaluate the appropriateness of admission and continued stay.
   g. Not all states have LTCH.

4. Inpatient Rehabilitation Facility
   a. Inpatient rehabilitation facility (IRF) or acute rehabilitation (AR) is also referred to as acute rehab. This is hospital level of care, which means that a patient may be directly admitted to the facility if he/she meets admission criteria. An IRF may be a distinct but connected part of an acute care hospital or a stand-alone facility.
   b. The criteria for admission, in addition to requiring hospital level of care, are that the patient requires rehabilitation and can tolerate 3 hours of combined rehabilitation services a day.
   c. There are diagnosis-specific criteria for this level of care as well. This means that at least 60% (previously 75%) of admitted patients must fall into 1 of 13 diagnoses. A Medicare Administrative Contractor (MAC) is responsible to determine if facilities meet the 60% rule requirement for payment under Medicare's IRF prospective payment system (CMS-IRF, 2015).
   d. The 13 diagnoses and associated descriptions may be used by hospital case managers to screen patients for this level of care (Table 13-1). These are compiled based on the CMS (CMS-IRF 60%, 2011).
   e. It is important to note that only 60% of patients must have one of these diagnoses. This means that access to an IRF should not be automatically denied if the hospital believes the patient will benefit from a referral to an IRF.
   f. The assessment tool used by the IRF is called the Inpatient Rehabilitation Facility–Patient Assessment Instrument (IRF-PAI) (CMS-IRF-PAI, 2015).

TABLE 13-1 Diagnoses Used for Patient Screening for Inpatient Rehabilitation

Diagnosis	Explanatory Note
Stroke	
Spinal cord injury	
Congenital deformity	
Amputation	
Major multiple trauma	
Fracture of the femur (hip)	
Brain injury	
Neurological disorders	Including multiple sclerosis, motor neuron diseases, polyneuropathy, muscular dystrophy, and Parkinson disease
Burns	
Active, polyarticular rheumatoid arthritis, psoriatic arthritis, and seronegative arthropathies	Resulting in significant functional impairment of ambulation and other activities of daily living that have not improved after an appropriate, aggressive, and sustained course of outpatient therapy services or services in other less intensive rehabilitation settings immediately preceding the inpatient rehabilitation admission or that result from a systemic disease activation immediately before admission but have the potential to improve with more intensive rehabilitation

continued

TABLE 13-1 Diagnoses Used for Patient Screening for Inpatient Rehabilitation, *continued*

Diagnosis	Explanatory Note
Systemic vasculitides with joint inflammation	Resulting in significant functional impairment of ambulation and other activities of daily living that have not improved after an appropriate, aggressive, and sustained course of outpatient therapy services or services in other less intensive rehabilitation settings immediately preceding the inpatient rehabilitation admission or that result from a systemic disease activation immediately before admission but have the potential to improve with more intensive rehabilitation
Severe or advanced osteoarthritis (osteoarthrosis or degenerative joint disease)	Involving two or more major weight-bearing joints (elbow, shoulders, hips, or knees but not counting a joint with a prosthesis) with joint deformity and substantial loss of range of motion, atrophy of muscles surrounding the joint, significant functional impairment of ambulation, and other activities of daily living that have not improved after the patient has participated in an appropriate, aggressive, and sustained course of outpatient therapy services or services in other less intensive rehabilitation settings immediately preceding the inpatient rehabilitation admission but have the potential to improve with more intensive rehabilitation. (A joint replaced by a prosthesis no longer is considered to have osteoarthritis, or other arthritis, even though this condition was the reason for the joint replacement.)
Knee or hip joint replacement or both	During an acute hospitalization immediately preceding the inpatient rehabilitation stay and also meet one or more of the following specific criteria: (A) The patient underwent bilateral knee or bilateral hip joint replacement surgery during the acute hospital admission immediately preceding the IRF admission. (B) The patient is extremely obese with a body mass index of at least 50 at the time of admission to the IRF. (C) The patient is 85 years or older at the time of admission to the IRF.

5. Skilled Nursing Facility
    a. A skilled nursing facility (SNF) is a service level in which patients receive skilled nursing 24 hours a day, 7 days a week, required therapies, room and board, a physician who oversees the care and is of relatively short stay. Patients referred to an SNF are expected to be able to return to a community setting.
    b. To be eligible for Medicare Part A extended care services in an SNF, the beneficiary must have an inpatient 3 consecutive day stay in a hospital either immediately before or within 30 days of

SNF admission. The type of hospital includes those listed above and the admission acute care requirement for Medicare Part A; in addition, the reason for admission to an SNF for the extended care benefit must be for the reason for the 3-day qualifying stay (Birmingham, 3 Midnight rule, 2008).

c. The physical location of SNF beds varies. Some are within nursing homes that maintain dedicated Medicare beds for extended care benefits or within facilities, which are dedicated to providing skilled level services.

d. It is important to note that patients who are in the hospital over the time of midnight must be classified as inpatient. Patients in observation status do not meet the three qualified midnight stay requirement and are not be eligible to receive Medicare Part A for extended care services. Although their health care needs may meet qualification criteria, qualifying to access Part A benefits is a challenge.

e. When a beneficiary is in observation status, the case manager should ask if the patient has been in any hospital for three consecutive midnights within the last 30 days. It does not need to be the same hospital, but does need to be within the last 30 days.

f. Any attempt to keep the patient in acute care for the third night without appropriate medical necessity is a fraud against Medicare. However, a case manager may work with the physicians to determine if the patient's second or third night qualifies under the rule that the stay was unnecessary only when hospitalization for 3 days represents a substantial departure from normal medical practice (CMS 3 day, 2014).

   i. For example: A patient is admitted with a hip fracture and appears medical necessity for 2 days, and the surgeon writes that the patient is stable or other such wording. In order to keep the patient for the third day, the patient should be assessed for other needs, and the case manager can work with all physicians to determine if discharging a patient with hip fracture at day two is a substantial departure for from normal medical practice. Review what the hospital medical staff considers as normal medical practice for patients. Document the patient needs and match those against inpatient criteria for all body systems.

g. Case managers must understand their state bed hold policies. When it is time for a patient to return to a nursing facility from which she/he was originally admitted, understanding bed hold regulations helps determine if the patient may return to the same facility.

   i. The patient and family need to be aware that the nursing facility may not place him/her in the exact same bed from which she/he was last located.

   ii. Search the term "bedhold" in the applicable jurisdiction, particularly for Medicaid beneficiaries.

h. Skilled nursing facilities use the minimum data set (MDS) as an assessment and care planning tool. They also use the MDS as a way to determine the Resource Utilization Groups (RUGs), which translate to payment for SNFs (CMS-MDS, 2015).

    i. Medicare maintains the Nursing Home Compare Web site to find and compare nursing homes quality indicators. Case managers should use this resource and refer patients and family members to use it as well (CMS NH Compare, 2015).

6. Home Health Agency
   a. The role of the case manager involves assessment of the patient for appropriateness for home health agency (HHA) level of care. One of the important steps that must be taken is to make a preliminary certification that the patient qualifies for home health.
   b. Although the certification rule applies to Medicare beneficiaries, the requirement has been tested and therefore can be used to apply to all patients as a tool to determine if home health is an option.
   c. Certifying patients for home health requirements make sense and is a good screening step for the patient as well as the payer. It helps determine if the patient can benefit from that service and encourages the patient to participate more in their care.
   d. Requirements for Medicare beneficiaries to be certified for home health care services include a number of eligibility criteria including those described in Box 13-5 and based on the CMS CoPs (CMS-MLN, 2015).
   e. The assessment tool used by Home Health Agencies is the Outcome and Assessment Information Set (OASIS) (CMS-OASIS, 2015).
   f. Home Health Quality Data, search functions, and other publicly reporting information about Medicare-certified HHAs are found on the Home Health Compare Web site (CMS-HHA Compare, 2015).

7. Hospice Care
   a. In hospice care, the focus in on palliation of symptoms with the goal of promoting comfort. Hospice care is palliative by nature, but the patient's illness has progressed to a point where curative treatment is no longer desired or beneficial.
   b. While focusing on relieving symptoms and offering comfort for symptoms that occur at the end of life, hospice offers support (e.g., physical, spiritual) to both the patient and family/caregiver. To qualify for hospice care, Medicare requires a physician to certify that

BOX

13-5 Eligibility Criteria for Home Care Services

- Patient must be confined to home, based on criteria established by Medicare (homebound).
- Need for skilled services on an intermittent basis with nursing and physical therapy (PT) as the prime skilled services and occupational therapy (OT) as the prime skilled service if the patient continues to need only OT in order to meet the therapy goals
- Be under the care of a physician
- Receive services under a plan of care established and reviewed by a physician
- For Medicare beneficiaries: face-to-face encounter with a physician or allowed nonphysician practitioner (NPP) and have services provided by a Medicare-certified agency

a patient's condition is terminal and that life expectancy is 6 months or less. The certification for hospice services may be renewed indefinitely. Beneficiaries enrolled in hospice agree to focus on palliative treatment and comfort measures. Medicare beneficiaries may "opt out" at any time and request curative treatment.

   c. For Medicare beneficiaries enrolled in a managed Medicare plan (Part C), payment for hospice services is based on a carve-out. Hospice benefits are paid for by Medicare, and service rendered for unrelated health care needs is paid by the managed care organization administering Part C benefits (CMS-Hospice, 2014).

   d. Hospice services may be rendered at home, at an inpatient hospice facility, or at an SNF that has a contractual arrangement with a hospice provider or with a hospice program. When the patient's symptom control is compromised and cannot be managed elsewhere, admission to an acute care hospital may be necessary for palliative purposes (CMS Hospice Compare, 2015).

8. Palliative Care

   a. Palliative care focuses on relieving symptoms that are related to chronic illnesses. This care level can be used at any stage of illness, not only the advanced disease stages. In palliation, treatments are not limited and may range from conservative to aggressive/ curative. Palliative care may be considered at any time during the course of a chronic illness.

9. Infusion Therapy

   a. Infusion therapy may be one of the most convoluted types of therapy for case managers to arrange as part of a transition plan. This is due to the rather confusing orders required to administer the infusion therapy. The provider orders required may include:

     i. To initiate infusion therapy

     ii. To obtain nursing services

     iii. Proper equipment and supplies necessary to administer the treatment

     iv. The drug, medication, and/or fluid to be administered

   b. The source of each ordered element may be different. For instance, the equipment and supplies come from one vendor, the nursing services are delivered through a home health agency, and the medication comes from a specialty pharmacy. In some cases, the cost of all three is in the bundled payment for skilled nursing facilities referred to as consolidated billing (CMS-Consolidated Billing, 2015).

   c. Commercial insurers and managed Medicare organizations may have different policies to pay for infusion therapy.

   d. Infusion therapy may be administered at a hospital outpatient clinic, a freestanding clinic, a physician's office, at home, or an SNF.

10. Assisted Living Facilities

   a. An assisted living facility (ALF) offers a housing alternative for older adults who need assistance with dressing, bathing, eating, and toileting but do not require the intensive or skilled medical and nursing care provided in residential nursing homes. Assisted living facilities may be part of a retirement community, nursing home, and senior housing complex or may stand alone.

13-6 Examples of Services Offered in ALFs

- Health care management and monitoring
- Help with activities of daily living such as bathing, dressing, and eating
- Housekeeping and laundry
- Medication reminders and/or help with medications
- Recreational activities
- Security
- Transportation

  b. Licensure requirements for ALFs vary by state. The official name of ALFs varies and includes residential care, board and care, congregate care, or personal care (HHS-Assisted Living, 2015).
  c. An ALF resident usually lives in an individual unit or apartment. In addition to support staff and meals, most ALFs offer residents a multitude of services such as those listed in Box 13-6.
  d. ALF services may be part of a program to prevent an individual from requiring inpatient custodial nursing home care and is sometimes an option for patients receiving Medicaid services. As the Medicaid program continues to evolve as a result of the PPACA, requirements and payment source eligibility will change. The case manager must remain informed as to benefits and eligibility for ALF level of care.

 11. Outpatient Clinics or Centers
  a. Outpatient centers may be operated by hospitals, freestanding facilities, or within an SNF. Hospital outpatient services have specific rules under the prospective payment system (PPS). In addition, there is specific information about outpatient observation services and outpatient dialysis services not covered under the end-stage renal disease (ESRD) program (CMS-HospOutpatient, 2015).
  b. Non–hospital-based outpatient program has specific rules and, in many states, licensure requirements. The organization that certifies outpatient Medicare and Medicaid rehabilitation facilities is called Comprehensive Outpatient Rehabilitation Facility (CORF).
  c. The following are considered core services that a CORF must provide: consultation with and medical supervision of nonphysician staff, establishment and review of the plan of treatment and other medical and facility administration activities, and physical therapy services and social or psychological services (CMS-CORF, 2015).

 12. Durable Medical Equipment, Prosthetics, Orthotics, and Supplies
  a. Durable medical equipment (DME) is equipment used in a patient's place of residence (e.g., home, ALF) for medical purposes. This means that the piece of equipment would be used by an individual for a medical purpose and is able to withstand repeated use. Examples of DME include hospital beds, walkers, oxygen delivery equipment, and assistive devices.

    b. A prosthetic is an artificial device attached or applied to the body to replace a missing part. It is an artificial replacement of a part of the body (e.g., hip, arm). A prosthetic is designed for functional and/or cosmetic reasons. It is a type of equipment that replaces a body part or allows the body part to function.

    c. An orthotic is a support, brace, or splint. It is used to support, align, prevent, or correct the function of movable parts of the body. Examples of orthotics include shoe inserts, neck braces, and wrist supports.

    d. Supplies are products required for treatment of a medical condition, like a surgical wound, a pressure ulcer. The way to distinguish prosthesis from a supply is to consider if the item (e.g., supply, device) replaces a normal body function. A urinary catheter replaces the patient's urethra and ability to void. An ostomy bag is used to replace the body function of elimination.

    e. Vendor selection is generally based on the patient's payer. Medicare uses a competitive bidding process to award specific DME companies a contract to supply selected DME products to patients (CMS-DME, 2015). The need to track the DME vendor for Medicare patients is a necessary task because of the potential denial and patient financial liability. Commercial payers, managed care organizations, accountable care organizations, and managed Medicare have contracts for vendors as with other postacute providers.

    f. Case managers must be mindful of individual benefit levels, as well as payer-specific requirements and patient preference when making arrangements for equipment, prosthetics, orthotics, and supplies.

13. Nonmedical Custodial Services

    a. Many community-based providers are able to provide and/or coordinate services to help maintain a patient in the least restrictive setting. A number of companies are available to provide care coordination that may include skilled services and nonmedical home services. These home services include activities, which supplement the patients' instrumental activities of daily living (IADL) (e.g., household chores, housekeeping, shopping, transportation, managing financial resources). Case managers are encouraged to explore these types of services and agencies that are contracted with Medicaid and/or commercial insurers.

The Role of the Case Manager in the Process of Transitional Planning

A. Transitional and discharge planning activities include those that aim to address the needs of the patient and patient's family/caregiver at every phase of care—preadmission to a hospital, facility, or episode of care; the admission process; the hospital stay or care provision; before discharge from the hospital or episode of care; and time of discharge.

1. Before admission to the hospital or episode of care, the case manager must collect all pertinent information about the patient's condition and family and caregiver's situation to identify the patient's and family/caregiver's needs and communicate such information to other care providers as necessary.

2. During the admission process, the case manager ensures the provision of care and services that are consistent with the patient's condition and makes appropriate referrals to other care providers as indicated by the patient's condition and treatment plan. The case manager also facilitates the transfer of the patient to the appropriate level of care and setting or to other facilities based on the patient's acuity and needs.

3. While in the hospital or in other specific care settings (e.g., a clinic), the case manager maintains continuity of services through the phases of assessment, treatment, and reassessment of the patient's condition. The case manager also ensures that care is well coordinated among all care providers involved, including the postdischarge services and resources.

4. Before discharge from the hospital or an episode of care, the case manager evaluates the patient's and family/caregiver's postdischarge needs and arranges for their availability to maintain continuity of care and prevent disruption of treatment. These activities also include referrals to other care providers and teaching the patient and family/caregiver in self-care management and the treatment regimen.

5. At the time of discharge from a hospital or other episode of care, the case manager reassesses the patient's condition and the patient's and family/caregiver's ability to manage self-care, as well as ensures that the arranged postdischarge resources and services continue to be appropriate for the patient. In addition, the case manager communicates pertinent information about the patient's condition and treatment plan to other agencies to be involved in the care of the patient postdischarge, such as skilled nursing facilities and home care agencies. In the end, the case manager ensures a safe discharge or transition to another level of care.

B. Case managers in the provider and payer organizations are involved in transitional and discharge planning activities. Although they may overlap in their involvement, roles and responsibilities are somewhat distinct and based on the organization or care setting.

C. The provider-based case manager are involved in transitional planning or discharge planning activities in any organization that is providing or managing care for a patient who is receiving medical or nursing services.

1. Examples of these organizations are acute care hospitals, nursing facilities, inpatient rehabilitation facilities, psychiatric and behavioral health facilities, home health care agencies, hospice and palliative care agencies, and others in specific markets (e.g., Indian Health Service, Critical Access Hospital).

2. Specific discharge and transitional planning functions of provider-based case managers are described in Box 13-7.

D. The payer-based case manager also is involved in transitional and discharge planning activities, however, to a lesser degree than a provider-based case manager. Both usually work in collaboration to assure patients' postdischarge needs and services are met in a timely fashion, especially ensuring safety and continuity of care (Box 13-8).

E. Case managers execute their discharge and transitional planning activities while involved in the case management process. These activities are part and parcel of the case management process. In fact, transitional

(text continues on page 341)

BOX 13-7   **Responsibilities of Provider-Based Case Managers in Discharge and Transitional Planning**

- Identification of individuals who are at risk for adverse outcomes during the transition or discharge from one level of care or setting to another.
- Evaluation of the patient's continuing care needs.
- Assessment of resources appropriate and available to the patient/family/caregiver.
- Planning for transition to the next level of care.
- Implementation of the plan.
- Monitoring and ongoing reassessment of the plan.
- Use of evidence-based guidelines for patients with specific care needs and where applicable.
- Documentation of all pertinent information related to the planning for discharge or transition and necessity of the admission including meeting the 2-Midnight Rule for Medicare beneficiaries.
- Knowledge of the admission criteria for various levels of care (e.g., home health care with the requirement that patient be homebound).
- Advocacy for patients' rights, needs, and values; ensuring that patients' ethnic, cultural, or religious values, beliefs, preferences, and needs are considered during the transition or discharge phase.
- Collaboration with the multidisciplinary health care team and in particular with the patient's attending physician.
- Coordination of the plan of care and discharge plan with other providers and payer-based case managers, where applicable.
- Communication of relevant information across the continuum.
- Knowledge of the roles and responsibilities of other members of the health care team, including nurses, social workers, therapists, pharmacists, dietitians, utilization review staff, and other case managers within the organization.
- Validation that the services ordered or arranged for at the next level of care are reasonably assured.
- Education and counseling of patients and their families/caregivers regarding the transition or discharge phase of care.
- Education of the patients and their families/caregivers about their roles and responsibilities in care, especially after discharge from an acute care setting.
- Protection of the privacy of health care information during the referral process (Health Information Privacy and Accountability Act—HIPAA).
- Participation in coordination of benefits for patients with more than one interested payer (e.g., Medicare and workers' compensation).
- Reporting of abuse, neglect, abandonment, or exploitation as mandated by the individual state laws and regulations.
- Participation in the evaluation of the patient's capacity for decision making.
- Engaging in quality assurance and quality improvement initiates and activities.
- Reporting any complaints or concerns about other providers to administration for appropriate follow-up.
- Participation in follow-up contact with patients per the organization's policy and protocol.
- Education of other health care professionals in the transition and discharge planning process and other relevant information (e.g., community resources).
- Compliance with all related regulations as applicable to one's own organization.
- Assurance of patient safety throughout the care process, especially during the handoff period.
- Assurance of open communication between health care providers at all levels during the handoff phase.
- Collection of data as required by the department for reporting purposes and completion of related reports as required by own organization or by law (e.g., referral patterns).

- Identification of at-risk members or populations within their membership (i.e., health plan members), with emphasis on risks associated with transition or discharge to a new level of care.
- Acting as a resource to provider-based staff during the evaluation of a member's transition or discharge planning needs.
- Advocating for patient's rights, needs, and values and for the patient's ethnic, cultural, or religious needs and preferences to be considered during the transition or discharge phase.
- Collaboration with the health care team and in particular with the patient's attending physician and, when possible, with the member's/patient's community-based primary care physician.
- Assessment of resources within the member's health care plan. This may also include an assessment of other public or private programs that can supplement the member's continuing care needs, for example, the American Cancer Society.
- Planning for the transition of the member to the next level of care.
- Determining the patient's health insurance benefits and participation in the coordination of benefits for members with more than one payer source. For example, HMO and workers' compensation claim.
- Determining providers that are contracted with the payer and that can meet the next level of care needs for the patient.
- Assuring availability of the contracted provider and communicating that information to the provider-based staff.
- Assisting the current provider in implementing the transition or discharge plan, keeping in mind that the responsibility for the implementation belongs to the direct care provider.
- Monitoring the progress of the transition or discharge plan with a focus on expected outcomes and relevancy to the patient's condition.
- Utilization of evidence-based protocols in working with members or populations.
- Use of established certain criteria, such as discharge criteria, as a guide during the transition or discharge phase.
- Collaboration with provider-based staff during the transition or discharge phase and knowing the roles and responsibilities of the provider-based members of the health care team including nurses, social workers, therapists, pharmacists, dietitians, utilization review staff, other case managers within the organization.
- Knowing the roles and responsibilities of other members of the payer-based health care team including nurses, social workers, therapists, pharmacists, dietitians, utilization review staff, and other case managers within the organization, such as disease management case managers, oncology case managers.
- Utilization of resources within the payer organization as needed, which requires an understanding of the role of the medical director and coverage determination procedures.
- Advocacy for members within the payer system and when requested outside the payer system.
- Discontinuing case management services when appropriate.
- Educating members on their benefits.
- Educating members on their responsibilities in participating in the transition or discharge phase of care.
- Assuring that there is opportunity for questions and responses between health care providers and payers at all levels during the handoff phase.
- Collecting data as required by the case management department or the organization for reporting purposes.
- Documenting according to the policies and procedures of the organization including the policy on transitional/discharge planning or continuity of care.
- Following mandatory reporting of abuse, neglect, abandonment, exploitation if and when applicable.
- Conforming to the HIPAA and privacy rules as applicable.

(or discharge) planning activities take place at every step of the case management process to a point that such activities may appear seamless.

1. Upon the patient's admission to a hospital, facility, or an episode of care, the case manager screens the patient for postdischarge needs and arranges for such services after obtaining agreement from the patient, the patient's family, the health care team, and the payer where appropriate.

2. The case manager identifies the patient's actual and potential problems and incorporates them in the transitional or discharge plan.

3. The case manager engages in interdisciplinary planning, implementation, and coordination activities that not only focus on the necessary treatment plan but also on the transitional plan as well. These activities include brokerage of services and referrals to other specialty care providers, such as rehabilitation medicine (physical and occupational therapy), and home care agencies.

4. The case manager also incorporates patient and family/caregiver education in the transitional plan as well as engages in ongoing assessments and reassessments of the patient and family to ensure that the plan is appropriate and they are able to assume responsibility for self-management after discharge.

5. The case manager prepares the patient and family/caregiver for discharge or transfer to another facility when expected outcomes and goals of care specific to the hospital stay or to the episode of care are met.

6. Throughout the episode of care, the case manager repeats the transitional planning process (i.e., the case management process) as indicated by the patient's condition, such as in the case of deterioration in the patient's condition that requires a drastic change in the plan of care.

Value-Based Purchasing and Impact on Transition Management and Readmissions

A. As part of the Patient Protection and Affordable Care Act (PPACA) of 2010, the concept of Value-Based Purchasing (VBP) was introduced. The principle behind this concept is to pay for services based upon quality rather than quantity. Medicare is the largest purchaser of health care services, so they set the pace for payment rules. Under the VBP program, Medicare makes incentive payments to hospitals based on either how well they perform on each measure or how much they improve their performance on each measure compared to their performance during a baseline period.

1. The clear priority is to place value and quality at the center of payment decisions. In the VBP programs, huge amounts of CMS data and analytics about past outcomes, value, and quality take precedence.

2. Another target of value-based payment involves the fact that Medicare pays more for the same service provided in different care settings. With VBP, the outcome becomes the driver and so addresses this inconsistency in current payment strategies. This leads to looking at both quality and financial outcomes.

3. A summary report by the RAND Corporation, Measuring Success in Health Care Value-Based Purchasing Programs, provides an overview of the VBP approach (RAND-VBP, 2014).

B. Financially, VBP payment works through withholding of a certain percent of Medicare payment to a hospital. At year-end, calculations demonstrate how hospitals compare to each other within each state and nationally. Medicare distributes the withheld monies to high performing hospitals on a percentage basis.

C. VBP payments are not considered a bonus structure. It redistributes payment to hospitals that perform best. The better a hospital performs, the greater the amount of withheld money is returned. Hospitals that are poor performers may receive no repayment. Financial stakes are high. Case manager impact on the bottom-line reimbursement has never been higher.

1. The VBP payment domain of most importance to case managers is the efficiency score. This is also referred to as Medicare Spending per Beneficiary (MSPB). This measure assesses Medicare Parts A and B payments for services provided to a beneficiary during a spending-per-beneficiary episode spanning from 3 days prior to an inpatient hospital admission through 30 days after discharge. The payments included in this measure are price standardized and risk adjusted (MLN-MSPB, 2013).

   a. Note that the efficiency score includes 3 days prior to admission. Poor use of resources prior to admission will impact scoring. The following elements factor into this formula:
      i. Time in the emergency department
      ii. Time in outpatient observation
      iii. Medical tests and imaging performed prior to admission

   b. The hospital efficiency score includes care the patient receives 30 days following discharge and expenditures that come under Medicare Parts A and B.
      i. This raises the importance on accurate assessment of postacute care needs as well as proper level of care selection on the financial impact on the hospital. For instance, a patient may require postacute rehabilitation services. The case manager is aware of three most likely options: IRF, SNF, and HHA. Home health is the least expensive for Medicare, but it may not be the right choice for the individual. If that patient ends up being readmitted, year-end metrics will reflect accordingly. When final calculations are complete, the overall MSPB will likely be higher when a case manager designs a successful postacute transition plan that is best for the patient and avoids a readmission to the hospital (Hunter, 2013).

2. Readmission rate is the measure receiving a lot of attention due to the associated financial penalties. Case managers should pay attention to readmissions because of the impact on the patient's continuity of care. Every unplanned readmission causes a disruption in the patient's care as well as with the caregiver's ability to cope with the complication of a backward step in the recovery path.

   a. The focus for readmissions has been on three diagnoses, selected because they were found to comprise a high percentage of readmission, and thus, regulators believed it would be logical to track those three for risk adjustment: heart attack, heart failure, and pneumonia.

  b. In looking back at the domains targeted for data collection, it is clear that reimbursement is moving toward an all-cause, unplanned hospital-wide readmission rate (HWR).

   i. HWR estimates the hospital-level, risk-standardized rate of all–cause unplanned readmissions, defined as an inpatient admission to any acute care facility, which occurs within 30 days of the discharge date for an earlier, eligible index admission, with any eligible condition (AHRQ-HWR, 2013).

   ii. Case managers may find a particular hospital's efficiency score at the Hospital Compare Web site (CMS-Hospital Compare, 2015). The Web site for information on hospital VBP is found at the CMS Web site. Search for Medicare Hospital Value-Based Purchasing (CMS-VBP, 2015).

 D. HHAs have a quality measure program by which they are evaluated. HHA measures for quality ratings are based on claims data. The following claims-based utilization measures are currently used in the home health QRP:

  1. Acute care hospitalization (ACH)
  2. Emergency department use without hospitalization
  3. Rehospitalization during the first 30 days of home health
  4. Emergency department use without hospital readmission during the first 30 days of home health (CMS-HHA Quality, 2015)

 E. Nursing facilities have active programs addressing readmission from nursing homes called the Initiative to Reduce Avoidable Hospitalizations Among Nursing Facility Residents (CMS: Reduce Readmits from NF, 2015).

  1. Case managers involved in transition planning must look at all readmissions and evaluate the circumstances to identify root cause(s).

  2. Considerations include whether the discharge plan was inadequate, if the patient's condition worsened following discharge, if the patient's environmental circumstances changed, if a particular nursing facility readmit more patients with the same condition.

Case Manager and Managing Care Transitions

 A. In addition to the knowledge, skills, and experience of nurses or social workers who function as case managers, the CMS has identified in their Interpretive Guidelines §482.43(b)(2) Discharge Planning (CMS: Discharge Planning Qualifications, 2014) other additional knowledge and skills that influence the value of the role to the patient and the organization.

  1. The rule states that "The patient's discharge planning evaluation must be developed by a registered nurse, social worker, or other appropriate qualified personnel, or by a person who is supervised by such personnel." East state law governs the qualifications required to be considered a registered nurse or a social worker so these recommended qualification are above and beyond the State Licensure Rules.

13-9   Requirements for the Discharge Planning Role

- Previous experience in discharge planning
- Knowledge of clinical and social factors that affect the patient's functional status at discharge
- Knowledge of community resources to meet postdischarge clinical and social needs and assessment skills
- Knowledge of clinical, social, or insurance/financial factors
- Knowledge of physical factors that must be considered when evaluating how a patient's expected postdischarge care needs can be met

NOTE: CMS also determined that it is acceptable for a hospital to include new staff who may not have had previous discharge planning experience, but who are being trained to perform discharge planning duties and whose work is reviewed by qualified personnel.

2. In addition to the CMS and State Rules, the hospitals must have written discharge planning policies and procedures, which specify the qualifications for personnel other than registered nurses or social workers who develop or supervise the development of the evaluation.

B. Additional qualifications noted by the CMS are that all personnel performing or supervising discharge planning evaluations, including registered nurses and social workers, must have appropriate and relevant knowledge and qualifications to assume the discharge planning role (Box 13-9).

C. The state surveyor will use the Survey Procedures for section §482.43(b)(2) of the discharge planning conditions of participation. Surveyor activities include:

1. Review a sample of cases to determine if the discharge planning evaluation was developed by an RN, social worker, or other qualified personnel, as defined in the hospital discharge planning policies and procedures or someone they supervise.

2. Review the hospital written policy and procedure governing who is responsible for developing or supervising the development of the discharge planning evaluation.

3. Does the policy permit someone other than an RN or social worker to be responsible for developing or supervising such evaluations?

4. If yes, does the policy specify the qualifications of the personnel other than an RN or social worker to perform this function?

5. Determine which individual(s) is(are) responsible for developing or supervising discharge planning evaluations.

6. Review their personnel folders to determine if they are an RN or social worker or meet the hospital's criteria for developing/supervising the discharge planning evaluation.

7. If not, are they supervised by an individual who is an RN or social worker or is qualified according to the hospital's policies?

8. Are their discharge planning evaluations reviewed by their supervisor before being finalized?

9. Ask personnel who supervise or develop discharge planning evaluations to give examples illustrating how they apply their knowledge of clinical, social, insurance/financial, and physical factors when performing an evaluation (CMS SOM-A, 2014).

References

ADA-Olmstead. (2015). *American with disabilities act: Title II*. Retrieved from Olmstead: Community Integration for Everyone: http://www.ada.gov/olmstead/olmstead_about.htm, on April 1, 2015.

AHRQ. (2015, March 29). *Healthcare cost and utilization project (HCUP)*. Retrieved from AHRQ-GOV: https://www.hcup-us.ahrq.gov/, on March 28, 2015.

AHRQ-HWR. (2013). *Agency for health care quality*. Retrieved from Endorsed measure: All cause hospital readmission rate: http://www.qualitymeasures.ahrq.gov/content.aspx?id=46502, on April 3, 2015.

Birmingham, J. (2007). Case management: Two regulations with co-existing functions. *Professional Case Management, 12*(1), 16–24.

Birmingham, J. (2008). Understanding the rule for extended care services—Aka the 3 Midnight Rule. *Professional Case Management, 13*(1).

Case Management Innovations. (2015). *Length of stay: What is the difference between "Average" and "Geometric Mean"?* Retrieved from http://www.casemanagementinnovations.com/length-of-stay-what-is-the-difference-between-average-and-geometric-mean/, on April 7, 2016.

CCMC. (2005). *Glossary of terms*. Retrieved from Commission for Case Manager Certification: http://ccmcertification.org/sites/default/files/downloads/2011/CCMC%20Glossary.pdf, on February 16, 2015.

CMS: DP Qualifications. (2014, September). *State operations manual*. Retrieved from Appendix A—Survey Protocol—Rev 122: https://www.cms.gov/Regulations-and-Guidance/Guidance/Manuals/downloads/som107ap_a_hospitals.pdf, on April 3, 2015.

CMS 3 day. (2014, April 4). *Medicare policy manual*. Retrieved from Chapter 8—Coverage of Extended Care (SNF) Services Under Hospital Insurance: http://www.cms.gov/Regulations-and-Guidance/Guidance/Manuals/downloads/bp102c08.pdf, on April 3, 2015.

CMS-COP HHA. (2015, January 9). *Conditions of participation for home health agencies*. Retrieved from PART 484—CONDITIONS OF PARTICIPATION: http://www.gpo.gov/fdsys/pkg/CFR-1999-title42-vol3/pdf/CFR-1999-title42-vol3-part484.pdf, on March 27, 2015.

CMS Hospice Compare. (2015). *Medicare.gov*. Retrieved from Hospice Quality Reporting: http://www.cms.gov/Medicare/Quality-Initiatives-Patient-Assessment-Instruments/Hospice-Quality-Reporting/, on April 6, 2015.

CMS IMPACT Act. (2014, September 18). *IMPACT Act 2014*. Retrieved from IMPACT Act of 2014 & Cross Setting Measures: http://www.cms.gov/Medicare/Quality-Initiatives-Patient-Assessment-Instruments/Post-Acute-Care-Quality-Initiatives/IMPACT-Act-of-2014-and-Cross-Setting-Measures.html, on March 27, 2015.

CMS NH Compare. (2015). *Medicare.gov*. Retrieved from Nursing Home Compare: https://www.medicare.gov/nursinghomecompare/?AspxAutoDetectCookieSupport=1, on April 6, 2015.

CMS-Reduce Readmits from NF. (2015, March 29). *Initiative to reduce avoidable hospitalizations among nursing facility residents*. Retrieved from http://www.cms.gov/Medicare-Medicaid-Coordination/Medicare-and-Medicaid-Coordination/Medicare-Medicaid-Coordination-Office/ReducingPreventableHospitalizationsAmongNursingFacilityResidents.html, on April 3, 2015.

CMS SOM-A. (2014, September 26). *Appendix A—Survey protocol and regulations and interpretive guidelines for hospitals*. Retrieved from SOM-A Rev.122: https://www.cms.gov/Regulations-and-Guidance/Guidance/Manuals/downloads/som107ap_a_hospitals.pdf, on March 22, 2015.

Case Management Society of America (CMSA). (1995, October). *Committee for standards of practice for case management*. Little Rock, AR: Case Management Society of America.

Case Management Society of America (CMSA). (2002). *Standards of practice for case management*. Little Rock, AR: Case Management Society of America.

Case Management Society of America (CMSA). (2010). *Standards of practice for case management*. Little Rock, AR: Author.

CMS-ACA. (2011, October 20). *The affordable care act: Helping providers help patients: A menu of options for improving care*. Retrieved from http://www.cms.gov/Medicare/Medicare-Fee-for-Service-Payment/ACO/downloads/ACO-Menu-Of-Options.pdf, on April 7, 2016.

CMS-BFCC. (2014, May 9). *CMS.gov*. Retrieved from CMS launches improved Quality Improvement Program: http://www.cms.gov/Newsroom/MediaReleaseDatabase/Press-releases/2014-Press-releases-items/2014-05-09.html, on March 31, 2015.

CMS-Consolidated Billing. (2015, March 31). *Skilled nursing facility PPS*. Retrieved from Consolidated Billing: https://www.cms.gov/Medicare/Medicare-Fee-for-Service-Payment/SNFPPS/ConsolidatedBilling.html, on March 31, 2015.

CMS-CORF. (2015, March 31). *CMS-comprehensive outpatient rehabilitation facilities*. Retrieved from CORF: http://www.cms.gov/Medicare/Provider-Enrollment-and-Certification/CertificationandComplianc/CORFs.html, on March 31, 2015.

CMS-DME. (2015, March 31). *Medicare.gov—What medicare covers*. Retrieved from Durable Medical Equipment: http://www.medicare.gov/what-medicare-covers/part-b/durable-medical-equipment.html, on March 31, 2015.

CMS-HHA Compare. (2015, March 31). *Home health compare*. Retrieved from CMS-Home Health Compare: http://www.medicare.gov/homehealthcompare/search.html, on March 31, 2015.

CMS-HHA Quality. (2015). *Home health quality reporting program*. Retrieved from Home Health Quality Measures: http://www.cms.gov/Medicare/Quality-Initiatives-Patient-Assessment-Instruments/HomeHealthQualityInits/HHQIQualityMeasures.html, on April 3, 2015.

CMS-Hospice. (2014, May 1). *Medicare benefit policy manual*. Retrieved from Chapter 9-Coverage of Hospice Services under Hospital Insurance—Rev 188: http://www.cms.gov/Regulations-and-Guidance/Guidance/Manuals/downloads/bp102c09.pdf, on March 2015.

CMS-Hospital Compare. (2015). *Hospital compare*. Retrieved from http://www.medicare.gov/hospitalcompare/search.html, on April 3, 2015.

CMS-HospOutpatient. (2015, March 31). *CMS*. Retrieved from Hospital Outpatient Services: http://www.cms.gov/Medicare/Medicare-Fee-for-Service-Payment/HospitalOutpatientPPS/index.html?redirect=/hospitaloutpatientpps, on March 31, 2015.

CMS-IM. (2015). *Beneficiary notice initiative*. Retrieved from Hospital Discharge Appeal Notices: https://www.cms.gov/Medicare/Medicare-General-Information/BNI/HospitalDischarge AppealNotices.html, on March 31, 2015.

CMS-IRF. (2015, March 31). *CMS.gov*. Retrieved from IRF Classification Criteria: https://www.cms.gov/Medicare/Medicare-Fee-for-Service-Payment/InpatientRehabFacPPS/Criteria.html, on March 31, 2015.

CMS-IRF 60%. (2011, October 1). *Code of Federal Regulations (CFR) Chapter IV*. Retrieved from Classification criteria for payment under the IRF PPS 412.29: http://www.gpo.gov/fdsys/pkg/CFR-2011-title42-vol2/pdf/CFR-2011-title42-vol2-sec412-29.pdf, on March 31, 2015.

CMS-IRF-PAI. (2015, January 15). *CMS.gov*. Retrieved from IRF Patient Assessment Instrument: http://www.cms.gov/Medicare/Medicare-Fee-for-Service-Payment/InpatientRehabFacPPS/IRFPAI.html, on March 31, 2015.

CMS-Jimmo. (2014). *Jimmo v Sebelius Program Manual Clarifications Fact Sheet*. Retrieved from CMS Fact Sheet: http://www.cms.gov/Medicare/Medicare-Fee-for-Service-Payment/SNFPPS/Downloads/jimmo_fact_sheet2_022014_final.pdf, on March 31, 2015.

CMS-LTCH. (2014, August). *What are long-term care hospitals*. Retrieved from https://www.medicare.gov/Pubs/pdf/11347.pdf, on March 29, 2015.

CMS-MDS. (2015). *Nursing home quality initiative*. Retrieved from MDS 3.0 RAI Manual: http://www.cms.gov/Medicare/Quality-Initiatives-Patient-Assessment-Instruments/NursingHomeQualityInits/MDS30RAIManual.html, on April 6, 2015.

CMS-MLN. (2015, January 20). *Medicare learning network*. Retrieved from Certifying Patients for the Medicare Home Health Benefit: http://www.cms.gov/Outreach-and-Education/Medicare-Learning-Network-MLN/MLNMattersArticles/Downloads/SE1436.pdf, on March 28, 2015.

CMS-OASIS. (2015, March 28). *Outcome and assessment information set*. Retrieved from CMS OASIS: http://www.cms.gov/Medicare/Quality-Initiatives-Patient-Assessment-Instruments/OASIS/index.html, on March 28, 2015.

CMS-Table 5. (2014). *Acute patient prospective payment system—TABLES*. Retrieved from Final Rule FY2015: http://www.cms.gov/Medicare/Medicare-Fee-for-Service-Payment/

AcuteInpatientPPS/FY2015-IPPS-Final-Rule-Home-Page-Items/FY2015-Final-Rule-Tables. html, on April 5, 2015.

CMS-VBP. (2015). *Hospital value based purchasing—HVBP.* Retrieved from http://www.cms. gov/Medicare/Quality-Initiatives-Patient-Assessment-Instruments/Hospital-Value-Based-Purchasing/, on April 4, 2015.

eCFR. (2015, March 15). *Electronic code of Federal Regulations.* Retrieved from Title 42 → Chapter IV → Subchapter G → Part 482: http://www.ecfr.gov/cgi-bin/text-idx?tpl=/ecfrbrowse/ Title42/42cfr482_main_02.tpl, on March 20, 2015.

Health Resources and Services Administration (HRSA). (2016). *What are critical access hospitals (CAH)?* Retrieved from http://www.hrsa.gov/healthit/toolbox/RuralHealthITtoolbox/ Introduction/critical.html, on April 7, 2016.

HHS-Assisted Living. (2015, March 31). *Department of Health and Human Resources.* Retrieved from Assisted Living: http://www.eldercare.gov/eldercare.net/public/resources/factsheets/ assisted_living.aspx, March 31, 2015.

HHS-SSA. (2015, March 29). *Complication of social security laws.* Retrieved from Sec. 1861. [42 U.S.C. 1395x]: http://www.ssa.gov/OP_Home/ssact/title18/1861.htm, on March 29, 2015.

HSAP. (2014, August 1). *Health Service Advisory Group.* Retrieved from Quality Improvement Organizations: http://www.hsag.com/medicare-providers/qio-program-changes/, on March 22, 2015.

Hunter, T. N. (2013, March/April). Preventing readmissions through comprehensive discharge planning. *Professional Case Management, 18*(2), 56–65.

Kramer, A. M. (2006). *Uniform patient assessment for post-acute care.* Aurora, CO: Division of Health Care Policy and Research, University of Colorado.

LII Cornell. (2015). *Legal Information Institute.* Retrieved from 42 CFR 424.13—Requirements for inpatient services of hospitals other than psychiatric hospitals: https://www.law.cornell. edu/cfr/text/42/424.13, on April 3, 2015.

McLaughlin Davis, M. (Ed.) (2014). *The Standards of Practice for Case Management, a Foundation for Care Coordination across the Entire Care Continuum (whitepaper).* Little Rock, AR: Case Management Society of America.

MLN—Dispo Codes. (2014, March 6). *Medicare learning network.* Retrieved from Clarification of Patient Discharge Status Codes and Hospital Transfer Policies: http://www.cms.gov/ Outreach-and-Education/Medicare-Learning-Network-MLN/MLNMattersArticles/downloads/SE0801.pdf, on March 31, 2015.

MLN-HIPAA. (2014, November). *Medicare learning network.* Retrieved from Medical Privacy of Protected Health Information: http://www.cms.gov/Outreach-and-Education/Medicare-Learning-Network-MLN/MLNProducts/Downloads/MedicalPrivacyTextOnlyFactSheet.pdf, on April 1, 2015.

MLN-MSPB. (2013, March). *Medicare learning network.* Retrieved from Hospital Value Base Purchasing Fact Sheet: http://www.cms.gov/Outreach-and-Education/Medicare-Learning-Network-MLN/MLNProducts/downloads/Hospital_VBPurchasing_Fact_Sheet_ ICN907664.pdf, on April 4, 2015.

Neumann, S. P. (2012, November 8). Medicare's enduring struggle to define "reasonable and necessary" care. *New England Journal of Medicine, 367,* 1775–1777.

OCR-ADA 504. (2015). *Section 504 of the Rehabilitation Act of 1973.* Retrieved from YOUR RIGHTS UNDER SECTION 504 OF THE REHABILITATION ACT: http://www.hhs.gov/ ocr/504.html, on March 1, 2015.

PASRR. (2015, March 22). *Preadmission screening and resident review.* Retrieved from Medicaid. gov: http://www.medicaid.gov/Medicaid-CHIP-Program-Information/By-Topics/Delivery-Systems/Institutional-Care/Preadmission-Screening-and-Resident-Review-PASRR.html, on March 22, 2015.

PTAC-PASRR. (2015, March 31). *PASRR Technical Assistance Organization.* Retrieved from PASRR: http://www.pasrrassist.org/, on March 31, 2015.

RAND-VBP. (2014). *Measuring success in health care value-based purchasing programs.* Washington, DC: Rand Corporation.

Rural Assistance Center. (2015, March 29). *CAH*. Retrieved from Critical Access Hospital: http://www.raconline.org/topics/critical-access-hospitals#beds, on March 29, 2015.

Shojania, K., McDonald, K., Wachter, R., & Owens, D. (2007, June). Closing the quality gap: A critical analysis of quality improvement strategies. In *AHRQ, Technical Reviews, No. 9, Vol. 7: Care Coordination*. AHRQ Publication No. 04(07)-0051-7. Rockville, MD: Agency for Healthcare Research and Quality.

Sprague, L. (2002, June 3). Contracting for quality: Medicare's quality improvement organizations. *National Health Policy Forum, 774*, 1–15.

Tahan, M. H. (2007, January/February). One patient, numerous healthcare providers, and multiple settings. *Professional Case Management, 12*(1), 37–46.

CHAPTER 14

Resource and Utilization Management

Michael B. Garrett and Teresa M. Treiger

LEARNING OBJECTIVES

Upon completion of this chapter, the reader will be able to:

1. Identify terms and concepts associated with utilization management.
2. Understand the utilization management process.
3. Describe clinical review criteria tools used in utilization management
4. Identify the areas of focused utilization management.
5. Review the outcomes and reporting of utilization management programs.
6. List key accreditation bodies associated with UM.

IMPORTANT TERMS AND CONCEPTS

Admission Certification
Alternative Level of Care
Appeal
Appropriateness of Setting
Case Management
Case Manager
Case Rates
Certification
Continued Stay Review
Continuum of Care
Denials
Discharge Outcomes
Discharge Planning
Fee for Service (FFS)
Focused/Targeted Utilization Management
Length of Stay (LOS)
Overutilization
Preadmission Certification
Prospective Payment System (PPS)
Quality Improvement Organization (QIO)
Resource Management (RM)
Retrospective Review Utilization Management (UM)
Utilization Review (UR)

Introduction

A. Utilization management (UM), as a program or process, has existed for more than 40 years.
1. UM functions began in the early 1970s with the creation of the professional standards review organization (now referred to as a Quality Improvement Organization or QIO), which evaluated health care services provided to Medicare and Medicaid beneficiaries
2. At first, UM was conducted after health care services were delivered (e.g., retrospective review), but gradually the process included precertification and concurrent review
3. The initial focus of UM was to review hospital care. This expanded to include outpatient services. By the 1980s, health maintenance organizations (HMOs) used UM processes as a means to control specialist provider access and gradually health care services utilization across the delivery continuum.
4. UM programs may be all-inclusive or focused on multiple areas including precertification, admission review, concurrent review, outpatient and ancillary services, imaging and x-ray, pharmacy management, therapies, and/or ambulatory surgery centers.
B. In the commercial sector, UM was conducted by insurance companies, managed care organizations, or third-party utilization review (UR) vendors. The industry is now seeing integrated delivery systems (IDSs), accountable care organizations (ACOs), and other forms of provider organizations performing UM due to risk-bearing contracts and/or pay-for-performance arrangements.
C. UM programs may be telephonic, onsite, and/or web-based. Each format has plus and minus arguments. As organizations move to web-based communication, special attention must be paid to security and privacy measures.
D. The validated clinical and outcome impact of UM is challenging to discern in a broad sense. The reasons for this include the absence of a specific methodology for measurement and the condition-specific nature of program reporting. In addition, outcomes are not consistently shared. This variation of methodology and lack of transparency make generalizations difficult.
E. Workers' compensation programs have dedicated UM standards and practices that are different from those required by Medicare, Medicaid, or commercial health insurance plans/third-party payers. Refer to Chapter 24 for more information about workers' compensation.
F. Social workers are rarely involved in UM. Sometimes, social workers may collaborate with nurse case managers in obtaining authorizations from the payer for postdischarge services and resources for a patient or in identifying which postdischarge service providers are part of the health insurance plan panel of providers.

 Descriptions of Key Terms

A. Admission certification—A form of utilization review in which an assessment is made of the medical necessity of a patient's admission to a hospital or other inpatient facility. Admission certification ensures that patients requiring a hospital-based level of care and length of stay appropriate for the admission diagnosis are usually assigned and certified as medically necessary according to care guidelines, but this is not necessarily a guarantee of payment for such services (payment is a benefit and/or claims determination).

B. Adverse determination—A decision by a health carrier, UM organization, or designee that a request for benefit coverage does not meet the requirements for medical necessity, appropriateness, health care setting, level of care, or effectiveness. It may also mean that the requested service or product is considered experimental or investigational and not a covered benefit. An adverse determination may be denial, reduction, termination, or failure to provide or make payment (National Association of Insurance Commissioners, 2012).

C. Alternative level of care—A level of care that can safely be used in place of the current level and is determined based on the acuity and complexity of the patient's condition and the type of needed services and resources.

D. Appeal—The formal process or request to reconsider a decision made not to approve an admission or health care services, reimbursement for services rendered, or a patient's request for postponing the discharge date and extending the length of stay.

E. Authorization—In the context of managed care, authorization is the need to obtain permission prior to coverage for specified services. This is common practice for gatekeeper-type health maintenance organizations. For instance, a primary care provider must authorize a member for a specialist provider visit in order for payment of said services (Kongstvedt, 2013).

F. Case rate—Rate of reimbursement that packages pricing for a certain category of services. Typically combines facility and professional practitioner fees for care and services.

G. Clinical practice guidelines—The Institute of Medicine (IOM) defined clinical practice guidelines as statements that include recommendations intended to optimize patient care that are informed by a systematic review of evidence and an assessment of the benefits and harms of alternative care options (Graham, Mancher, Wolman, Greenfield, & Steinberg, 2011). These guidelines should include the following characteristics: founded in systematic evidence review, developed by multidisciplinary expert panel, provide a clear explanation of the relationship between care options and health outcomes, and provide ratings of both the quality of evidence and the strength of the recommendations (National Heart, Blood, and Lung Institute, 2015).

H. Clinical review criteria—The written screens, decision rules, medical protocols, or guidelines used by the UM organization as an element in the evaluation of medical necessity and appropriateness of requested admissions, procedures, and services under the auspices of the applicable health benefit plan (URAC, 2010). Examples of clinical review criteria include InterQual, Managed Care Appropriateness Protocol (MCAP), and Milliman Care Guidelines (now known simply as MCG).

I. Continued stay review (also known as concurrent review)—A type of review used to determine whether each day of the hospital stay is necessary and that care is being rendered at the appropriate level. This

UM process takes place during a patient's hospitalization for care to evaluate the medical necessity of continued acute care.

J. Continuum of care—The continuum of care matches ongoing needs of individuals being served by the case management process with the appropriate level and type of health, medical, financial, legal, and psychosocial care for services within a setting or across multiple settings.

K. Denials (also called noncertifications)—A determination that the requested health care services do not meet medical necessity criteria, resulting in the issuance of a notice of noncertification decision.

L. Diagnostic-related groups (DRGs)—A patient classification scheme that provides a means of relating the type of patient a hospital treats to the costs incurred by the hospital. DRGs include groups of patients using similar resource consumption and length of stay.

1. The prospective payment system implemented as DRGs was designed to limit the share of hospital revenues derived from the Medicare program budget. Use of DRGs also is known as a statistical system of classifying any inpatient stay into groups for the purposes of payment.

2. DRGs may be primary or secondary; an outlier classification also exists. This is the form of reimbursement that the Centers for Medicare and Medicaid Services (CMS) uses to pay hospitals for Medicare beneficiaries.

3. Some Medicaid agencies also use this payment methodology; additionally, it is used in few states for all payers and by many private health insurance plans for contracting purposes.

M. Discharge criteria—Clinical criteria to be met before or at the time of the patient's discharge. They are the expected or projected outcomes of care that indicate a safe discharge.

N. Discharge planning—The process of assessing and evaluating the patient's needs of care after discharge from a health care facility and ensuring that the necessary services are in place before discharge.

1. A registered nurse, social worker, or other appropriately qualified personnel must develop, or supervise the development of, the evaluation.

2. The discharge plan must be discussed and developed with the patient and family. This process ensures a patient's timely, appropriate, and safe discharge to the next level of care or setting including appropriate use of resources necessary for ongoing care.

O. Evidence-based medicine (EBM)—A systematic approach to clinical problem solving, which allows the integration of the best available research evidence with clinical expertise and patient values. Evidence-based implies that the recommendation has been created using an unbiased and transparent process of systematically reviewing, appraising, and using the best clinical research findings of the highest value to aid in the delivery of optimum clinical care to patients.

P. Length of stay (LOS)—The number of days that a health plan member/patient stays in an inpatient facility, home health, or hospice.

Q. Level of care (LOC)—The intensity of effort required to diagnose, treat, preserve, or maintain an individual's physical or emotional status.

R. Overutilization review—Using established criteria as a guide, determination that the patient is receiving services that are redundant, unnecessary, or in excess of what is determined to be medically necessary.

S. Preadmission certification (also known as prospective review)—An element of utilization review that examines the need for proposed services before admission to a health care facility to determine the appropriateness of the setting, procedures, treatments, and length of stay.

T. Precertification/prospective review—The process of obtaining and documenting advanced approval from the health plan by the provider before delivering the medical services needed. This is required when health care services are of a nonemergent nature.

U. Prospective payment system (PPS)—A health care payment system used by the federal government since 1983 for reimbursing health care providers/agencies for medical care provided to Medicare and Medicaid participants. The payment is fixed and based on the operating costs of the patient's diagnosis.

V. Quality Improvement Organization (QIO)—A federal program established by the Tax Equity and Fiscal Responsibility Act of 1982 that monitors the medical necessity and quality of services provided to Medicare and Medicaid beneficiaries under the prospective payment system. QIOs also are involved in the discharge appeals process, especially for Medicare beneficiaries when they disagree with their discharge plans (and/or date) from various health care facilities including acute/hospital, rehabilitation, skilled nursing, and long-term acute care.

W. Resource management (RM)—A quality improvement activity that analyzes resources used in patient care processes to improve quality, efficiency, and value (Brown, 2015).

X. Retrospective review—A form of medical records review that is conducted after the patient's discharge to track appropriateness of level of care, quality of care, and consumption of health care resources.

Y. Utilization management (UM)—UM is the evaluation of the medical necessity, appropriateness, and efficiency of the use of health care services, procedures, and facilities under the provisions of the applicable health benefits plan, sometimes referred to as utilization review (URAC, 2015).

Z. Utilization review (UR)—UR is a safety mechanism that guards against unnecessary and/or inappropriate medical care. It is also used to establish circumstances where underutilization is problematic. It allows for the review of patient care through the use of evidence-based guidelines, expert consensus statements, to determine a variety of care elements (e.g., medical necessity, quality of care, decision making, place of service, length of hospital stay) (Spector, 2004).

Applicability to CMSA'S Standards of Practice

A. The Case Management Society of America (CMSA) describes in its standards of practice for case management (CMSA, 2010) that case management practice extends across all health care settings, including payer, provider, government, employer, community, and home environment.

Factors Affecting the Complexity of Case Management Practice

- The context of the care setting (e.g., wellness and prevention, acute, subacute, rehabilitative, or end of life)
- The health conditions and needs of the patient population(s) served including those of the patients' families
- The reimbursement method applied for services rendered (payment), such as managed care, workers' compensation, Medicare, or Medicaid
- The health care professional discipline assuming the role of the case manager such as registered nurse, social worker, or rehabilitation counselor

B. The CMSA (2010) in its standards of practice for case management explains that case management practice varies in degrees of complexity and comprehensiveness based on four factors described in Box 14-1.

C. This chapter describes utilization and resource management across the continuum of care with special focus on the role of the case manager and the case management services provided.

D. This chapter addresses case management practice, which requires knowledge of and proficiency in the following practice standards: client assessment, monitoring, facilitation/coordination/collaboration, legal, advocacy, resource management and stewardship.

 UM Program and Process

A. A UM program is a comprehensive, systematic, and ongoing effort. UM review activities are conducted through telephonic, fax, mail, on-site, and Web methods of communication with providers. Increasingly, health plans are interacting with providers through Web-based platforms that results in a more efficient and timely UM process. The UM process includes the evaluation of the appropriateness, quality, and level of care for health care services, equipment, and supplies across the delivery system.

B. UM programs focus on a variety of goals such as those summarized in Box 14-2.

C. UM review process: Web based
  1. Provider logs into the health plan's UM portal, which could be through a single sign-on process.
  2. Provider enters basic demographic information, so that the system can confirm the patient is eligible under the health plan and that the requested health care services require the UM review process.
  3. Some Web-based processes have the clinical review criteria or guidelines embedded into the system, so that the system requests specific clinical information for the particular health care service being requested. This is typically an algorithm based on the applicable clinical review criteria or guidelines.
     a. At the end of that process, the system will either generate an authorization or inform the provider that the requested service cannot be approved.
     b. In the event the provider does not receive an approval, the provider will usually need to communicate with the health

14-2 Goals of Utilization Management

- To ensure effective utilization of health care resources through application of clinical review criteria or clinical practice guidelines
- To determine medical necessity and appropriateness of care
- To identify patterns of overutilization, underutilization, and inefficient scheduling of resources
- To promote quality patient care, appropriate sequencing of health care services, and optimal outcomes
- To assist in the identification of coordination of care options for members and providers
- To facilitate appropriate, safe, timely, and effective discharge to the most appropriate level of care (LOC)
- To provide education concerning the UM program to providers and department staff
- To identify potential participants in chronic care management, case management, and other appropriate programs
- To profile providers' adherence to clinical guidelines
- To identify psychosocial needs that may not be already addressed, yet affecting utilization of resources. This is helpful in executing appropriate referrals to social services, community-based supportive programs, and behavioral health.

plan regarding the next steps in the UM process, such as filing an appeal, telephonic communication, or submission of supplementary medical information.

4. Other Web-based processes allow for open narrative information to be submitted regarding the requested service. Through this process, the health plan must have clinical reviewers evaluate the information to validate that the case meets clinical criteria or guidelines. The health plan can then communicate through the Web-based platform the decision at the conclusion of the clinical review process.

D. UM review process: Not conducted through the Web.

1. Verification of the patient's eligibility for services—This can be accomplished by a nonclinical customer service representative who can access the eligibility database of the health plan

2. Determination of whether the requested service is a covered benefit and requires a review—This can also be done by a nonclinical customer service representative by accessing the benefit plan for covered services and the UM review requirements description.

3. Collection of demographic and clinical information necessary to certify a requested service or length of stay, including history of prior health care services, current medical situation, and anticipated treatment plan (including surgeries, therapies, and other treatment modalities).

4. Selection of the applicable clinical criteria or guidelines to evaluate the requested services.

5. Clinical information is reviewed against evidence-based decision support criteria or guidelines for a review determination. The UM clinical reviewer evaluates, based on the information provided, whether the case meets criteria or guidelines.

E. Peer review process.
 1. If the clinical review criteria or guidelines are not met, then the review will be sent for peer review by an appropriate physician peer reviewer or medical director.
 2. The physician reviews the clinical information and may choose to approve the case based on medical judgment. The physician reviewer must request additional clinical information to evaluate the appropriateness of the requested health care service. If the physician reviewer believes the request should not be approved, then an offer is made to communicate with the attending physician about the case (sometimes called a peer-to-peer conversation or reconsideration). At the end of the discussion with the attending physician (or at the end of the time frame available for the discussion), the physician advisor makes a determination as to whether the request is approved or denied. If the request is denied, the provider or member can initiate the appeal process.
F. UM review types.
 1. Prospective review/precertification admission
 2. Continued stay/concurrent review
 3. Retrospective review
 4. Second surgical opinion
 5. Pharmacy benefit management
 6. Referral review to chronic care management, case management, and/or other available programs

UM Team

A. A staff responsible for performing UM may include:
 1. Initial clinical reviewer
 2. Medical director or clinical director
 3. Physician peer reviewer
 4. Administrative and nonclinical staff
 5. Case manager or UM specialist
B. Personnel who conduct the initial clinical review are usually registered nurses, licensed behavioral health specialists, licensed practical/vocational nurses, social workers, occupational therapists, physical therapists, or other health care professionals qualified to review the service requested by providers. Some health care organizations have health information management professionals provide the initial clinical review.
C. Medical director serves as the clinical leader of the UM team. This person may have supervisory oversight of physician advisors as well as managerial oversight of the clinical review department (e.g., clinical review policy, clinical review criteria selection, information system) used by the UM program.
D. Physician peer reviewer provides professional evaluation of the medical necessity and quality of care when a case fails the initial clinical review criteria, guidelines, or screens.
E. Administrative and nonclinical staff member can collect administrative and demographic information, and they can conduct scripted clinical screening. However, the administrative and nonclinical staff cannot engage in unscripted clinical dialogue.

Certifications Related to UM and UR

A. The American Board of Quality Assurance and Utilization Review Physicians, Inc. (ABQAURP) offers certification for Health Care Quality and Management (HCQM) for physicians, nurses, and other health care professionals. ABQAURP also offers subspecialty certifications in transitions of care, managed care, patient safety/risk management, case management, workers' compensation, and physician advisor.
B. The American Association of Medical Audit Specialists is the parent organization of the Certification Council for Medical Audit Specialists and is the sole credentialing authority for Certified Medical Audit Specialists (CMAS).
C. The National Association for Healthcare Quality (NAHQ) administers the Certified Professional in Healthcare Quality (CPHQ) certification.

 ## UM Criteria and Strategies

A. Clinical decision support tools, such as guidelines, protocols, algorithms, and pathways, are used by health plans and providers in evaluating the utilization, quality, and appropriateness of health care services.
B. The application of these tools helps determine if a proposed service is clinically indicated, appropriate, and provided in the right care setting.
C. Criteria may be developed by organizations that specialize in the development of clinical criteria, specialty providers through the coordination of their associations, or internally by a health plan or health care organization.
D. Criteria must be current, clinically sound, objective, reviewed and approved annually, and grounded in evidence-based medicine or systematic consensus-based processes.
E. Health plans provide providers and patients with access to the criteria tools for decision-making in an effort to promote transparency and shared decision-making.

 ## UM Clinical Review Criteria and Guidelines

A. The major sources for clinical review criteria include
   1. McKesson's InterQual products include level of care criteria, planning criteria, and behavioral health criteria as well as coordinated care and procedure content.
   2. MCG features evidence-based guidelines for the assessment, treatment, and management of conditions across the continuum of care.
   3. MCAP Clinical Review Criteria and CritView products may be used concurrently and retrospectively to determine appropriate care levels based on medical necessity and best practices.
B. Some medical societies and associations produce clinical guidelines specific to their specialty practice, such as the American College of Obstetrics and Gynecology, American Society of Addiction Medicine, and the American Academy of Pediatrics.
C. The Agency for Healthcare Research and Quality (AHRQ) provides the National Guidelines Clearinghouse (NGC) as a public resource for evidence-based clinical practice guidelines. The case manager may find these helpful when discussing the delivery of care and possible variances with providers.

Focused UM

A. Many UM programs and organizations have restructured to narrow their focus on certain providers and/or health care services. This results in a migration away from broad-based UM programs requiring reviews from all providers for all services to a more focused program.
1. The focused UM is typically based upon data analysis. Health plans evaluate data to determine if the providers are consistently adhering the clinical review criteria or guidelines. For those providers who demonstrate substantial adherence to clinical review criteria or guidelines, then the health plan may lift the UM review requirements.
2. A health plan may determine that certain health care services are nearly always approved and lift the UM review requirements.
3. A health plan may evaluate data and discover that a wide variation for certain health care services across providers. In those instances, a health plan may intensify the UM review process, especially for high cost/high utilization services.
4. A health plan may modify its program. Instead of requiring a clinical review process, the plan may only require notification of certain health care services.
B. Data indicate that this type of focused intervention reduces the overall administrative cost of a traditional UM program and improves the overall organizational management of patient care.
C. The case manager's role in focused UM is particular to the health plan.
1. UM may be integrated in the case manager's responsibilities to his/her caseload clients or may be relegated to an entirely separate team of clinical reviewers.
2. Due to the lack of job title consistency, positions may be inaccurately classified as case management and, close review of the job description is important.

 Denials of Admissions and Services

A. A denial, also termed a lack of certification or adverse determination, may be issued when admission to or continued stay in the facility cannot be justified as medically necessary. Denial notice is also issued in the event that a procedure, service, product, or device is rejected.
B. There are different types of denials. Regulations governing the issuance of denial determinations vary by payer (e.g., Medicare, Medicaid, commercial plan) as well as by state and other regulatory authorities
1. Private review agencies maintain policies and procedures for denials in accordance with specific payer groups.
2. The US Department of Labor (USDOL) issued claims regulations, which apply to UM decisions for fully insured and self-funded health plans.
3. Medicare and Medicaid issue copious regulations pertaining to the processing of authorization and adverse determinations.
C. UM organizations must remain compliant with the standards by which they are granted accreditation status (e.g., National Committee for Quality Assurance [NCQA], URAC).

Adverse Review Determination

A. A health insurance carrier maintains written policies and procedures detailing its UM and benefit determination processes.
B. URAC and NCQA consider nonauthorization decisions that are based on either medical appropriateness or benefit coverage or experimental treatments to be denials.
C. The partial or total denial, reduction, and termination are considered adverse determinations, as is a rescission of a previously approved product or service.
D. If the UM review does not meet clinical decision support criteria or there is no criterion for a particular diagnosis, procedure, or imaging procedure, the next steps may include:
   1. Supervisor review and referral to a physician advisor for medical review
   2. Medical review, which may involve a second-level medical review in circumstances where the requested product or service is outside the knowledge or practice of the medical reviewer.
E. Each payer source issues written notifications for adverse determination (inclusive of potential adverse determination) as well as for end of authorization period notices. Regulation outlines notification requirements including time frames, which are designated by federal, state, or accreditation agencies. Organizational policy provides more specific guidance to its respective staff.
   1. These notifications are referred to by a variety of names depending upon the payer. The names of these notifications may change as policies and regulations are redefined.
   2. The case manager must maintain knowledge as to each payor's general process and regulations, which pertain to both verbal and written requirements.
   3. In the event a payer shares a determination verbally with a case manager, the payer is required to communicate the determination in writing regardless of the verbal alert of such.
F. Only physician reviewers may deny care (e.g., product or service). However, physicians may seek the input of others involved (e.g., case managers) in the determination process.
G. Case managers must maintain knowledge of UM laws and regulations applicable to their respective jurisdiction, organizational policies and procedures governing clinical review process, organization accreditation standards, individual certification standards, and licensure regulations specific to their scope of practice.

 Medical Review Outcomes

A. Medical review determinations are based on the peer reviewer's judgment and expertise after reviewing the case for medical appropriateness. The health plan may deny a product or service because it is not a covered benefit by the individual's health insurance plan or policy or is considered to be experimental or investigational. Outcomes of medical reviews may include but are not limited to four options/ determinations (Box 14-3).

14-3 Classification of Medical Review Outcomes

1. Approval
2. Partial approval (e.g., procedure is approved on an outpatient basis, but the request was for an inpatient stay). This may also be considered as a partial denial.
3. Administrative denial (e.g., failure to provide requested information within the designated time frame)
4. Medical necessity denial
5. Clinical denial

B. Case managers are often part of the UM process leading up to a medical review. It is important that the case manager educate the provider, client, caregiver, and colleagues as to the review process and available resources. In addition, the case manager should strive to facilitate the review process by ensuring that the information necessary for a complete review is available to the medical reviewer.

Appeal Process

A. The appeal process is the formal mechanism by which a provider or member (or both) requests reconsideration of an adverse determination (e.g., denial). An appeal is the due process available for providers and members when there has been an adverse determination.
B. The process to file any kind of appeal is specific to the payer. The information presented herein represents a general representation of an appeal process. The case manager must verify the specific requirements for filing/adjudicating an appeal based on the payer involved.
C. The goal of the appeal process is to reach a mutually acceptable solution to the benefit coverage request.
D. Non-Medicare appeals are generally defined into the following levels:
1. Reconsideration (e.g., peer-to-peer discussion)—An additional review for a request, which is going to be denied. A reconsideration is completed prior to issuance of a formal adverse UM determination.
   a. It is generally performed by the reviewer responsible for the original review and is based on the inclusion of additional information or discussion with the requesting provider.
   b. For example, a request for a biologic agent to treat rheumatoid arthritis is pending. The prescribing provider reaches out of the reviewer with additional information regarding the patient's adverse reaction to a previously attempted oral medication, which makes a trial of the parenteral form less desirable.
   c. Some organizations consider reconsideration as the first level of appeal.
2. Appeal—A request for additional review of a decision to not certify imminent or ongoing services, requiring a review conducted by a clinical peer physician reviewer who was not involved in the original decision to not certify.
   a. The appeal is completed according to request timeframe
      i. Standard appeal—Completed within 30 days of the request.
      ii. Expedited or urgent appeal—Completed 24 to 72 hours from the request (dependent on the type of review).

BOX 14-4 Five Levels of Medicare Fee-For-Service–Related Appeals

1. First level of appeal is a redetermination by a Medicare carrier, fiscal intermediary (FI), or Medicare Administrative Contractor (MAC).
2. Second level of appeal is a reconsideration performed by a Qualified Independent Contractor (QIC).
3. Third level of appeal is an administrative law judge (ALJ) hearing, which takes place in the office of Medicare Hearings and Appeals.
4. Fourth level of appeal is a review by the Medicare Appeals Council.
5. Fifth level of appeal is a judicial review in federal district court.

    b. Clinical review conducted by appropriate clinical peers, who were not involved in peer clinical review, when a decision not to certify a requested admission, procedure, or service has been appealed (URAC, 2010).
    c. Accreditation organizations (e.g., NCQA, URAC) maintain standards by which health plans are assessed as part of its respective accreditation program. Standards are reviewed and updated regularly. The case manager should be knowledgeable of the accreditation expectations, which impact his/her performance.
       i. Standards look at the existence of policies, procedures, and processes as well as performance measurement as compared to the plan's declared expectation.
    3. Independent review organization (IRO)—An IRO is an independent group that a payor contracts with to provide external review services. The IRO examines denials based on medical necessity. The IRO has been a requirement in many states. PPACA mandates all payers and health plans to have IRO arrangements (Kongstvedt, 2013). Some acute care facilities also are using IROs today.
E. Medicare appeals
    1. Traditional Medicare (fee-for-service) appeals, which are applicable to both Parts A and B, are defined by five levels (Box 14-4) according to the CMS (2015a).
    2. Medicare-managed care (Part C) appeals must meet the requirements for grievance and appeals processing defined within the Medicare advantage regulations (Box 14-5). As these are updated regularly, the case manager is advised to seek current information directly from the CMS Web site.

BOX 14-5 Medicare Part C Appeal Determinations

1. Organization determination
2. First-level appeal (health plan reconsideration)
3. Second-level appeal (independent review)
4. Third-level appeal (administrative law judge)
5. Fourth-level appeal (Medicare Appeals Council)
6. Judicial review (federal district court)

   a. If a Medicare health plan denies service or payment, in whole
      or in part, the plan is required to provide a written notice of its
      determination (CMS, 2015b).
   b. Medicare health plan enrollees receiving covered services from an
      inpatient hospital, skilled nursing facility, home health agency,
      or comprehensive outpatient rehabilitation facility have the right
      to a fast, or expedited, review if they think their Medicare-covered
      services are ending too soon (CMS, 2015b).
   c. Plans and providers have responsibilities related to notifying
      beneficiaries of Medicare appeal rights (CMS, 2015b).
F. Inadequate, untimely, and incomplete communication and/
   or documentation are often factors that contribute to a denial
   determination.
   1. The case manager's should ensure that the request for health care
      authorization and/or certification be submitted with all required
      documentation and information in order to justify coverage.
      a. Health plans share authorization criteria on request. This provides
         staff with the specific information and/or documentation required
         for approval of the request.
      b. The case manager advocates for appropriate resources and
         resource utilization in order that the patient reaches his/her
         optimal level of wellness and function as efficiently and cost-
         effectively as possible.
G. The case manager should maintain knowledge of resources and tools,
   which may support or refute UM determinations.
   1. The Effective Health Care Program (EHCP), positioned within the
      Agency for Healthcare Research and Quality, creates summaries regarding
      the benefits and risks of different health conditions and treatments.
      a. Although not considered clinical recommendations or care
         guidelines, these effectiveness reviews are helpful in understanding
         the benefit of various treatments as compared to each other.
      b. These summaries are useful for policymakers, providers,
         colleagues, and patient/caregivers.
   2. The National Guideline Clearinghouse (NGC) is a database
      containing evidence-based clinical practice guidelines and associated
      documentation.
      a. It is a service, which falls under the auspices of AHRQ.
      b. NCG's intent is to provide an organized and accessible means for
         interested parties (e.g., providers, patients) to obtain objective,
         detailed information regarding current clinical practice guidelines
         and to support evidence-based practice.
      c. The database contains national and international clinical practice
         guidelines.
H. Quality Improvement Organizations (QIOs)—A group of health quality
   experts, clinicians, and consumers organized to improve the care
   delivered to people with Medicare. QIOs work under the direction of the
   Centers for Medicare and Medicaid Services to assist Medicare providers
   with quality improvement and to review quality concerns for the
   protection of beneficiaries and the Medicare Trust Fund (CMS, 2015c).
   The core functions of a QIO are:
   1. Improving quality of care for beneficiaries

2. Protecting the integrity of the Medicare Trust Fund:
   a. Ensure Medicare only pays for goods and services and goods that are reasonable and necessary.
   b. Ensure Medicare pays for goods and services that are provided in the most appropriate setting.
3. Protecting beneficiaries by expeditiously addressing individual complaints including
   a. Beneficiary complaints
   b. Provider-based notice appeals
   c. Violations of the Emergency Medical Treatment and Labor Act (EMTALA)
   d. Other related responsibilities as articulated in QIO-related law (CMS, 2015c)
4. The case management department should partner with the QIO to ensure all documentation is available to demonstrate Medicare beneficiary health care services.
5. The case management department should seek constructive CIO feedback to consider as part of program and process improvement.

UM Performance Reporting

A. Transparency, accountability, and performance measurement have long been a part of the health care environment. Although various settings and payer types dictate metrics and desired outcomes, case managers play a pivotal role in many of them.
B. Accreditation organizations (e.g., NCQA, URAC, TJC) look for organizations to manage quality improvement through continuous measurement and outcomes-driven actions. Understanding accreditation standards pertaining to UM and case management's part in the overall process is important.
C. Healthcare Effectiveness Data and Information Set (HEDIS) is used by more than 90% of health plans. HEDIS consists of 81 measures across 5 domains of care (NCQA, 2015a).
   1. HEDIS measures are developed using a multistep process, involving the identification of a clinical area requiring evaluation, literature review, measurement development, expert review, stakeholder comment period, field testing, and final decision whether to institute or deactivate (NCQA, 2015b).
D. Organizations review a variety of measurements, which are specific to the type of organization, mandated reporting, accreditation requirements, internal performance improvement programs, and other variables. A sampling of health care provider reports is provided in Box 14-6.

Key Regulatory and Accreditation Bodies Associated with the UM Process

A. The CMS is a federal regulatory agency that oversees the Medicare program and oversees the states' administration of Medicaid programs.

BOX 14-6   Health Care Provider Reports

The following is a list of utilization-related reports generated within health care provider organizations. This is not intended to be an all-inclusive list.
- Admissions (e.g., total, by payment class)
- All-cause readmission
- Average length of stay (ALOS)
- Procedures per thousand
- Alternative LOC transition (e.g., cost per day, savings per day)
- Delays in services (e.g., days delayed, cost per day delayed)
- Emergency department visits
- Number and type of denials (e.g., inpatient days, procedures, services)
- Reconsiderations
- Appeals of denials (based on a statistic, such as percentage of denied cases brought to appeal)
- Denials (based on a statistic, such as percentage of all reviews that result in a denial)
- Peer reviews (based on a statistic, such as percentage of all reviews that are referred to a physician advisor for clinical peer review)
- Case referrals to chronic care management, case management, and other services
- UM statistics may be reported by facility within a network, provider, and/or payer class (e.g., Medicare, Medicaid, commercial).
- Appeal overturn rate (the percentage of appeals that resulted in overturning the original denial or noncertification decision)

B. The Joint Commission (TJC) is an independent, not-for-profit organization. The Joint Commission accredits and certifies more than 20,500 health care organizations and programs in the United States. Joint Commission accreditation and certification are recognized nationwide as a symbol of quality that reflects an organization's commitment to meeting certain performance standards (TJC, 2015).

C. URAC is a not-for-profit organization that promotes health care quality through its accreditation, education, and measurement programs. URAC offers a wide range of quality benchmarking programs and services that provides health care organizations a method for validating their commitment to quality and accountability. Previously known as the Utilization Review Accreditation Commission, this organization formally changed its name to URAC (URAC, 2015).

D. National Committee for Quality Assurance (NCQA) is an independent nonprofit organization dedicated to improving health care quality through review, recognition, and accreditation of a wide range of health care organizations. It also recognizes clinicians and practices in key areas of performance (NCQA, 2015c).

UM Regulatory and Accreditation Processes

A. For organizations performing UM, it is important to seek accredited status because it ensures that the process of conducting utilization review is clinically sound and respects both the patient's and provider's rights and at the same time providing a reasonable framework within which payers are able to function in an efficient and consistent manner. Accreditation demonstrates an organization meets regulatory requirements and supports a commitment to quality improvement.

14-7   Common Phases of the UM Accreditation Process

1. Preparing/building the application
2. Desktop/remote review of application by accrediting body
3. On-site review
4. Committee review/determination
5. Accreditation status determination and notification
6. Renewal submission, determination, and notification

B. The accreditation process varies according to the organization from which recognition is sought (Box 14-7). Requirements change over time. It is the responsibility of the seeking organization to understand its obligations when seeking accreditation and to maintain operational adherence with the awarded accreditation.
C. There are multiple accreditation and recognition programs offered by a variety of organizations. Each program's specific requirements vary. The case manager must maintain knowledge of accreditation requirements of their organization as well as individual specifications pertaining to their job's role, function, and individual scope of practice.

Certification Programs in UR or UM

A. Certification programs in UR and UM have undergone significant changes. Two previously available certifications, CPUR and CPUM offered by McKesson, no longer exist.
B. The American Board of Quality Assurance and Utilization Review Physicians (ABQAURP) offer the Health Care Quality and Management (HCQM) credential. This certification demonstrates that diplomates have the practical knowledge and the tools that can reduce medical errors, ensure patient safety, and eliminate waste and unnecessary services, while avoiding potentially harmful delays in care (ABQAURP, 2015). There are additional subspecialty certifications also offered (e.g., Risk Management, Workers' Compensation, Transition of Care).
C. The American Board of Managed Care Nurses (ABMCN) offers the Certification in Managed Care Nursing (CMCN). The certification offers nurses and social workers a credential promoting excellence and professionalism in managed health care and recognizes individuals who demonstrate an acquired body of knowledge and expertise in managed care through voluntary certification (ABMCN, 2015).

References

American Board of Managed Care Nurses. (2015). *The value of certification*. Retrieved from http://www.abmcn.org/index.htm, on July 22, 2015.
American Board of Quality Assurance and Utilization Review Physicians (ABQAURP). (2015). *Certification*. Retrieved from http://www.abqaurp.org/ABQMain/Certification/Overview_of_HCQM_Certification/ABQMain/Certification.aspx?hkey=b6edc3b2-6da9-49d0-a824-3399badf629e, on July 22, 2015.
Brown, Janet A. (2015). *The health care quality handbook: A professional resource and study guide* (28th ed.). Pasadena, CA: JB Quality Solutions.

Case Management Society of America. (2010). *Standards of Practice for Case Management*. Little Rock, AR: Author.

Centers for Medicare and Medicaid (CMS). (2015a). *Original medicare (fee-for-service) appeals*. Retrieved from http://www.cms.gov/Medicare/Appeals-and-Grievances/OrgMedFFSAppeals/index.html?redirect=/OrgMedFFSAppeals, on July 21, 2015.

Centers for Medicare and Medicaid (CMS). (2015b). *Medicare managed care appeals and grievances*. Retrieved from http://www.cms.gov/Medicare/Appeals-and-Grievances/MMCAG/index.html, on July 21, 2015.

Centers for Medicare and Medicaid (CMS). (2015c). *Quality improvement organizations*. Retrieved from http://www.cms.gov/Medicare/Quality-Initiatives-Patient-Assessment-Instruments/QualityImprovementOrgs/index.html?redirect=/QualityImprovementOrgs, on July 21, 2015.

Graham, R., Mancher, M., Wolman, D. M., Greenfield, S., & Steinberg, E. (Eds.). (2011). *Clinical practice guidelines we can trust*. Washington, DC: National Academies Press.

Kongstvedt, P. R. (2013). *Essentials of managed health care* (6th ed.). Burlington, VT: Jones & Bartlett.

National Association of Insurance Commissioners. (2012). *Utilization review and benefit determination model act*. Retrieved from http://www.naic.org/store/free/MDL-73.pdf, on July 20, 2015.

National Committee for Quality Assurance (NCQA). (2015a). *HEDIS and performance management*. Retrieved from http://www.org/HEDISQualityMeasurement.aspx, on July 21, 2015.

National Committee for Quality Assurance (NCQA). (2015b). *HEDIS measurement development process*. Retrieved from http://www.ncqa.org/tabid/414/Default.aspx, on July 21, 2015.

National Committee for Quality Assurance (NCQA). (2015c). *About NCQA*. Retrieved from http://www.ncqa.org/AboutNCQA.aspx, on July 22, 2015.

National Heart, Blood, and Lung Institute. (2015). *About systematic evidence reviews and clinical practice guidelines*. Retrieved from http://www.nhlbi.nih.gov/health-pro/guidelines/about#cpg, on July 20, 2015.

Spector, R. A. (2004). Utilization review and managed health care liability. *Southern Medical Journal, 97*(3). Retrieved from http://www.medscape.com/viewarticle/472608, on July 22, 2015.

The Joint Commission (TJC). (2015). *About The Joint Commission*. Retrieved from http://www.jointcommission.org/about_us/about_the_joint_commission_main.aspx, on July 22, 2015.

URAC. (2010). *Definitions for health accreditation*. Retrieved from http://www.naic.org/documents/committees_b_consumer_information_100706_urac_definitions_hca.pdf, on July 22, 2015.

URAC. (2015). *What is health utilization management?* Retrieved from https://www.urac.org/accreditation-and-measurement/accreditation-programs/all-programs/health-utilization-management, on July 22, 2015.

CHAPTER 15

Case Management and Use of Technology

Teresa M. Treiger

LEARNING OBJECTIVES

Upon completion of this chapter, the reader will be able to:

1. Describe health information technology and case management information systems (CMIS).

2. State the goals, benefits, and limitations of CMIS.

3. Discuss the role of case management informatics in practice consistency and standards of care.

4. Describe how CMIS support case management outcomes and process improvement.

5. Describe telehealth as it pertains to case management.

6. Explore the benefits and barriers of telepractice.

7. Discuss the evaluation of health-related Web sites for professional and patient use.

8. Discuss telephonic case management and remote telehealth monitoring technology.

9. Discuss case management's role in the evolution and delivery of telehealth interventions.

10. Discuss technology tools available to the case manager.

NOTE: This chapter is a revised version of Chapters 15 and 16 in the second edition of *CMSA Core Curriculum for Case Management*. The contributor wishes to acknowledge the work of Dee McGonigle, Kathleen Mastrian, and Robert Pyke, as some of the timeless material was retained from the previous version.

IMPORTANT TERMS AND CONCEPTS

Case Management
Information System
(CMIS)
Clinical Decision
Support Software
(CDSS)
Committee for Nursing
Practice Information
Infrastructure (CNPII)
Decision Support
Software (DSS)

Health Information
Technology (HIT)
Health Information
Technology for
Economic and
Clinical Health Act
of 2009 (HITECH)
Health Level Seven
International (HL7)
Interoperability
Meaningful Use

Nursing Information
and Data Set
Evaluation Center
(NIDSEC)
Systematized •
Nomenclature of
Medicine (SNOMED)
Telehealth (TH)
Telemedicine (TM)
Telemental Health
(TMH)

 Introduction

A. Health care includes some of the most complex business models across all industries in the United States. In response to the passage of the Health Information Technology for Economic and Clinical Health (HITECH) Act in 2009, health care organizations began to actively migrate traditional paper-based systems to computer-based systems. Until the financial incentives pushed hospitals to computerize its medical records and support systems, implementation of case management technology solutions was spotty at best.

B. Contemporary case managers must appreciate and use the functionality of these increasingly sophisticated health information technology (HIT) and case management information systems (CMIS). Case managers must also be knowledgeable of health care informatics principles in order to maximize the benefits of these systems. It is important to actively engage in technology advances and to leverage technology to its maximum potential in support of quality, safe, efficient, and effective care.

C. CMIS enhances the ability to gather information and provide indicators of case management's contribution to positive patient outcomes and health care quality improvement.

1. Case managers encounter heavier caseloads, in both the quantity and the complexity. Justifying case management's value in the care delivery chain is essential and ongoing. The return-on-investment (ROI) issue will always need to be addressed.

2. Informatics and electronic tools must continue to evolve to support the effectiveness of case management practice and to consistently record and measure its impact, especially on patient care outcomes and adherence to regulatory and accreditation demands.

D. Usability is a key factor in the success of any CMIS. Users who work with the systems are the most important resource in helping developers understand current needs as well as new and innovative approaches to enhance the work of the case manager and to meet the ultimate goal—successful patient outcomes.

E. Career opportunities are available for case managers to work in or collaborate with developers of information systems (IS) and with organizations wishing to expand their use of technology. Case managers, as primary users, generate ideas to improve and enhance these systems.

F. This chapter discusses the progression of HIT and CMIS as is designed to bring efficiencies to case management workflow; eliminating activities that subtract from case management's value to the health care team and clients. It also addresses case management–specific aspects of telehealth (TH) and other technologies, which extend the reach of case management intervention. As an integral part of healthcare, case management is part of the electronic wave.

Descriptions of Key Terms

A. Aggregated data—data that represent the same element of information or variable for many different records such as a list of surgeries and length of stay for all patients for the month of April. The purpose of studying data in the aggregate is to determine patterns, turn information into knowledge, and then act on it with the purpose of decision making and improvement. The data may be from any size of database, from just a few records to millions of records (Sewell & Thede, 2013).

B. Algorithms—a set of unambiguous steps for accomplishing a defined task. The algorithm has a definite starting and stopping point. It may contain decision points, but finite choices are given and the results of each choice clearly stated (Sewell & Thede, 2013).

C. Application program—a computer program designed for an end user such as a word processor or database. This is separate from systems software, which interacts with the computer (Sewell & Thede, 2013).

D. App—an abbreviation of the word application frequently associated with mobile computer technology and/or smartphones. It is a software program.

E. Audit trail—a record made by a system or software in which all actions of the user are recorded and stored. For example, when Ellen accesses the medical record of Patient Lynn, there is an electronic recording of the access and of everything Ellen views while in Lynn's record. The audit trail is how a system administrator is able to determine whether a user complied with security measures during his/her time in the medical record or if a breach occurred.

F. Biometric identification—the use of physiological characteristics such as fingerprints or voiceprint to authenticate that a user is who she/he says she/he is. Biometric devices are those that are capable of making an identification based on a specific human train that is unique to the individual. For example, a mobile phone allows a user to scan fingerprints in order to authenticate access to the device instead of manual password entry.

G. Bluetooth—a standard for the short-range wireless interconnection of cellular phones, computers, and other electronic devices. It replaces or is used in addition to hardwires or cables connecting devices (e.g., mobile phones to headsets).

H. Clinical decision support system (CDSS)—a computer system that links health observations (e.g., signs, symptoms, laboratory results) with a knowledge repository, which gives feedback to the provider in order to influence diagnostic and treatment options of the user clinician. See decision support system.

I. Clinical information system (CIS)—information technology applied at the point of clinical care. It includes electronic medical records, clinical data repositories, decision support programs (e.g., clinical guidelines, drug interaction verification), handheld devices for collecting data and viewing reference material, imaging modalities, and communication tools such as electronic messaging systems (Sewell & Thede, 2013).

J. Computerized Provider Order Entry (CPOE)—although sometimes translated to mean Computerized Physician Order Entry, CPOE includes licensed independent clinical professionals with prescriptive authority (e.g., nurse practitioners). CPOE describes the use of a computer to enter prescriptions and other health care orders. These systems are designed to catch prescribing errors, drug interactions, allergies, and other contraindications, which could result in a problem or complication for the patient (Sewell & Thede, 2013).

K. Database—a collection of data or records that is stored in a systematic fashion that allows you to search through the data for specific aims. You can run a query (ask or request information) from the database. For example, you could ask: how many people have asthma? How many people have been readmitted following an appendectomy?

L. Data mining—searching for meaningful patterns and relationships among data. For example, data mining could help to identify patients at risk based on their lifestyle/behaviors, frequency of access to avoidable services (e.g., emergency department visits), and medical history.

M. Data warehouse—a data warehouse is a collection of diverse data from sources that one would not think of relating that is specifically structured for query and analysis. Developing a data warehouse involves processes that extract the data and then clean, scrub, and date them. Large health care databases would produce volumes of information if put into a warehouse and subjected to data mining (Sewell & Thede, 2013).

N. Decision support system (DSS)—part of an information system that correlates information from many different sources including specific patient data and the literature to provide suggestions to the clinician (Sewell & Thede, 2013). DSS and CDSS enrich a case manager's professional judgment by quickly verifying or refuting business decisions. The user has at his or her fingertips all of the pertinent elements required for evaluation. See clinical decision support system (CDSS).
1. The heart of a DSS system is a medical information warehouse containing all of the information about the patient (e.g., health, clinical, and demographics), as well as data and outcomes of patients identified as having similar medical conditions (Dietzen, 1997).
2. Data come from a variety of sources (e.g., laboratories, pharmacy, authorizations), although the majority of information may come from claims. Data must be organized in a way that facilitates easy retrieval for meeting the identified business needs.

O. Electronic health record (EHR)—similar to personal health record described below. The complete record of an individual's health care and integrates information and documentation from many sources. Often, it is created based on information gathered cumulatively from more than one health care agency. This term is often erroneously used to mean an electronic medical record (Sewell & Thede, 2013).

P. Electronic medical record (EMR)—the electronic record of patient care created and owned by one health care agency or health care provider's office. It is different from electronic and personal health records (Sewell & Thede, 2013).

Q. Health care informatics—the science of managing health care information that draws on information and computer science, health care discipline knowledge, and theories such as sociotechnical theory, change theories, cognitive theory, usability principles, learning theories, and diffusion and chaos theories (Sewell & Thede, 2013).

R. Health information exchange (HIE)—the electronic exchange of health-related data between health care agencies not under the same ownership using agreed protocols, standards, and other criteria. May also be referred to as a Regional Health Information Organization (Sewell & Thede, 2013).

S. Health information technology (HIT)—technology applied in health care, generally meant to refer to electronic records. Sometimes, the name of the department that has the responsibility for the electronic records (Sewell & Thede, 2013).

T. Meaningful use—a set of criteria in electronic records that must be met by health care agencies to gain Medicare or Medicaid incentive payments. They are staged with a given year to meet each of the levels. The goal is to promote electronic records that can interchange data (Sewell & Thede, 2013).

U. Patient portal—a portal specific to an individual that is tied to the patient's electronic health record. A patient portal may offer one- or two-way communication for a patient to interact with his/her provider(s) but the information will be specific to that individual (Sewell & Thede, 2013).

V. Personal health record (PHR)—a compilation of health care information from many sources for a consumer. This system allows a person to access their electronic health records from any location. The owner of the PHR determines who can see what part of their record. Some health care agencies now provide these for patients but will only contain information from within their agency. A full PHR requires providers and agencies to have electronic medical records that communicate with each other as part of an EHR system (Sewell & Thede, 2013).

W. Telehealth (TH)—using communications networks to provide health services including but not limited to direct care, health prevention, consulting, and home visits to patients in a geographical location different than the provider of these services. Any delivery of health services to a client in a geographical location different than the provider (Sewell & Thede, 2013).

X. Telemedicine (TM)—a part of telehealth that is defined as a health professional in one location using electronic technologies for the diagnosis and/or treatment of a patient in another location (Sewell & Thede, 2013).

Applicability to CMSA'S Standards of Practice

A. The Case Management Society of America (CMSA) describes in its standards of practice for case management (CMSA, 2010) that case management practice extends across all health care settings, including payer, provider, government, employer, community, and home environment.

B. This chapter introduces basic technology concepts and usage, of which a professional case manager should be aware and knowledgeable. Of specific importance are the issues of use of Internet resources for both personal and professional purposes.

C. Although this chapter discusses how technology supports case management practice standards (e.g., identification and selection, assessment, monitoring, outcomes), the professional case manager is especially mindful of how technology supports CMSA's practice standards on facilitation, coordination, and collaboration by allowing more consistent and structured case management practice.

D. Technology is especially important to CMSA's Research and Research Utilization standards when leveraging technology for the purpose of seeking out educational material for oneself and for the use of clients and caregivers. The use of consistent Web site evaluation methodology helps to ensure the use of timely, accurate, and unbiased material as well as guidance to clients as they use the Internet to learn more about health, self-management skills, support groups, and other available options.

 ## Health Information Technology and Case Management Information Systems

A. An information system (IS) is a combination of hardware, software, telecommunications networks, and the Internet. These interconnected elements collect, manipulate, store, and disseminate data and information.

1. IS is a purposefully designed system bringing people, data, and procedures together for the purpose of managing information in order to support important operations, management, and decision functions.

2. IS are everywhere in our lives—at the bank, grocery store, etc. With few exceptions, our interaction with these systems is now routine and seamless. We regularly provide feedback as to system improvements.

B. Health information technology is technology applied in the health care context. Availability of HIT enhances the effectiveness of case managers and contributes to better care outcomes.

C. Functional capabilities of CMIS are important in enhancing the role of the case manager and the execution of the case management process. The broader the system functionalities are, the more desirable the system is to ultimately contribute to an efficient and cost-effective case management practice.

D. It is important that CMIS is able to integrate both clinical and nonclinical components and workflows. Such characteristic allows case managers easy access to important information for use in the case management process and care provision. Examples of functionalities are as follows:

1. Assessments and plans of care—The responses to any individual question can be tracked over time. Responses also can trigger entries on the case manager's to-do list (tickler feature) or generate a goal or problem.

   a. For example, if the case manager asks the patient whether he or she is able to tolerate mild activity and the patient responds negatively, the CMIS can generate a problem on the patient's problem list that states "patient has poor tolerance to activity."

   b. The system also should be able to automatically trigger a care goal focusing on improvement in physical activity. The system can also generate a reminder when the time is appropriate to perform a reassessment.

2. Goal setting—CMIS can automatically remind the case manager when the target date for a goal is approaching and track the progress toward the goal.

   a. Problems—Electronic linking of problems and goals with plans to resolve each problem.

   b. Milestones—Electronic tracking of the status of a patient's care milestones. Is the patient reaching the milestones by the target dates?

3. Rule-based alerts, messages, and reminders based on information gathered or clinical recommendations—Structured data entry with discrete data elements allow for this functionality. Reminder rules used in the system assess patient states, determine what issues need attention, and then generate the system reminders regarding these key issues.

   a. Rules can be related to overlooked treatments (e.g., variances and delays in care), preventive care (reducing complications and exacerbations), addressing value-based purchasing core measures, proper follow-up, or monitoring of current treatment and interventions.

   b. Reminder rules usually consist of a decision point/issue (e.g., a particular patient condition such as heart failure readmission) and a predetermined required response to the issue (e.g., complete a readmission quality review).

   c. The success of reminder rules depends on an organization's ability to identify, analyze, and select a set of simple principles for building them.

4. Electronic transfer or sharing of key documents—Ability to use the CMIS for discharge and transitional planning activities such as sharing specific patient documents (e.g., summary of care, requests for durable medical equipment from a vendor, or application for a skilled care facility placement) across care settings or providers as the patient transitions between care settings.

5. Communication tools to support meaningful dialogue among health care providers and with patient and family caregiver—The CMIS must enhance collaboration in real time through data sharing and text, audio, and/or video interchanges.

   a. It should be able to send electronic messages, referrals, and review requests to other users of the system.

   b. It must provide timely communication among varied levels of personnel involved in the care of the patient.

   c. It must facilitate patient activation and engagement to ultimately enhance patient's self-management abilities and adherence to care regimen.

6. Utilization management—Focus on reimbursement through electronic communications with the patient's health insurance plan. For example:

   a. Notification of admission

   b. Provision of clinical/concurrent reviews

    c. Denials and appeals management
    d. Tracking and reporting on utilization management activities including financial savings as a result of case management interventions
  7. Automated tracking of services and activities—This feature is instrumental in generating productivity reports that can be used in demonstrating the value of case management services, for example, tracking admissions, readmissions, discharge and disposition, use of durable medical equipment, transportation service requests, variances, and delays in care.

 ## Goals, Benefits, and Limitations of Case Management Information System (CMIS)

A. The goals of a CMIS are derived from the general goals of case management and the organization's mission, vision, and goals.
  1. Case management strives to create a collaborative partnership between providers of health care products and services and consumers to ensure the focus on promotion of quality cost-effective outcomes (CMSA, 2010).
  2. The system used to manage case information must allow for efficient and effective assessment, planning, facilitation, care coordination, evaluation, advocacy, and outcome measurement.
B. Case managers need timely, usable information about the client from as many sources as are available and feasible. Although case managers rely heavily on the individual and/or caregiver as the main source of information, modern interconnectivity means data are available from a variety of sources.
  1. Data are discrete facts or details. Data may not have meaning in and of themselves.
  2. Information is data interpreted to mean something in the context of a specific patient or population.
C. A CMIS should be designed for usability such that a beginning intermediate-skilled user requires minimal start up training in order to improve in proficiency level.
D. Optimally, CMIS meets or exceeds the user needs to facilitate both individual and population management care coordination needs.
  1. The traditional individual-level system includes such features as clinical workstations, physician ordering systems, clinical decision support, and drug dispensing.
  2. The population-level system is designed to support the collection and analysis of aggregate data through clinical registries, data warehouse development, provision of benchmarking data, and pharmaceutical surveillance (Weiner, Savitz, Bernard, & Pucci, 2004).
E. A well-designed CMIS will:
  1. Eliminate double-data entry by the same user; that is, data can be viewed in several places within the system and in several formats.
  2. Eliminate double-data entry by multiple users; permit data-sharing capabilities for all users with appropriate access security in place.

3. Provide the ability to run in tandem with other systems and communicate with other systems either in real time (data are accessible as soon as they are entered anywhere in the system or in a legacy system with which the CMIS is integrated) or in batch mode (data are updated on a preset timed periodic schedule); make decision-making data available in real time.
4. Provide users with the ability to access the information that is most important to them and to filter out messages, reminders, and other prompts that are not directed to them.
5. Act as central repository for all the information about a patient. Patient-centered data/information:
   a. Encompass the entire continuum of the illness or disability, such as medical history, psychosocial history, financial status, goals and problems, plan of treatment, and intervention target dates.
   b. Support the key elements of case management, including assessment, problem and goal definition, planning, monitoring, and evaluation.
   c. Are easily transmitted among different service providers.
6. Act as a central repository for population-level data for many purposes such as those described in Box 15-1.
7. CMIS allows objective, standardized reporting across the managed population by all case managers through consistent use of terminology, documentation, data management practices, outcome measurement, and reporting.
   a. A limitation in this area is a dependency because the organization must configure its CMIS in a logical and methodical manner for optimal output.
   b. Poorly thought out CMIS programming leads to work-arounds, which skew report consistency and inability to verify input.
8. CMIS provides the ability to document and retrieve case manager interventions and cost of care information and directly relate these activities to patient outcomes and cost savings. Additionally, it allows case management leaders to ascertain whether the outcomes are a direct result of the case manager coordinating the appropriate level of care, at the appropriate site, in the appropriate time frame.

BOX
15-1 **Purpose and Benefits of Population-Level Central Data Repository**

- Provide for long-term population trending and enhance outcome analysis.
- Provide health care cost details.
- Allow for better understanding of the clinical causes of patient variances including trends and patterns.
- Simplify accreditation and regulatory updates by tracking the minute details required by accreditation and regulatory agencies.
- Generate specific user-designed reports and charts to facilitate evaluation of case management goals and outcomes, aggregate relevant data and information, and set milestone reminders for regulatory agency interactions.
- Provide patient census data and case manager's caseload volume.
- Allow for automated tracking of key outcome measures (e.g., value-based purchasing core measures) and electronic reporting to regulatory agencies.

9. CMIS links the financial aspects of care with clinical data, giving organizations the advantage of knowing what the cost of care is and where specifically dollars are spent.
   a. A limitation is access to the CMIS documentation system. Such limitations may include the following:
      i. Too few input devices
      ii. Lack of or limited mobile access to CMIS
      iii. Limited technology in remote locations
10. CMIS capabilities are tailored to practice settings as documentation and reporting needs differ accordingly (Box 15-2).
11. Provide a DSS that turns data into actionable information, potentially providing additional cost savings mechanisms.
    a. Data inputs (e.g., admission reports, pharmacy utilization) must be timely in order for the resulting information to be easily retrieved and provide insights, which are usable for effective intervention.

F. The benefits of using a CMIS are divided into the categories of workflow, patient care, and organization.
   1. Workflow benefits include the following:
      a. Support of the case management process (allowing the case manager to focus on the patient and patient outcomes and not be overwhelmed by clerical tasks)

BOX 15-2   Specific CMIS Capabilities Based on Care Setting

- Hospital CMIS
  - Patient management systems (e.g., admission notification)
  - Electronic discharge/transition planning software integration supporting postacute level of care placement through sharing of information (e.g., client data, bed availability).
  - EMR integration
- Payer CMIS
  - Tracking clients across care settings and leverages claims information for triggering screening process
  - Utilization management automates authorization and continued stay reviews and procedure approval
  - High-risk trigger (e.g., multiple admissions, emergency department visits, polypharmacy)
  - Admission notification from inpatient facilities
- Long-term postacute CMIS
  - Applicability to private case management practice
  - Maintaining long-term client management records across care settings (e.g., traumatic brain injury)
- Worker's compensation and disability CMIS
  - Integration of case management with document management and data systems
  - Supporting claims management
- Accountable care organization and patient-centered medical home CMIS
  - Integration of EMR allowing cross-continuum care management
  - Secure patient–provider messaging
  - Timely receipt of discharge/transition summary
  - Personal health record connectivity

      b. Reduction of documentation duplication; elimination of double-data entry; generation of reminders or ticklers when a case manager intervention is required

      c. Improving data entry and storage

      d. Improving data access for sharing and reporting

      e. Simplifying and streamlining routine tasks

  2. Patient care benefits include the following:

      a. Mechanisms to keep patients from falling through the cracks

      b. Monitoring and recording the progress of the patient throughout the health continuum

      c. Promoting a consistent, best practice approach to managing patients with similar medical conditions

      d. Incorporating national standards and reducing the variability of case management practices

  3. Organizational benefits focus on:

      a. Enhancing the value chain by improving efficiency in the case management process

      b. Improving case manager job satisfaction; increasing staff accountability and empowerment

      c. Improving patient satisfaction

      d. Improving relationships with providers; increasing consistency in providing care

      e. Providing the ability to document and report outcomes

  4. Evaluation of the organization's capacity results from the documentation being integrated, streamlined, simplified, standardized, and reportable.

G. Limitations of the CMIS reflect not only internal limitations such as software, interfacing, and enhancements that may be lacking but also external factors such as decreased data transmission rates or bandwidth that can compromise data sharing and communication.

  1. When dealing with people, health care professions are intuitive at times as to the patient's status, and the system cannot replicate or take the place of what is sometimes called the gut factor. Guidance provided by DSS or CMIS must be carefully considered by the health care professional.

  2. Health care lags behind other industries in information management. Despite considerable progress, standardization of data across the entire health continuum has not come to fruition.

      a. In an accountable care organization (ACO) or integrated delivery system (IDS), data sharing is less of a challenge because there are fewer issues pertaining to information ownership and security.

  3. Until standardization of terminology and architecture are used throughout the care continuum, seamless information flow across the patient care continuum remains challenging.

      a. Use of Health Level Seven International (HL7) facilitates standardization.

         i. HL7 was founded in 1987 as a not-for-profit, American National Standards Institute (ANSI)–accredited standard-developing organization.

    ii. HL7 is dedicated to providing a comprehensive framework and related standards for the exchange, integration, sharing, and retrieval of electronic health information that supports clinical practice and the management, delivery, and evaluation of health services.

    iii. HL7 is supported by more than 1,600 members from over 50 countries, including 500+ corporate members representing health care providers, government stakeholders, payers, pharmaceutical companies, vendors/suppliers, and consulting firms (HL7 International, 2015).

    b. Committee for Nursing Practice Information Infrastructure (CNPII) and the Nursing Information and Data Set Evaluation Center (NIDSEC) are two American Nurses Association committees whose work concerns informatics and information system standardization.

    c. CNPII and NIDSEC are important to case management because many organizations place case management under the Department of Nursing umbrella. As software was developed, many vendors turned to NIDSEC for their seal of approval for endorsement. NIDSEC criteria are no longer in use, but it was an important step in the progression of consistency (Murphy, 2010). Table 15-1 lists accepted terminologies and classifications.

    d. The Systematized Nomenclature of Medicine (SNOMED)— SNOMED is a complete dictionary of medical terms containing the relationships between the SNOMED terms and other coding systems, such as billing codes and diagnostic codes. Requiring care providers to use the same medical terminology dictionary to capture data allows analyses to compare apples to apples. Conventions such as NANDA, Nursing Interventions Classification (NIC), and the Nursing Outcomes Classification (NOC) codes are mapped to SNOMED.

TABLE 15-1 Accepted Terminologies and Classifications

Classification	Acronym
North American Nursing Diagnosis Association, Inc.	NANDA
Nursing Interventions Classification System	NIC
Nursing Outcomes Classification System	NOC
Nursing Management Minimum Data Set	NMMDS
Clinical Care Classification (formerly HHCC)	CCC
Omaha System	
Patient Care Data Set	PCDS
Perioperative Nursing Data Set	PCDS
Systematized Nomenclature of Medicine Clinical Terms	SNOMED CT
Nursing Minimum Data Set	NMDS
International Classification of Nursing Practice	ICNP
ABC Codes	
Logical Observation Identifiers Names and Codes	LOINC

     e. The Health Insurance Portability and Accountability Act (HIPAA) mandates development of standards to facilitate the safe and protected exchange of patient information.

   4. There is no single centralized database for all patient data as the patient moves across the health care continuum and between providers. The lack of standardization makes integration, interfacing, and maintenance difficult or in some cases impossible.

 ## CMIS and Case Management Informatics in Support of Consistency and Standards of Care

A. CMIS and health care informatics for case managers support practice from identification, selection, and assignment of patients through patient assessment, identification of problems, planning, monitoring, and evaluation.

   1. Identification, selection, and assignment of patients

     a. Case managers are assigned patients according to identification and selection criteria. Additional considerations applicable in various work settings include existing caseload, area of expertise, medical unit/hospital floor, physician, or medical group practice.

     b. Case identification and selection begin the patient's enrollment into case management. However, with few exceptions (e.g., worker's compensation), case management is a voluntary intervention and a patient may refuse enrollment regardless of perceived benefits.

     c. The CMIS automatically identifies individuals eligible for case management based on predefined triggers. The individual is then screened using criteria or a brief interview to determine the suitability and willingness to participate in case management.

     d. Risk stratification software allows the grouping of patients into risk categories such as low, moderate, and high. It also supports prioritization of potential clients based on variety of information rather than simple diagnosis or event trigger, which creates more efficient screening and selection process. Prioritization is based on the risk category information generated automatically by the system, despite that case managers have the ability to override a patient's category.

     e. Predictive modeling supports risk stratification of potential clients prior to actual major health events based on artificial intelligence, algorithmic logic, or combination of technologies.

   2. Patient assessment

     a. Provides the case manager with a method of conducting a thorough and objective analysis of the patient's status. The case manager performs baseline and ongoing assessments, utilizes evidence-based specialty assessment tools, administers patient satisfaction surveys, and performs clinical status reviews with the patient's care team.

     b. CMIS provides a mechanism for data entry and tracks changes in patient status and response to case management interventions over the period of time that a case manager is involved in care coordination.

   c. An integral part of the selection and assessment process is to move patients with a particular disease or condition into homogeneous subgroups, called stratification groups.
     i. The system guides the user through the stratification process, applying criteria as appropriate and available, to reduce subjectivity and variability.
     ii. Patients move from one stratification group to another as the illness progresses. This reclassification may be a background function of the CMIS based on information input to the CMIS.
     iii. The CMIS alerts the case manager to stratification changes for their patients. The CMIS also alerts the case manager to patient assessment results that require immediate attention.
3. Identification of problems
   a. Problems are issues, circumstances, or barriers affecting the health and/or functioning of the patient or causing a detrimental effect on their care.
     i. Default problems may automatically generate to a patient record based on the patient's illness or response to an assessment question.
     ii. Patient problems may filter through an artificial intelligence (AI) system built into the CMIS, which further refines appropriate case management strategies for the individual.
     iii. AI may be a computer or IS. An expert system processes huge amounts of data (or information) and draws conclusions based on the input.
     iv. Patient problems may be aggregated into a database to evaluate appropriate interventions and desired outcomes. This helps establish the case-specific return on investment (ROI).
4. Planning
   a. The identification of short-, intermediate-, and long-term as well as ongoing needs. Planning is completed with prioritization of needs and a timeline in which to address them.
   b. CMIS allows for coordination of patient-centered goals that are devised in many ways. For example:
     i. Return to work with occupational therapy
     ii. Endurance improvement to complete simple housekeeping chores and meal preparation with comprehensive therapies
     iii. Stabilization of diabetic status with condition education including proper use and administration of insulin
   c. CMIS tracks the status of goal achievement.
     i. By using AI, goals may be defined by the system based on the patient's diagnosis and the subgroup to which they have been assigned.
     ii. The AI-generated plan is closely evaluated and monitored by a case manager to verify that actual patient's needs are addressed appropriately and in a timely manner.
5. Monitoring
   a. The case manager employs ongoing assessment and documentation to measure the client's response to the case management plan (CMSA, 2010).

    b. Throughout the continuum of care, the case manager monitors and assesses the patient's status as well as collects information regarding the delivery of services.

    c. Sometimes, patients fall through the cracks due to a lack of provider follow-up as well as lack of patient understanding as to the importance of his/her treatment (e.g., medication, medical care).

       i. The case manager plays a vital role in proactively monitoring the patient as he or she progresses through critical junctures in the course of the disease.

       ii. The AI-generated case management plan uses preset parameters to define and schedule time-critical interventions.

       iii. The case manager actively monitors and verifies that planned interventions are implemented in a timely manner.

6. Evaluation

    a. The case management process requires continuous evaluation. Ongoing evaluation and response to interventions and medical treatment help to refine case management goals.

    b. Failure to meet anticipated milestones provides the opportunity to re-evaluate interventions and may result in modification of goals or new problems, which require action.

    c. The CMIS supports evaluation of the case management plan. Evaluation is more meaningful and effective when status and outcomes can be measured consistently and objectively.

    d. Upon each evaluation, the intervention plan is validated as accurate when milestones and goals are deemed accomplished. If milestones are missed, the CMIS allows for modification to the plan.

    e. This is a dynamic process through which the case manager, patient, and care team work together. The CMIS is a valuable tool in this regard.

    f. The case manager must constantly review and evaluate the process because the CMIS is a tool. It requires a knowledgeable professional case management to carry out the proposed interventions.

    g. When the CMIS misses targets or proposes interventions, which are not applicable for a patient, it is the case manager who reports occurrences in an objective manner and including evidence of the issue (e.g., supportive documentation like screenshots). The case manager is instrumental in ensuring necessary changes are made within the CMIS to enhance and improve patient care quality.

B. CMIS and health care informatics support the tracking and analysis of outcomes.

1. Patient outcomes are defined in a variety of ways, depending on what elements of the patient's health status the case manager has the ability to affect.

2. The same data provide different views of a situation depending upon the user and the way in which the data are presented.

    a. A CMIS reports how many patients have met a particular goal (e.g., understanding their disease process) within the target date period. Tracking and analysis occur at various levels within the organization:

       i. The case manager looks at the data to determine whether his or her intervention strategy with the patient was appropriate.

      ii. The medical director looks at the results of assessments. For example, because the patient was unable to recite the basic aspects and goals of his or her treatment, it is determined that the providers were not adequately explaining the disease to the patient or involving him or her in the treatment plan.

     iii. The case management director identifies that the target date of the goal was too aggressive, based on the target population.

     iv. The health plan uses the data to support the development of a disease management program for the specific disease to promote patient education and improve outcomes.

3. There are different ways a CMIS measures patient outcomes (Box 15-3). The most important measures come from the client and caregiver, their involvement in goal setting, perception of the outcome, health status improvement, satisfaction with care, and level of self-sufficiency.

4. Value-based purchasing concerns

    a. CMS requires hospitals to attain performance levels in order to obtain optimal reimbursement. Evaluation measures highlight process of care, patient experience, efficiency, and outcomes.

BOX 15-3   CMIS Contribution to Measuring Patient Care Outcomes

- Medical
  - Readmission rates
  - Emergency department visits signifying treatment failure
  - Exacerbations of condition and symptoms
  - Complications
  - Clinic visit interval and length
  - Lengths of stay (LOS)
  - Mortality
- Case management
  - Defined processes followed
  - Goals met/not met
  - Variance/delays in care reporting
  - Time-dependent interventions completed (turnaround time)
  - Adherence to health regimen improved (patient and provider)
  - Patient's health knowledge improved
- Patient
  - Improved quality of life
  - Satisfaction with provider and the care received
  - Empowerment and engagement
  - Activation
- Organizational
  - Value chain evaluation
  - Cost savings
  - Population profiling
  - Improved working relationships
  - Improved image and reputation in the community

b. Integrated software (e.g., calculators) analyzes a facility's clinical quality measures, performance scores, and other outcomes to provide VBP feedback for required measures. This also allows for mock testing of various scenarios, which provide possible solutions and improvement suggestions.

Using CMIS to Measure Effectiveness of Case Management Interventions

A. Technology makes it possible to measure the effectiveness of case management outcomes. Consumer demand for high-quality affordable care, organizational return-on-investment assessments, and the reality that health care resources are finite, makes it necessary for the case manager to become an active contributor to revenue goals through knowledgeable, responsible, efficient, and effective practice.

B. Health care is about providing outcome-based care and sharing evidence to build the basis for further investments in technology, staffing, and other tools and resources.

C. In order to succeed, an organization needs buy-in at all management levels and belief in the value of outcome-based practice. This does not mean that everything that came before should be discarded.
   1. The contrary, the value of existing tools must be identified and integrated into the overall strategy.
   2. Automated tools facilitate evidence-based practice through integration of the various pieces (e.g., clinical pathways, protocols, patient data, case manager data, physician data, financial data, evaluative strategies, criteria)

D. Dollar amounts linked to the patient data and case management practice, which apply financial formulas automatically in the system.

E. Cost–benefit analysis is an approach that demonstrates the benefits of case management involvement in patient care. Cost should not drive practice; however, in a world that is cost-containment oriented, case managers are aware that their involvement in a patient's care must reflect a benefit, which is demonstrated in tangible savings.

F. Organizations focus on the high-cost, high-risk, complex cases to show the most benefit; but the day-to-day benefit on all case-managed patients may be considered using a cost–benefit analysis methodology.

G. Organizations must establish a dollar amount for the tangible and intangible benefits of case management as well as the costs. This process can be automated using technology thus eliminating the time-consuming process of manual tracking and calculation.

H. Cost–benefit analysis and other ROI methodologies are vital to promoting case management and improving patient care. These strategies should be automated using CMIS technology.

The Evolution and Delivery of Telehealth Interventions

A. Telehealth (TH) is the use of electronic information and telecommunications technologies to support long-distance clinical health care, patient and professional health-related education, public health, and health administration. Technologies may include videoconferencing, the Internet, store-and-forward imaging, streaming media, and terrestrial and wireless communications (Health Resources and Services Administration [HRSA], 2015).

B. For the purpose of this text, TH is meant as inclusive of telemedicine (TM) and telemental health (TMH).

C. By 2000, health care videoconferencing was more common in rural areas, but far from routine. The spread of TH has been impeded by a number of factors, the most oppressive influences were as follows:
  1. Restrictions in Medicare, Medicaid, and private insurance reimbursement
  2. Requirement to purchase a dedicated, hardware-based videoconferencing system
  3. Reliance on grants to launch and sustain programs

D. TH efforts continue to flourish because it brings primary care physicians to locations, which would otherwise lack clinical care because of the difficulties associated with individuals traveling great distances. Telemental health promises to take a similar path, but slower. Some argue this is an even more urgently needed expansion.

E. TH enables specialty care access where clinical expertise does not exist. It also addresses the cost of health care in that the cost of the tele-encounter requires less consumption of resources associated with having multiple satellite offices.
  1. The Internet, as well as wireless technology, have evolved and become less costly.
  2. Legislation and regulations around meaningful use of electronic health records have spurred more rapid development and deployment. Payment for non–face-to-face encounters and care coordination activities has finally started to become more the norm rather than the exception.
  3. Accountable care organizations and other initiatives pushed the quality care agenda forward, which recognizes the importance of care continuity through various means of communication.
  4. The general public's demand for improved connectivity to health care providers has also influenced progress in use of TH.

F. For the case manager, TH may include simple telephonic contact (e.g., telephone triage, a monitoring call pertaining to medication adherence, a blood pressure or blood sugar check) for the purpose of following up on care and monitoring of patient's condition.
  1. Incorporating long-term monitoring into the case manager's repertoire enhances patient care outcomes and offers patients with support along the continuum of care.
  2. Monitoring also provides valuable information for the case manager to clearly document outcomes and return on investment.

G. In addition to traditional means (e.g., hard copy letters, telephone), case managers use various HIPAA-compliant means to contact the client and other members of the health care team. For example:
  1. E-mail and online messaging
  2. Text messaging using mobile phones
  3. Video-chats (e.g., Skype).

Telehealth Legislation

A. As of February 3, 2016, there were over twenty pieces of legislation introduced in the 114th US Congress addressing a variety of initiatives inclusive of TH activity (American Telemedicine Association, 2016). The 113th US Congress saw over 55 pieces of legislation introduced.

    1. Listing the current inventory of TH-related legislation herein not only is unreasonable but also becomes quickly outdated. The informed case manager is encouraged to investigate legislative and regulatory updates pertinent to his/her area of practice to maintain current knowledge.

    2. Special interest areas, which have been included in legislation, highlight:

        a. Reimbursement of TH services

        b. Parity of reimbursement for TH services

        c. Removal of geographic barriers in place for currently recognized TH services

        d. Removal of licensure limitations for recognized Medicare providers to treat beneficiaries across state lines

           i. This would allow providers to practice across state lines without requiring separate licensure in each state and enhances patient choice for which provider to choose for obtaining services.

           ii. A bill known as TELEmedicine for MEDicare Act of 2013 (TELE-MED Act of 2013) is an example of bills that address the issue of licensure and practice across state lines. This particular bill died in the 113th Congress. It was reintroduced in the 114th Congress and was referred to subcommittees in both House and Senate (Congress.gov, 2016).

        e. Requirement that TM services be cost neutral or provide savings in order to seek reimbursement from CMS

B. With few exceptions (e.g., military, veteran health), there is a lack of national policy for the use of TH. This highlights licensure and scope of practice limitations plaguing licensed clinical professionals for decades.

    1. Congress considered legislation to allow Medicare-recognized providers to practice TH services across state lines without requiring separate state licensure.

        a. A case manager is not a Medicare-recognized provider unless she/he meets defined criteria and has an individual billing number. The majority of today's case managers are registered nurses and social workers and are not considered Medicare-recognized providers.

        b. As required by the Balanced Budget Act of 1997, all nurse practitioners, clinical nurse specialists, and physician assistants must have their own billing number in order to bill Medicare, even if they are employed and even if their employer has always billed for their services using the employer's billing number (American Association of Nurse Practitioners, 2013).

        c. Case managers, not Medicare-recognized providers, were not included in the scope of this proposed legislation. Therefore, issues of licensure-related barriers to practice affecting thousands of case managers working in managed care and other settings, which require interstate contact with clients, remain in place.

C. Many practice issues need to be addressed in legislation and regulation, including the following:
   1. Interstate and international practice
   2. Reimbursement schema for independent case managers
   3. Protection from fraud and abuse

 Barriers to Telehealth

A. Early on, the barriers to TH were higher-level concerns such as the following:
   1. Potential breakdown in the relationship between health professional and patient (especially depersonalization) and among health professionals
   2. Issues related to the accuracy and quality of health information
   3. Organizational (resistance to change) and bureaucratic issues (Hjelm, 2005)
B. Because HITECH pushed technology implementation forward, contemporary barriers are more in the form of usability concerns, such as those listed in Box 15-4 and based on Foster and Sethares (2014).
C. Telehealth Security and Privacy
   1. The success of TH could be undermined due to security and privacy risks. Failing adequate protections, providers and patients do not trust TH solutions. No federal agency has authority to enact TH privacy and security requirements.
   2. Highlights of privacy and security risks of telehealth are described in Box 15-5 and based on Hall and McGraw (2014).
   3. HIPAA routinely requires implementation of security precautions. However, privacy and security measures are not consistently observed, for example, when one end of the communication is a device that sends signals to a physician or a health app that endpoint falls outside of HIPAA-regulated clinical care.
   4. The case manager's role with regard to TH security and privacy is focused on ensuring that the means used to communicate with a client are secured and in compliance with organizational policy.
   5. Education of the patient and caregiver as to privacy and security issues relating to use of technology may be included in any applicable discussion.

BOX 15-4   Contemporary Usability Concerns of Health Technology

1. Font size, unusual characters (difficult to read).
2. Graphics and poor color contrast.
3. Using devices requiring fine motor eye–hand coordination.
4. Use of hand-operated mouse is difficult to use with arthritic hands.
5. Lack of experience or skill in the use of a smartphone or a computer.
6. Too many screen transitions to complete a task.
7. Menu bars that contain several layers.
8. Inappropriate size of a smartphone (too big or too small; frail patients who have diminished grip strength may have problems handling the device).

BOX 15-5 Privacy and Security Risks in Telehealth

Privacy risks of TH
- Lack of controls or limits on the collection, use, and disclosure of sensitive personal information.
- Sensors that are located in a patient's home or that interface with the patient's body to detect safety issues or medical emergencies may inadvertently collect sensitive information about household activities.
- Routine transmissions from a medical device may be collected and stored by the manufacturer rather than a health care provider.
- Device or application information may feed information to a third-party advertiser for directed marketing based on patient use.

Security risks of TH
- Provider-to-provider communication may have limited security.
- Breach of confidentiality during collection or transmission of sensitive data.
- Unauthorized access to the functionality of supporting devices as well as to data stored on them.
- Distribution of software and hardware to the patient from untrustworthy sources.

D. The Digital Divide
   1. Equality of access to computers and the Internet and the acquisition of skills necessary to become proficient may be barriers to the implementation of TH.
   2. The case manager inquires about use of computers and electronic communication as part of patient assessment to ensure information intended for the patient is communicated using the most appropriate means available.
   3. There is a temptation to make all educational materials available via secure Web site or sent through electronic mail. These materials should be available in hard copy form in the event that an individual does not have reliable Internet access.
E. Cost
   1. TH equipment and service costs are borne by health care providers (e.g., individuals, institutions).
   2. Vendor rates must be evaluated prior to installing equipment in a patient's home.
   3. Many smartphone apps downloaded by patients are free or very low cost. However, the cost in security and privacy of personal information has not yet been quantified.
   4. The case manager may be asked to provide patient education with regard to the use of TH applications or devices. Seek guidance from organizational policy before providing specific details.
F. Reimbursement for services
   1. TH services are increasingly reimbursed by major payers. While some geographic limitations remain in place, legislation has been introduced to remove such barriers.
   2. Reimbursement parity and the budget neutrality for all new reimbursement requests are drivers in the expansion of TH utility.
   3. Continued payer adaptation is necessary as technology surges forward.

G. Licensure concerns for telehealth for case managers
1. The lack of national policy for interstate practice affects the use of TH technology in case management practice. The case manager's individual licensure (or certification in some jurisdictions) is the primary driver for TH practice limitation.
2. Regardless of one's employment status, the case manager must maintain current knowledge regarding licensure status and requirements pertaining to clinical practice.
3. The case manager should consult the Board of Registration (or like regulatory body) within their license jurisdiction for specific information pertaining to TH and interstate practice issues.
H. Standard of care issues
1. Individual licensure, certification, or professional association affiliation are the most frequent drivers of practice standards. However, care standards are driven by evidence-based guidance.
2. Community standards vary more widely and should be of concern to the prescribing provider whereas the case manager should be cognizant of care standards, which are applicable in the patient's geographic region.
3. Liability is an issue. Clinical professionals maintain individual licensure and/or certification. The case manager must understand his/her individual liability for TH practice apart from their employer's guidance. Failing to comply with one's practice act risks one's licensure. This becomes especially important in malpractice issues. TH practice outside of one's scope of practice = practicing without a license. It is likely that one's personal liability protection would not cover such practice.

Evaluation of Web Sites for Professional and Patient Use

A. The Health On the Net Foundation (HON) promotes and guides the deployment of useful and reliable online health information and its appropriate and efficient use. Created in 1995, HON is a nonprofit, nongovernmental organization, accredited to the Economic and Social Council of the United Nations (Health On the Net Foundation, 2015).
B. HONcode certification demonstrates a Web site's intent to publish transparent information. The transparency of the Web site improves its usefulness and the objectivity of the information.
1. There is an initial certification process to which each Web site subjects itself. There is ongoing monitoring conducted as well.
2. The HONcode is the most widely accepted reference for online health and medical publishers. As of August 2015, the HONcode is used by over 7,300 certified Web sites, more than 10 million pages, covering 102 countries (Health On the Net Foundation).
C. The evaluation process for health-related Web sites follows a consistent process. Box 15-6 lists the focus of the validation process when using a Web site or considering one for patient reference (Sewell & Thedes, 2013).
D. The case manager may have to comply with organizational policy pertaining to use of Web sites in patient education. However, it is

BOX
15-6 **Areas of Focus in the Evaluation of Health Web sites**

- Source
    - Who sponsors the Web site?
    - Who owns the Web site?
- Funding
    - Who authors the content? Credentials? Expertise on topic? Is author qualified to write on topic?
    - Author affiliation(s)? Able to contact author?
    - Commercially funded site? Conflict of interest present? Advertisers on site? Advertisers clearly labeled?
- Validity and quality
    - Date of last information update?
    - Clear purpose of site?
    - Is information accurate and appropriately referenced to scholarly sources?
    - Is information peer-reviewed or verified by a qualified editor?
    - Is information free from bias and opinion?
    - Do all links function properly?
- Privacy
    - Does site include a privacy statement that is easy to understand?
    - Does site include a recognized privacy standard (e.g., Health On The Net)?

essential that each case manager maintains professional approach to evaluating the Web site sources he/she refers to for clinical information. The HONcode provides a seal of approval but individual verification using a consistent approach to evaluation is important as well.

HIT Solutions in Support of Case Management

A. The expansion of technology throughout health care delivery is supported by the HITECH, a section within the American Recovery and Reinvestment Act of 2009 (ARRA). One of the most important concepts within ARRA was that in order to qualify for the financial incentive, providers had to demonstrate meaningful use of technology.

B. The Centers for Medicare and Medicaid Services define meaningful use as using certified EHR technology to achieve health and efficiency goals. However, the definition of meaningful use was modified in different stages of the EHR Incentive Program. Basically, meaningful use intent was that providers were able to demonstrate they were using certified EHR technology in ways that could be measured in terms of quality and quantity.

C. HIT is not foolproof and, as a result, will require human oversight and clinical implementation as part of its adoption: completely safe technology is not assured.

D. There are two areas where adherence management and technology users intersect:

   1. Provider use of clinical guidelines in monitoring and prescribing treatment

      a. Clinical algorithms and other tools built into the EHR support evidence-based decision making for prescribing the most appropriate treatment for each patient.

2. Patient use technology to learn about health conditions and adhere to prescribed treatment, such as the following:
   a. Use of the Internet to investigate health condition and medication information
   b. Use of tools to assess and monitor health and treatment
      i. Keeping an activity log
      ii. Tracking blood pressure or blood sugars
      iii. Review provider and/or hospital quality ratings
      iv. Use of mobile applications to manage diet, exercise, blood sugars, etc.
3. People track tremendous amount of health-related information (e.g., exercise, diet) to which providers have limited if any access or knowledge. Patient-centered care where the individual is an equal member of their own care team will begin to leverage this, and other patient-generated information, in order to actively engage with the individual's health activities.
4. An astute case manager inquires as to these activities in order to document patient engagement and incorporate patient-provided findings in the case management plan.

E. Medication reconciliation is a process where all medications taken by a patient are reconciled, that is, examined and monitored for compatibility, necessity, and safety across the continuum of care. The goal is to reduce the number of adverse drug events and resulting avoidable health care costs.
1. Technology prompts the case manager to complete list of all medications (including over-the-counter and herbal supplements and vitamins) as part of an initial assessment.
2. This record is compared to pharmacy records, prescription bottles, physician orders, and other source of information to evaluate accuracy in the patient's medication regimen. A sophisticated EHR also identifies discrepancies, potential medication interactions, and other issues requiring attention and possible resolution and brings the information to the attention of the user.
   a. The case manager utilizes this information to communicate medication issues to other care team members in support of medication reconciliation.
   b. It may be the responsibility of a pharmacist to complete the reconciliation process; however, the case manager should be vigilant of medication-related issues in order to provide appropriate patient education and care team communication.

References

American Association of Nurse Practitioners (AANP). (2013). *Medicare update.* Retrieved from http://www.aanp.org/legislation-regulation/federal-legislation/medicare/68-articles/326-medicare-update, on August 9, 2015.

American Telemedicine Association. (2016). *Telemedicine/telehealth bills in the 114th Congress.* Retrieved from http://www.americantelemed.org/docs/default-source/policy/ata-doc-114th-congress-bills.pdf?sfvrsn=2, on April 8, 2016.

Case Management Society of America. (2010). *Standards of practice for case management.* Little Rock, AR: Author.

Congress.gov. (2016). *TELEmedicine for MEDicare Act (TELE-MED Act)*. Retrieved from https://www.congress.gov/bill/114th-congress/house-bill/3081, on April 8, 2016.

Dietzen, J. (1997). Decision support systems: Technology enhancing case management. *The Journal of Case Management, 3*(6), 12–17.

Foster, M. V., & Sethares, K. A. (2014). Facilitators and barriers to the adoption of telehealth in older adults: An integrative review. *Computers, Informatics, and Nursing, 32*, 523–533. Retrieved on August 9, 2015. doi: 10.1037/0003-066X.59.1.29

Hall, J. L., & McGraw, D. (2014). For telehealth to succeed, privacy and security risks must be identified and addressed. *Health Affairs, 33*(2), 216–221. Retrieved from http://content.healthaffairs.org/content/33/2/216.full.pdf, on August 9, 2015.

Health On the Net Foundation. (2015). *Health on the net*. Retrieved from https://www.healthonnet.org, on August 9, 2015.

Health Resources and Services Administration. (2015). *What is telehealth?* Retrieved from http://www.hrsa.gov/ruralhealth/about/telehealth, on August 9, 2015.

Hjelm, N. M. (2005). Benefits and drawbacks of telemedicine. *Journal of Telemedicine and Telecare, 11*(2), 60–70. doi: 10.1258/1357633053499886.

HL7 International. (2015). *About HL7*. Retrieved from http://www.hl7.org/about/index.cfm?ref=common, on August 7, 2015.

Murphy, J. (2010). Nursing informatics: The intersection of nursing, computer, and information sciences. *Nursing Economics, 28*(3), 204–207. Retrieved from http://search.proquest.com.contentproxy.phoenix.edu/docview/577364695?accountid=458, on August 5, 2015.

Sewell, J., & Thede, L. Q. (2013). *Glossary of informatics and nursing: Opportunities and challenges* (4th ed.). Retrieved from http://dlthede.net/informatics/glossary.html, on August 4, 2015.

Weiner, B., Savitz, L., Bernard, S., & Pucci, L. (2004). How do integrated delivery systems adopt and implement clinical information systems? *Health Care Management Review, 29*(1), 51–66. Retrieved ABI/INFORM Global database (Document ID: 543097111).

CHAPTER 16

Case Manager's Role Leadership and Accountability

Suzanne K. Powell and Hussein M. Tahan

LEARNING OBJECTIVES

Upon completion of this chapter, the reader will be able to:

1. Define leadership and leadership style.
2. List four essential components of effective leadership.
3. Explain how case managers demonstrate role accountability.
4. Differentiate between aggressive and cooperative negotiation.
5. Describe components of emotional intelligence.
6. Identify key critical thinking strategies and skills for case managers.
7. Describe the role of the case manager in delegation and supervision.
8. Compare and contrast hard and soft savings.
9. Discuss the role of the case manager as an agent of change.
10. Describe motivational interviewing and its use in case management.

IMPORTANT TERMS AND CONCEPTS

Accountability
Change Agent
Communication
Conflict Management
Cost–Benefit Analysis
Critical Thinking

Delegation
Emotional Intelligence
Empowerment
Hard Savings
Leadership

Motivational
Interviewing
Negotiation
Soft Savings
Succession Planning

Introduction

A. Case management requires a wide array of management skills: accountability, delegation, conflict resolution, crisis intervention, collaboration, consultation, coordination, communication, motivational interviewing, advocacy, and documentation. However, case managers are no longer just managers of care.
   1. Case managers are leaders, and there is a difference. *Managers manage systems; leaders lead people.*
   2. Case managers do both; they manage cases (a number of clients) and lead, or guide, people.
   3. Leadership is one step up the ladder of professional growth and development. As case management responsibilities continue to grow, leadership qualities will necessarily be presumed (Powell, 2000a).
B. Management and leadership are *not* the same thing; they are not synonyms, and case managers must recognize the difference.
   1. A *manager* is an individual who holds an office—attached to which are multiple roles.
   2. *Leadership* is one of those roles (Shortell & Kaluzny, 2000).
C. Leadership is about the ability to influence people (e.g., clients, health care professionals) to accomplish goals. Leaders can be *formal* (by their position in the organization or society) or *informal* (by the amount of influence they have on others). Case managers are constantly in a position to influence people to accomplish health care goals, and sometimes they are leaders by virtue of their positions.
D. Leadership is defined as a process by which an individual exerts influence over other people and inspires, motivates, supports, and directs their activities to help achieve individual, group, or organization goals. Effective leadership is demonstrated when a leader assists others to realize their potential and creates opportunities for them to excel and contribute to a higher purpose or bigger cause.
E. Six core components within the definition of leadership expound on the description (Shortell & Kaluzny, 2000) (Box 16-1).
F. How the above definition and criteria relate to case management roles and responsibilities:

BOX 16-1 Core Components of Leadership

1. Leading is a *process,* an action word, a verb.
2. The *locus* of leadership is a person; only individuals (as opposed to corporations or inanimate objects) can lead.
3. The *focus* of leadership is other people or groups. This connection must exist for leadership to take place.
4. Leadership necessitates *influencing.* It is the leader's ability to influence others that sets apart an effective leader from an ineffective one. This may be the most critical of the leadership components.
5. The object of leadership is *goal accomplishment.*
6. Leadership is *intentional,* not accidental.
7. Leadership is about *inspiring* others to achieve their maximum potential.

1. Case management is a process where the case manager (the leader) must assess multiple variables that relate to the patient, the family, the disease process, the treatment, the insurance, the psychosocial situation, the desired goals and outcomes, and the interdisciplinary health care team.
2. The goals chosen are the road map for the creation of best outcomes; the case manager must intentionally influence the situation to bring about the best outcomes for the patient and family.
3. The ability to influence others may be the case manager's "center of gravity" and most critical skill. Influence is a multipronged concept. On a daily basis, case managers intentionally influence patients/ families, for example, to take appropriate medications, to think carefully about possible treatment choices, or to eat a diet that is best for their disease state. Case managers also influence insurance companies, and other important health care team members.

Descriptions of Key Terms

A. Accountability—Feeling, having the willingness to, and acting with a true sense of obligation toward others, one's role, organization, and society.
B. Critical thinking—Purposeful, outcome-directed thinking that aims to make judgments based on facts and is based on scientific principles. It is an intellectually disciplined process of actively and skillfully conceptualizing, applying, analyzing, synthesizing, and/or evaluating information gathered or generated from observation, experience, reflection, reasoning, or communication, as a guide to belief and action.
C. Delegation—The process of assigning tasks to a qualified person and supervising that individual as needed.
D. Emotional intelligence—Also called EI or EQ; describes an ability, capacity, or skill to perceive, assess, and manage the emotions of one's self, of others, and of groups.
E. Empowerment—Allowing employees or subordinates to make decisions with support from the leader or manager.
F. Hard savings—Occur when costs can be measurably saved or avoided.
G. Leadership—A process by which an individual exerts influence over other people and inspires, motivates, and directs their activities to help achieve group or organization goals.
H. Motivational interviewing—A counseling-like and purposeful style of interaction that aims to facilitate and engage intrinsic motivation and desire within the client in order to change behavior. This method is goal-oriented, client-centered communication that is able to elicit lifestyle behavior change by assisting the client to explore and resolve existing ambivalence or fear of uncertainty.
I. Negotiation—Essentially a communication exchange for the purpose of reaching agreement.
J. Soft savings—Also called potential savings (or potential costs or charges); are less tangibly measurable than are hard savings (see hard savings, above).
K. Succession planning—Is a process for identifying and developing internal people with the potential to fill key leadership positions in

an organization or department. Succession planning increases the availability of experienced and capable professionals who are prepared to assume leadership roles as they become available.

Applicability to CMSA's Standards of Practice

A. The Case Management Society of America (CMSA) describes in its standards of practice for management that case management extends across all health care settings (e.g., preacute, acute, postacute) and various professional disciplines such as nursing, social work, pharmacy, vocational rehabilitation counseling, and others (CMSA, 2010).
   1. Leadership, responsibility, and accountability for effective practice are then a priority for every involved health care professional, especially case managers, and in every care or work setting.
   2. Leadership and accountability in areas of change management, performance improvement, communication, emotional intelligence, motivational interviewing, negotiation, and conflict resolution are among important skills of successful case managers. These allow case managers to have productive and effective relationships with patients, families, other health care professionals, and peers.
B. The CMSA standards of practice for case management describe a number of case manager's roles, functions, and activities where the topics addressed in this chapter are necessary for case manager's success in these roles. Examples of these functions and activities are the following:
   1. Conducting a comprehensive assessment of the client's health and psychosocial needs, including health literacy status and deficits
   2. Development of a case management plan collaboratively with the client and family or caregiver, as well as other health care professionals
   3. Planning care with the client, family or caregiver, other health care professionals, and the payer to maximize quality, safety, cost-effective outcomes, and access to services
   4. Assisting the client in the safe transition of care to the next most appropriate level or provider
   5. Promotion of the client's self-determination, self-advocacy, informed and shared decision-making, and autonomy (CMSA, 2010)
C. Leadership and accountability are necessary for effective facilitation of communication and coordination among members of the health care team, involving the client in the decision-making process in order to minimize fragmentation in the services.
D. Leadership and accountability are also important traits of case managers for use in empowering the client to problem-solve and explore options of care and alternative plans to achieve desired outcomes.
E. The CMSA standards of practice cite "advocating for both the client and the payer to facilitate positive outcomes for the client, the health care team, and the payer" (CMSA, 2010, p. 14) as a case manager's role.
   1. Leadership and accountability are important skills for case managers to be effective in executing this responsibility.
   2. These skills are even more important when a conflict arises and case managers are expected to resolve it while advocating for the patient

and placing the patient's interests above all. The standards state "if a conflict arises, the needs of the client must be the priority" (CMSA, 2010, p. 14).

F. "The case manager should be aware of, and responsive to, cultural and demographic diversity of the population and specific client profiles" (CMSA, 2010, p. 22). Communication and conflict resolution skills, discussed in this chapter, are necessary for meeting the expectation of cultural competency in the provision of care, especially delivery of patient-centered care.

G. Motivational interviewing (MI) is an essential skill case managers must possess to influence patient's healthy lifestyle behavior. It is an approach case managers should use to impact patient's self-management skills and abilities and to overcome undesired situations or behaviors patients may exhibit, such as those included in the CMSA standards of practice for case management. For example:
   1. Nonadherence to plan of care (e.g., medication adherence)
   2. Lack of health education or understanding by patients in areas such as disease processes, medication lists, insurance benefits, and community resources
   3. Lack of a support system or presence of a support system, especially when under stress
   4. Patterns of care or behavior that may be associated with increased severity of condition (CMSA, 2010)

H. The case manager should maximize the client's health, wellness, safety, adaptation, and self-care through quality case management, client satisfaction and optimal care experience, and cost-efficiency. Case managers' leadership and accountability enhances performance in this role responsibility.

Accountability

A. Case managers cannot lead or influence others without accountability. They are able to demonstrate accountability in many ways, such as those shared in Box 16-2.

B. Case managers in their roles as managers, facilitators, and coordinators of care and client advocates pay careful attention to and apply the

BOX 16-2   Examples of How Case Managers Exhibit Role Accountability

- Accepting responsibility to act
- Owning their actions and their impact on achieving desired outcomes
- Willingness to collaborate with the client/support system and other members of health care teams
- Obligation to answer, respond to, or report on the outcomes of their own actions
- Safeguarding the client and public interest: quality, safety, cost-effectiveness, and timely access to necessary health care services
- Taking initiative, identifying opportunities for improvement in systems of care, and effective desirable change
- Advocating for clients and their support systems

> **BOX 16-3**   **Aspects of Accountability in Case Management**
>
> - Leadership
> - Moral
> - Ethical
> - Legal
> - Relationships
> - Quality and safety
> - Cost-effectiveness
> - Professional
> - Organizational
> - Political
> - Health and public policy

various aspects of role accountability to effect desirable outcomes (quality, safety, cost, and access to care) and maintain successful relationships with fellow health care professionals and clients/families (Box 16-3).

C. Successful case managers are accountable for own professional development, advancement, and growth. They are also responsible for promoting an environment of professional practice.

D. As part of their accountability, case managers assure the provision of care in accordance with ethical, regulatory, accreditation, and evidence-based standards. They also adhere to the scope and standards of their professional organizations such as CMSA.

E. Case management leaders and executives have an obligation for succession planning. Because of the continued lack of academic programs that prepare health care professionals for the roles of case managers and case management leaders, it is important for those in leadership positions to develop mentoring and coaching programs to create new talent and assure succession planning.

Leadership Styles

A. A leader's style is often based on a combination of beliefs, values, personal traits, and preferences, in addition to the leader's organization's culture and norms, which will encourage some styles and discourage others.

B. There are several styles of leadership (Box 16-4). Case managers use these styles differently, depending on the situation and the role they are playing at the time. However, personality traits may make one or two styles predominant (or nonexistent).

C. Authentic leadership—An approach to leadership that emphasizes building the leader's legitimacy through honest, open, and transparent relationships with followers, which value their input and are built on an ethical foundation. Generally, authentic leaders are positive people with truthful self-concepts who promote openness (Wikipedia, 2015b).

1. Characteristics of authentic leaders include the following (Kruse, 2013):

16-4 **Various Leadership Styles Case Managers May Use**

- Authentic leadership
- Charismatic leadership
- Participative leadership
- Situational leadership
- Transactional leadership
- Transformational leadership
- Quiet leadership
- Servant leadership

    a. Self-awareness and genuine attitude. Authentic leaders are self-actualized individuals who are aware of their strengths, their limitations, and their emotions. They also show their real selves to their followers. They do not act one way in private and another in public; they don't hide their mistakes or weaknesses out of fear of looking weak.

    b. Being mission driven and focused on results. Authentic leaders are able to put the mission and the goals of the organization ahead of their own self-interest.

    c. Leading with the heart, not just with the mind. Authentic leaders are not afraid to show their emotions and their vulnerability and to connect with their employees. This does not mean authentic leaders are "soft." In fact, communicating in a direct manner is critical to successful outcomes, but it's done with empathy; directness without empathy is cruel.

    d. Focus on the long-term goals and vision, and be future oriented in actions and plans.

  2. Key components of authentic leadership are self-awareness, relational transparency, balanced processing, and internalized moral perspective. These allow leaders to have the capacity to understand personal strengths, limitations, opportunities for improvement or further development, and impact on others (Shirey, 2015).

    a. Self-awareness requires the leaders to pursue self-discovery, self-improvement, reflection, and renewal. These demonstrate the leader's understanding of the world around them.

    b. Relational transparency refers to the leader's ability to present his/her true self when engaging with others, be genuine, and share openly.

    c. Balanced processing focuses on maintaining objectivity, seeking out pertinent insights, and ensuring nothing important is missing before making final decisions.

    d. Internalized moral perspective allows the leader to adhere to ethical and moral standards; to demonstrate integrity, self-regulation, and alignment of own behaviors with personal values; and to assure that actions are consistent with spoken words (Shirey, 2015).

D. Charismatic leadership—The word *charisma* is derived from a Greek word meaning "divinely inspired gift."

  1. Charismatic leaders feel that charm and grace are all that is needed to create followers and that people follow others that they personally admire.

2. Charismatic leaders pay a great deal of attention in scanning and reading their environment and are good at picking up the moods and concerns of both individuals and larger audiences. They then will hone their actions and words to suit the situation ("Leadership Styles," 2006).

E. Participative leadership—Participative leaders believe that involvement in decision-making improves the understanding of the issues concerned by those who must carry out the decisions. Further, people are more committed to actions when they have been involved in the relevant decision-making, and are less competitive and more collaborative when they are working on joint goals ("Leadership Styles," 2006) (Table 16-1).

F. Situational leadership—Situational leaders use a range of actions and styles that depend on the situation. This style may be *transactional* or *transformational* (see below) or any of the leadership styles discussed.[1]

G. Transactional leadership—Transactional leaders believe that people are motivated by reward and punishment. Social systems work best with a clear chain of command. When people have agreed to do a job (the transaction), a part of the deal is that they cede all authority to their manager. The prime purpose of the subordinates is to do what their manager tells them to do ("Leadership Styles," 2006).

H. Transformational leadership—While transactional leadership attempts to preserve and work within the constraints of the status quo, transformational leadership seeks to subvert and replace it and looks at the greater good (Shortell & Kaluzny, 2000).
   1. Transformational leaders believe people will follow a person who inspires them, has vision and passion, and can achieve great things. The way to get things done is by injecting enthusiasm and energy.
   2. Transformational leadership starts with the development of a vision (by the leader or by the team)—a view of the future that will excite and convert potential followers ("Leadership Styles," 2006).
   3. Transformational leadership is about the leader developing other leaders from the followers and creating opportunities for them to expand and recognize their potential.

I. Quiet leadership—The quiet leader believes that the actions of a leader speak louder than his or her words. People are motivated when you give them credit rather than take it yourself. Ego and aggression are neither necessary nor constructive ("Leadership Styles," 2006). Quiet leaders

TABLE 16-1 Participative Leadership Styles

Not Participative			**Highly Participative**
Autocratic decision by leader	Leader proposes decision, listens to feedback, and then decides	Joint decision with team as equals	Full delegation of decision to team

Source: http://changingminds.org/disciplines/leadership/styles/leadership_styles.htm

---

[1]One caution of situational leadership: The leader's *perception* of the follower and the situation will affect what they do rather than the *truth* of the situation. The leader's perception of themselves and other factors such as stress and mood will also modify the leader's behavior ("Leadership Styles," 2006).

promote a sense of calm, peace, and comfort in their environment and people around them.

J. Servant leadership—The servant leader believes the leader has responsibility for the followers and toward society and those who are disadvantaged. The servant leader serves others, rather than others serving the leader ("Leadership Styles," 2006).

 ## Leadership Skills

A. The jury is still out about whether leaders are born or made. However, experts have noticed specific actions that successful leaders share, regardless of the type of organization they lead.

B. Qualities of effective leaders are listed below. Note the similarities between effectively working with patients/clients and leaders working within their organizations. Effective leaders:

1. *Promote empowerment.* They emphasize the strengths and utilize the talents of others in the organization. Leaders share decision-making with others, allowing those people at the point of care or service to be the key decision makers. Then they share in the success and give credit where it is due.

2. *Promote a vision.* People need a vision of where they are going. Leaders provide that vision.

3. *Follow the golden rule.* Anyone who has been demeaned or treated with disrespect knows what effect that treatment has on the work.

4. *Admit mistakes.*

5. *Praise others in public.* And criticize others only in private.

6. *Stay close to the action.* In case management, this is the administrator who goes to the "front lines" occasionally to stay in touch with the reality of the working situation. This also means that the leader is visible and accessible (Powell & Tahan, 2010).

7. Say *"I don't know"* when confronted with a case management problem, and then assist with a solution (Powell & Tahan, 2010).

8. Focus on *what* is right, not *who* is right (Powell & Tahan, 2010).

9. *Motivate others* by demonstrating a number of behaviors such as those shared in Box 16-5.

10. *Hold their staff accountable,* but also let them do their jobs.

C. Conflict management is an important skill for leaders. Five strategies can be employed, from less desirable to most desirable.

BOX 16-5 Ways of Motivating Others

- Establishing credibility
- Improving one's communication skills—outstanding communication
- Being a role model
- Taking an interest in others
- Rewarding positive behaviors
- Sharing in decision-making
- Offering constructive criticism
- Forwarding others
- Inspiring others to pursue a cause
- Rewarding and recognizing others
- Supporting, guiding, and helping others

      1. Avoidance
      2. Competition ("I win, you lose")
      3. Accommodation ("You win, I lose")
      4. Negotiation (also known as compromise) (see next section)
      5. Collaboration ("You win, I win") (the best strategy)
         a. Takes more time to use
         b. Saved for complex or emotional issues

  D. Another necessary leadership skill is succession planning. Astute case management leaders develop and execute on a strategy for workforce planning. This applies to both case managers involved in care of the patients and for leaders of case management programs. This is even more important today because of the limited pool for case management roles/positions and the continued need to develop talent on the job. This is even more complicated due to the aging case management workforce, impending large numbers of retirees and lack of academic programs to prepare young talent for these roles.

 ## Negotiation Skills

  A. In the current health care environment of scarce resource availability and declining health insurance benefits, the art of negotiation is extremely important.

  B. Negotiation serves several important purposes (Powell, 2000a):
      1. It has the capacity to control costs. This is one of the primary reasons case managers negotiate.
      2. It has the capacity to gain medically necessary benefits for the patient that the patient would otherwise not receive. This is the other primary reason case managers negotiate.
      3. It can avoid chaos. Many case managers have lived through the frustration and chaos that results when a patient's condition deteriorates, at least partly because the negotiation for the requested service or equipment was denied.
      4. Negotiation can be a learning experience. Case managers may learn why the request is denied (sometimes there is a valid reason). They may also reveal weaknesses in the "No!" argument that could lead to further strengths in the case manager's negotiation stance.

  C. Successful negotiation steps include:
      1. Being optimally prepared. Before negotiation begins, it is wise to do some research; understand the other side before negotiation, for example, if you are negotiating the price of a resource or service, research current prices of the same service offered by competitors.
      2. Negotiation starts by stating the problem or problems and the goal and stating what is needed to solve the problem. State the request in a positive and thorough way. Areas in which there is agreement can be put aside; then begin to search for a mutual compromise where there is disagreement.
      3. Use of the three Cs—communication, communication, communication. Common mistakes can create a defensive environment that is not conducive to negotiation. Some behaviors that may be problematic include poor listening skills, poor use

of questions, improper disclosure of ideas, mismanagement of issues, inappropriate stress reactions, rejecting alternatives too quickly, misusing a negotiating team member, not disclosing true feelings, improper timing, and being aggressive rather than assertive.

4. Being realistic. Attempting to negotiate for a service or a price that absolutely will not be covered or met wastes everyone's time and energy.

5. Putting things in writing. Once an agreement has been reached, write it down and have all parties sign it.

D. There are two types of negotiators: aggressive and cooperative. Aggressive negotiators use psychological maneuvers such as intimidation and threats to make their "opponent" feel disparaged. Cooperative negotiators try to establish trust.

1. The aggressive negotiator:

   a. Moves psychologically against his or her opponent. Note the key word *psychologically*. If the case manager feels that something is amiss—that is, that he or she is being toyed with—he or she should bring the case back to facts.

   b. Common tactics include intimidation, accusation, threats, sarcasm, and ridicule.

   c. There is an overt or covert claim that the aggressive negotiator is superior.

   d. The aggressive negotiator will make extreme demands and few concessions.

   e. There will be frequent threats to terminate negotiations.

   f. False issues will be brought up time and again. This is another opportunity to bring the case back to facts.

2. Weaknesses of the aggressive method:

   a. It is more difficult to be a successful aggressive.

   b. Tension and mistrust that develop may increase the likelihood of misunderstandings.

   c. Deadlock over one trivial issue may escalate other issues.

   d. The opponent may develop righteous indignation and pursue the case with more vengeance.

   e. The reputation as an aggressive hurts future negotiations.

   f. Aggressive tactics increase the number of failed negotiations.

   g. The trial rate for aggressive negotiators is more than double.

3. The cooperative negotiator:

   a. Moves psychologically toward his or her opponent.

   b. This negotiator establishes a common ground. For case managers, the common ground is the patient.

   c. This negotiator is trustworthy, fair, objective, and reasonable. This is very important. Respect and trustworthiness are critical for negotiations and for self-respect as a case management professional.

   d. This negotiator works to establish credibility and unilateral concessions. The attitude is one of "win–win."

   e. This negotiator seeks to obtain the best joint outcome for everyone. This requires respect, empathy, and active listening, as described in other sections of this text.

  4. Strengths of the cooperative method:
   a. Promotes mutual understanding.
   b. Generally produces agreement in less time than does the aggressive approach.
   c. Produces agreements in a larger percentage of cases than does aggressiveness.
   d. Often produces a better outcome than do aggressive strategies.
   e. There is a much higher percentage of "successful" negotiations.
   f. Future negotiations are made easier.
  5. Weaknesses of the cooperative method:
   a. Aggressive negotiators view cooperative negotiators as weak, so they push harder.
   b. Cooperative negotiators risk being manipulative or exploitive because of the assumption that "if I am fair and trustworthy and make decisions with all parties in mind, then the other side will feel an irresistible moral obligation to reciprocate."
E. A critical trait to possess when negotiating (or dealing with humanity) is *emotional intelligence.*
F. Emotional intelligence, also called EI or EQ, describes an ability, capacity, or skill to perceive, assess, and manage the emotions of one's self, of others, and of groups. However, being a relatively new area, the definition of emotional intelligence is still in a state of flux (Wikipedia, 2006).
G. The Mayer-Salovey model defines emotional intelligence as the capacity to understand emotional information and to reason with emotions. More specifically, in their four-branch model, they divide emotional intelligence abilities into four areas (Wikipedia, 2006):
  1. The capacity to accurately perceive emotions
  2. The capacity to use emotions to facilitate thinking
  3. The capacity to understand emotional meanings
  4. The capacity to manage emotions
H. Goleman divides emotional intelligence into the following five emotional competencies, all essential in case management work (Wikipedia, 2006):
  1. The ability to identify and name one's emotional states and to understand the links among emotions, thought, and action
  2. The capacity to manage one's emotional states—to control emotions or to shift undesirable emotional states to more adequate ones
  3. The ability to enter into emotional states (at will) associated with a drive to achieve and be successful
  4. The capacity to read, be sensitive to, and influence other people's emotions
  5. The ability to enter and sustain satisfactory interpersonal relationships

Delegation Skills

A. Some case managers see delegation as a loss of power and control.
B. Some case managers simply do not trust others to do the job correctly. They live by the credo, if you want something done correctly, do it yourself.

16-6 **Examples of Delegation Standards for Case Managers**

- Always act in a reasonable and prudent manner.
- Ensure that the delegate is qualified to perform the tasks.
- Assign tasks that are within the person's scope of practice and licensure.
- Provide proper supervision (guidance and monitoring) to the person to whom the task was delegated. However, let the delegate put his or her "spin" on the task (it may be better than your idea).
- Assign a due date or time for activity completion.
- Explain expectations.
- Remain available to the delegate in case of questions or needed support.
- Follow up on state of the delegated activity with the delegate.
- Address issues or concerns as they arise.
- Communicate, communicate, communicate.

   C. Some case managers feel a legal liability when delegating responsibility.
   D. Delegation standards that will minimize risk may include those listed in Box 16-6 (Powell, 2000a).
   E. Effective delegation recommendations:
     1. Stress results, not details. Make it clear that you are more concerned with the final outcome than with all of the day-to-day details. This provides autonomy to the one who is responsible for the results.
     2. Do not always become the solution to everyone's problems. Teach others how to solve problems rather than just providing the answers. Again, this builds confidence and independence and provides autonomy.
     3. When an employee or peer comes to you with a problem and a question, ask him or her for possible solutions. Be there to brainstorm when needed.
     4. Establish measurable and concrete objectives and expected outcomes. Make them clear and specific. This is the road map that others can follow.
     5. Develop reporting systems. Obtain feedback from written reports, statistical data, and planned face-to-face meetings. This does not always work in case management if a particularly tough problem arises; teach employees when to come to you with details, and when to come to you after exhausting other avenues.
     6. When appropriate, give strict but realistic deadlines. This gives the task credibility and gives the person accountability.
     7. Keep a delegation log. This is especially important for very busy people or those with many employees.
     8. Recognize and use the talents and personalities of the people you work with. Being a good delegator is very much like being a good coach.

Communication Skills for Quality and Patient Safety

   A. Poor communication skills can have ramifications that range from stressful working environments to unsafe patient environments and ultimately poor outcomes up to a patient's death or permanent injury.

B. Unsafe patient environments can have many causes and take many forms. Clearly, communication plays a large role, and communicating clearly and completely is essential.

   1. The transfer of timely and accurate information across settings (e.g., transitions of care and handoffs) is critical to the execution of effective care transitions.

   2. One definition of care transfers includes transfers to or from an acute hospital, skilled nursing or rehabilitation facility, or home with or without home health care.

   3. Not all patients undergoing transitions are at high risk for adverse events; however, those with poor transitional care plans are particularly likely to "fall through the cracks" (HMO Workgroup on Care Management, 2004).

   4. Processes for accurate and complete transitions of care must be developed by health care organizations and case management programs. However, at this time, there is often a lack of agreement about what comprises the core clinical information that all practitioners require irrespective of setting.

   5. The care transition measure (CTM) was developed by researchers at University of Colorado Health Sciences Center to assess the quality of care transitions from the perspective of the patient or his or her proxy.

      a. CTM scores have been shown to be significantly associated with a patient's return to a hospital or emergency department after discharge (HMO Workgroup on Care Management, 2004).

      b. CTM scores are now part of value-based purchasing and incorporated into the consumer assessment of health care providers and systems (CAHPS) required by the Centers for Medicare and Medicaid Services (CMS). Case managers play an important role in achieving desirable scores and improving the patient's experience of care transitions including discharge from the acute care/hospital setting.

C. Stressful working environments are often a result of poor communication skills that lead one to "act out" rather than "talk it out" when the topic is one of high stress/high stakes (Patterson et al., 2002).

   1. In the "Silence Kills" study, it was found that the ability to hold crucial conversations is key to creating a culture of safety in health care; conversely, the prevalent culture of poor communication and faulty collaboration among health professionals relates significantly to continued medical errors and patient complaints.

   2. Crucial conversations occur when (Patterson et al., 2002):

      a. Opinions vary (e.g., what is the *best* course of treatment or discharge plan for this client?).

      b. The stakes are high (e.g., there is an imminent danger to patient safety).

      c. Emotions are strong (e.g., adrenaline is already flowing, so thought processes are impaired).

      d. Responsibility and accountability are missing (e.g., this is not my job, and as a result, something important does not get done in a timely manner).

16-7	Strategies for Positive Dialogue

- Figure out what you really want: for yourself and for others.
- People often act out (go to "silence or violence") when they do not feel *safe*. Learn to notice when the other party does this.
- Make it safe. Conditions/dialogue that promotes *mutual respect* is one place to start.
- Apologize when appropriate. Agree when appropriate.
- Consider that what YOU think is happening may not be exactly correct (i.e., what "story" are you telling yourself?). If you are telling a negative "story" about the other person, go back to "just the facts." And ask what part you play in the scene.
- *Ask* others questions, and consider that they have good information to add to the pool of knowledge.
- Seek *help* and *support* when you face a situation you are unable to resolve alone.
- Understand and recognize your limitations and do not *overcommit or overpromise*.

D. Dialogue skills are learnable and can be used in nearly every case management encounter. For positive dialogue, case managers may apply specific strategies such as those described in Box 16-7 (Patterson et al., 2002).

 ## Critical Thinking and Decision-Making

A. Critical thinking is broader than problem solving. It is more than finding a single solution to a problem.
B. In health care, critical thinking may be referred to as clinical reasoning; in nursing, it is sometimes equated to the nursing process. In case management, critical thinking equates with the global thinking necessary to appropriately put all the pieces of the client/patient puzzle together.
C. Critical thinking is being creative and/or "connecting the dots." In general, it is the ability to:
   1. Put together the known components of the problem or situation
   2. Research all possible solutions
   3. Find a way to improve the condition (Powell, 2000a)
D. Critical thinking is focused on outcomes, not tasks. It is purposeful, outcome-directed thinking that aims to make judgments based on facts. It is reflective and reasonable thinking about client problems and is focused on deciding what to do.
E. Good critical thinkers demonstrate a number of skills (Box 16-8).
F. Variables that affect critical thinking:
   1. Thinking styles
   2. Personal factors, such as age, gender, and education
   3. Situational factors, such as available time, resources, peer support, and administrative support
   4. Urgency of need to manage the situation at hand
   5. Availability, importance and credibility of relevant information
   6. Number of parties involved in a situation
G. Levels of critical thinking
   1. Basic level—knowing right from wrong
   2. Complex level—identifying all possible alternatives or solutions (e.g., "It depends.")

BOX 16-8   Examples of Skills of Critical Thinkers

- Flexibility
- Creativity
- Outstanding communication
- Generous listening
- Contextual or situational thinking
- Open-mindedness
- Willingness to change
- Outcome focused
- Ability to see "the big picture"
- Caring
- Empathy
- Ownership and responsibility
- Leadership

3. Committed level—selecting the most reasonable alternative ("Plan A") and having one or more backup plans in case Plan A is unsuccessful

H. Critical thinking strategies and cognitive skills based on an American Philosophical Association (APA) study (Facione & Facione, 1996). Some of these are characteristic of emotional intelligence.
   1. Interpretation (clarifying meaning)
   2. Analysis (examining ideas, data)
   3. Evaluation (assessing outcomes)
   4. Inference (drawing conclusions)
   5. Explanation (justifying actions)
   6. Self-regulation (self-examination and correction)

I. Critical thinking process case managers may apply in their roles may consist of the following action steps:
   1. Analyze all of the problems or issues in a situation.
   2. Determine the expected outcomes.
   3. List all possible alternatives and solutions to the problems.
   4. Select the best or highest-priority alternative.

J. Determine if the plan worked (i.e., were the outcomes met?).

The Ethics of Decision-Making

A. The ethics of decision-making includes how to recognize ethical issues, make ethical judgments, and then convert them into *action*.

B. Consider the following:
   1. Identify which stakeholders will be affected by the decision(s).
   2. Identify costs/benefits of the decision(s) *alternatives* for these stakeholders.
   3. Consider any moral expectations of the decision(s) (look at norms, regulatory issues, laws, organizational ethics, codes of conduct, principles related to honest communication and fair treatment).
   4. Be familiar with ethical dilemmas that leaders in your organization/ profession commonly face.

5. Discuss ethical matters with those affected.
6. Convert your ethical judgments into appropriate action (Jones, 1996).

 Financial/Cost–Benefit Analysis

A. Not only is a solid knowledge of financial methodologies important to case management, but the above leadership skills will help the case manager discuss the financial issues that follow when the stakes are high and the potential conflicts may be intensified. Case managers *and especially* case management leaders must thoroughly understand—and judiciously manage—individual cases, staff resources, departmental resources, and organizational resources.
B. Case management leaders must understand and be savvy about budgetary issues.
C. Many case managers will be asked to conduct a cost analysis of a case or of parts of a case. For example:
   1. Case management client and family members request comparative financial information. This is more common in private/independent case management than in other work settings.
   2. Health insurance companies who are inclined to refuse payment for a requested plan of care or service if they believe that a less cost-intensive solution is available may request prices.
   3. Many case managers are required to make a formal documentation of savings per case for accounting purposes, especially in independent, private, and disability management case management.
   4. Case managers in primary care, patient-centered medical home, accountable care organizations, and disease management care settings are able to contribute to the quality, safety, and cost outcomes and savings for an entire population of disease-specific patients.
D. Some case managers shun this responsibility. There may be several reasons for the dislike (Powell, 2000b), such as the following:
   1. We did not go into the helping professions to do accounting work. We are case managers to improve the quality of a patient's life.
   2. We already know that we improve quality and decrease costs per case; justifying our existence is another's responsibility.
   3. It is difficult to understand accounting and budgeting concepts.
   4. It is often tedious and time consuming to address and report financial details.
E. Case managers are as real an expense to the payers and facilities who employ them as are physician services, hospital costs, and medications expenses. Cost analysis is one method used to prove case managers' worth and value in the business world.
F. Hard savings or avoided costs are costs that can be measurably saved or prevented. Examples of hard savings facilitated by the case manager include those listed in Box 16-9 (Powell, 2000b).
G. Soft savings, or potential savings, costs, or charges, are less tangibly measurable than are hard savings. If no case manager is assigned to a particular patient, the potential costs incurred could be much higher without than with case management services and oversight. Soft savings represent costs that are avoided most likely because of case management intervention, especially those that are preventive in nature.

BOX 16-9 Examples of Situations of Hard Savings

- Change in the client's level of care
- Change in the client's length of stay or number of home care visits during an episode of care
- Change in primary care provider to someone from the contracted preferred provider organization panel
- Negotiation of price of services, supplies, equipment, or per diem rates
- Negotiation of frequency of services
- Negotiation of duration of services
- Prevention of unnecessary bed days, supplies, equipment, services, or charges
- Identifying unauthorized charges that are not warranted
- Conversion of denials as a result of appeal process
- Consumer experience of care surveys today and their role in value-based purchasing. These impact financial reimbursement and contribution can be quantifiable.

H. Examples of soft savings include avoidance of potential care concerns such as those described in Box 16-10 (Powell, 2000b).
I. Other soft savings relate to quality, safety, experience of care, and satisfaction. It is challenging to put a dollar amount on improved:
   1. Quality of care
   2. Patient and family satisfaction with and experience of case management
   3. Patient adherence
   4. Quality of life
J. With the advent of value-based purchasing, some traditional soft savings can be translated to hard savings and case management is able to impact on these savings, therefore demonstrating case management value.
   1. Core measures included in the value-based program are examples of soft savings converted to hard savings today. Examples are

BOX 16-10 Examples of Situations of Soft Savings

Soft savings related to prevention and avoidance of specific services, resources, and/ or core measures with associated financial risk such as the following:
- Hospital readmissions
- Emergency department visits
- Medical complications
- Mortality
- Legal exposure and risk management
- Use of unnecessary equipment and supplies
- Extended or prolonged acute care days
- Extended or prolonged home health visits
- Implementation of services without insurance authorizations despite their requirement

patient experience with care score, transitions of care measure score, reduction in rate of readmissions to acute care, and avoidance or prevention of incidence of health care–associated infections.
2. This shift is attributed to reduction in financial risk and increase in potential reimbursement from CMS due to improved performance and meeting performance targets including national benchmarks.

Case Management Outcomes in the Supervisory Role

A. Leaders/supervisors must look at outcomes in their department, staff, or organization. Well-chosen outcomes give case management leaders knowledge of *where* they currently are and act as a compass for future improvement.
B. First attempts at evaluating outcomes should be easily and concretely measurable.
   1. Begin by looking at only one or two outcomes.
   2. Traditionally, cost savings have been one of the most common measurements used for case management outcomes. Hard savings are more tangible and easily measured; soft savings are more obscure.
   3. Quality of life issues are also more nebulous and require careful consideration when turning them into something that is measurable (Powell, 2000b).
   4. Measure outcomes based on what is required in the value-based purchasing program, patient experience with care, safety, and reduction in avoidable readmissions to acute care.
C. Defining an "outcomes" budget when beginning an outcomes management program is important.
   1. Measuring outcomes is an important marketing tool, but the process requires resources of time, money, and personnel.
   2. It is important to assess what resources will be needed and to define a budget for the project that is acceptable to the organization. Consider the following (Powell, 2000b):
      a. What resources are *available* to plan, select, modify or develop, and implement an effective case management intervention?
      b. What resources are *required* to plan, select, modify or develop, and implement a case management intervention?
      c. In some projects, other people or organizations are asked to commit resources to the project. In those instances, determine what resources will be required of others. Are they willing and able to provide the resources? Some resources to consider are provider staffing, physician time, and beneficiary co-payments or deductibles.
      d. Can the improved outcome be translated into projected cost savings? If the cost of the case management intervention exceeds the amount of projected cost savings, is this still acceptable to the organization?

   e. Data collection and analysis is complex and costly. Does the
      case management organization have the necessary resources and
      information systems to execute these tasks, or can the organization
      secure appropriate data elements from other avenues that will
      provide the information necessary to record outcome measurements?
      Put a dollar amount on this and assess whether it is feasible.
   f. Selecting measures that assist in demonstrating the value and
      contribution of case management to organizational success is
      important place to focus on.
D. One aspect of outcomes is demonstrating value of case management
   programs. The ability to do so is a leadership role and skill required
   of case managers and leaders. This is more important today than ever
   due to the interest in the financial return on the investment in case
   management programs in a health care organization.
   1. The quantity of work completed by case managers (e.g., number of
      patients seen, number of assessments completed on a given day)
      is no longer the desired approach to articulate the value of case
      management.
   2. More contemporary approach is capitalizing on the value-based
      purchasing and Hospital Readmissions Reduction programs and
      quantifying the contribution of case managers financially (e.g.,
      revenue, reduction in financial risk, avoidable reimbursement
      denials), which adds to the organization's bottom line.

Case Managers as Change Agents

A. Although some people embrace change, most find it intimidating.
   Because of the unpredictable nature of change, some people respond to
   it with fear. Change is often at the core of stress.
B. New and fast-changing managed care and financial constraints must be
   managed.
C. Case management is more important than ever before in managing these
   changes in the best interests of the patients; case managers are essentially
   change agents.
D. There are three components of the change process case managers as
   leaders must be familiar with and apply in their practice (Box 16-11).

BOX 16-11   Three Components of Change

1. Unfreezing the current behavior or situation
   a. Determine driving forces (supportive forces for the change)
   b. Determine restraining forces (opposing forces for the change)
   c. Develop a plan to overcome resistance to change.
2. Implementing the change
   a. Enable the change
   b. Monitor the change
3. Freezing the new change
   a. Sustain and support the change
   b. Evaluate the change

E. Attitudes of change agents (i.e., case managers) are important for effective coping with the change process and its related experience.
   1. Sometimes these methods fail. You have worked hard with the case and used the most appropriate clinical pathways or plan of care possible. Then, it seems the case is falling off the path at every turn, and variances are winning. There is no shortage of problems.
      a. First, assess whether you could have done anything differently for a better outcome.
      b. If so, learn from it to apply in similar future situations.
      c. If not, realize that sometimes these methods fail.
      d. Identify any knowledge or skill gaps and fill these gaps so that you are more prepared in the future.
   2. Choose your battles carefully. Many aspects of case management are completely out of the case manager's realm of control. Assess whether the problem is really something over which you have influence. Seek others' support and guidance as appropriate.
   3. Consider that one approach to change includes a resistance to change, as though the ones who need to change are passive and sitting down instead of being active, moving where we want them to be. Instead, create attractors to promote change.
   4. Remember this wise adage—Robert Eliot, a cardiologist at the University of Nebraska, has developed two rules for keeping things in perspective (Charlesworth & Nathan, 1984):
      a. Don't sweat the small stuff.
      b. It's all small stuff.
   5. Remember that change is risk. Being vulnerable in assuming the change agent role is a sign of courage and responsibility.
   6. It is OK to disagree. Not everyone has to be in agreement to move forward. Use the continuous quality improvement (CQI) tool of "consensus."
   7. Anticipate changes. Do not wait for changes to happen. Be proactive with other possibilities.
F. The Eight-Stage Change Process (Table 16-2)—Successful transformations are neither easy nor linear. Still, some change experts believe that a general sequence of change *does* occur, that no steps should be missed, and that—at times—multiple phases occur at once. The Eight-Stage Change Process (Kotter, 1996) includes timeless concepts that can help case managers in many aspects of their work (both at the patient level and at the corporate level).
G. Succession planning—One of the key roles case manager leaders must plan for is succession planning. Succession planning is a process for identifying and developing internal people with the potential to be case management leaders.
   1. This process starts with recruitment of talented people who have all the attributes listed in this chapter.
   2. Provide critical development experiences to those that can move into key roles.
   3. Engage the top management in supporting the development of high-potential leaders (Wikipedia, 2015a).

TABLE 16-2 Eight Stages of Kotter's Change Process

Stage	Highlights
1. Establish a sense of urgency.	This can be accomplished by examining the market and competitive realities or the patient's clinical trajectory, identifying crises or potential crises, and/or identifying major opportunities.
2. Create a guiding coalition.	Put together a group with enough power to lead the change; then, get the group to work together like a team (leadership is needed here). In case management, this may be the essential patient care team.
3. Develop a vision and strategy.	The vision created will direct the change effort. Then, develop strategies to achieve the vision. What does the team want? More importantly, what does the patient/family want?
4. Communicate the change.	Use all vehicles to communicate the vision and strategies. Have the guiding coalition to role model the behavior.
5. Empower broad-based action.	Remove obstacles (from the team, the patient, the case, if possible). Change systems or structures that undermine the change vision. Encourage risk taking and nontraditional ideas.
6. Generate short-term wins.	Plan for visible improvements early in the process. Visibly recognize and reward the people who made the "win" possible. From a patient perspective, this may help the patient/family become more autonomous.
7. Consolidate the gains and produce more change.	As the patient/family becomes more knowledgeable or independent, use this progress to instill more sense of autonomy and produce more results.
8. Anchor the new approaches in the culture.	Last step and perhaps most important for a department /organization. Create better performance through customer service and excellent leadership. Articulate the connection between new behaviors and organization success. And develop ways to ensure leadership development and succession.

 ## Case Managers and Motivational Interviewing

A. Motivational interviewing (MI) is a technique case managers use during the comprehensive assessment of patients/clients and their families, at every step of the case management process, and at every interaction possible between the case manager and patient or family.

B. MI is known to elicit sensitive and important information for effective case management planning and lifestyle behavior change including enhancement in patient/family engagement in self-management and adherence to health regimen.

C. Motivational interviewing as a concept and strategy evolved from the experiences of psychologists and counselors in the field of mental health, behavioral health, and substance and alcohol abuse counseling and recovery programs (Miller & Rollnick, 2012).

1. MI is a method that works on facilitating and engaging intrinsic motivation within the client in order to change behavior, especially promoting healthy lifestyle and adherence to health regimen, including challenging medication schedules.

2. MI is a goal-oriented, client-centered, and counseling style of communication that aims to elicit desire and motivation for health behavior change by helping clients to explore and resolve their own ambivalence about the change including barriers and challenges (US Department of Health and Human Services, Substance Abuse and Mental Health Services Administration, 2015).

3. MI is focused and goal directed. It uses influence to entice clients to consider making necessary changes in their lives, embody a healthy life style, and prevent avoidable disease progression (Miller & Rollnick, 2012).

D. Clients may approach the lifestyle behavior change process with different levels of readiness and motivation. Case managers should focus on, and be able to recognize, such readiness during the comprehensive assessment and care planning steps of the case management process. They must then incorporate the change goals and strategies in the client's plan of care.

E. During the assessment, case managers may identify the patients who may have thought about healthy lifestyle behavior change but either have not taken steps to change yet or attempted in the past, however, unsuccessfully. Case managers then engage in a change talk with their patients and use MI to elicit interest in the pursuit of necessary change.

F. There are a number of basic interaction skills and principles case managers may exhibit for effective MI; some examples are listed in Box 16-12 (Miller & Rollnick, 2012). Case managers may use these skills

---

BOX 16-12 Essential Skills and Principles in Motivational Interviewing

Skills:
1. The ability to ask the client open-ended questions to allow inquiry, exploration, and personal talk
2. The ability to provide the client with affirmations to encourage desirable behavior and promote progression
3. The capacity for reflective listening, which communicates empathy
4. The ability to periodically provide summary statements to the client to ensure understanding, clarity, and mutual agreement on next steps

Principles:
1. Obtaining client's agreement or permission to engage in the change talk
2. Expression of empathy through reflective thinking and generous listening
3. Developing discrepancy between client's goals or interests and current state or behaviors—revealing the gap
4. Supporting client's optimism, enthusiasm, and self-efficacy
5. Understanding to the client's resistance rather than directly opposing it
6. Avoidance of arguments, confrontation, judgment, and coercion

and principles strategically and intentionally while focusing on the client's past experiences, current state and interest in the change, and future outlook on life without the current behaviors of concern. Such an approach allows the client to recognize the value of change.

G. Motivational interviewing is nonjudgmental, nonconfrontational, and nonadversarial (Miller & Rollnick, 2012). The approach attempts to increase the client's awareness of the potential consequences of the current state such as progression of disease state that is avoidable if the client's lifestyle and risk behaviors were addressed.

H. When case managers engage in change talk with their clients, they use "MI" to assist them in envisioning a better future, creating urgency for change, and increasing their motivation to achieve the envisioned future.

   1. Change talk can be elicited by asking the client questions, such as "How might you like things to be different?" or "How does smoking interfere with things that you would like to do?"

   2. Based on the clients' answers to above questions, case managers determine whether the clients are ready for change and if they are, a plan for change is developed. If clients express ambivalence, hesitation, or resistance, case managers then focus on supporting their clients, reassure them, counsel them, and explore their interest and agreement to continue addressing the risk behavior in future sessions and interactions.

I. Case managers recognize that MI is characterized by collaboration with clients/support systems, maintaining and protecting clients' autonomy, and exploration of readiness for change, agreement with clients on realistic, practical, and achievable change goals, and that there process varies based on the clients and encounters (Box 16-13).

BOX 16-13

Key Characteristics of the Motivational Interviewing Interaction between Case Managers and Their Clients

1. Establishing client's agreement and willingness to talk about a specific lifestyle behavior and explore the benefit of change.
2. Motivation to change behavior is elicited from within the client and is not imposed externally from the case manager.
3. The client and not the case manager articulates and resolves own ambivalence about the change. The case manager creates the opportunity for change and influences, facilitates, and supports the client's efforts to change.
4. The case manager uses a counseling-like communication style to elicit sensitive information from the client, especially in relation to health condition, barriers to change, past attempts, and reasons for lack of enthusiasm or for nonadherence to healthy lifestyle behavior.
5. Coercion, direct persuasion, and critical judgment are not effective methods for resolving ambivalence or motivating the change.
6. Readiness to change is a result of effective motivational interviewing and working interpersonal interactions and relationships between the case manager and the client/family/support system.
7. The motivational interviewing relationship is like a trusting and respectful partnership between the case manager and the client/family/support system.

J. When using MI, case managers may follow six general processes to support their clients in achieving and sustaining successful lifestyle behavior change. These are:

1. Engaging: used to make the client feel comfortable and supported and to elicit information about issues, concerns, interests, preferences, hopes for different future, and goals. It also is used to establish a trusting relationship with the case manager.

2. Focusing: used to narrow the conversation to lifestyle behaviors, habits, or patterns that clients want to change. Here, the case managers act in an intentional manner to generate dialogue about how the future may look for the client, identify gap between current and future states, and recognize the needed change.

3. Evoking: used to elicit client motivation for change. Case managers here attempt to increase the clients' understanding and recognition of the importance of change, become aware of their own confidence about change, and identify their level of readiness to change.

4. Planning: used to develop the practical and realistic steps and tactics clients desire to take to achieve the changes they declare.

5. Supporting and affirming: used to follow up on the clients' ability to change, actual accomplishments, what is working, and challenges and barriers faced. This talk allows case managers to examine where the clients compared to the change plan, identify opportunity to affirm the change or address barriers to change and ultimately to assist clients revise their change plans where needed.

6. Normalizing: used to establish dialogue with clients about their successes in both achieving their change goals and recognizing the strategies that have worked so that they continue to apply routinely in their lives. This allows what worked to become the norm for the clients. Case managers here assist their clients recognize what worked and explore effective ways to sustain it long term.

References

Case Management Society of America. (2010). *Standards of practice for case management.* Little Rock, AR: Author.

Charlesworth, E., & Nathan, R. (1984). *Stress management: A comprehensive guide to wellness.* New York, NY: Atheneum.

Facione, N. C., & Facione, P. A. (1996). Externalizing the critical thinking in knowledge development and clinical judgment. *Nursing Outlook, 44*(3), 129–136.

HMO Workgroup on Care Management. (2004). *One patient, many places: Managing health care transitions.* Washington, DC: AAHP-HIAA Foundation.

Jones, G. (1996). *Organizational behavior: Understanding and managing life at work* (4th ed.). New York, NY: HarperCollins College Publishers.

Kotter, J. P. (1996). *Leading change.* Boston, MA: Harvard Business School Press.

Kruse, K. (2013). *Forbes. What is authentic leadership.* Retrieved from Website: http://www.forbes.com/sites/kevinkruse/2013/05/12/what-is-authentic-leadership/, on April 11, 2015.

Leadership Styles. (2006). Retrieved from Website: http://changingminds.org/disciplines/leadership/styles/leadership_styles.htm, on March 19, 2006.

Miller, W. R., & Rollnick, S. (2012). *Motivational interviewing* (3rd ed.). New York, NY: Guilford Press.

Patterson, K., Grenny, J., McMillan, R., & Switzler, A. (2002). *Crucial conversations: Tools for talking when the stakes are high.* New York, NY: McGraw-Hill Publishers.

Powell, S. K. (2000a). *Case management: A practical guide to success in managed care*. Philadelphia, PA: Lippincott Williams & Wilkins.

Powell, S. K. (2000b). *Advanced case management: Outcomes and beyond*. Philadelphia, PA: Lippincott Williams & Wilkins.

Powell, S. K., & Tahan, H. A. (2010). *Case management: A practical guide for education and practice*. Philadelphia, PA: Lippincott Williams & Wilkins.

Shirey, M. (2015). Self awareness: Enhance your self-awareness to be an authentic leader. American Nurse Today, *10*(8). Retrieved from http://www.americannursetoday.com/enhance-self-awareness-authentic-leader/, on August 17, 2015.

Shortell, S. M., & Kaluzny, A. D. (2000). *Health care management: Organization design and behavior* (4th ed.). Albany, NY: Delmar.

US Department of Health and Human Services (USDHHS), Substance Abuse and Mental Health Services Administration (SAMHSA). (January 28, 2014). Motivational interviewing. *National Registry of Evidence Based Practice and Programs. USDHHS SAMHSA*. Retrieved from http://nrepp.samhsa.gov/ViewIntervention.aspx?id=346, on August 10, 2015.

Wikipedia. (2006). *Emotional Intelligence*. Retrieved from Website: http://en.wikipedia.org/wiki/Emotional_intelligence, on March 19, 2006.

Wikipedia. (2015a). *Succession Planning*. Retrieved from Website: http://en.wikipedia.org/wiki/Succession_planning, on April 11, 2015.

Wikipedia. (2015b). *Authentic Leadership*. Retrieved from Website: http://en.wikipedia.org/wiki/Authentic_leadership, on April 11, 2015.

CHAPTER 17

Professional Development, Certification, and Accreditation in Case Management

Marietta P. Stanton and Hussein M. Tahan

LEARNING OBJECTIVES

Upon completion of this chapter, the reader will be able to:

1. Identify those organizations and standards that exert an influence over case management education, training, certification, and accreditation.

2. Describe key components of the case manager's initial education and clinical preparation.

3. Describe competency-based approaches to case management education and training.

4. Examine the relationship between various certifying agencies in case management and case management education and training curriculum development.

5. Delineate topics appropriate for training and continuing education or staff development in case management.

6. Determine the differences in academic preparation and how these relate to basic and advanced levels of case management practice.

7. Define credentialing, certification, and accreditation.

8. List the components of the credentialing process employed for accreditation of case management organizations, programs, or services.

IMPORTANT TERMS AND CONCEPTS

Academic Preparation
Accreditation
Accreditation
  Standards
Case Management
Case Management
  Philosophy

Center for Case
  Management
Certificate
Certification
Core Components of
  Case Management
Credentialing

Licensure
Professional
  Development
  (Standards of Care
  and Practice)

 Introduction

A. Essential information related to the education, clinical preparation, and work–life experience of case managers comes from several important sources.
  1. Professional organizations, case management certification organizations, regulatory bodies, and accreditation agencies provide an overview of the knowledge areas required for case management education and training.
  2. Certification in and accreditation of case management are valued and therefore are powerful forces in shaping training and educational requirements for case management preparation.

B. Educational preparation of case managers is critical to the success of the case manager's role in the health care system. Consensus information about core areas of knowledge needed by case managers for basic, intermediate, and advanced levels of practice and competence have been delineated in the literature.

C. Because case management preparation is dependent on both the experience and educational preparation, using competency standards for case management in the clinical area is an effective mechanism for training, continuing education, and ongoing professional development.

D. Academic preparation and clinical experience are determinants of knowledge, competence, and skill levels of the case manager. There are case management skills that appear to be at the basic or entry level of practice, while there are others that appear to be at the advanced level of practice, for example, master's-degree level of academic preparation.

E. Necessary training and education in specialty areas may vary according to the specialty itself and related certifications.

F. Certifications in case management have been in existence since the early 1990s. Currently, there are more than 30 different certifications in case management or its related practices. Despite the popularity, this presents a challenge for the interested case manager in deciding which one best fits her or his specialty practice or professional discipline.

G. *Certification, accreditation,* and *credentialing* are three terms that tend to be confused and often used interchangeably. These terms are different and professionals in the case management field should be clear about their meaning and intent and should use these terms appropriately (*see key definitions section*).

Descriptions of Key Terms

A. Accreditation—A process in which a nationally recognized agency (other than a health care provider organization), usually nongovernmental, assesses a health care organization's operations and performance to determine whether it meets a set of nationally recognized and accepted standards, mainly designed to demonstrate quality and safe care.

B. Case manager—A health care professional who is responsible for coordinating the care delivered to a group of patients based on diagnosis or need. Other responsibilities may include patient and family education, advocacy, management of delays in care, utilization management, transitional planning, and outcomes monitoring and management. Case managers work with people to get the health care services and other community resources they need, when they need them, and for the best value (quality, safety, and cost).

C. Certificate—A document awarded to affirm that an individual participated or attended a given educational program. It can be provided by any professional agency (private or public, for-profit and not-for-profit), university, or college. Usually, a certificate is not nationally recognized in any form other than an educational credit.

D. Certification (individual)—An official form of credential that is provided by a nationally recognized governmental or nongovernmental certifying agency (i.e., credentialing body) to a professional who meets a set of predetermined eligibility criteria and requirements of a particular field, practice, or specialty. It usually signifies the achievement of a passing score on an examination prepared by the certifying agency for that purpose. It also denotes an advanced degree of competence.

E. Certification (organization or program)—An official form of accreditation that is provided by a nationally recognized governmental or nongovernmental agency to an organization or a program within an organization (e.g., center of excellence) that meets nationally recognized requirements or standards of quality and safe performance.

F. Consensus—Agreement in opinion of experts. Building consensus is a method used when developing case management plans.

G. Credentialing (individual)—The process used to protect the consumer and to ensure that individuals hired to practice case management are providing quality case management services. This involves a review of the provider's licensure, certification, insurance, evidence of malpractice insurance (if applicable), performance, knowledge, skills and competencies, and history of lawsuits/malpractices.

H. Credentialing (organization or program/service)—The process used in the review of a case management program or organization to ensure that it meets nationally recognized industry standards of quality. This is necessary for the provision of quality case management services and to protect the consumer.

I. Credentials—Evidence of competence, current and relevant licensure, certification, education, and experience.

J. Licensure—A mandatory and official form of validation provided by a state governmental agency affirming that an individual has acquired the basic knowledge and skill, and minimum degree of competence required for safe practice in one's profession such as nursing, medicine, and social work. This is usually conducted in compliance with a statute for a given occupation and carries the expectation that the licensed individual act in an unsupervised way.

K. Standard (individual)—An authoritative statement by which a profession defines the responsibilities for which its practitioners are accountable.

L. Standard (organization)—An authoritative statement that defines the performance expectations, structures, or processes that must be substantially in place in an organization to enhance the quality of care.

M. Standards of care—Statements that delineate care that is expected to be provided to all clients. They include predefined outcomes of care that clients can expect from providers and that are accepted within the community of professionals, based on the best scientific knowledge, current outcomes data, and clinical expertise.

N. Standards of practice—Statements of acceptable level of performance or expectation for professional intervention or behavior associated with one's professional practice. They are generally formulated by practitioner organizations based on clinical expertise and the most current research findings.

Applicability to CMSA's Standards of Practice

A. The Case Management Society of America (CMSA) explains that case management practice extends across all health care settings and professional disciplines (CMSA., 2010). This results in availability of case managers in virtually every practice setting along the continuum of health and human services. It also indicates that case managers come from diverse health care and professional backgrounds.

B. In its standards of practice for case management, CMSA describes the requirements for the case manager role including education, licensure, or certification and other qualifications.

C. The standards emphasize that case managers should maintain knowledge, skills, and competence in their area of practice. It states that they possess:

1. Current, active, and unrestricted professional licensure or certification in a health or human services discipline that allows the case managers to conduct an assessment independently as permitted within the scope of practice of the discipline they belong to (e.g., nursing, social work).

2. Baccalaureate or graduate degree in social work, nursing, or another health or human services field that promotes the physical, psychosocial, and/or vocational well-being of the persons being served (CMSA, 2010).

3. The educational degree must be from an institution that is fully accredited by a nationally recognized educational accreditation organization, and the case manager must have completed a supervised field experience in case management, health, or behavioral health as part of the degree requirements (CMSA, 2010).

D. Case managers according to CMSA must demonstrate professional standing and maintain their qualifications at all times. They are expected to meet the requirements described in Box 17-1.

E. This chapter focuses on the training and education of case managers and how to seek certification or accreditation. These topics support the CMSA

BOX 17-1   CMSA's Requirements for the Case Manager Role

- Possession of the education, experience, and expertise necessary for the case manager's area(s) of practice
- Adherence to national and/or local laws and regulations that apply to the jurisdictions(s) and discipline(s) in which the case manager practices
- Maintenance of competence through relevant and ongoing continuing education, study, and consultation
- Practicing within the case manager's area(s) of expertise, making timely and appropriate referrals to, and seeking consultation with, others when needed
- Pursuing professional excellence and maintaining competence in practice
- Promotion of quality outcomes, including safety, and measurement of those outcomes
- Supporting and maintaining compliance with federal, state, local, organizational, and certification rules and regulations

From Case Management Society of America (CMSA). (2010). *Standards of practice* (2nd ed.). Little Rock, AR: Author.

standards of case management practice and assist case managers and organizations in the implementation or use of the standards.

F. The CMSA standards of practice for case management are an excellent source for the development of professional development, training, and educational programs. They also are beneficial in guiding the development and implementation of formal academic programs. In this regard, the standards clearly identify a list of topics that can be addressed in the training and educational programs.

Education and Training of Case Managers

A. Education and training programs for case managers are developed based on the standards of practice, evidence-based outcomes, accreditation and credentialing criteria, and certification examination content.

B. URAC in its case management accreditation standards describes the key elements of case management education and training programs. These standards state that case managers must be educated in the specific areas that are relevant to the case management practice in the individual organization or work setting (Box 17-2). URAC also explains that training does not need to be completed on an annual basis; however, it encourages ongoing professional development (URAC, 2013).

C. Education should include knowledge of the organization's policies and procedures, case management process, state requirements, professional roles, organizational ethics and confidentiality, health care requirements of specific populations, URAC standards, CMSA's standards of practice, knowledge domains of the CCMC certification in case management, and certification examination blueprints of other certifying agencies.

D. URAC encourages case managers to engage in annual training and recognizes major case management certifications.[1]

E. The Commission for Case Management Certification (CCMC, 2015) has identified eight essential activities of case management that may be included in training and education programs:

[1]https://www.urac.org/wp-content/uploads/URAC_Recognized_Case_Management_Certifications.pdf

17-2   Topics of Case Management Training Programs According to URAC

1. The health care organization's case management–specific policies, procedures, evidence-based plans of care, and quality management program
2. The laws and regulations that apply to the case management program and based on the appropriate jurisdiction (i.e., local, state, and federal)
3. Case management roles, responsibilities, and accountabilities
4. Scope and standards of case management practice reflective of national and widely accepted or recognized knowledge domains
5. Cultural competence, health literacy, and motivational interviewing and principles for client engagement
6. Any special requirements based on the particular clients the organization and the case management program serve
7. Available resources to support case managers in their roles
8. Professional conduct and ethical practice
9. Coordination and transitions of care
10. Case management evaluation and measurement of outcomes

---

    1. Assessment
    2. Planning
    3. Implementation
    4. Coordination
    5. Monitoring
    6. Evaluation
    7. Outcomes
    8. General (across all activities)

F. The CCMC has also delineated five core components of case management knowledge necessary for effective performance.[2] These core components provide a basic foundation for case management education, training and continuing education, and competencies (Tahan, Watson, & Sminkey, 2016):
    1. Care delivery and reimbursement methods
    2. Psychosocial concepts and support systems
    3. Rehabilitation concepts and strategies
    4. Quality and outcomes evaluation and measurements
    5. Ethical, legal, and practice standards
G. The CCMC also specifies criteria for validating practice for certification as a certified case manager (CCM). For example, an individual can practice under the auspices of a CCM for 12 months or 24 months under the supervision of a case manager. There is a mechanism for validating experience as a self-employed case manager.
H. The Center for Case Management (CFCM) delineates specific content for the Case Management Administrators Certification (CMAC).[3] Topics covered in the exam include (CFCM, 2015) those described in Box 17-3.
I. The CMAC demonstrates professional recognition of the knowledge required to be a case/care management administrator, director, manager,

---

[2]Detailed descriptions of these core components and subtopics are available at the CCMC Website (www.ccmcertification.org).
[3]http://www.cfcm.com/wordpress1/cmac/

17-3 | Domains of the CMAC Certification Examinations

1. Identification of at-risk populations
2. Assessment of clinical systems' components
3. Development of strategies to manage at-risk populations
4. Leadership for change
5. Market assessment and strategic planning
6. Human resource management
7. Program evaluation through outcomes management

educator, or supervisor of any case management service or independent practice throughout the continuum of health care. This certification is also offered to case management faculty in the academic setting (CFCM, 2015).

J. Case management administrators and faculty lead organizations in the development and implementation of strategies to achieve clinical quality, financial, and satisfaction outcomes. Their activities may include education, program design and collaboration, direct supervision, consultation, and evaluation.

K. CMSA provides a foundation for education of case managers with the specification of their standards of practice (2010). The standards for care and the related "performance evidence specifications" are essential elements in case management education and training.

   1. Educational components include client identification and selection for case management services, assessment and problem or opportunity identification, development of the case management plan, implementation and coordination, evaluation of the case management plan, and termination of the case management process (CMSA, 2010).

   2. Each step in the case management process provides measurement guidelines that give direction for education and training.

   3. Performance evidence prescribed by CMSA in the area of quality of care, qualifications of case managers, collaboration with patients and providers, as well as legal, ethical, and advocacy considerations for case management practice also provide direction for education and training.

   4. CMSA's standards of practice address resource management and stewardship, as well as provide measurement guidelines for each of the performance evidence, resulting in a comprehensive overview of the requirements for the training, education, and ongoing continuing development of case managers.

   5. The CMSA standards specify the educational preparation and certification qualifications for case managers, including professional licensure, specific training related to case management and a minimum number of years of experience related to the health needs of the target population, appropriate continuing education, and maintaining certifications. These specifications regarding preparation have laid the groundwork for consideration of case management as advanced practice in nursing (CMSA, 2010).

L. The American Nurses Association (ANA), through its credentialing arm (the American Nurses Credentialing Center [ANCC]), has identified five components of case management practice reflected in the certification examination. These are

1. Fundamentals of practice
2. Resource management
3. Quality management
4. Legal and ethical practice
5. Education and health promotion (ANCC, 2013)

M. The education and training for case management has included extensive experience as a licensed professional and past practice as a case manager. The practice element in case management should be coupled with education and training.

N. Areas of specialization, like workers' compensation, disability case management, or maternal child case management, also provide additional foundational areas for case management education and training. Many of these are similar to the CCM in terms of content and focus.

Consensus Areas for Case Management Education: Core Components

A. The literature in case management provides an indication of what needs to be included in case management education and training programs.

B. Reviewing previous research studies and other published materials on case management education and training provides insight into topics that should be included in both formal and informal educational programs. This also promotes the development of evidence-based training and education curricula.

C. Research in this area is lacking; however, findings from past old surveys are still relevant today. Examples are the following:

1. A large survey of case managers conducted by Leahy et al. (1997) provides an in-depth description of case management services in a variety of work settings. Foundational elements were abstracted and five core areas were identified:
   a. Coordination and service delivery
   b. Physical and psychosocial issues
   c. Benefit systems/cost–benefit analysis
   d. Case management concepts
   e. Community re-entry

2. In another survey of nurse educators, content areas for case management were grouped into four levels of complexity as well as by content (Kulbok & Utz, 1999). These were
   a. Background in history and trends
   b. Case management process (basic levels)
   c. Ethical and legal issues (intermediate level)
   d. Case management research (advanced)

D. Benner and colleagues (Kulbok & Utz, 1999) categorized the stages of skill development as novice, advanced beginner, competent, proficient, and expert.

1. Applying these levels to case managers, a new graduate would be an advanced beginner.
2. Through experience, maturity, and formal and informal learning, the case manager would progress through the experience levels to expert level within the role of the case manager.

3. For some expert-level case managers with advanced education, a natural progression into a leadership position as a case management director responsible for educating and mentoring other beginning or intermediate case managers may occur.
4. Based on this notion, much of the content that is appropriate for nursing administrators is also appropriate for case management administrators.

E. In social work, graduate courses in case management assist social workers in preparing for advanced practice. Core elements that have been integral to graduate coursework for social workers include five content areas that give case management a transdisciplinary character (Moxley, 1996). These content areas are:
   1. Policy environment and problem formulation
   2. Diverse purposes, aims, and models of case management
   3. Context of case management practice
   4. Role definitions and staffing implications
   5. Ethical challenges to practice

F. Not all case management is advanced practice, nor does it require graduate education. However, it is becoming abundantly clear that in the past several years, case managers are performing more complex duties that appear to match the competencies and skill levels of other advanced practice roles.

G. Case managers perform their roles at individual, group, and system levels. Case management at the system level requires advanced practice skills that are traditionally not found in entry-level professional education (Stanton, Swanson, Sherwood, & Packa, 2005).

H. The differences between basic and advanced case management skills are depicted in Tables 17-1 and 17-2 (Stanton & Dunkin, 2002).

(*text continues on page 429*)

TABLE 17-1 Case Management at the Basic Practice Level: An Overview of the Role of the Nurse Case Manager

Aspect	Content
Practice	• Uses basic knowledge of physiology and pathophysiology
	• Uses basic health assessment skills
	• Designs, implements, and evaluates health promotion and disease prevention programs for selected individuals
	• Uses knowledge and understanding of ethical standards of practice according to ANA
	• Coordinates case management services for individual clients/family
	• Participates in disease management programs
	• Fulfills practice standards outlined by AACN, CMSA, and CCM
	• Collects outcomes data
	• Participates in the development of evidence-based practice guidelines
	• Collaborates with utilization and resource management in the coordination of patient case management services
	• Screens patients for case management
	• Collaborates with discharge planners, social workers, and other internal and external resources to coordinate case management services

TABLE 17-1 Case Management at the Basic Practice Level: An Overview of the Role of the Nurse Case Manager, *continued*

Aspect	Content
Research	• Participates in research studies under the direction of an advanced practice nurse or other professionals • Uses published research to apply to case management practice • Participates on multidisciplinary teams in the provision of case management services
Administration	• Uses basic knowledge in the policy, organization, and financing of health care and case management systems • Uses tools under the supervision of a graduate level to collect data for assessing clinical, financial, humanistic/satisfaction, quality, and functional outcomes for patients, families, disease management populations, and communities • Participates in case or disease management systems • Participates in continuous quality improvement (CQI) programs
Education	• Participates in professional organizations and staff development programs related to case management • Maintains certification as case manager

TABLE 17-2 Case Management at the Advanced Practice Level: An Overview of the Role of the Case Manager

Aspect	Content
Practice	• Uses advanced knowledge of pathophysiology • Uses advanced health assessment skills • Synthesizes theories from natural, behavioral, social, and applied sciences to support advanced practice and role development for case management • Uses community development and intervention processes to design, implement, and evaluate health promotion and disease prevention programs for patient populations and communities • Collaborates with providers and consumers in designing, implementing, and evaluating innovative health programs and community services for patient populations • Assumes accountability of ethical values, principles, and personal beliefs that acknowledge human diversity and influence professional practice decisions and nursing interventions • Designs and administers quality case management services at the individual, disease management, and/or community level • Designs case management systems that address human diversity and social issues • Becomes "expert" generalist in terms of dealing with health care issues • Provides leadership in coordinating, managing, and improving health programs and health services to culturally diverse individuals and populations • Develops and/or accesses evidenced-based practice guidelines

continued

TABLE 17-2 Case Management at the Advanced Practice Level: An Overview of the Role of the Case Manager, *continued*

Aspect	Content
Research	• Initiates research to address case management issues and practices in rural areas • Acts as a consultant to other researchers and providers regarding case management • Provides research consultation to members of multidisciplinary team on all aspects of case management for patient populations • Supervises interdisciplinary research on case management requirements for patient populations • Develops research proposals for external funding • Assesses and accesses pre-existing data bases to facilitate case management processes at all levels • Contributes through research to elaboration of case management conceptual frameworks
Administration	• Uses advanced knowledge in health policy, organization, and financing of health care and case management systems to design, coordinate, and evaluate case management systems • Designs cost-effective intervention/strategies collaboratively with multiple disciplines to provide quality health care for patient populations • Assumes leadership in professional role definition and development for case managers • Develops informational and organizational systems for assessing clinical, financial, humanistic/satisfaction, quality, and functional outcomes for all levels of case management within patient populations • Designs, implements, and evaluates methods for efficient and effective use of human and material resources to support case management services • Organizes and evaluates case management systems • Organizes CQI programs that address unique characteristics of case management • Advocates for patient populations in policy formulation, organization, and financing of health care
Education	• Acts as a facilitator and mentor to advanced practice case management students • Serves as case management expert for staff development processes in area of rural case management • Provides leadership in professional organizations • Educates consumers and health care professionals about the role of case manager • Provides leadership in the design, implementation, and evaluation of education for patient populations • Disseminates research findings at professional meetings

1. Basically, case management at the baccalaureate level focuses on the basic concepts and principles of case management practice including care coordination and transitions of care and how these topics apply to caring for individual clients.
2. Case management at the graduate level focuses not only on the knowledge areas covered in baccalaureate programs but also on use of evidence-based practice guidelines or plans of care, quality management, ethical and legal practice, chronic care management, and research. It also assists the case manager student in understanding the application of these knowledge areas in the care of cohorts of clients or a larger population with the intent to improve the health of a community.
3. Outcomes at the basic level focus on clinical, satisfaction, or care experience, cost, safety, and functional outcomes for the individual client.
4. Outcomes at the systems level focus on a roll-up and analysis of these individual outcomes for the entire group of patients, a population, or a community.

Approaches to Case Management Education and Training

A. Professional licensure is the basic mechanism for credentialing of case managers. Certification in case management has become increasingly available and is thought to demonstrate advanced knowledge, experience, and competence.
B. There is a growing list of distinct certification examinations in case management practice. Some of the better known and well regarded have been influential in determining content for case manager education and training programs and curricula. They also provide entry level for case management clinical knowledge and skills acquisition.
C. Competency in case management is paramount. Individual competence is the foundation or backbone for the case management process and for effecting desirable outcomes (i.e., quality, safety, care experience, and cost-effectiveness).
   1. A variety of methods can be used to assess, develop, and evaluate competency, including self-assessment tools, orientation curricula, competency and skills checklists, and/or on-site/online education (Stanton, Swanson, & Baker, 2005).
   2. Assessing competence can be used to determine beginning competence or increasing knowledge and skills, and as a mechanism for ongoing performance appraisal.
D. There are continuing education and certificate programs available as preparation courses in case management practice. The better educational programs have core accreditation from URAC and/or continuing education approval by the CCMC or other professional organizations.
E. There is a large number of graduate-level programs in nursing and social work that include case management content, especially in the preparation of clinical nurse specialists, nurse practitioners, and master's degree–prepared social workers. Some schools also include case management courses in their undergraduate curriculum.

BOX 17-4 Types of Case Management Training and Education Programs

1. Noncertificate programs offered by health care organizations as part of orientation or inservice education sessions.
2. Certificate programs offered by independent agencies through conferences conducted for the purpose of continuing education in case management, such as those offered by Contemporary Forum, CMSA, and American Health Consultants.
3. Multiple-credit certificate courses offered by colleges and universities.
4. Postbaccalaureate certificate programs also offered by universities and colleges.
5. Master's degree–granting programs; that is, graduate-level educational programs offered by universities or colleges.

   F. Several graduate programs in nursing focus on case management as a specialty at the graduate level of nursing practice. Although limited, there are also programs that combine nursing and social work with a focus on case management and in the form of interprofessional education.
   G. The case management literature describes a variety of training and education programs for preparing case managers for their roles:
     1. Degree- or non–degree-granting programs
     2. Programs offered by health care organizations in the practice sector, independent continuing education agencies, or colleges and universities
   H. The case management training and education programs are classified by Cesta and Tahan (2003) into five types or levels (Box 17-4).
   I. Case management training programs that are offered by health care organizations may include topics such as those described in Box 17-5.
   J. Case management educational programs offered by colleges and universities are considered formal programs and may include courses that cover topics such as those listed in Box 17-6.

BOX 17-5 Topics Addressed in Informal Case Management Training Programs

- Leadership
- The change process
- Communication and interpersonal skills
- Case management concepts, principles, and models
- The case management process
- The role of the case manager
- Care coordination and interdisciplinary rounding
- Utilization review and management
- Transitional and discharge planning
- Case management plans and tools
- Legal and ethical considerations
- Patient and family/caregiver engagement, education, and patients' rights
- Motivational interviewing
- Risk stratification
- Quality management and safety

BOX 17-6   Topics Addressed in Formal Case Management Educational Programs

- Health care delivery systems and models
- The continuum of care and settings including community resources and the transitional planning process
- Integrated health care delivery systems
- Health care finance and reimbursement concepts including resource allocation, utilization review, and management
- Implementation of case management systems and the role of the case manager
- Research and program evaluation including outcomes management
- Ethical and legal issues of health care delivery and case management practice
- Leadership concepts including systems theory, change theory, multidisciplinary collaboration, negotiation, conflict resolution, and delegation
- Client advocacy
- Client activation and engagement and client identified caregiver involvement in care
- Cultural competence, health literacy, and health education
- Case management tools and plans
- Health care policy and legislation
- Quality and performance improvement including working in teams

K. Educational programs that grant academic degrees usually include clinical courses or practicum.
   1. Clinical courses consist of the case manager student spending a few hundred hours in a clinical setting practicing with a case manager mentor.
   2. Examples of colleges or universities that offer academic degrees in case management are College of Nursing at Seton Hall University, NJ, and Capstone College of Nursing at University of Alabama, AL.
L. Case management training and education programs that are offered by professional organizations or continuing education agencies include specific topics that are related to case management practice, especially those that are based on practical experiences, and tell the success stories or learned lessons of some health care organizations, research findings, and innovations/advances.
   1. Generally, each topic is addressed over a 45-minute to 3-hour period. Some programs are one day long; others vary and may extend up to 5 days.
   2. Topics addressed in these sessions aim to build the knowledge, skills, and competencies of case managers, leaders of case management programs, and health care professionals associated with case management practice.
   3. These programs offer continuing education credits and are of the ongoing professional development activity type.

Credentialing in Case Management

A. Credentialing is an essential activity in case management and aims to protect the consumer of health care services—to ensure that the individuals hired to practice case management are qualified, knowledgeable, and competent, as well as able to provide quality services.

B. Certification is but one aspect of credentialing. Others may include a review of knowledge, skills, performance, competence, licensure, work history, and experience.

C. Credentialing is the process of evaluating a person's education and experience against a standard to determine whether he or she is qualified to perform the job, taking into consideration community standards; national standards; and state practice acts, statutes, and liability.

D. Credentialing also is a dynamic process in determining the qualifications of a person compared with standards to perform a given responsibility safely, effectively, and legally.

E. URAC has developed accreditation standards for case management organizations and programs and offers case management program accreditation to interested organizations.

1. URAC advocates in its accreditation standards that case managers must be licensed or certified in a health care discipline that, in the applicable jurisdictions, allows them to conduct an assessment independently within their scope of practice.

2. URAC requires case managers to have 2 years of experience in direct clinical care provision to the consumer.

3. URAC also states that case managers must have either of the following qualifications: health-related bachelors' degree, or CM certification, or a license as an RN.

F. Standards of practice for case management, adopted by CMSA in 1995 and the revised in 2002 and 2010, are authoritative statements defining the behaviors expected of case managers, that is, qualifications, roles, functions, and responsibilities.

G. There are many components to credentialing in case management. They are usually embedded in the form of credentialing standards and may include the meaning of case management, philosophy, roles and responsibilities of case managers, client selection, evaluation measures, and other topics.

1. CMSA defines case management as "a collaborative process which assesses, plans, implements, coordinates, monitors and evaluates options and services to meet an individual's health needs through communication and available resources to promote quality cost-effective outcomes" (CMSA, 2010, p. 6).

2. The CCMC defines case management as "a collaborative process that assesses, plans, implements, coordinates, monitors, and evaluates the options and services required to meet the client's health and human services needs. It is characterized by advocacy, communication, and resource management and promotes quality and cost-effective interventions and outcomes" (CCMC, 2015, p. 3).

3. Philosophy of case management: A philosophy is a statement of belief, setting forth principles that guide case management programs and the case manager in his or her practice.

a. CMSA's philosophy of case management highlights the underlying premise that the practice is based on the fact that when a client reaches optimal level of functioning and wellness, everyone involved (i.e., stakeholders) benefits, for example, the client's support system, the payer, the provider, and the employer.

    i. Case management serves as a means for achieving client's wellness and autonomy through advocacy, communication, health education or instruction, and facilitation of access to services and resources needed.

    ii. Case management optimizes the achievement of outcomes through a practice environment that promotes open communication among all parties involved.

    iii. Provision of holistic and client-centered care to those in need and who benefit most from case management services such as clients with catastrophic illnesses or injuries.

    iv. Provision of care in collaboration with other health care professionals with special attention to enhancing integration, eliminating fragmentation and duplication, and promoting quality, safety, and cost-effectiveness (CMSA, 2010).

  b. Philosophy of case management as developed by the CCMC (2015, p. 3) indicates that case management:

    i. Is an area of specialty practice within one's health and human services profession. Its underlying premise is that everyone benefits when clients (e.g., patients, employees) reach their optimum level of wellness, self-management, and functional capability—the clients being served, their support systems, the health care delivery systems, and the various payer sources.

    ii. Facilitates the achievement of client wellness and autonomy through advocacy, assessment, planning, communication, education, resource management, and service facilitation.

    iii. Based on the needs and values of the client, and in collaboration with all service providers, the case manager links clients with appropriate providers and resources throughout the continuum of health and human services and care settings, while ensuring that the care provided is safe, effective, client centered, timely, efficient, and equitable. This approach achieves optimum value and desirable outcomes for all—the clients, their support systems, the providers, and the payers.

    iv. Provides services that are optimized best when offered in a climate that allows direct communication among the case manager, the client, the payer, the primary care provider, and other service delivery professionals. The case manager is able to enhance these services by maintaining the client's privacy, confidentiality, health, and safety through advocacy and adherence to ethical, legal, accreditation, certification, and regulatory standards or guidelines (CCMC, 2015).

4. Certification, which determines that the case manager possesses the education, skills, knowledge, and experience required to render appropriate and effective services according to sound principles of practice.

5. The case manager's job description is an important part of credentialing. It is used as the day-to-day working document delineating the roles and responsibilities of the case manager (activities and role relationships) and requirements for practice (knowledge, skills, abilities, educational degrees, licensure, and certification).

| BOX 17-7 | Key Components of a Case Manager's Job Description |

- Job title
- Department
- Reports to whom
- Summary of position
- Specific duties, functions, and responsibilities
- Required knowledge
- Qualifications, including education, experience, licenses, and certifications

6. There are a number of key components the case manager's job description must address to assure role clarity and avoid role conflict and/or confusion (Box 17-7).
7. The employment application or contract, which sets forth in writing the education, work experience, and skills of the individual.
8. The applicant (candidate for the case manager job) interview conducted by a supervisor, peers, and subordinates, if any.

H. Credentialing occurs usually upon hire and annually thereafter.
   1. Upon hire: Verification of licenses, good standing, educational degree(s), past experience, and certifications.
   2. Annually: Competency-based performance appraisal. This process focuses on the ability of the case manager to perform his or her roles and responsibilities as described in the job description. It is a measure of maintaining continued competence especially for the protection of the consumer and to ensure the provision of quality care.

I. Recredentialing ensures that case managers continue to meet professional standards in their performance. It is also a process for identifying the areas of knowledge or performance case managers need to improve in, and therefore, it identifies continuing training and education needs.

 ## Overview of Certification in Case Management

A. Certification is a process of validation of knowledge, skills, and abilities of individual practitioners. It is usually provided by a nationally recognized agency such as the CCMC or the ANCC.
B. Certification is based on predetermined standards, including licensure, education, acceptable past experience, and examination. It builds on an existing and defined health license such as registered nurse (RN), medical doctor (MD), or licensed clinical social worker (LCSW).
C. The CCMC has developed a certification process for case managers since 1992. The CCMC is the first multidisciplinary and largest organization to certify case managers in the practice of case management. The credential used by the CCMC is called the *certified case manager* (CCM). Today, however, there are more than 30 different certifications in case management offered by varying professional organizations and agencies.
D. Certification is governed by independent bodies created to define and set standards for certification and administer the certification and the recertification process.

E. Certification-governing bodies are composed of individuals certified by that body and a variety of other individuals who represent the broad spectrum of individuals served, including consumers (public members), academicians, researchers, and other experts in the field.

F. Certification is for an initial period, which is typically 3 to 5 years on average, at which time recertification is required to maintain the certification or credential.

G. Recertification is completed in either of two ways:
   1. Based on continued acceptable employment in the field and a predetermined number of continuing education requirements
   2. By retaking the certification examination itself

H. Individuals who are certified have a specific credential (designation) they are allowed to use after their name, such as CCM or Care Manager Certified (CMC), for as long as their certification is active and they are in good standing in the community.

I. Certification is voluntary. However, some accreditation standards recommend certification.

J. Certifying bodies/agencies have a code of professional conduct for the individuals they certify. CCMs are expected to abide by the codes of professional conduct of their own professional specialty (e.g., nursing, social work, rehabilitation counseling) and that of case management.
   1. A code of professional conduct protects the public interest and delineates the behavioral expectations of case managers.
   2. Codes of professional conduct contain
      a. Principles
      b. Rules of conduct
      c. Guidelines or standards for professional and ethical conduct
   3. Individuals may have more than one code of professional conduct if they are licensed or a member of a profession.

K. Certification examinations should be free of bias and nondiscriminatory. There should be validity of the examination established through a job analysis survey and ongoing scientific research that helps maintain the currency of the examination and its representation of current case management practice.

L. There are many certifications in case management; however, credible ones employ research in the development of the examination items and in identifying the domains of knowledge and practice the examination must reflect. Another criterion of credibility is recognition by the National Organization for Certifying Agencies (NOCA). For example, the CCMC is recognized by the NOCA.[4]

M. The benefits of certification in case management are many, of which those described in Box 17-8 are of prime importance.

N. A case manager should choose a specific certification depending on his or her job function and responsibilities and the care or work setting, matched to the requirements of the certification and certifying agency.

---

[4]For information on how to assess the credibility of case management certifying agencies, refer to the CCMC Website (www.ccmcertification.org).

BOX
17-8 **Benefits of Certification in Case Management**

- Provides a standard of knowledge, skills, and competence for employers of case managers
- Assures the consumer and public that the case manager has a sufficient level of knowledge, skills, and competence
- Demonstrates ability to safeguarding the public interest
- Provides a recognized benchmark for health care workers and consumers of case management services
- Indicates that the person certified is knowledgeable, informed, and current in his or her area of practice
- Keeps the certification holder competitive and marketable

 Select Certifications in Case Management

A. The oldest certification in case management is the CCM that is offered by the CCMC.

1. The CCM is the first certification developed specifically for case managers regardless of professional specialty; that is, it is multidisciplinary.

2. In 1992, the National Case Management Task Force organized a meeting with representatives of various national organizations (stakeholders of case management) with interest in case management. This meeting was organized because of the growing concern that there were no standards or qualifications for people calling themselves case managers.

3. Consensus was reached in the 1992 meeting to appoint the Commission of Insurance Rehabilitation Specialists (now known as the Commission for Disability Management Specialists) to develop a certification for individual case managers, based on the work of the National Task Force.

4. The work of the National Task Force culminated in the creation of the CCMC and the certification for individual case managers (the CCM).

5. Certification requirements for the CCM are as follows (CCMC, 2015):

a. Good moral character, reputation, and fitness for the practice of case management

b. Licensure and certification requirements:

i. License or certification must be based on a minimum educational requirement of a post–secondary-degree program in a field that promotes the physical, psychosocial, or vocational well-being of the persons being served.

ii. The license or certification awarded on completion of the educational program must have been obtained by passing an examination in the area(s) of specialization.

iii. The license or certification process must grant the holder the ability to legally and independently practice without the supervision of another licensed professional and to perform

the following eight essential activities of case management—assessment, planning, implementation, coordination, monitoring, evaluation, outcomes, and general (e.g., case management actions that span all of the essential activities, such as advocacy).
  iv. All licenses and certifications must be current.
  c. Employment experience falls into three categories. The candidate must meet one of them to be eligible for the certification examination:
   i. Twelve months of acceptable full-time case management employment or equivalent under the supervision of a CCM for the 12 months.
   ii. Twenty-four months of acceptable full-time case management employment or equivalent. Supervision by a CCM is not required under this category.
   iii. Twelve months of acceptable full-time case management employment or its equivalent as a supervisor, supervising the activities of individuals who provide direct case management services.
  d. All experience must be verifiable by a manager, supervisor, or employer. Self-employment is acceptable but also must be verified.
  e. To qualify as acceptable employment, the applicant must demonstrate as part of his or her employment the eight essential activities of case management (listed earlier).
6. The CCM examination is administered multiple times online per year. This certification is the most widely held certification by case managers—more than 37,000 case managers have been certified by the CCMC since the inception of the certification. Applicants who successfully pass the examination use the designation CCM.
B. Board certification (BC) in nursing case management is another certification/credential available in case management and offered by the ANCC (ANCC, 2013). This certification is limited to registered nurses (RN) only.
  1. The credential designation is RN-BC, nurse case manager.
  2. Eligibility requirements to sit for the RN-BC case management examination are as follows:
   a. Hold an active RN license in the United States or its territories
   b. Currently hold an associate, a diploma, baccalaureate, or higher degree in nursing
   c. Have functioned within the scope of a registered nurse, equivalent to 2 years of full time
   d. Have practiced in the capacity of a nurse case manager for a minimum of 2,000 hours within the last 3 years
   e. Have completed 30 hours on continuing education in nursing case management within the last 3 years
  3. The RN-BC nurse case manager computer-based examination is administered year round by the ANCC. The first examination was offered in 1997.

4. Applicants who successfully pass the examination use the designation RN-BC. The person must be recertified every 5 years.

C. Another certification is the Care Manager Certified (CMC) offered by the National Academy of Certified Care Managers.

1. Eligibility requirements to sit for the CMC examination are as follows:

   a. A master's degree in social work, nursing, gerontology, counseling, or psychology.

   b. Two years of supervised, paid, full-time care/case management experience.

   c. Experience must include personal, face-to-face interviewing, assessment, care planning, problem solving, and follow-up.

   d. Applicants with a bachelor's degree in social work, nursing, gerontology, counseling, or care management.

   e. Four years of paid, full-time work experience with clients in practice settings of social work, nursing, mental health, counseling, or care management. Two of those years must be supervised, paid, full-time care management experience.

   f. Applicants with a high school diploma or any degree in an area not related to care management.

   g. Six years of paid, full-time, direct experience with clients in social work, mental health, nursing, counseling or care management; 2 of those years must be supervised.

2. The first examination for Care Manager Certified was administered in 1996. The person must be recertified every 3 years.

D. The Certified Case Management Administrator (CCMA) is offered by the Center for Case Management and focuses on case managers in leadership positions (Center for Case Management, 2015).

1. Candidates for the CCMA are case management administrators who supervise employees or who perform the functions listed below. If applying as an experienced case manager, candidates must perform at least eight of the functions described in Box 17-9 on a daily basis (Center for Case Management, 2015).

BOX 17-9

Functions Covered in the Certified Case Management Administrator Certification Examination

1. Identifying cases/clients for case management services
2. Comprehensively assessing a client's situation
3. Evaluating and coordinating the plan of care
4. Matching client resources to client needs
5. Monitoring delivery of services
6. Using critical thinking skills, prioritizing appropriately, and managing time wisely
7. Measuring and evaluating financial, clinical, functional, and satisfaction outcomes
8. Maintaining accountability for financial, clinical, functional, and satisfaction outcomes
9. Displaying effective leadership in the performance of current role
10. Communicating effectively
11. Evaluating and responding to the needs of clients, clinicians, and the community

2. Eligibility requirements to sit for the CCMA examination are a master's degree and 1 year of experience in case management administration, a master's degree and 3 years of experience as a case manager, or a bachelor's degree and 5 years of experience as a case manager.
3. Recertification is required every 5 years.
4. The examination for case management administrators was first administered in 1998. Individuals who successfully pass the examination use the designation CMAC (Case Management Administrator Certified).
E. Recently, CMSA collaborated with the American Board of Quality Assurance and Utilization Review Physicians (ABQAURP) to offer a subspecialty certification in transitions of care. This certification is available through ABQAURP's Health Care Quality Management Board Certification (HCQM).
1. Eligibility criteria for the transitions of care subspecialty certification include the following:
   a. Current diplomate status with ABQAURP.
   b. Current, nonrestricted licensure and/or certification appropriate to the individual's profession in each state or territory in which the individual is licensed or certified (if applicable to individual's profession).
   c. Documentation of active involvement in the subspecialty within the past 4 years. A minimum of 312 hours must be devoted to the subspecialty.
   d. The experience must be verified by a reference.
   e. A minimum of 24 hours of ABQAURP-approved continuing education pertinent to the subspecialty (i.e., transitions of care).
2. Transitions of care (TOC) involve patient transfers from one level of care to another, including a patient's movement from primary to specialty care or from a hospital setting to home or another care facility.
3. The ABQAURP also offers a subspecialty certification in case management. Requirements are the same as those of transitions of care.
4. When candidates are credentialed and successfully complete the HCQM board examination, they are certified in both health care quality and management and in the subspecialty of transitions of care and may use the designation CHCQM-TOC.
F. There are many other certifications for individuals working in health care. To determine credibility of certification, refer to the section Certification for Case Managers presented earlier in this chapter. See Table 17-3 for a select listing of certifications and contact information.
G. Persons supervising case managers for 12 months may be able to sit for the CCMC certification exam. Similarly, the CMAC exam acknowledges length of experience as a master's degree–prepared case manager and case management administrator as a criterion for application to sit for the examination.
H. There are many credentials case managers use after they obtain certification in case management practice and related areas. Table 17-4 lists some examples of these credentials.

(*text continues on page 443*)

TABLE 17-3 Select Certifications in Case Management

Certification	Sponsoring Organization	Web site	Phone Number
ACM, Accredited Case Manager	American Case Management Association	http://www.acmaweb.org	501-907-2262
CCM, Certified Case Manager	Commission for Case Manager Certification	www.ccmcertification.org	856-380-6836
CDMS, Certified Disability Management Specialist	Certification of Disability Management Specialists Commission	www.cdms.org	847-944-1335
CMAC, Case Management Administrator, Certified	The Center for Case Management	www.cfcm.com	781-446-6980
CMC, Case Management Certified	American Institute of Outcomes Care Management	www.AIOCM.com	562-945-9990
CRC, Certified Rehabilitation Counselor	Commission on Rehabilitation Counselor Certification	www.crccertification.com	847-944-1325
CRRN, Certified Rehabilitation Registered Nurse	Association of Rehabilitation Nurses	www.rehabnurse.org	800-229-7530
COHN, Certified Occupational Health Nurse	American Board for Occupational Health Nurses, Inc.	http://www.abohn.org	630-789-5799
COHN-S, Certified Occupational Health Nurse—Specialist	American Board for Occupational Health Nurses, Inc.	http://www.abohn.org	630-789-5799
RN-BC Registered Nurse Case Manager	American Nurses Credentialing Center	www.nursecredentialing.org	800-284-1278

TABLE 17-4 Examples of Credentials in Case Management Certifications

AAOHN **American Association of Occupational Health Nurses**
Primary focus: Occupational health nurses
Provided by: American Association of Occupational Health
                   Nurses
Web site: https://www.aaohn.org/

ABDA **American Board of Disability Analyst**
Primary focus: Rehab, medicine, case management
Provided by: American Board of Disability Analysts
Web site: http://www.americandisability.org/certifications.
                   html

ACM **Accredited Case Manager**
Primary focus: A certification for hospital/health system case
                   management professionals
Provided by: American Case Management Association (ACMA)
Web site: http://www.acmaweb.org/section.asp?sID=16

AOCN **Advanced Oncology Certified Nurse**
Primary focus: Nurses
Provided by: Oncology Nursing Certification Corporation (ONCC)
Web site: http://www.oncc.org

CASWCM **Certified Social Work Case Manager**
CSWCM
Primary focus: MSW social workers
                   BSW social workers
Provided by: National Association of Social Workers (NASW)
Web site: http://www.socialworkers.org

CCM **Certified Case Manager**
Primary focus: Multiple-practice setting case managers
Provided by: Commission for Case Management Certification
Web site: http://www.ccmcertification.org

CCP **Chronic Care Professionals**
Primary focus: Health coaching and chronic care certification
                   program; focus is on all members of the health care
                   team.
Provided by: Health Sciences Institute
Web site: http://www.healthsciences.org/information-about-
                   ccp-certification.html

CCRNS **Certification in Critical Care Nursing (as granted by the AACN Certification)**
Primary focus: Nurses
Provided by: American Association of Critical Care Nurses
Web site: http://www.healthsciences.org/information-about-
                   ccp-certification.html

continued

TABLE 17-4 Examples of Credentials in Case Management Certifications, *continued*

CDMS	**Certified Disability Management Specialist**	
	Primary focus:	Disability managers
		Insurance based
		Rehab specialists
		Vocational counselors
	Provided by:	Certified Disability Management Specialist Commission
	Web site:	http://www.cdms.org
CHCQM	**Certified Health Care Quality Management**	
	Primary focus:	Certification in five subspecialty areas:
		• Transitions of care
		• Patient safety/risk management
		• Case management
		• Managed care
		• Workers' compensation
		This certification is over and above the HCQM board certification.
	Provided by:	American Board of Quality Assurance and Utilization Review Physicians (ABQAURP)
	Web site:	http://www.abqaurp.org
CMAC	**Case Management Administrator Certification**	
	Primary focus:	Case management administration
	Provided by:	The Center for Case Management
	Web site:	http://www.cfcm.com/resources/certification.asp
CMC	**Certification for Case Managers**	
	Primary focus:	All health care professionals
	Provided by:	The American Institute of Outcomes Case Management (AIOCM)
	Web site:	http://www.aiocm.com
CMC	**Care Manager Certified**	
	Primary focus:	Gerontology, counseling care management
	Provided by:	National Academy of Certified Care Managers
	Web site:	http://www.naccm.net
CMCN	**Certified Managed Care Nurse**	
	Primary focus:	Nurses in managed care
	Provided by:	American Board of Managed Care Nursing
	Web site:	http://www.abmcn.org
COHN/CM COHN-S/CM	**Certified Occupational Health Nurse/ Case Manager**	
	Primary focus:	Occupational health case management
	Provided by:	American Board of Occupational Health Nursing— Case Manager
	Web site:	http://www.abohn.org

TABLE 17-4 Examples of Credentials in Case Management Certifications, *continued*

CPHQ	**Certified Professional in Healthcare Quality**
	Primary focus: Quality managers
	Utilization managers
	Risk managers
	Provided by: Healthcare Quality Certification Board of the National Association for Healthcare Quality
	Web site: http://www.cphq.org
CPON	**Certified Pediatric Oncology Nurse**
	Primary focus: Oncology nurses
	Provided by: Oncology Nursing Certification Corporation (ONCC)
	Web site: http://www.oncc.org
CRC	**Certified Rehabilitation Counselor**
	Primary focus: Rehab counselors
	Provided by: Commission on Rehabilitation Counselor Certification (CRCC)
	Web site: http://www.crccertification.com
CRRN	
CRRN-A	**Certified Rehabilitation Registered Nurse Certified Rehabilitation Nurse—Advanced**
	Primary focus: Rehab nurses
	Provided by: Rehabilitation Nursing Certification Board
	Web site: http://www.rehabnurse.org
RN-BC	**Registered Nurse Case Manager**
	Primary focus: Nurse case manager
	Provided by: American Nurses Credentialing Center (ANCC)
	Web site: http://www.nursingworld.org
RN-C	**Certified Nurse Case Manager**
	Primary focus: Nurse case manager
	Provided by: American Nurses Credentialing Center (ANCC)
	Web site: http://www.nursingworld.org

URAC Accreditation of Organizations Performing Case Management

A. Accreditation is the process of reviewing all aspects of an organization, program, or service for the purpose of evaluating whether it meets published and nationally recognized standards of providing quality services.

B. Accreditation is a voluntary process and applies specific standards determined by the credentialing agency.

C. In June 1999, URAC adopted accreditation standards for organizations performing case management.

1. URAC used an expert panel/advisory committee with representatives from all case management stakeholders to develop the standards.
2. Organizations represented included the CMSA, CCMC, ANA, American Medical Association, American Association of Health Plans, URAC-accredited companies, Association of Managed Healthcare Organizations, health care business representatives, Washington Business Group on Health, American Health Quality Association, American Hospital Association, Blue Cross Blue Shield Association, Centers for Medicare and Medicaid Services (CMS), and representatives from the Department of Defense.
3. The resulting URAC standards are the first to specifically address case management organizations and to set what constitutes a quality case management organization, program, or service.

D. To date, URAC has accredited over 150 of organizations that provide all types of case management services. These include health insurance plans, payers, employers, and federal and state agencies.

E. URAC case management accreditation is considered a catalyst in boosting care coordination, quality, and overall excellence of client-centric services. URAC continuously improves this accreditation program through research and best practices to keep pace with health care reform and demands of the Patient Protection and Affordable Care Act (PPACA) (URAC, 2015).

F. URAC notes that this accreditation program helps build organizational excellence in managing transitions of care, which result in reducing readmissions and poor health outcomes and enhance meeting the value-based purchasing expectations. The accreditation standards reflect the latest advances in case management techniques and industry best practices (URAC, 2015).

G. URAC designed the standards to fit organizations that provide telephonic or on-site case management services in conjunction with a privately or publicly funded benefits program across settings and specialties. Accreditation or certification is available depending on the type of organization and services being offered.

H. URAC's accreditation process addresses a set of standards that are considered core to all URAC accreditation programs.
1. These standards address several key organizational management functions that are important for any health care organization.
2. The core standards provide the basic structures and processes any organization must have to maintain a level of quality expected in a URAC-accredited organization.
3. Each accreditation program also includes additional standards specific to the program. For example, case management programs must meet the core standards as well as the specific case management standards.

I. The URAC core standards address several critical areas of basic structure and processes including organizational structure, personnel management, operations, quality improvement, oversight of delegated responsibilities, and consumer protection (URAC, 2016a). Specifics of the general standards are described in Box 17-10.

1. Organizational structure standard requires the organization to define:
   a. Its structure and oversight responsibility and how it maintains policies and procedures that govern all aspects of the operation
   b. The job descriptions
   c. Licensure required for certain personnel
   d. A regulatory compliance program that ensures it is conducting business in accordance with applicable federal and state laws
   e. Confidentiality and conflict of interest policies
   f. Other requirements such as a structured quality management program and processes to protect the safety and welfare of consumers
2. The personnel standard requires the organization to ensure that:
   a. Written job descriptions for all staff clearly define the following qualifications—education, training, professional experience, expected professional competencies, appropriate licensure/certification requirements, and scope and role of responsibilities.
   b. Credentials of licensed or certified personnel are verified.
   c. A clear orientation, training, and evaluation program exists and that staff members are given the necessary guidelines to do their job.
3. The operations and process standard expects the organization to:
   a. Establish communication methods across all departments and disciplines to promote collaboration
   b. Coordinate internal activities
   c. Provide quality services
   d. Have systems and processes in place for information management, business relationships, clinical oversight, regulatory compliance, and incentive programs
4. The quality improvement standard requires the organization to:
   a. Maintain a quality management program that promotes objective and systematic monitoring and evaluation of consumer and client and health care services
   b. Implement its own quality management program that assists the organization in focusing its unique needs and efforts
5. The delegation of responsibilities standard requires the organization to:
   a. Maintain responsibility and oversight for any function it delegates to another entity
6. The consumer satisfaction and protection standard expects the organization to:
   a. Communicate with consumers and clients clearly and accurately
   b. Represent information about the organization's services and how to obtain these services
   c. Have a complaint or grievance mechanism in place
   d. Have a process to respond quickly in situations that create an immediate threat to the safety or welfare of consumers

J. The URAC standards that are specific to case management program accreditation cover several critical operational categories. These standards are referred to as core standards and described in Box 17-11 (URAC, 2016b).

K. The URAC accreditation standards assist organizations in the development of policies and procedures that include a definition of case management, the types of consumers served, the delivery model for case management services, case management staff qualifications and continuing education, and evaluation of the program.

(*text continues on page 447*)

17-11   URAC's Core Standards for Case Management Accreditation

1. Case management program components:
   a. Program overview
   b. Written policies and procedures
   c. Definition and philosophy of case management
   d. A description of types of consumers served
   e. A description of the delivery model for case management services
   f. Guidelines or criteria for identifying clients for case management services
   g. Guidelines for discharge planning and client's transitions of care
   h. Guidelines for case manager's caseload
   i. Clinical practice and evidence-based guidelines
   j. Development of the plan of care
   k. Use of information support systems
   l. Shared decision-making involving the client/consumer of care
   m. Collaborative communication with all stakeholders
   n. Client's consent for case management including documentation of the client's oral or written consent to services (written consent is preferred.)
   o. Accessing physicians and other consultants including a list of licensed physicians available for consultations with case managers
   p. Health information and education materials
   q. Internal performance monitoring and quality committee
   r. Tools that enable the case manager to collect the information necessary to carry out the case management process
   s. Implementation of a policy and procedure to protect the confidentiality of individually identifiable health information and to protect the welfare and safety of consumers and case managers
   t. Implementation of policies and procedures to promote the autonomy of consumer and family decision-making
   u. Support for consumer and family decision-making by respecting the rights of the consumer to have input into the case management plan, refuse treatment or services, obtain information regarding the criteria for case closure, and so on
2. Case management client education and engagement:
   a. Consumer motivation and engagement policy
   b. Consumer health education policy
   c. Health education packets and materials
   d. Case management disclosure policy
   e. Disclosure to patients information concerning the nature of the case management relationship, the circumstances under which information will be disclosed to third parties, the availability of a complaint process, the availability of written notification of case management activities, any incentive compensation system for case managers based on utilization rates, and, upon request, a description of the rationale for selecting case management services
   f. Policy for resolving disagreements within the organization regarding consumer care options
   g. Policies and procedures through which consumers and providers may submit a complaint
3. Case management staff training and qualifications:
   a. Sufficient personnel to provide services to consumers.
   b. Job descriptions of case management supervisors. These are encouraged to have a bachelor's (or higher) degree in a health-related field; licensure as a health professional, certification as a case manager, or professional certification in a clinical specialty; and five years' experience as a case manager.
   c. Job description of case managers including a description of qualifications.

BOX 17-11 URAC's Core Standards for Case Management Accreditation *continued*

    d. Case management staff roles and responsibilities.
    e. Job descriptions of case management support staff.
    f. Scope of practice and attestation for such.
    g. A process or program for training and education of case managers that focuses on:
       i. Current principles, procedures, and knowledge of case management based on nationally recognized standards
      ii. Knowledge of the organization's policies and procedures, state requirements, professional roles, health care requirements of specific populations, and URAC standards
     iii. Annual professional education for case managers and the organization to encourage professional development
4. Case management assessment and plans of care:
    a. Policies to conduct and document an assessment for each consumer
    b. Policy for client-centered plan of care; case management plan of care for each client must lay out short-term and long-term goals, time frames for re-evaluation, resources to be used, and collaborative approaches to be used
    c. Medications safety assessment policy
    d. Clearly defined roles of case managers and support staff in provision of care
5. Care coordination:
    a. Policy for care coordination
    b. Tools and templates used for care coordination and transitions of care
    c. Ways of communicating with providers and other stakeholders
    d. Policy for provider selection; must be executed based on client's assessed needs and goals of care
6. Transitions of care (optional or organization may pursue specific accreditation for this):
    a. Transitions of care policy
    b. Criteria for the discharge of consumers or the termination of case management services
    c. Use of personal health records
    d. Use of individualized health care tools
    e. Transitions of care information sharing process and communication across settings and providers
    f. Accountabilities of staff involved in transitions of care (clinical and nonclinical)
    g. Transitions of care follow-up and client outreach
7. Measurement and reporting:
    a. Measures used to evaluate the outcomes of case management services such as hospital readmission rates, clients return to work rates, complaints response time, client satisfaction, and care experience
    b. Use of patient activation tools and patient activation measure
    c. Care transitions measure
    d. Conduct of case reviews to promote achievement of case management goals and use of the information for quality management purposes

  L. The URAC case management accreditation standards provide a solid foundation for effective case management programs. They build on core accreditation standards to enable organizations to successfully:
    1. Train case managers
    2. Identify individuals for case management

3. Manage and conduct case management activities in an efficient and professional manner
4. Promote the autonomy of consumer and family decision-making
5. Maintain confidentiality
6. Delegate responsibility

M. URAC defines a case management organization as an organization or program that provides telephonic or on-site case management services in conjunction with a private or publicly funded benefits program. All such organizations are eligible to apply for accreditation.

N. Case management organizations applying for accreditation participate in a process that entails a rigorous review of four phases as described in Box 17-12 (URAC, 2006).

O. URAC's executive committee makes a final accreditation determination. Applicants who successfully meet all requirements are awarded a full accreditation, and an accreditation certificate is issued to the organization.

P. Full URAC accreditation lasts 2 years. The accredited case management organization must remain in compliance with the standards throughout the accreditation period.

Q. Because there are no other generic case management organization standards, the standards developed by URAC are the standards all organizations—both accredited and nonaccredited organizations—are evaluated against and held to.

BOX 17-12   Phases of URAC's Case Management Accreditation Process

1. The initial phase, *building the application,* consists of completing the application forms and supplying supporting documentation, and payment of the application and base fee.
2. In the second phase, *desktop review,* the applicant's documentation is analyzed in relation to the URAC standards by one or more URAC reviewers. Documents include the organization's formal policies and procedures, organizational charts, position descriptions, contracts, sample template letters, and program descriptions and plans for departments such as quality management and credentialing.
3. In the third phase, *on-site review,* the accreditation review team (the same team involved in the desktop review) conducts an on-site review to verify adherence to the URAC standards. The management and leadership team of the case management organization is interviewed about the organization's programs, and staff is observed performing its duties. Audits are conducted and personnel and credentialing files analyzed. Education and quality management programs are reviewed in detail as well.
4. The fourth phase, *committee review,* entails a review of the accreditation process by two URAC committees that include professionals from a variety of areas in health care as well as industry experts selected from or chosen by URAC's member organizations. The process begins with a written summary documenting the findings of the desktop and on-site reviews. This summary is submitted to URAC's accreditation committee for evaluation. An accreditation recommendation is then forwarded to URAC's executive committee, which has the authority to grant accreditation.

NCQA Accreditation in Case Management

A. The National Committee for Quality Assurance (NCQA) is another organization that credentials case management and care coordination programs. It places special attention on transition of care practices.

B. NCQA's case management accreditation is a comprehensive, evidence-based program dedicated to quality improvement and can be applied for case management programs in provider, payer/health insurance plans, population health management, or community-based organizations including accountable care organizations (ACOs) and patient-centered medical homes (PCMHs).

C. NCQA's case management accreditation focuses on the following main areas:
   1. How case management services are delivered, not just the organization's internal administrative processes
   2. Transitions of care
   3. The core of care coordination and quality of care
   4. The client's experience of care (NCQA, 2012a)

D. NCQA notes that the quality and effectiveness of case management programs vary among organizations and that independent assessments of organizational and program capabilities assist case management organizations in assuring key program elements are in place to deliver the highest quality and safe care (NCQA, 2012b).

E. NCQA developed its case management accreditation program drawing on considerable expertise it previously had in evaluating health insurance plans (including Medicare Special Needs Plans) and other practices such as the PCMH.

F. NCQA's case management accreditation standards address how case management programs operate and enhance quality and safety for the clients they serve (Box 17-13).

BOX 17-13   Focus of NCQA's Case Management Accreditation Standards

- Identify people/clients who are in need of case management services.
- Target the right services to clients and monitor their care and needs over time.
- Develop personalized and individualized patient-centered case management plans of care.
- Monitor clients to ensure care goals are achieved and to make adjustments as needed.
- Manage communication among health care providers and share information effectively when clients transition between care settings, especially when they move from hospital or facility-based to community or home care settings. This assures client's safety and optimal care experience.
- Build in consumer protections and ensure clients have access to knowledgeable, well-qualified case management staff.
- Work toward continuous improvement of patient outcomes and satisfaction.
- Keep personal health information safe and secure.

From NCQA. (2012a). *NCQA case management accreditation.* Washington, DC: Author.

G. NCQA describes its accreditation standards for health insurance plans in its quality improvement and management manual in the form of standards and guidelines. Case management, care coordination, and continuity of care, among other aspects of case management practice are included in these standards. They function as guidelines health plans may use in their case management improvement efforts (Box 17-14).

17-14 NCQA Health Plans Accreditation Standards

Complex Case Management
- Population Assessment
- Program Description
- Identifying Members for Case Management
- Access to Case Management
- Case Management Systems
- Case Management Process
- Initial Assessment
- Case Management–Ongoing Management
- Experience with Case Management
- Measuring Effectiveness
- Action and Remeasurement

Disease Management
- Program Content
- Identifying Members for Disease Management Programs
- Frequency of Member Identification
- Providing Members with Information
- Interventions Based on Assessment
- Eligible Member Active Participation
- Informing and Educating Practitioners
- Integrating Member Information
- Experience with Disease Management

Continuity and Coordination of Medical Care
- Identifying Opportunities
- Acting on Opportunities
- Measuring Effectiveness
- Notification of Termination
- Continued Access to Practitioners
- Transition to Other Care

Continuity and Coordination Between Medical Care and Behavioral Health Care
- Data Collection
- Collaborative Activities
- Measuring Effectiveness

Practice Guidelines
- Adoption and Distribution of Guidelines
- Adoption and Distribution of Preventive Health Guidelines
- Relation to Disease Management Programs
- Performance Measurement

Quality Improvement Program Structure
- Program Structure
- Annual Evaluation

BOX

17-14   NCQA Health Plans Accreditation Standards *continued*

Quality Improvement Program Operations
• Quality Improvement Committee Responsibilities
• Informing Members and Practitioners

Health Services Contracting
• Health Services Contracting
• Affirmative Statement
• Provider Contracts

Availability of Practitioners
• Cultural Needs and Preferences
• Practitioners Providing Primary Care
• Practitioners Providing Specialty Care
• Practitioners Providing Behavioral Health Care

Accessibility of Services
• Assessment Against Access Standards
• Behavioral Health Care Access Standards
• Behavioral Health Care Telephone Access Standards

Member Experience
• Annual Assessment
• Opportunities for Improvement
• Annual Assessment of Behavioral Health Care and Services
• Behavioral Health Care Opportunities for Improvement

Marketplace Network Transparency and Experience
• Network Design Criteria for Practitioners
• Network Design Criteria for Hospitals
• Marketplace Member Experience

Delegation of Quality Improvement
• Written Delegation Agreement
• Provision of Member Data to the Delegate
• Provisions for Personal Health Information
• Predelegation Evaluation
• Review of Quality Improvement Program
• Opportunities for Improvement

From NCQA. (2015). *NCQA quality management and improvement: Health plans standards and guidelines.* Washington, DC: author.

H. Case management organizations that pursue accreditation by NCQA can earn any of three accreditation status levels based on their performance against the NCQA's case management standards and guidelines (Box 17-15).
I. NCQA accreditation standards emphasize the need for case management program staff (e.g., case managers) to stay current on the latest evidence and care management techniques and work toward continuous improvement, especially in the areas of quality, safety, and satisfaction with the care experience (NCQA, 2012b).
J. NCQA's focus on managing transitions of care is critical to its case management accreditation program. It believes that managing care transitions effectively can:

BOX 17-15 NCQA's Levels of Case Management Accreditation

1. *Accredited—3 years*: Awarded to organizations that demonstrate strong performance of the functions outlined in the accreditation standards.
2. *Accredited—2 years*: Awarded to organizations that demonstrate acceptable performance of the functions outlined in the accreditation standards.
3. *Denied*: Accreditation is denied in organizations found not to meet the requirements during the accreditation survey.

From NCQA, Case Management Accreditation Levels. Retrieved from http://www.ncqa.org/Programs/Accreditation/CaseManagementCM/CaseManagementAccreditationLevels.aspx, on August 14, 2015.

1. Improve patient safety by reducing or completely preventing errors that could occur as patients transition between settings and care providers.
2. Improve communication between caregivers and health care providers so that changes in care settings or providers maintain continuity of care.
3. Ensure continuity of critical services as patients travel through often fragmented health care delivery systems (NCQA, 2012a).

Differentiating Individual from Organizational Certification

A. The field of case management has been experiencing a rise in the number of certified case managers and certified (or accredited) programs in case management. This has resulted in confusion about the difference between *individual* and *institution* certification; sometimes they are erroneously used as interchangeable terms (Tahan, 2005).
B. Certification of an individual means that a professional such as a case manager has achieved an advanced level of competence in an area of specialty or practice such as case management.
   1. Certifying an individual care provider/professional is based on the individual meeting certain eligibility criteria prior to sitting for the certification exam provided by a nationally recognized certifying agency, such as the CCMC.
   2. Individuals are certified based on their ability to achieve a passing score on the certification exam.
   3. Certifications recognized by URAC.
C. Certification of a program/institution means that an organization has met nationally accepted and recognized standards set forth by a nationally recognized agency, such as URAC.
   1. An institution pursuing certification of a program or service is not obligated to meet any eligibility criteria prior to engaging in the accreditation process.
   2. Certification of a program or service affirms that the institution has a center of excellence in that program or service.
   3. The decision of certification is made based on the institution's ability to demonstrate compliance with the certification (accreditation) standards.

17-16   Characteristics of an Individual Certification

- Offered by a nationally recognized agency.
- Credentialing is in the form of "certification."
- Certifies individual professionals/care providers.
- Uses an exam as the basis for certification.
- The decision to certify is made based on the individual achieving a passing score on the examination.
- Uses nationally recognized standards that focus on the certification exam.
- Individuals who pursue certification must meet eligibility criteria first to be able to sit for the exam.
- Is science based.
- The offering agency tends to engage in ongoing research activities regarding the certification exam.
- Certification of an individual does not extend to the institution where he or she works.
- Certification recognizes the individual care provider as competent in the area of specialty.

D. Although the credential *certification* is used for both individual case managers and institutions, credentialing an individual case manager (Box 17-16) takes place in the form of a "certification" and credentialing a program (Box 17-17) or service occurs in the form of "accreditation" (Tahan, 2005).

E. Agencies that provide certifications for programs do not normally certify individual professionals; if they happen to do so, different departments within the agency assume responsibility for either of the certifications.

F. There are several agencies that offer accreditation or certification for organizations or case management programs—for example:
 1. ACHC—Accreditation Commission for Health Care
 2. CARF—Commission on Accreditation of Rehabilitation Facilities
 3. TJC—The Joint Commission
 4. NCQA—National Committee for Quality Assurance
 5. URAC—Utilization Review Accreditation Commission

17-17   Characteristics of an Organizational Certification/Accreditation

- Offered by a nationally recognized agency.
- Credentialing is in the form of "accreditation."
- Certifies a specific program or service in an organization.
- Uses a national set of standards as the basis for certification.
- The decision to certify is made based on the institution's ability to demonstrate compliance with the set of standards; a review is completed through a survey process.
- Uses nationally recognized standards that focus on practice/health care delivery.
- Institutions may pursue credentialing (certification) at any time—there are no prerequisites.
- There is no obligation to be science based; however, the offering agency may use research outcomes in the design of its standards.
- Certification of the institution/program does not extend to those who work in it.
- Certification recognizes the program as a center of excellence.

References

American Nurses Credentialing Center (ANCC). (2006). *Specialty nursing certifications, nursing case management.* Silver Spring, MD: American Nurses Association. Retrieved from Website: http://www.nursingworld.org/ancc/certification/certs/specialty.html, on March 13, 2015.

Case Management Society of America (CMSA). (2010). *Standards of practice* (2nd ed.). Little Rock, AR: Author.

Cesta, T. G., & Tahan, H. A. (2003). *The case manager's survival guide: Winning strategies for clinical practice* (2nd ed.). St. Louis, MO: Mosby.

Center for Case Management. (2015). *Certification for case management administrators.* Retrieved from Website: http://www.cfcm.com/wordpress1/cmac/, on August 17, 2015.

Commission for Case Manager Certification (CCMC). (2015). *Certification Guide to the CCM® Examination.* Mount Laurel, NJ: Author. Retrieved from http://ccmcertification.org/sites/default/files/downloads/2013/Cert%20Guide.pdf, on August 14, 2015.

Kulbok, P. A., & Utz, S. W. (1999). Managing care: Knowledge and educational strategies for professional development (electronic version). *Family and Community Health, 22*(3), 1–11.

Leahy, M., Chan, Fong, Shaw, L., & Lui, J. (1997). Preparation of rehabilitation counselors for case management practice in health care settings. *Journal of Rehabilitation, 63*(3), 53–59.

Moxley, D. (1996). Teaching case management: Essential content for the preservice preparation of effective personnel. *Journal of Teaching in Social Work, 13*(1/2), 111–139.

National Committee for Quality Assurance (NCQA). (2012a). *NCQA Case Management Accreditation, Program Brochure.* Washington, DC: Author.

National Committee for Quality Assurance (NCQA). (2012b). *NCQA Case Management Accreditation, Program Fact Sheet.* Washington, DC: Author. Retrieved from http://www.ncqa.org/Programs/Accreditation/CaseManagementCM.aspx, on August 14, 2015.

Stanton, M., & Dunkin, J. (2002). Rural case management: Nursing role variations. *Lippincott's Case Management, 7*(2), 48–58.

Stanton, M., Swanson, C., & Baker, B. (2005a). Development of a military competency checklist for case management. *Lippincott's Case Management, 10*(3), 128–135.

Stanton, M., Swanson, M., Sherrod, R. A., & Packa, D. (2005b). Case management evolution: From basic to advanced practice role. *Lippincott's Case Management, 10*(6), 274–284.

Tahan, H. A. (2005). Clarifying certification and its value for case managers. *Lippincott's Case Management, 10*(1), 14–21.

Tahan, H. A., Watson, A. C., & Sminkey, P. V. (2015). What case managers should know about their roles and functions: A National Study from the Commission for Case Manager Certification- Part I. *Professional Case Management, 21*(1), 3–24.

URAC. (2006). *Case management accreditation and certification program overview.* Washington, DC: American Accreditation Health Care Commission/URAC. Retrieved from http://www.urac.org/prog_accred_CM_po.asp?navid=accreditation&pagename5prog_accred_CM, on March 13, 2015.

URAC. (2016a). Core Standards, Version 3.0. Retrieved from https://www.urac.org/wp-content/uploads/STDGlance_CORE.pdf, on April 17, 2016.

URAC. (2016b). Case Management Accreditation, Version 5.1. Retrieved from https://www.urac.org/wp-content/uploads/CaseMgmt-Standards-At-A-Glance-10-9-2013.pdf, on April 17, 2016.

URAC. (2015). *Accreditation programs: Case management.* Retrieved from https://www.urac.org/accreditation-and-measurement/accreditation-programs/all-programs/case-management/, on August 14, 2015.

Professional Obligations in Case Management

CHAPTER 18

Ethics and General Case Management Practice

John D. Banja

IMPORTANT TERMS AND CONCEPTS

Advocacy
Autonomy
Beneficence
Client
Code of Professional
 Conduct for Case
 Managers
Competence
Confidentiality

Conflict of Interest
Deontologism
Dignity
Ethical Dilemma
Ethics
Impartiality
Justice
Moral Character
Morality

Nonmaleficence
Normative Guidelines
Unprofessional
 Behavior
Utilitarianism
Values
Veracity
Virtue Ethics

Introduction

A. Changes in the American health care delivery system, such as the increased complexity of financing health care costs, the need for authorizations for services prior to care provision, and the demands for cost-effectiveness, client safety, and quality of care, have resulted in a rising number of ethical concerns for health care professionals including case managers.

B. These changes have also resulted in the expectation that the case manager, as a client advocate, will prevent ethical conflicts from occurring—or at least manage them when they arise—and especially reduce their impact on health care outcomes, the experience of the patient/family, the providers of care, and any others who may be involved.

C. Ethical theories attempt to explain what it means to act ethically by:
  1. Addressing key ethical terminologies and concepts
  2. Offering proofs or arguments that explain or justify certain actions as ethical and others not
  3. Describing the four familiar ethical theories or models:
     a. Virtue ethics
     b. Deontologism
     c. Utilitarianism
     d. Contractualism (Beauchamp & Childress, 2001; Banja, 2003)

D. Ethical principles are derived from ethical theories and constitute important values and moral beliefs that inform or serve as guidelines for ethical conduct.

E. There are five (5) common ethical principles case managers must be aware of and must incorporate into their practice. These include the following:
  1. Autonomy
  2. Nonmaleficence
  3. Beneficence
  4. Justice
  5. Veracity (Beauchamp & Childress, 2001; Case Management Society of America [CMSA], 2010)

F. Ethical ambiguity or conflict occurs when an ethical principle that might inform behavior is absent, unclear, or controversial.
  1. Conflict also happens when guidelines or principles clash with each other, that is, when satisfying one principle—such as honoring a client's right to make his or her own decisions—collides with another principle—such as working to provide a benefit rather than a harm for the client (Banja, 1999).
  2. Unethical behavior would therefore connote actions that violate ethical standards, such as the ones that are enumerated among the CMSA Standards of Practice.

G. Ethics and law share certain similarities and differences (Lo, 2000).
  1. Both ethics and law are concerned with right behavior and sustaining a social order wherein people can settle their differences reasonably and respectably.
  2. Law sets only a minimally acceptable standard of conduct and, through enforced regulation (e.g., fines, licensure suspension or

revocation, or imprisonment), can insist that its rules and regulations are followed.

3. A violation of an ethical rule (e.g., respect for a client's inherent dignity) need not necessarily result in a legal sanction.

4. Whereas law tolerates minimally acceptable behavior, ethics aspires to ideal behavior or focuses on securing the right or best decision or action in a situation.

5. Controversies exist over certain laws being unethical (e.g., capital punishment) and whether certain illegal acts might sometimes be ethically acceptable (e.g., active euthanasia). These controversies nevertheless illustrate how legal intuitions look to ethical beliefs and values for their justification.

H. Codes of ethics, such as the Code of Professional Conduct for Case Managers advocated for by the Commission for Case Manager Certification (CCMC), attempt to do the following:

1. Protect the public interest by providing guidance to the profession's members on what constitutes ethical conduct and on the kind of conduct required from the profession's members (or certificants or licensees).

2. While such codes of conduct can be helpful, their primary shortcoming consists in the difficulty in applying them to the oftentimes complex and multifactorial nature of many ethical dilemmas (Lo, 2000).

I. Advocacy is a fundamental duty in the ethical case manager's practice. It can be accomplished through a process that promotes a client's self-determination, independence through education, resource and service facilitation, informed decision making, and elimination of disparities (CMSA, 2010).

Descriptions of Key Terms

A. Advocacy—A process that fosters clients' independence by educating them about their rights, health care and human services, resources, and benefits. Advocacy entails securing informed consent and includes considerations of the client's values, beliefs, and interests (CCMC, 2015).

B. Advocate—The individual or groups involved in advocacy activities.

C. Autonomy—A form of personal liberty whereby an individual possesses sufficient mental ability and an absence of external constraint to determine his or her behavior in accordance with a plan chosen and developed by himself or herself (CCMC, 2015).

D. Beneficence—Promoting the other's good or taking steps that further the other's legitimate interests (CCMC, 2015).

E. Client—The individual to whom, or on whose behalf, a case manager provides services (CCMC, 2015).

F. Code of Professional Conduct for Case Managers—A document consisting of principles, rules of conduct, and standards for professional conduct, as well as procedures for processing complaints, that the CCMC offers by way of providing ethical guidelines for case managers (CCMC, 2015).

G. Competence—The domain of skills, behaviors, practices, obligations, and responsibilities that are defined and bounded by the professional's training and qualifications, licensure(s), or certification(s) (Banja, 2006).

H. Confidentiality—A nondisclosure responsibility that connotes refraining from divulging client information to individuals who have neither a need nor a right to know it (Jonsen, Siegler, & Winslade, 2002).

I. Conflict of interest—A set of conditions in which professional judgment concerning a primary interest, such as a patient's welfare or the validity of research, tends to be unduly influenced by a secondary interest, such as financial gain (Thompson, 1993).

J. Contractualism—A model for resolving ethical dilemmas, usually bearing on the distribution of benefits or objects of value, that looks to a formal agreement among the principles where formal rules, principles, and procedures for settling disputes have been settled and adopted (Banja, 2003).

K. Deontologism—Popularized by Immanuel Kant (1724 to 1804): An ethical theory that is grounded in reason and bases decisions on the moral acceptability of the principles that are used to resolve a dilemma; the best principles are the ones that have the widest applicability (to similar cases) and that are performed from a sense of obligation (Beauchamp & Childress, 2008).

L. Dignity—A characteristic of human beings, largely deriving from their rational capacities to self-legislate their moral and legal rules and obligations, that explains their inherent value and their enjoying fundamental rights.

M. Ethical dilemma—A situation wherein the ethically correct course of action is unclear, usually arises due to lack of clarity regarding which ethical principle is appropriate to apply or because multiple ethical principles are in conflict (Banja, 1999).

N. Ethics—A word that can refer to the literature of moral philosophy, the development of a virtuous character, or the analysis of principles, rules, or language that characterize an action or judgment bearing on human welfare as right or good, or wrong, harmful, evil, beneficial, burdensome, etc. (Beauchamp & Childress, 2008).

O. Impartiality—Treating others similarly; making decisions that do not discriminate against individuals or groups on the basis of irrelevant differences such as ethnicity, race, age, gender, or lifestyle (Jansen, 2003).

P. Justice—Providing someone with his or her right or due, providing what a person is owed, and treating another fairly (Beauchamp & Childress, 2008).

Q. Moral character—A habituated response or repertoire of responses to situations bearing on human welfare (Beauchamp & Childress, 2008).

R. Morality—A term that refers to conduct that represents the customs, practices, or conventions that define and characterize people's moral behavior. Unlike ethics, which tends to be critical, analytical, and inquiring toward beliefs, customs, and social conventions, morality is simply the compendium of a society's or a community's sensibilities bearing on acceptable versus unacceptable behavior (Lo, 2000).

S. Nonmaleficence—Refraining from harming, preventing harm from occurring, or, if only harm can occur from an inevitable act or decision, ensuring that the least amount of harm occurs (Beauchamp & Childress, 2008).

T. Normative guidelines—Guidelines that are nationally accepted and considered or looked upon as recommendations or maxims that inform choices and justify action.

U. Privacy—Protecting or securing sensitive information from persons who have no need or right to it.

V. Publicity—The act of making decisions based on standards and rules that are not only available publicly but also accessible by those influenced by the decisions (Jansen, 2003).

W. Unprofessional behavior—Behavior that unreasonably deviates from norms, guidelines, standards, and ethical codes that inform professional behavior.

X. Utilitarianism—An ethical theory popularized by John Stuart Mill (1806 to 1873). It recommends right actions are the ones that produce the greatest amount of happiness for the greatest number of people (Beauchamp & Childress, 2008).

Y. Values—Ascriptions of worth, significance, or importance that inform the bases of standards, goals, or attitudes (Banja, 1997).

Z. Veracity—The act of telling the truth, or the truthfulness of one's statements.

AA. Virtue ethics—Popularized by Aristotle (384 to 322 B.C.), an approach to moral behavior that emphasizes the development of good character by education and training that concentrates on developing virtuous habits, dispositions, and sensibilities (Beauchamp & Childress, 2001).

Applicability to CMSA's Standards of Practice

A. The Case Management Society of America (CMSA) describes in its standards of practice for case management (CMSA, 2010) that case management practice extends across all health care settings, including payer, provider, government, employer, community, and home environment.

B. This chapter introduces ethics concepts and applicability to general case management practice reflective of CMSA standards. Ethical practice overlays each of the practice standards.

C. This chapter discusses how ethics underpins case management practice and the case manager is especially mindful of ethical frameworks, which transcend his/her achieved licensure(s) and certification(s). The ethical standards and practices described here apply to all care settings and professional disciplines involved in case management.

D. The Ethics Standard described in the CMSA standards of practice for case management recognizes that case managers should behave and practice ethically while adhering to the tenets of the ethical code, which underlies the individual case manager's professional credential (e.g., nursing, social work).

Ethical Decision Making and the Case Manager

A. Case managers are expected to act based on case management–related ethical principles and professional codes as well as those of their original profession or specialty, such as the American Nurses Association's Code of Ethics or the National Association of Social Workers' Code of Ethics.

B. Examples of specific ethical principles in case management can be found in the CCMC's Code of Professional Conduct for Case Managers and the CMSA's statement on case management ethics. These principles:

1. Require case managers to place clients' interests above their own, respecting the client's rights and inherent dignity and maintaining objectivity.

2. Expect case managers to act with integrity, maintain competency, and obey relevant laws and regulations.

C. Ethically competent case managers according to Taylor (2005) are able to practice according to ethical standards and protect the patient/client and support system at all times (Box 18-1).

D. Taylor (2005) describes a process for ethical decision making that case managers may apply in their handling of patient care issues. This process is especially important in situations that present potential for ethical conflicts and includes the following steps:

1. Assessment—Gathering and documenting pertinent medical and nonmedical information

   a. Medical may include information about the patient's health condition, past medical history, and any treatment regimens.

   b. Nonmedical information addresses the patient's and family's situation including its characteristics: financial, social, values, beliefs, interests, guardian, including the names of persons who have the authority to make decisions and responsibility for the consequences.

   c. Pay special attention to factors creating or fueling conflict.

2. Diagnosis—Identifying ethical issues and differentiating ethical problems (e.g., termination of life support measures) from those that are nonethical (e.g., shortness of breath).

3. Planning—Identifying goals and desired outcomes. This includes listing and exploring options and courses of actions that are likely to resolve the ethical issue/conflict.

4. Implementation—Putting a course of action into effect and assessing the consequences. This may require calling for an ethics consult from the clinical or organizational ethics committees.

5. Evaluation—Critiquing the decision, goals, and course of action, including the consequences.

BOX

18-1   Ways Case Managers Demonstrate Competence in Ethical Practice

- Act in ways that protect or advance the best interests of their patients
- Be accountable for their practice and its associated outcomes
- Act as effective patient advocates, especially for those who cannot speak for themselves
- Mediate ethical conflicts when they occur or prevent their occurrence altogether
- Recognize the ethical dimension of their practice and adhere to ethical practice standards at all times
- Abide by their professional code of conduct and ethical principles

Ethical Theories

A. Ethical theories try to explain, usually at an abstract level, how right action or goodness should be understood or what the properties of right action or goodness are. Ethical theories generate principles and reasons that help individuals arrive at an ethically appropriate course of action (Beauchamp & Childress, 2008).

B. There are four major ethical theories case managers should be familiar with and incorporate into their practice. These are:

1. Deontologism—A theory that stipulates doing one's "duty" as morally obligatory.

   a. *Duty* might be understood as what any reasonable person would consistently do in that situation or in others like it such that a client's welfare is respected and maintained. Alternatively, duty might be defined in terms of ethical standards, codes, or regulations. Often, when a case manager carries a caseload of patients, such responsibility sometimes is referred to as "duty" to provide care for a number of patients.

   b. Two principles of the CCMC's Code of Professional Conduct for Case Managers (CCMC, 2015) are deontological in nature. The first principle states that "Certificants will place the public interest above their own at all times," and the second principle notes that "Certificants will respect the rights and inherent dignity of all of their clients."

2. Utilitarianism—A theory that defines "right action" as that which produces the most happiness or benefits for the most people. A common example of utilitarian reasoning is determining how to allocate scarce health care resources, such as in organ transplantation and triage situations, or determining coverage or benefits in a health insurance plan.

3. Virtue ethics—An ethical model that bases action on what a reasonable person would do who acts prudently and in accordance with the laws, regulations, and ethical standards of her/his society or profession. Some prominent virtues among health care professionals including case managers might be caring, faithfulness, justice, beneficence, nonmaleficence, humility, courage, practical wisdom, and subordinating one's self-interest to caring for others.

4. Contractualism—An ethical model that derives from the marketplace. It seeks to define values and principles, especially as they might affect the distribution of benefits (or property and resources), as a result of negotiation or contract. The distribution of coverage under a private insurance policy is an example, where one might argue that what the insured is entitled to are the benefits he or she has purchased in the contract, for example, the health insurance policy (Banja, 2003).

 Ethical Principles and Decision Making

A. Ethical *theory* is often presented in an abstract and formal way. It provides a broad perspective or framework that seeks to explain ethical practice and decision making. However, it occasionally is not helpful in informing real-life dilemmas, which can be extremely complex.

Sometimes, it is more useful for case managers to apply ethical *principles* to their decision making in order to reach acceptable outcomes.

B. Four ethical principles are derived from the work of Beauchamp and Childress (2001) that are much discussed and are often helpful in assisting persons (e.g., case managers) in doing what ethics requires. Each principle can be read as a professional duty or as a right the patient or client enjoys. These are:

1. Autonomy—An ethical principle that connotes individual liberty, individual rights, self-determination, my "being my own person," personal inviolability, and antipaternalism. It is the right to make own decisions, self-governing and self-directing, especially in moral independence.

   a. In medicine, a frequent demonstration of autonomy is the patient's right to refuse treatment.

   b. In case management, an instance of autonomy would be the client's right to refuse case management services or to choose a treating or evaluating physician. Case managers also encourage patients to make informed decisions through health instruction and counseling activities.

2. Nonmaleficence—An ethical principle that is fundamental to health care ethics in that the professional is obligated "to do no harm."

   a. Case management examples of harming patients would be where the case manager loses objectivity and writes reports that bias the treating health care professional or the payer (insurer) for health care services against the patient.

   b. Other examples might include the case manager's practicing outside the scope of his or her credentialing or licensure, failing to protect confidential communications, or not acting on certain important information or events such as delays in care.

3. Beneficence—An ethical principle that obligates the health professional to do as much good as is reasonable.

   a. Problems with achieving beneficence occur when the case manager differs with the client as to what constitutes the client's best interest, such as a return to work versus collecting unemployment benefits for as long as possible.

   b. In instances of concern, case managers should be guided not only by their client advocacy obligations but also by what a "reasonable and prudent" case manager would likely do.

4. Justice—An ethical principle requiring that the patient/client receives what he or she is owed, or is treated fairly. Problems with justice occur when:

   a. The client's policy language regarding benefits is unclear

   b. The client demands services the case manager believes are excessive

   c. The case manager believes the client is noncompliant and finds it difficult to advocate for him or her

5. Veracity—An ethical obligation to be truthful to clients and to resist paternalistically based concealments of information, especially in instances where the professional is tempted to justify such concealment with rationalizations like the client will be made worse by having such information.

   a. Veracity honors the client's decision-making skills, assuming the client can exercise those skills in a reasonably competent manner.

b. Case managers may violate this principle when they promise clients they will be calling back or returning to check, or they will be contacting the client's primary care provider, but never do or act in a timely manner as they have promised.

C. The Four-Quadrant Model can be used for ethical decision making by case managers. This model is a method popularized by Jonsen et al. (2002) that helps in identifying and grouping ethically important aspects of a case.

    1. The model, however, does not resolve cases nor does it prioritize which ethical elements in a case merit the most attention or weight. The case manager must still exercise critical thinking and judgment.

    2. The four quadrants or groups are described in Box 18-2.

BOX 18-2   The Four-Quadrant Model of Ethical Decision Making

1. Medical indications, which include the answers to the following questions:
   a. What is the patient's medical problem and history?
   b. Diagnosis and prognosis?
   c. Is the problem acute, chronic, critical, emergent, incurable, or reversible?
   d. What are the goals of treatment?
   e. What are the probabilities of success?
   f. What is the plan in case of therapeutic failure?
   g. How can the patient be benefited and how can harm be prevented?
2. Patient preferences, which include answers to the following questions:
   a. Is the patient mentally capable and legally competent?
   b. If competent, what are the patient's preferences for treatment?
   c. Has the patient been informed of benefits and risks?
   d. Has he or she given consent?
   e. If incapacitated, who is the appropriate decision maker?
   f. Is the patient's surrogate or proxy making decisions as the patient would wish (which is ethical) or as the surrogate prefers (which is unethical)?
   g. Has the patient expressed prior preferences, such as by an advance directive (e.g., living will, durable power of attorney for health care)?
   h. Is the patient's right to choose being respected to the greatest extent possible in ethics and law?
3. Quality of life, which includes answers to the following questions:
   a. What are the prospects, with or without treatment, for a return to a normal life?
   b. What physical, mental, and social deficits is the patient likely to experience if the treatment succeeds?
   c. Are there biases that might prejudice the professional's evaluation of the patient's quality of life?
   d. Does the patient's present or future condition potentially result in poor quality of life and well being such that his or her continued life might be judged undesirable?
   e. Is there any plan or rationale to forego treatment?
   f. Are there plans for comfort and palliative care?
4. Contextual features, which include answers to the following questions:
   a. Are there family issues, financial and economic factors, or religious or cultural factors that might unjustly influence treatment decisions?
   b. Are there legal issues or clinical trial (research) involvement that might compromise the patient's welfare?
   c. Is there any conflict of interest on the part of the providers or the institution?

BOX 18-3 CCMC's Values of Case Management Practice

- Case management is a means for achieving client wellness and autonomy through advocacy, communication, education, and services facilitation.
- Board certified case managers must recognize the dignity, rights, and worth of all individuals.
- Board certified case managers must commit to safety and quality outcomes, appropriate use of resources, and empowerment of clients and their families.
- Case management practice must be guided by the ethical principles of autonomy, beneficence, nonmaleficence, justice, veracity, and distributive justice.
- Case management practice focuses on achieving quality outcomes and facilitates the individual's ability to reach optimal level of wellness and functional capability (patient-centeredness); thus, everyone benefits—the individuals being cared for and their support system, the health care delivery system, and the various reimbursement systems.

   D. CMSA has summarized the following ethical principles in its statement on ethical case management practice (CMSA, 2010).
   1. Case managers must adhere to the code of ethics of their profession of origin, that is, nursing, social work, rehabilitation counseling, and so on.
   2. Case management practice must be guided by the principles of autonomy, beneficence, nonmaleficence, justice, and veracity. It also must preserve the dignity of the client and family.
   3. Case managers foster the client's autonomy, independence, and self-determination.
   4. Case managers support the client and family in their self-advocacy and self-direction and in their options and decisions related to health care services and treatments.
   5. Case managers must not discriminate based on social or economic status, personal attributes, or the nature of the health problem. They must show respect for the individual and deal with their clients with dignity and fairness.
   6. Case managers refrain from doing harm to others and emphasize quality outcomes.
   7. Case managers must advocate for their clients to receive needed care and promote access to services, especially when they are rare or limited.
   E. CCMC has identified several values of case management practice described in Box 18-3 (CCMC, 2015).

BOX 18-4 Violations Board Certified Case Managers Must Avoid

1. Intentionally falsify an application or other documents
2. Conviction of a felony that involves moral turpitude
3. Violation of the code of ethics governing the original profession of the case manager (e.g., nursing, rehabilitation counseling)
4. Loss of primary professional credential (e.g., nursing, social work)
5. Violation or breach of the guidelines of professional conduct
6. Failure to maintain eligibility requirements once certified
7. Violation of the rules and regulations governing the taking of the certification examination
8. Lack of documentation or subjective, untruthful, or judgmental documentation

F. CCMC has also identified several rules of conduct for case managers (CCMC, 2015). These are written in terms of violations that result in sanctions up to revocation of certification (the CCM credential). Case managers must avoid these violations at all times (Box 18-4).

Ethical Responsibilities Particularly Affecting Case Managers

A. Ethical conflicts can arise despite a case manager's best intentions and efforts (Tahan & Stolte-Upman, 2006).
B. The case manager must advocate for his/her clients and ensure that their needs are comprehensively addressed, service options are provided, and access to resources that meet their individual needs and interests is also made possible (CCMC, 2015).
C. According to Tahan and Stolte-Upman (2006), important ethical responsibilities for case managers may include the following:
   1. Advocacy—Ensuring that client's needs are reasonably and justly met. The case manager must never handle or neglect a case in a grossly negligent fashion, for example, in a manner that fails to meet the case management standard of care and practice.
   2. Professional behavior—The case manager must maintain honesty and desist from acts of fraud, deceit, discrimination, or sexual intimacy with a client.
   3. Representation of practice—Practicing within the boundaries of competence and never misrepresenting the case manager's role or competence to clients.
   4. Client advocacy and voiding conflict of interest—Ensuring that secondary interests (especially bearing on financial gain) do not compromise the case manager's primary responsibility of client advocacy.
      a. Although some conflicts of interest might be ethically manageable, they should be fully disclosed to all parties affected by them.
      b. If, after full disclosure, an objection is made by any party, the case manager should attempt to manage the objection; if all fails, withdrawal from further participation in the case is necessary.
   5. Reporting misconduct—Case managers who are aware of ethical violations committed by other case managers should report that knowledge to the appropriate party or to the CCMC if the alleged violator is a certificant. All such reports must be based in fact and not be malicious or unwarranted.
   6. Description of services—Case managers should provide information to clients about the services offered, the risks that might be associated with those services, the alternatives to services, and the client's right to refuse services.
   7. Termination of services—Case managers should provide written notification of service discontinuation to all parties involved in a case consistent with applicable statutes, regulations, and guidelines.
   8. Objectivity—Case managers will refrain from imposing their personal (e.g., political, philosophical, cultural) values on their clients; they will respect their clients rights, liberties, and autonomy; they will provide care as dictated by professional case management standards.

Case managers will also be objective in reporting the results of their professional activities to third parties and avoid exerting any undue influence on the decision-making process.

9. Disclosure—Case managers who perform services at the request of a third party must disclose their dual relationship, and their role and responsibilities in it, at the outset of establishing a relationship with the client.
   a. Case managers are also ethically required to inform clients who are receiving services that any information obtained through the case management relationship might be disclosed to third parties (e.g., health care providers, third party payers, etc.) who have a legal or ethical right or need to know it.
   b. Disclosure should be limited only to what is necessary and relevant, except in instances to prevent the client from (1) committing acts likely to result in bodily harm, either to the client or to others, and (2) committing criminal, illegal, or fraudulent acts.
10. Records keeping and protection—Case managers must maintain records in a manner designed to ensure privacy, that is, to protect and secure the information from individuals who have no right to it.
11. Refraining from solicitation—Case managers should refrain from rewarding, paying, or compensating anyone who directs or refers clients to them for case manager services.
12. Refraining from funneling referrals—Case managers must not direct referrals for follow-up care or for postdischarge services and while the patient/client is back in the community after an episode of illness to select providers for financial or other gains (e.g., kickbacks). Such practice does not adhere to ethical and legal standards.

Strategies for Maintaining Ethical Behavior

A. It is important for health care organizations and administrators of case management programs to consider the implementation of an ethics group, patient services, or professional advisory committee charged to address ethical conflicts or dilemmas as they arise.
   1. The group/committee, which presumably can be comprised of persons who are known for their expertise and professional integrity and for maintaining ethical and legal standards, can be convened for hearing ethical issues and offering ethical recommendations.
   2. The group/committee can also initiate ethics roundtables or informal meetings to discuss ethical and professional issues and concerns (Banja, 1999).
B. It is important for case managers to understand the types of ethical conflicts they may face and how to handle them.
   1. Jansen (2003) differentiates between two types of ethics consults that one could translate into the need for two types of ethics groups or committees; these are clinical and organizational.
      a. *Clinical* ethics committees—Usually handle ethical conflicts that are clinical in nature and related to the medical treatment. Examples of these conflicts are:
         i. End-of-life matters and termination of care
         ii. Lack of understanding by patient/family of the medical treatment

         iii. Conflicts between patient, family, and provider regarding decisions made (or that need to be made) about best treatment and options

         iv. Dilemmas surrounding care decisions, for example, saving a mother's life versus the fetus or protecting at-risk caregiver versus discharging the patient to the same at-risk caregiver

     b. *Organizational* ethics committees—Usually handle ethical conflicts that pertain to an organization's behaviors as they relate to the individuals represented by that organization (including patients, health care providers, and other employees), the community served by the organization, and other organizations with which it interacts and collaborates. Examples of these conflicts are:

         i. Utilization management and allocation of resources

         ii. Denial of services

         iii. Delays in care

         iv. Conflicts of interest

  2. Jansen (2003) also identified five subcategories of potential ethical conflicts case managers must be well aware off and implements strategies to avoid their occurrence (Box 18-5).

  C. Case managers must remember that being able to justify an act as ethical is crucial. They should therefore be able to analyze the reasons for their behaviors and decisions and ask themselves whether or not those reasons can withstand public or professional scrutiny (Banja, 1999).

  D. Case managers should pay careful attention to their own moral feelings.

    1. Often, the first symptom of an ethical dilemma is an affective one, as in, "This situation makes me professionally uncomfortable. What I'm doing (or being asked to do) doesn't feel right."

    2. Ethical behavior and ethical learning tend to be associated with particular feelings about right and wrong.

    3. The case manager who experiences moral anxiety or distress should have some mechanism to have it addressed (Tahan & Stolte-Upman, 2006), for example, seeking the assistance, guidance, or counsel of ethics groups/committees.

  E. Case managers must be aware of and attend to their ethical and racial biases (e.g., racial stereotyping or profiling). They must excuse themselves from cases where conflicts arise and result in feelings impairing the level and quality of care they deliver to patients. In these

---

BOX
18-5) Five Types of Ethical Conflicts

1. Unethical business practices such as fraud and abuse
2. Societal and public health violations such as denying care, concealment of medical errors, and discrimination
3. Health care advertising such as making unrealistic promises and endorsing specific medical products or service agencies
4. Scientific misconduct such as poorly conducted clinical trials
5. Unethical business practices such as shady relationships with vendors, employees, payers, and other outside agencies

cases, they must seek the attention and assistance of supervisors or ethics experts. Case managers must respect cultural diversity at all times.

F. Case managers should attend conferences on ethics and/or keep abreast of the case management ethical literature.

G. Whether they are certified or not, case managers should be familiar with the CCMC's Code of Professional Conduct for Case Managers and the CMSA's Standards of Practice for Case Management just as they should be familiar with the ethical code of their profession and licensing organization such as those of nursing, social work, rehabilitation counseling, and so on.

H. Case managers should examine the literature available in libraries, on the Internet, and at various state chapters of case management professional organizations/societies. They also should access the ethical resources available from these professional organizations/societies either online or during annual conferences, for example, the CMSA's online resources and annual conference.

I. Case managers should review the ethical codes and standards regularly— Perhaps each time the case manager renews his or her certification or licensure requirements (Tahan & Stolte-Upman, 2006).

J. Case managers may seek advisory opinions from the CCMC regarding ethical dilemmas. Such activities are important for case managers to ensure compliance with ethical codes and principles.

K. Case managers may request a change of assignment from a supervisor, especially in cases that present ethical distress or conflict (Tahan & Stolte-Upman, 2006).

L. Case managers should work within the case management scope of practice and professional guidelines. They should examine their job description for consistency with applicable ethical standards and modify it as necessary.

M. Case managers should maintain professional objectivity and ethical astuteness in creating records and documentation. The case manager must recognize the admissibility of certain of these documents in litigation, and she/he must realize that documentation is a direct reflection of one's ethical sensibilities and behaviors (Tahan & Stolte-Upman, 2006).

References

Banja, J. (1997). Values, function, and managed care: An ethical analysis. *Journal of Head Trauma Rehabilitation*, 12(1), 60–70.

Banja, J. (1999). Ethical decision-making: Origins, process, and applications to case management. *The Case Manager*, 10(5), 41–47.

Banja, J. (2003). Antifoundationalism and morality by contract: The case of managed care. In O. Ferrell, S. True, & L. Pelton (Eds.), *Rights, relationships & responsibilities, Vol. 1* (pp. 73–86). Kennesaw, GA: Kennesaw State University, Michael Coles College of Business.

Banja, J. (2006). Case management and the standards of practice. *The Case Manager*, 17(1), 21–23.

Beauchamp, T., & Childress, J. F. (2001). *Principles of biomedical ethics* (5th ed.). New York, NY: Oxford University Press.

Beauchamp, T., & Childress, J. F. (2008). *Principles of biomedical ethics* (6th ed.). New York: Oxford University Press.

Case Management Society of America. (2010). *Standards of practice for case management*. Little Rock, AR: Author.

Commission for Case Manager Certification (CCMC). (2015). *Code of professional conduct for case managers with standards, rules, procedures and penalties*. Mount Laurel, NJ: CCMC.

Jansen, L. A. (2003). Ethical issues in case management. In T. G. Cesta & H. A. Tahan (Eds.), *The case manager's survival guide: Winning strategies for clinical practice* (2nd ed., pp. 324–335). St. Louis, MO: Mosby.

Jonsen, A. R., Siegler, M., & Winslade, W. J. (2002). *Clinical ethics: A practical approach to ethical decisions in clinical medicine* (5th ed.). New York: McGraw-Hill.

Lo, B. (2000). *Resolving ethical dilemmas: A guide for clinicians*. Philadelphia, PA: Lippincott Williams & Wilkins.

Tahan, H. A., & Stolte-Upman, C. (2006). *Code of professional conduct for case managers: Establishing standards for ethical practice*. Mount Laurel, NJ: CCMC.

Taylor, C. (2005). Ethical issues in case management. In E. L. Cohen & T. G. Cesta (Eds.), *Nursing case management: From essentials to advance practice applications* (pp. 361–379). St. Louis, MO: Elsevier Mosby.

Thompson, D. (1993). Understanding financial conflicts of interest. *New England Journal of Medicine, 329*(8), 573–575.

CHAPTER 19

Ethical Use of Case Management Technology

Ellen Fink-Samnick

LEARNING OBJECTIVES

Upon completion of the chapter, the reader will be able to:

1. Define key terms specific to the use of electronic communication and social media.

2. Explain how to apply case management's ethical tenets to the interventions involving electronic communication and social media.

3. Identify relevant professional guidelines, standards, principles, and codes guiding use of electronic communication and social media.

4. Determine how to use relevant resources to continue to advance the evolving knowledge base and promote ethical parameters.

IMPORTANT TERMS AND CONCEPTS

Blogs	Encryption	Professional Networking
Boundary	Friend	Security
Boundary Crossing	Information Technology	Skype
Boundary Violation	Internet	Social Media
Cloned Medical Records	Internet of Things	Social Network
Conflict of Interest	Media Sharing Sites	Technology
Crowdsourcing	Mobile Device	Text Message
Digital Health	Netiquette	Tweet
Distance Counseling	Online	Virtual Relationship
Dual Relationships	Podcast	Wiki
Electronic	Privacy	World Wide Web
Electronic Technology	Privacy Setting	

Introduction

A. Most professionals would agree that technology has added value to the patient and health care professional's experience, including that of the case manager. A segment of this value stems from the innovative modes and expanded options by which health care professionals can communicate and engage with clients, clients' support systems, caregivers, professional colleagues, and industry stakeholders alike.

B. The unique ways in which access to care has been enhanced through technology extend from remote health and telemedicine to electronic health records and personal health portals. There are an abundance of positive outcomes to reflect the merits of this generation of innovation on the health care delivery process along with return on investment across the transitions of care (Free et al., 2013; Koivunen, Niem, & Hupli, 2014; Moorhead et al., 2013).

C. Technology's leveraged presence and utilization have yielded a new generation of ethical dilemmas for case managers to maneuver. Health care professionals strive to stay proficient with a constant flow of evolving products and programs in their work place, while reconciling updated federal and state regulations with organizational policies.

D. The speed at which this innovation occurs can be exacerbated by an atmosphere of business competition, one where organizations strive to incorporate new technologies to obtain their requisite market share. There are a variety of programs and products to meet their expanding target patient populations.

E. However, implementation processes to digitalize patient information and other health information technology are often rushed. These efforts leave end users, especially health care professionals contributing to unintended casualties (Daly, 2011). What results for case managers is increased vulnerability for ethical as well as potential legal sanction for their practice.

F. The ethical tenets of case management practice (also discussed in Chapter 18) serve as foundational pillars for the workforce (Box 19-1). They are the one constant for all professional case managers independent of discipline of origin, practice setting, and amid swift industry change.

G. Rapidly shifting societal constructs and contexts influence the way in which case managers interpret how each tenet is adhered to (Fink-Samnick, 2013a).

H. This chapter focuses on the alignment of case management's ethical tenets with two of these constructs, electric communication and social

---

BOX 19-1 **Ethical Tenets of Case Management Practice**

- Beneficence: To do good
- Nonmalfeasance: To do no harm
- Autonomy: To respect individuals' rights to make their own decisions
- Justice: To treat others fairly
- Fidelity: To follow through and to keep promises

media. Each has revolutionized while challenging each facet of a case manager's practice. For the application of ethical standards in the general practice of case management, refer to Chapter 18.

I. With case management and technology at the apex of case management, care coordination, and transitions of care, the stakes rise for the workforce. Varying interpretations of professional regulations and scope of practice by employers find case managers wrestling to which direction their ethical compass should point. This chapter provides guidance to that end.

 ## Descriptions of Key Terms

A. Blogs—A Web site on which someone writes about personal opinions, activities, and experiences. It contains online personal reflections, comments, and often hyperlinks provided by the writer (Merriam-Webster, 2015a).

B. Boundary—The edge of appropriate or professional behavior (Gutheil & Simon, 2002). They allow for a safe personal connection between patients and their health care providers (Baca, 2011).

C. Boundary crossing—A deviation from classical therapeutic activity that is harmless, nonexploitive, and possibly supportive of the therapy itself (Gutheil & Simon, 2002).

D. Boundary violation—When the health care provider displaces or confuses his or her own needs with the patient's needs (Gutheil & Simon, 2002).

E. Cloned medical records—The ability to carry forward old clinical information into the latest note—an explicit feature of some electronic health records (EHRs)—is often referred to as cloning. The problem lies in copying forward old information, such as patient complaints from an earlier visit or results of certain tests or old blood pressure readings that have been resolved, resulting in care activities that otherwise are unnecessary and potentially may pose safety concerns (Lowes, 2012).

F. Conflict of interest—A conflict of interest is a set of circumstances that creates a risk that professional judgment or actions regarding a primary interest will be unduly influenced by a secondary interest (Lo & Field, 2009).

G. Crowdsourcing—The practice of obtaining needed services, ideas, or content by soliciting contributions from a large group of people and especially from the online community rather than from traditional employees or suppliers (Merriam-Webster, 2015b).

H. Digital health—The ability to digitize human beings, by a variety of means (e.g., sequencing, sensors, imaging) fully exploiting our digital infrastructure of ever-increasing bandwidth, connectivity, social networking, the Internet of all things, and health information systems (Topol in Nosta, 2013).

I. Distance counseling—The provision of counseling services by means other than face-to-face meetings, usually with the aid of technology (American Counseling Association [ACA], 2014).

J. Dual relationships—Any situation in which a health care professional–patient/client relationship may be contaminated by a second co-occurring relationship (e.g., business or financial relationships, romantic involvement, blood ties, marital relatedness) (Segen's Medical Dictionary, 2011). They exist when there are other personal or professional demands, stresses, or considerations in the relationship in addition to the provider–patient relationship (Baca, 2011).

K. Electronic—A mode of communication and information acquisition, transmission, and storage, such as used in computers, telephones, cell phones, personal digital assistants, facsimile machines, etc. (National Association of Social Workers & Association of Social Work Boards, 2005).

L. Electronic technology—The digital or Internet-based technologies and devices. The following kinds of devices and tools are of special importance because of the growing concern related to vulnerability and risk in their use. These include but are not limited to laptops; home-based personal computers; personal digital assistants (PDAs) and smartphones; hotel, library, or other public workstations and Wireless Access Points (WAPs); USB flash drives and memory cards; CDs; DVDs; backup media; e-mail; smart cards; and remote access devices (including security hardware) (Certification of Disability Management Specialists' Commission [CDMS], 2010).

M. Encryption—Process of encoding information in a way that limits access to authorized users (ACA, 2014).

N. Friend—To add a person to one's list of contacts on a social networking Web site (Dictionary.com, 2015a).

O. Information technology (IT)—The overarching term to describe technologies that process information, most often in electronic form (National Association of Social Workers & Association of Social Work Boards, 2005).

P. Internet—A worldwide network of computer networks that share information (National Association of Social Workers & Association of Social Work Boards, 2005).

Q. Internet of Things—a computing concept that describes a future where everyday physical objects will be connected to the Internet and be able to identify themselves to other devices (Techopedia, 2015).

R. Media sharing sites—A Web site that enables users to store and share their multimedia files (e.g., photos, videos, music) with others. Such sites provide a modest amount of free storage and paid subscriptions for greater storage. The media is played/viewed from any Web browser and may be selectively available via password or to the general public. A media sharing site can also be used to back up files (PC Magazine, 2015).

S. Mobile device—A portable computing device such as a smartphone or tablet computer (Oxford Dictionaries, 2015). Today's mobile devices are multimodal and are used for multiple purposes such as taking pictures, text messaging, e-mailing, video calling, and accessing the Internet and health care organization–based (case management employers) clinical applications such as electronic medical records.

T. Moral distress—A human response to conflict, which is created by on-the-job ethical conflicts (Moffat, 2014).

U. Netiquette—Etiquette governing communication on the Internet (Merriam-Webster, 2015c).

V. Online—A mode of communication where the user is in direct contact with the computer network to the extent that the network responds rapidly to user commands (National Association of Social Workers & Association of Social Work Boards, 2005).

W. Podcast—A program (as of music or talk) made available in digital format for automatic download over the Internet (Merriam-Webster, 2015d).

X. Privacy—The right of an individual to withhold her/his information from public scrutiny or unwanted publicity (National Association of Social Workers & Association of Social Work Boards, 2005).

Y. Privacy setting—Privacy settings are controls available on many social networking and other Web sites that allow users to limit who can access your profile and what information visitors can see (IT Law Wiki, 2015).

Z. Professional networking—A type of social network service that is focused solely on interactions and relationships of a business nature rather than including personal, nonbusiness interactions (Vacellaro, 2007).

AA. Social media—Technology-based forms of communication of ideas, beliefs, personal histories, etc. (e.g., social networking sites, blogs) (ACA, 2014).

BB. Security—The protection of hardware, software, and data by locks, doors, and other electronic barriers such as passwords, firewalls, and encryption (National Association of Social Workers & Association of Social Work Boards, 2005).

CC. Social network—An online community of people with a common interest who use a Web site or other technologies to communicate with each other and share information, resources, etc. It may also be a Web site or online service that facilitates this communication (Dictionary. com, 2015b).

DD. Skype—A computer program that can be used to make free voice calls over the Internet to anyone else who is also using Skype (Webopedia, 2015).

EE. Technology—A set of prescribed events that are embedded in hardware, software, or telecommunications and that direct activities, decisions, or choices. Sometimes, technology is divided into hard technologies, such as switches and electronics, and soft technology such as the processes and procedures associated with accounting or risk assessment (National Association of Social Workers & Association of Social Work Boards, 2005).

FF. Text message—An electronic message sent over a cellular network from one cell phone to another by typing words, often in shortened form, as "18t" for "late," on the phone's numeric or QWERTY keypad (Dictionary. com, 2015c).

GG. Tweet—A very short message posted on the Twitter Web site: the message may include text and keywords, makes reference to specific users, links to Web sites, and links to images or videos on a Web site (Dictionary.com, 2015d).

HH. Videoconference—Use of electronic media to conduct client-related case conference in a virtual environment and to connect with multiple health care providers who are not necessarily in the same location, however involved in the client's care. In such environment, client-related personal health information is exchanged, which warrants adherence to ethical (e.g., privacy, confidentiality) and legal (e.g., HIPAA) standards.

II. Virtual relationship—A non–face-to-face relationship (e.g., through social media) (ACA, 2014).

JJ. Wiki—A Web site that allows users to add and update content on the site using their own Web browser. This is made possible by Wiki software that runs on the Web server. Wikis end up being created mainly by a collaborative effort of the site visitors (TechTerms.com, 2015).

KK. World Wide Webb (WWW)—A subset of the Internet that allows access using a standard graphical protocol (National Association of Social Workers & Association of Social Work Boards, 2005).

Applicability to CMSA'S Standards of Practice

A. The Case Management Society of America (CMSA) describes in its standards of practice for case management (CMSA, 2010) that case management practice extends across all health care settings, including payer, provider, government, employer, community, and home environment. Use of digital communication and other technologies apply to all these settings, and therefore, adhering to ethical standards is an expectation.

B. The use of technology has influenced all areas of case management. The ethical use of social medial and digital technology overlay all of the case management practice standards. This chapter introduces ethics concepts in context with a case manager's use of technology.

C. This chapter discusses how ethics underpins case management use of technology. The ethics standard recognizes that case managers should behave and practice ethically while adhering to the tenets of the ethical code, which underlies his/her professional credential (e.g., nursing, social work).

D. Some of the standards for case management practice described by CMSA (2010) apply in important ways to the use of digital media and communication technologies, especially those that pertain to privacy and confidentiality. Case managers should be well aware of how best to maintain client's privacy and confidentiality while using such tools in provision of care and resources.

E. Case managers use remote monitoring technology as well as social networking, medical information technology, and digital tools in order to enhance client self-management skills and abilities and improve client health knowledge. The Ethics standard described in the CMSA standards of practice is especially applicable in this regard. Case managers shall adhere to said standard at all times while caring for their clients/support systems.

Transition in Modes of Patient and Professional Interaction

A. Information and communication technology in health care are rapidly evolving, courtesy of the fast growing penetration of the Internet and mobile device use (Koivunen et al., 2014).
  1. At the time of this writing, 64% of Americans own a smartphone of some type, up 35% from 2011 (Smith, 2015). Globally, this number is over 80% (Tech.Firstpost.com, 2015).

2. By 2020, 90% of the world's population is expected to have a mobile phone (Woods, 2014).

3. Over 70% of clinicians use mobile screens to view patient-related data (Pai, 2014).

4. Over 3 million patients worldwide are connected to some remote monitoring device that is monitored by a professional caregiver. That number is expected to exceed 19 million persons by 2018 (Baum, 2014).

B. A vast learning curve accompanies the latest generation of technology, including what is now referred to as the Internet of Things (IOT). The pressure to quickly attain a minimal standard of understanding, let alone mastery, yields concerns by the workforce regarding information security, lack of technical skills, unworkable technology, and decreasing social interaction (Koivunen et al., 2014).

1. Case managers are exposed to an onslaught of innovative product implementation from electronic health portals, remote health and telehealth initiatives, plus mobile devices.

2. Professionals frequently misuse, misinterpret, and/or abuse regulations they do not fully comprehend (e.g., the Health Information Portability and Accountability Act [HIPAA]).

   a. Staff members' fear of the consequences of an unintended HIPAA violation is often overblown (Span, 2015).

3. Many of the breaches posted on the Health and Human Services Office of Civil Rights Web site occurred on the part of professionals who do not understand how to properly secure data, whether on the device itself or remotely (U.S. Department of Health & Human Services, 2015).

4. One of the most challenging ethical and legal areas of focus for case managers involves the critical connection between state-to-state licensure and technology and innovation, which now allows for diagnosis, assessment, and treatment intervention across via remote and telehealth means (Treiger & Fink-Samnick, 2016).

5. Challenges with technology proficiency manifest across the workforce and practice settings. These include but are not limited to those listed in Box 19-2.

6. The Economic Cycle Research Institute's (ERCI) top patient safety concern for 2014 is for data integrity failures with health IT (Manchitanti & Hirsch, 2015).

   a. Case managers are on the front lines of direct interface with these issues.

BOX 19-2   Challenges of Technology Proficiency

- Poor password protection and management
- Limited knowledge of and/or compliance with encryption
- Downloading of applications (apps), which do not meet guidelines for security and health care–related ethical standards
- Poor organizational oversight for education and training of staff prior to implementation of new programs, products, etc
- Practicing across state lines without the requisite licensure and/or certification

Electronic Communication

A. Effective communication is critical to information transfer and patient safety (Koivunen et al., 2014).
B. Case managers are able to engage with patients and industry stakeholders with increasing frequency across technology.
   1. Electronic communication is heavily utilized to facilitate and intervene about the patient experience.
   2. The scope and range of activities extends across all job functions of the case manager (Box 19-3).
C. Transition from traditional modes of communication (e.g., in-person, letters) to use of mobile devices, videoconferencing platforms, and Web portals has meant a considerable adjustment for the workforce, patients, and other industry stakeholders.
D. The ease of communication using technology has been a double-edged sword.
   1. Electronic communication has accelerated the speed at which decisions about treatment can be discussed, while promoting ease of access to care (Koivunen et al., 2014).
   2. Electronic devices promote the management of patient data, improve staff cooperation and competence, and make more effective use of working time (Koivunen et al., 2014). These factors are assets amid a health care atmosphere where speed and efficiency are critical to both treatment and case management success.
   3. On the other hand, experts argue how purely electronic dialogues lack the personal touch.
      a. Increased use of communication across devices, blogs, and social media has led to a generation plagued by inadequate social and emotional development (Ossola, 2015).
      b. In this age of overcommunication, a new kind of social order is being developed that is strengthening public and mass communication but weakening interpersonal communication (Bala, 2014).
      c. New media has contributed to changes in intrapersonal, interpersonal, group, and mass communication processes and content (Bala, 2014).

BOX 19-3   Examples of Use of Electronic Technology in Case Management

- Documentation
- Completion of clinical reviews and/or authorization for treatment
- Notification to patients about treatment concerns and test results
- Clarification of treatment orders and/or plans of care
- Conference with and/or conducting meetings with members of the care coordination team
- Communication with patients and their support systems who do not reside in the same geographic areas
- Evaluation of patients by treatment specialists and providers in rural regions and/or situations where the patient is otherwise unable to obtain care

4. Patients and families expect immediate response to texts, e-mails, and other modes of communicating, adding pressure to the already overburdened workforce.
   a. The new instant contact communication culture finds professionals pressured to use modes, which may not comply with standard rules and regulations for privacy, security, and confidentiality (e.g., personal mobile devices for professional calls).
   b. The result is case managers are at increasing risk of violating ethical and legal standards of practice (e.g., privacy and confidentiality, dual relationships).

 ## Social Media

A. Through social media, health care professionals are provided a variety of tools to enhance both their professional practice and the patient experience. Case managers engage with social media for a variety of professional reasons, including to:
   1. Explore and/or access resources
   2. Complete referrals
   3. Professional networking
   4. Professional education
   5. Seek employment opportunities
   6. Organizational promotion
   7. Patient care
      a. Track client treatment adherence through portals.
      b. Patient education and health monitoring.
      c. Convey patient reminders for appointments and prescription notifications.
      d. Patient education.
   8. Public health alerts and programs (Ventola, 2014)
B. Health care consumers are increasingly comfortable in communicating with providers and practitioners across social media and online communities. The use of social media fosters the ability of clinicians and health care institutions to be more engaged with their patients (Househ, 2013).
   1. Searching for health information online has become one of the most popular online activities (Househ, 2013).
   2. Health care consumers use social media sites to share sensitive health information (e.g., behavioral health, mental illness, and genetic) (Househ, 2013).
   3. More than 40% of patient consumers report that information they found via social media impacted their treatment of illness and overall health (Honigman, 2013).
      a. Poor quality and reliability of information is a main limitation of the information found on social media (Ventola, 2014).
C. Increasing use of and reliance on protected social networks and digital technology has transformed all relationships, especially between the clinical professional and consumer. The wait time between intervention (e.g., laboratory test, CAT scan, biopsy) and results has been abbreviated from days and weeks down to almost simultaneous access in light of personal health record innovations.

D. Any dialogues between patients and practitioners, though done with the best intent, can easily cross the lines of legal regulations and existing ethical standards. The list of the common ethical challenges includes those described in Box 19-4 (Dejong, 2012).

E. It is understood across the industry how easily dual relationships can and will occur between professionals and patients. However, social media has elevated this concept to new heights.
1. It is not uncommon for patients and former patients to extend invitations to connect with providers through online portals (Ventola, 2014).
2. Engaging with patients, former patients, and their caregivers through one of four types of social networking (Baker, 2014).
   a. Friending—As experienced through social media sites.
   b. Listening—Reading texts or visual cues to help engage in dialogue.
   c. Reinventing or communicating—Analysis of the context and relationship is explored.
   d. Sharing—Linking or typing (posting) in the social networking environment.
3. Ultimate accountability to maintain professional boundaries and adhere to professional regulations, standards, and ethical codes lies with the practitioner.
4. US licensing authorities have reported numerous professional violations by health care professionals on social media that resulted in disciplinary action (Ventola, 2014).

F. Patients and families who experience chronic illnesses can be especially vulnerable to online interactions. They will seek to find comfort, kinship, and helpful medical information through social media. This can occur with:
1. Professionals they are engaged with, including case managers
2. Other patients
3. Those who claim to be patients (Kolbasuk McGee, 2014)

G. Another major hazard associated with the use of social media is the posting of unprofessional content that can reflect unfavorably on health care professionals, students, and affiliated institutions. A more liberal feeling of expression can accompany an individual's online persona,

BOX 19-4   Common Ethical Challenges and Social Media

- Clinical care and liability of online intervention (e.g., prescribing medications and treatments without an established patient relationship)
- Practitioner and patient relationship boundaries (e.g., dual relationships, conflict of interest)
- Privacy and confidentiality
- Mandated reporting concerns (e.g., accuracy of social media reports of patients)
- Libelous claims of practitioners and providers (e.g., misrepresentation of professional, fraudulent credentials)
- Netiquette challenges (e.g., use of profanity, bold font and/or capitals)
- Technology proficiency

prompting behaviors that can be misconstrued as unprofessional. These include
1. Violations of patient privacy
2. Use of profanity or discriminatory language
3. Images of sexual suggestiveness or intoxication
4. Negative comments about patients, an employer, or a school (Peck, 2014)

H. Risks involving breaches of patient privacy can also occur. Infractions expose health care professionals and their employers to liability under federal HIPAA and state privacy laws (Ventola, 2014). They can also prompt ethical sanctions involving confidentiality and privacy.

I. Health care organizations should develop and institute social media policies and guidelines to assure employees appropriately manage any interface with the Internet (Ventola, 2014).

J. Social media is a positive force for patient advocacy and education as well as a resource for evidence-based practice and research (Baker, 2013). Yet, with the popularity and positioning of social media across society, case managers can walk a fine line between utilization for personal as opposed to professional reasons.
1. Licensed and/or certified professionals are accountable to regulations, which underlie their discipline.
   a. Licensing and certification boards define the scope of the practitioner and patient relationship and the importance of professional boundaries.
2. By the same token, ethical codes and standards denote clear guidelines for the latitude of the professional relationship. The onus is on the practitioner to be accountable for the appropriate use of social media on the job.

K. Health care consumers use social media to express their public displeasure over unauthorized treatments or plans by insurance companies as well as other payers.
1. Case managers may become the targets of online complaints by patients and/or their families.
2. Families and patients engage in social media sites to obtain public support.
   a. This includes seeking financial support through crowdfunding sites to pay for treatments and/or services.

L. Case managers often engage in professional groups, media sharing sites, list serves, and other types of portals, which allow for communication posts. When posting comments on social media, all professionals should observe social media communication tips noted in Figure 19-1.

M. Case managers should manage their online profile, always considering the following:
1. What do others want to know about you?
2. What do you want others to know?
3. Maintain a solid profile that is:
   a. Current
   b. Accurate
   c. Informative
   d. Promotes a professional presence

Be focused	Be authentic	Demonstrate competence
Avoid power struggles	Keep comments about problems and processes as opposed to other posters or specific people	Use the highest privacy settings for all social media sites
Review connections at least one a quater	Remove people you no longer wish to have access to you and/or your updates	Do not connect and/or friend everyone
	Do not gripe about an employer, clients, colleagues or the workplace	

FIGURE 19-1. Social media communication tips.

4. Use professional profile pictures only.
   a. Do not use selfies or pictures that present as informal (e.g., those that include family members, pets, peers, and/or potentially unethical professional behaviors including drinking alcohol).
5. Maintain a current vCard.
N. With respect to passwords, case managers may often have all or some of the following security strategies managed by their employer. Often, systems prompt case managers to adhere to their requirements for password creation and the frequency of changing passwords. A list of pointers is provided in Table 19-1. This may

TABLE 19-1 Password Pointers

Should	Should not
• Have at least eight characters. • Include symbols, punctuation marks, digits, and letters. • Use combinations of upper case letters, lower case letters, and numbers. • Use combinations that are easy to remember. • Be different for each machine • Change anywhere from 1 to 3 mo.	• Use password combinations found in any dictionary. • Use keyboard patterns (e.g., qwerty or ouipy). • Repeat characters more than once in a row. • Use phone numbers; names of friends, relatives, and/or pets; proper nouns; or dates. • Write passwords down or be careful of using autoremember for devices. Instead, try to memorize. • Reverse or reuse passwords.

Adapted from Marson, S. M., & Bishop, O. (2008). *Addressing NASW standard 1.07m privacy and confidentiality*. The New Social Worker Online. Retrieved from http://www.socialworker.com/feature-articles/ethics-articles/Addressing_NASW_Standard_1.07m_Privacy_and_Confidentiality, on July 18, 2015.

be helpful especially for those in independent or private case management practice.

O. When the risks are managed well, social media can be a positive force for patient advocacy and education as well as a resource for evidence-based practice and research (Baker, 2013).

 ## To Where Should Your Ethical Compass Point?

A. Managing the diverse types of ethical dilemmas wrought by social media and electronic communication can easily overwhelm case managers.
   1. Case managers strive to assure ethical and legal adherence to professional practice while ascertaining the impact of conflicting organizational policies (Treiger & Fink-Samnick, 2016).
   2. Struggling to interconnect the organizational, clinical, and personal ethics manifesting from these situations can contribute to moral distress.
   3. Moral distress for case managers is further compounded by the addition of the current legal concerns related to professional liability and adherence to laws and regulations (e.g., privacy and confidentiality, scope of practice, licensure portability).
      a. These relentless experiences combine to create an environment of conflict and constraint that are common risk factors for moral distress (Moffat, 2014).
   4. Case managers must recognize that laws, rules, policies, insurance benefits, and regulations will sometimes be in conflict with ethical principles.
      a. In such situations, case managers are bound to address such conflicts to the best of their abilities and/or seek appropriate consultation (CMSA, 2010).
   5. Case managers are beholden to the licensure regulations, which underlie their professional discipline, plus standards of practice and ethical codes.
B. There are established resources to ground the ethical practice of cases managers for the situations discussed in this chapter.
   1. These resources extend from professional standards and codes of ethical and professional conduct to decision-making models. All are understood as serving to guide rather than prescribe one's necessary interventions (Fink-Samnick, 2013b).
   2. The last decade has witnessed the revision of existing professional resources to now include content providing guidance with respect to practice extending across technology, inclusive of managing social media and electronic communication (ACA, 2014; Commission for Case Manager Certification [CCMC], 2015; CDMS, 2010; Commission on Rehabilitation Counselor Certification [CRCC], 2010).
   3. In addition, new standards, statements, white papers, and guidelines have been developed (American Nurses Association [ANA], 2014; American Society of Health System Pharmacists [ASHP], 2012; American Telemedicine Association [ATA], 2015; Case Management Society of America [CMSA], 2014; National Association of Social Workers [NASW], 2005; Association of Social Work Boards [ASWB], 2005; National Council of State Boards of Nursing [NCSBN], 2011). A listing of relevant established professional resources can be found in Table 19-2.

TABLE 19-2 Established Professional Resources—Social Media and Electronic Communication (Data from References as Noted)

Organization	Date	Title	Standard, Code, and/or Principle (as Relevant)
American Counseling Association (ACA)	2014	Code of Ethics	• Section H—Distance Counseling, Technology, and Social Media
American Medical Association (AMA)	2011	Professionalism in the Use of Social Media	
American Nurses Association (ANA)	2011	Principles for Social Networking and the Nurse	
American Nurses Association (ANA)	2015	Code of Ethics for Nurses	• Provision 3—The nurse promotes, advocates for, and protects the rights, health, and safety of the patient. ○ 3.1—Protect for the Rights of Privacy and Confidentiality
American Physical Therapy Association (APTA)	2012	Standards of Conduct in the Use of Social Media	
American Speech-Language-Hearing Association (ASHA)	2015	Telepractice Resources	
American Telemedicine Association (ATA)	2013	Practice Guidelines for Video-Based Telemental Health	
American Telemedicine Association (ATA)	2014	Core Operational Guidelines for Telehealth Services Involving Provider–Patient Interactions	
Case Management Society of America (CMSA)	2014	CMSA Group Policy for LinkedIn	
Commission for Rehabilitation Counselor Certification (CRCC)	2010	Code of Professional Conduct for Rehabilitation Counselors	• Section J—Technology and Distance Counseling
Federation of State Medical Boards (FSMB)	2014	Model Policy Guidelines for the Appropriate Use of Social Media and Social Networking in Medical Practice	
National Council of State Boards of Nursing (NCSBN)	2011	White Paper: A Nurse's Guide to the Use of Social Media	

TABLE 19-2 Established Professional Resources—Social Media and Electronic Communication (Data from References as Noted), *continued*

Organization	Date	Title	Standard, Code, and/or Principle (as Relevant)

The Certification of Disability Management Specialists' Commission (CDMS)	2010	The CDMS Code of Professional Conduct	• Definitions: Electronic technology
			• Section 1—Relationship with all Parties
			  ◦ RPC 1.10—Records: a–d
			  ◦ RPC.1.12—Misconduct a–e,
			  ◦ RPC 1.14—Conflict of Interest
			• Section 2—Provision of Services to Individual Clients
			  ◦ RPC 2.01—Dual Relationships
			  ◦ RPC 2.03—Confidentiality a–f

The Commission for Case Management Certification (CCMC)	2014, 2015	Professional Code of Conduct	• Section 2—Professional Responsibility
			  ◦ S6—Conflict of Interest
			• Section 3—Case Manager/ Client Relationships
			  ◦ S10—Relationships with Clients
			• Section 4—Confidentiality, Privacy, Security, and Recordkeeping
			  ◦ S16—Electronic Media
			  ◦ S17—Records: Maintenance/ Storage and Disposal
			• Section 5—Professional Relationships
			  ◦ S19—Dual Relationships
			  ◦ S20—Unprofessional Behavior

The National Association of Social Workers (NASW) and the Association of Social Work Boards (ASWB)	2005	Technology Standards and Social Work Practice	
The American Occupational Therapy Association, Inc. (AOTA)	2015	Social Media Tips and Resources	
The American Society of Health System Pharmacists (ASHP)	2012	Statement on the Use of Social Media by Pharmacy Professionals	

C. Formal ethical decision-making models serve as a template to guide a case manager's ethical analysis and problem-solving actions. Along with Taylor's Process and the Four Quadrant Model developed by Jonsen, Siegler, and Winslade (2010) that are presented in Chapter 18, the following paradigms offer a strategic means to resolve the loud rumblings of a case manager's ethical clinical gut:

1. Dolgoff, Loewenberg, and Harrington (2009) developed a three-step sequential model to provide distinct cues to professionals in order to guide ethical and legal decision-making.
   a. First, case managers should engage the Ethical Assessment Screen (EAS), which provides a series of self-checks or reminders for the practitioner. It takes into account the fact that most professionals strive to minimize the irrational, impulsive, and the unplanned consequences of their actions. Fundamental elements of the EAS include those described in Box 19-5.
   b. Next, the Ethical Rules Screen (ERS) offers the basic reminder for case managers to check the requisite codes, which underlie their unique professional licensure.
      i. Examine the Codes of Ethics for application of rules.
      ii. If code applies, follow code rules.
      iii. If code does not address specific problem or poses conflicting guidance, use the Ethical Principles Screen.
   c. If a case manager is unable to obtain the needed guidance from the ERS, proceed to the Ethical Principles Screen (EPS). This screen offers a rank ordering of ethical principles for consideration when assessing the alternatives for action. The principles (Box 19-6) are not listed in order of importance; however, it is not uncommon for health care professionals to refer to the protection of life in many risk assessment models (Treiger & Fink-Samnick, 2016).
2. E-ACTS is a framework for difficult decision-making that provides a template of five steps to guide a case manager's objective assessment and analysis. This expert level of critical thinking is particularly essential in mandatory reporting and/or duty to warn situations.
   a. Engage in the moment—Assure objectivity, remove distractions, and then get in an objective zone of thought.

BOX

19-5   Fundamental Elements of the Ethical Assessment Screen

- Identify relevant professional values and ethics, your own relevant values, and societal values relevant to the ethical decision to be made in relation to the ethical dilemma.
- What can you do to minimize conflicts between personal, societal, and professional values?
- Identify alternative ethical options that you may take.
- Which of the alternative ethical options will minimize conflicts between your client's, others', and society's rights and protect to the greatest extent your client's and others' rights and welfare and society's rights and interests?
- Which alternative action will be most efficient, effective, and ethical, as well as result in your doing the "least harm" possible?
- Have you considered and weighed both short- and long-term ethical consequences?
- Final check—Is the planned action impartial, generalizable, and justifiable?

	Elements of the Ethical Principles Screen

BOX 19-6

- Protection of Life—The protection of human life applies to all persons, both to the life of a client and to the lives of all others.
- Equality and Inequality—All persons of the same circumstances should be treated in the same way.
- Autonomy and Freedom—All practice decisions should foster a person's self-determination, autonomy, independence, and freedom.
- Least Harm—When faced with dilemmas that have the potential for causing harm, a case manager should attempt to avoid or prevent such harm. If harm is unavoidable, the professional should always choose the option that will cause the least harm, the least permanent harm, and/or the most easily reversible harm.
- Quality of Life—The option should be chosen that promotes the best quality of life for all people, the client, and the community.
- Privacy and Confidentiality—Practice decisions should be made by professionals that strengthen every client's right to privacy and confidentiality.
- Truthfulness and Full Disclosure—Practice decisions must be made by the professional that permit one to fully disclose all relevant information to clients and others.

   b. Assess Risk—Reflect on the patient's intent of risk, lethality, and immediacy of harming, plus safety for all involved.
   c. Contemplate then Act—Consider and engage in critical thinking.
   d. Transcribe notes—Document actions accurately in the available mode (e.g., electronic and/or hard copy).
   e. Seek to Process—Actively use supervision, mentoring, and/or peer support (Fink-Samnick, 2015).

References

American Counseling Association (ACA). (2014). *Code of ethics.* Alexandria, VA: Author.

American Medical Association (AMA). (2011). *AMA policy on social media, opinion 9.124—professionalism in the use of social media.* American Medical Association. Retrieved from http://www.ama-assn.org/ama/pub/physician-resources/medical-ethics/code-medical-ethics/opinion9124.page?, on July 17, 2015.

American Nurses Association (ANA). (2015). *Code of ethics for nurses with interpretive statements.* Washington, DC: American Nurses Association Nursebooks.org.

American Physical Therapy Association (APTA). (2012). Standards of conduct in the use of social media HOD P06-12-17-16 (position). *Social Media Tips and Best Practices.* Retrieved from http://www.apta.org/SocialMedia/Tips, on July 17, 2015.

American Speech and Language Association (ASHA). (2015). *Telepractice.* Retrieved from http://www.asha.org/PRPSpecificTopic.aspx?folderid=8589934956&section=Resources, on July 17, 2015.

American Telemedicine Association (ATA). (2013). *Practice guidelines for videoconferencing-based telemental health.* Washington, DC: Author.

American Telemedicine Association (ATA). (2014). *Core operational guidelines for telehealth services involving provider-patient interactions.* Washington, DC: Author.

American Telemedicine Association (ATA). (2015). *Telemedicine practice guidelines, American Telemedicine Association.* Retrieved from http://www.americantelemed.org/resources/telemedicine-practice-guidelines/telemedicine-practice-guidelines#.Vx4rPGM3ePo, on September 1, 2015.

Baca, M. (2011). Professional boundaries and dual relationships in clinical practice. *Journal for Nurse Practitioners, 7*(3), 195–200.

Baker, J. D. (2013). Social Networking and Professional Boundaries, AORN Journal, May 2013; *Elsevier, 97*(5), 501–506.

Bala, K. (Summer Issue, June 2014). Social media and changing communication patterns. *Global Media Journal-Indian Edition, 5*(1), 1–6. University of Calcutta.

Baum, S. (2014). Report: 19 Million will use remote patient monitoring by 2018. *MedCity News, June 26, 2014.* Retrieved from http://medcitynews.com/2014/06/biggest-market-remote-patient-monitoring, on July 18, 2015.

Case Management Society of America (CMSA). (2010). *CMSA standards of practice for case management.* Little Rock, AR: Author.

Case Management Society of America (CMSA). (2014). *CMSA Group Policy for LinkedIn, CMSA individual member page.* Retrieved from http://www.cmsa.org/Home/CMSA/SocialMediaPolicy/tabid/818/Default.aspx, on July 10, 2015.

Certification of Disability Management Specialists' Commission (CDMS). (2010). *The CDMS code of professional conduct.* Chicago, IL: Author.

Commission for Case Manager Certification (CCMC). (2015). *Code of professional conduct for case mangers with standards, rules, procedures and penalties.* Mount Laurel, NJ: Commission for Case Manager Certification.

Commission on Rehabilitation Counselor Certification (CRCC). (2010). *Code of ethics.* Schaumberg, IL: Commission on Rehabilitation Counselor Certification.

Daly, R. (2011). Not so fast. *Modern Healthcare, November 14, 2011.* Retrieved from http://www.modernhealthcare.com/article/20111114/MAGAZINE/311149967, on July 18, 2015.

Dejong, S. (2012). Networking, professionalism, and the internet. *Psychiatric Times.* Retrieved from http://www.psychiatrictimes.com/networking-professionalism-and-internet, on July 12, 2015.

Dictionary.com. (2015a). *Friend.* Retrieved from http://dictionary.reference.com/browse/friend?&o=100074&s=t, on June 4, 2015.

Dictionary.com. (2015b). *Social network.* Retrieved from http://dictionary.reference.com/browse/social+network, on June 4, 2015.

Dictionary.com. (2015c). *Text message.* Retrieved from http://dictionary.reference.com/browse/text+message, on June 4, 2015.

Dictionary.com. (2015d). *Tweet.* Retrieved from http://dictionary.reference.com/browse/tweeting?s=t, on June 4, 2015.

Dolgoff, R., Loewenberg, F. M., & Harrington, D. (2009). *Ethical decisions for social work practice* (8th ed.). Belmont, CA: Thomson, Brooks/Cole Publishing.

Fink-Samnick, E. (2013a) Case management's ethical eight: Preparing for the next wave. *Case In Point, 11*(11), 1–5.

Fink-Samnick, E. (2013b). Duty to act®: A comprehensive process in proceeding with duty to warn. Legal and regulatory column. *Professional Case Management, 18*(3), 151–154.

Fink-Samnick, E. (2015). E-ACTS®: A framework for difficult decision-making, case management matters. *Professional Case Management, 20*(4), 206–210.

Free, C., Phillips, G., Watson, L., Galli, L., Edwards, P. Patel, V., & Haines, A. (2013). The effectiveness of mobile-health technologies to improve health care delivery processes: A systematic review and meta-analysis. *PLoS Medicine, 10*(1), Retrieved from http://www.ncbi.nlm.nih.gov/pubmed/23458994, on July 18, 2015.

Gutheil, T. G., & Simon, R. I. (2002). Non-sexual boundary crossings and boundary violations: the ethical dimension. *The Psychiatric Clinics of North America, 25*(3), 585–592.

Honigman, B. (2013). 24 outstanding statistics and figures of how social media has impacted the health care industry. *ReferralMD.* Retrieved from https://getreferralmd.com/2013/09/healthcare-social-media-statistics, on July 10, 2015.

Househ, M. (2013). The use of social media in healthcare: Organizational, clinical, and patient perspectives. In K. L. Courtney, et al. (Eds.), *Enabling Health and Healthcare Through ICT* (pp. 244–248). Amsterdam: IOS Press.

IT Law Wiki. (2015). *Privacy settings.* Retrieved from http://itlaw.wikia.com/wiki/Privacy_settings, on June 2, 2015.

Jonsen, A., Siegler, M., & Winslade, W. (2010). *Clinical ethics: a practical approach to ethical decision-making* (7th ed.). New York, NY: McGraw Hill.

Koivunen, M., Niemi, A., & Hupli, M. (2014). The use of electronic devices for communication with colleagues and other healthcare professionals-nursing professionals' perspectives. *Journal of Advanced Nursing, 71*(3), 620–631.

Kolbasuk McGee, M. (2014). Social media: Teach patients the risks. *HealthcareInfo Security, January 31, 2014*. Retrieved from http://www.healthcareinfosecurity.com/blogs/social-media-teach-patients-risks-p-1616, on July 12, 2015.

Lo, B., & Field, M. J. (Eds.); Committee on Conflict of Interest in Medical Research, Education, and Practice, Institute of Medicine. (2009). *Conflict of interest in medical research, education, and practice*. Washington, DC: National Academies Press.

Lowes, R. (2012). *Cloned EHRs jeopardize medical payment, Medscape Medica*. Retrieved from http://www.medscape.com/viewarticle/771548, on August 12, 2015.

Manchitanti, L., & Hirsch, J. (May–June 2015). A case for restraint of explosive growth of health information technology: First, do no harm. *Pain Physician Journal, Health Policy Review, 18,* 293–298. Retrieved from http://www.painphysicianjournal.com/2015/may/2015;18;E293-E298.pdf, on July 18, 2015.

Marson, S. M., & Bishop, O. (2008). Addressing NASW standard 1.07m privacy and confidentiality. *The New Social Worker Online*. Retrieved from http://www.socialworker.com/feature-articles/ethics-articles/Addressing_NASW_Standard_1.07m_Privacy_and_Confidentiality, on July 18, 2015.

Merriam-Webster. (2015a). *Blog*. Retrieved from http://www.merriam-webster.com/dictionary/blog, on June 3, 2015.

Merriam-Webster. (2015b). *Crowdsourcing*. Retrieved from http://www.merriam-webster.com/dictionary/crowdsourcing, on June 3, 2015.

Merriam-Webster. (2015c). *Netiquette*. Retrieved from http://www.merriam-webster.com/dictionary/netiquette, on June 3, 2015.

Merriam-Webster. (2015d). *Podcast*. Retrieved from http://www.merriam-webster.com/dictionary/podcast, on June 2, 2015.

Moffat, M. (2014). Reducing moral distress in case managers. *Professional Case Management, 19*(4), 173–186.

Moorhead, A. S., Hazlett, D. E., Harrison, L., Carroll, J. K., Irwin, A., & Hoving, C. (2013). A new dimension of health care: Systematic review of uses, benefits, and limitations of social media for health communication. *Journal of Medical Internet Research, 15*(4), e85. Retrieved from http://www.jmir.org/2013/4/e85, on July 18, 2015.

National Association of Social Workers (NASW) & Association of Social Work Boards (ASWB). (2005). *Standards for technology and social work practice*. Washington, DC: Author.

National Council of State Boards of Nursing (NCSBN). (2011). *The nurses guide to use of social media, August 2011*, Chicago, IL: National Council of State Boards of Nursing.

Ossola, A. (2015). *A new kind of social anxiety in the classroom, The Atlantic*. Retrieved from HYPERLINK "http://www.theatlantic.com/education/archive/2015/01/the-socially-anxious-generation/384458/"http://www.theatlantic.com/education/archive/2015/01/the-socially-anxious-generation/384458, January 14, 2015.

Oxford Dictionaries. (2015). *Mobile device*. Retrieved from http://www.oxforddictionaries.com/us/definition/american_english/mobile-device, on June 2, 2015.

Pai, A. (2014). Survey: Almost 70% of clinicians at US hospitals use smartphones, tablets. *Mobihealthnews, December 9, 2014*. Retrieved from http://mobihealthnews.com/38859/survey-almost-70-percent-of-clinicians-at-us-hospitals-use-smartphones-tablets, on May 15, 2015.

PC Magazine. (2015). Media sharing site. *ENCYCLOPEDIA, PC Magazine.com*. Retrieved from http://www.pcmag.com/encyclopedia/term/63612/media-sharing-site, on June 4, 2015.

Peck, J. L. (2014). Social media in nursing education: responsible integration for meaningful use. *Journal of Nursing Education, 53*(3), 164–169.

Segen's Medical Dictionary. (2011). *Dual relationship*. Retrieved from http://medical-dictionary.thefreedictionary.com/Dual+Relationship, on June 4, 2015.

Smith, A. (2015). U.S. Smartphone use in 2015. *Pew Research Center: Internet, Science & Tech, April 1, 2015*. Retrieved from http://www.pewinternet.org/2015/04/01/us-smartphone-use-in-2015, on May 20, 2015.

Span, P. (2015). Hipaa's use as code of silence often misinterprets the law. *The New York Times—Health*. Retrieved from http://www.nytimes.com/2015/07/21/health/hipaas-use-as-code-of-silence-often-misinterprets-the-law.html?ref=health&_r=0, on July 17, 2015.

Tech.firstpost.com. (2015). More than half of the world's population owns a smartphone. *News & Analysis, January 12, 2015.* Retrieved from http://tech.firstpost.com/news-analysis/more-than-half-of-the-worlds-population-owns-a-smartphone-report-249361.html, on July 19, 2015.

Techopedia. (2015). *Internet of things.* Retrieved from http://www.techopedia.com/definition/28247/internet-of-things-iot, on June 18, 2015.

TechTerms.com. (2015). *Wiki.* Retrieved from http://techterms.com/definition/wiki, on June 2, 2015.

The American Occupational Therapy Association, Inc. (AOTA). (2015). Social media tips and resources. *Manage Your Practice.* Retrieved from http://www.aota.org/Practice/Manage/Social-Media.aspx, on July 17, 2015.

The American Society of Health System Pharmacists (ASHP). (2012). ASHP statement on the use of social media by pharmacy professionals. *Practice and Policy Statements: Automation and Information Technology.* Retrieved from http://www.ashp.org/menu/PracticePolicy/PolicyPositionsGuidelinesBestPractices/BrowsebyTopic/Automation.aspx, on July 17, 2015.

Topol, E. in Nosta, E. (2013). The STAT Ten: Eric Topol, MD speaks out on digital health. *Forbes Tech, January 30, 2013.* Retrieved from http://www.forbes.com/sites/johnnosta/2013/01/30/the-stat-ten-eric-topol-md-speaks-out-on-digital-health, on June 2, 2015.

Treiger, T., & Fink-Samnick, E. (2016). *COLLABORATE for professional case management: A universal competency-based paradigm* (1st ed.). Philadelphia, PA: Lippincott Wolters Kluwer.

U.S. Department of Health & Human Services' Office for Civil Rights. (2015). Breaches affecting 500 or more individuals. *Breach Portal.* Retrieved from https://ocrportal.hhs.gov/ocr/breach/breach_report.jsf, on July 10, 2015.

Vacellaro, J. E. (August 28, 2007). Social networking goes professional. *The Wall Street Journal.* Retrieved from http://www.wsj.com/articles/SB118825239984310205, on June 2, 2015.

Ventola, C. L. (2014). Social media and health care professionals: Benefits, risks, and best practices. *Pharmacy and Therapeutics, MediMedia USA, 39*(7), 491–499, 520. Retrieved from http://www.ncbi.nlm.nih.gov/pmc/articles/PMC4103576, on May 27, 2015.

Webopedia. (2015). *The STAT Ten: Eric Topol, MD speaks out on digital health.* Retrieved from http://www.webopedia.com/TERM/S/Skype.html, on June 3, 2015.

Woods, B. (2014). By 2020, 90% of world's populations aged over six will have a mobile phone: Report. *The Next Web, Insider, November 18, 2014.* Retrieved from http://thenextweb.com/insider/2014/11/18/2020-90-worlds-population-aged-6-will-mobile-phone-report, on May 19, 2015.

CHAPTER 20

Legal Considerations in Case Management

Lynn S. Muller

LEARNING OBJECTIVES

Upon completion of this chapter, the reader will be able to:

1. Understand a wide range of legal terms and identify sources for additional resources.
2. Gain an appreciation for the interaction of conflicting areas of law and ethical practice.
3. Discuss the role of the case manager in relation to the legal community.
4. Recognize and understand patients' rights and case managers' responsibilities.
5. Identify several strategies for case management practice that facilitate adherence to relevant laws or regulations.

IMPORTANT TERMS AND CONCEPTS

Advocate	Codify	Discovery
Agent	Common Law	Duty
Battery	Compensable	Expert Witness
Breach	Conflict of Interest	Fundamental Right
Breach of Contract	Contract	Harm
Business Associate	Contribution	Informed Consent
Agreement	Damages	Intentional Tort
Case Law	Decision	Interrogatories
Causal Connection	Defendant	Joint Liability
Civil Law	Deposition	Law

Lawyer	Proximate Cause	Standard of Care
Liability	Regulation	Statutory Law
Liable	Regulatory Compliance	Subpoena
Malpractice	Remedy	Tort
Medical Malpractice	Res Judicata (Latin	Verdict
Negligence	term meaning "a	Waiver
Opinion	thing [already]	Witness
Professional	adjudicated")	
Negligence	Several Liability	

 Introduction

A. In our litigious society, case managers are concerned with an ethical–legal conflict in which they want to provide quality case management services, obey the law, meet licensing requirements and regulations, please their employers or contractors, and still act as advocates for their patients. The good news is that it is possible.

B. Legal issues affecting case management are interwoven in the complex matrix that is case management practice. Just as each patient is an individual who presents with uniquely different life experiences, expectations, and health outcomes potential, so the interplay of the law is unique and will affect decision making and ultimately the practice of the case manager.

C. Case managers have recognized the need for greater understanding in this area but must always be mindful of the parameters of practice. It is in knowing those parameters of practice or knowing the sandbox that reduces liability (Garner, 1996) exposure for the case manager.

D. It is important for case managers to be knowledgeable about the health and case management practice-related laws and regulations in the jurisdiction where they practice. It is also as important for them to be familiar about how, where, and when to seek information that pertains to these laws and regulations when uncertain or unsure or consult with a specialized person such as legal counsel when necessary.

 Descriptions of Key Terms (Garner, 1996)

A. Advocate—A person who assists, defends, or pleads for another.
B. Agent—One who is authorized to act for or in place of another.
C. Battery—In tort law (civil law), an intentional and offensive touching of another.
D. Breach of contract—Violation (failure to perform) of a contract obligation.
E. Breach—Violation or infraction of a law or obligation. A failure on one's part to conform to the standard required.
F. Business Associate Agreement—A mandatory written contract between a covered entity and a business associate.
G. Case law—The collection of reported cases that form the body of jurisprudence within a given jurisdiction.
H. Causal connection—The relationship between cause and effect.
I. Civil law—The law of civil or private rights.

J. Codify/codification—The process of compiling, arranging, and systematizing the laws of a given jurisdiction into an ordered code.

K. Common law—The body of law derived from judicial decisions and opinions, rather than from statutes or constitutions, also known as *case law.*

L. Compensable—A situation a person encounters that entitles the person for compensation, usually financial in nature. Often in the workers' compensation arena, it is a work-related injury or death, which deems the injured worker or the deceased's family eligible for financial compensation.

M. Conflict of interest—A real or seeming incompatibility between one's private interests and one's fiduciary duties.

N. Contract—A set of promises, for breach of which the law gives a remedy, or the performance of which the law in some way recognizes as a duty.

O. Contribution—The right to demand that another, who is jointly responsible for a third-party injury, supply part of what one is required to compensate a third party.

P. Damages—Monetary compensation for loss or injury to person or property.

Q. Decision—A court's (judge's) ruling in a case.

R. Defendant—The party being sued in a civil lawsuit.

S. Deposition—A witness' out-of-court testimony that is reduced to a writing, usually by a court reporter, for later use in court or for discovery purposes.

T. Discovery—The act or process of finding and learning something that was previously unknown. (Each state's court rules govern the discovery process.)

U. Duty—An obligation recognized by the law, requiring a person to conform to a certain standard of conduct, for the protection of others against reasonable risks.

V. Expert witness—A witness qualified by knowledge, skill, experience, training, or education to provide scientific, technical, or other specialized opinions about the evidence or a fact issue.

W. Fundamental right—(1) A right derived from natural or fundamental law. (2) Fundamental rights as enumerated by the Supreme Court, including the right to vote, interstate travel, along with various rights of privacy.

X. Harm—Actual loss or damage resulting from the actions or inactions of another.

Y. Informed consent—(1) A person's agreement to allow something to happen, made with full knowledge of the risks involved and the alternatives. (2) A patient's intelligent choice about treatment, made after a physician discloses whatever information a reasonably prudent physician in the medical community would provide to a patient regarding the risks involved in the proposed treatment.

Z. Intentional tort—A tort committed by someone acting with general or specific intent; examples are battery, false imprisonment, and trespass. May also be termed a *willful* tort and is distinguished from negligence.

AA. Interrogatories—A numbered list of written questions submitted in a legal context, usually to an opposing party in a lawsuit as part of discovery.

BB. Joint liability—Liability shared by two or more parties (persons, agencies, or organizations).

CC. Law—(1) A set of rules that order human activities and relations. (2) The collection of legislation and accepted legal principles; the body of authoritative grounds of judicial action.

DD. Lawyer—One who is designated to transact business for another; a legal agent, attorney.

EE. Liability—The quality or state of being legally obligated or responsible.

FF. Liable—(1) Legally obligated or responsible. (2) To have a duty or burden.

GG. Malpractice—Negligence or incompetence on the part of a professional.

HH. Medical malpractice—A tort that arises when a doctor (or other health professional, including registered nurses, dentists, or social workers) violates the standard of care owed to a patient and the patient is injured as a result (often shortened to med mal).

II. Medical Marijuana—Provision in a state that has approved its use through legislation, by way of a prescription by a physician licensed to practice in that state, of cannabis for the treatment of a known diagnosis. Some recognized diagnoses include AIDs, seizure disorders, anorexia, glaucoma, migraines, etc.

JJ. Negligence—(1) The failure to exercise that standard of care that a reasonably prudent person would have exercised in the same situation. (2) A tort (civil wrong) grounded in this failure.

KK. Opinion—The court's (a judge's) written statement explaining its decision in a given case, including statements of fact, points of law, rationale, and dicta.

LL. Plaintiff—The party who brings a lawsuit in a civil action.

MM. Professional Negligence—See Malpractice above.

NN. Proximate cause—A cause that directly produces an event and without which the event would not have occurred.

OO. Regulations—Rules and administrative codes issued by governmental agencies at all levels, municipal, county, state, and federal. Although they are not laws, regulations have the force of law, since they are adopted under authority granted by statutes and often include penalties for violations (LAW.COM, 2015).

PP. Remedy—The enforcement of a right or the redress of an injury, usually in the form of monetary damages that a party asks of a court.

QQ. Res judicata (Latin term meaning "a thing [already] adjudicated")—An issue that had been definitively settled by judicial decision.

RR. Several liability—Liability that is separate and distinct from another's liability, so that the plaintiff may bring a separate action against one defendant without joining the other liable parties.

SS. Standard of care—In the law of negligence, the degree of care that a reasonable person would exercise.

TT. Statutory law—The body of law derived from statutes rather than from constitutions or judicial decisions.

UU. Subpoena—A court order commanding the appearance of a witness, subject to penalty for noncompliance.

VV. Tort—(1) A civil wrong for which a remedy may be obtained, usually in the form of damages. (2) Breach of a duty that the law imposes.

WW. Verdict—A jury's findings or decision on the factual issues of a case.

XX. Waiver—(1) To voluntarily relinquish or abandon. Waiver may be expressed or implied (by one's actions). A person who is alleged to have waived a right must have had both knowledge of the existing right and intention to relinquish it. (2) Waiver may also refer to the document by which a person relinquishes a right.

YY. Witness—(1) One who sees, knows, or vouches for something. (2) One who testifies under oath or affirmation, either orally or by affidavit or deposition. (3) Someone unrelated to a case but sometimes is brought into the case to share own expert view on the issue, referred to as expert witness.

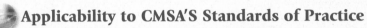

Applicability to CMSA'S Standards of Practice

A. The Case Management Society of America (CMSA) describes in its standards of practice for case management (CMSA, 2010) that case management practice extends across all health care settings, including payer, provider, government, employer, community, and home environment.

B. Health care and the law are inextricably intertwined. The practice of case management has become more complex with the expansion of practice across the care continuum. The case manager is strongly advised to remain aware of the evolving legal and regulatory landscape affecting health care and the implication to case management practice.

C. One of the CMSA's standards of practice for case management addresses the legal obligations of case managers and others involved in the provision of care and services to clients and their support systems. In this regard, the standards state that the case manager should adhere to applicable:
1. Local, state, and federal laws
2. Employer policies and procedures governing all aspects of case management practice, including client privacy and confidentiality rights (CMSA, 2010, p. 19)

D. CMSA also emphasizes that it is the responsibility of the case manager to work within the scope of the licensure he/she holds (e.g., nursing). It directs the case manager, in the event that the employer's policies and procedures or those of other entities involved in the care of a client are in conflict with applicable laws and regulations, to seek clarification from an appropriate and reliable expert resource, such as the employer, government agency, or legal counsel (CMSA, 2010).

E. According to the CMSA standards of practice, the case manager is expected to adhere to applicable laws and organizational policies governing the client, client's privacy, and confidentiality rights and protect the client's best interest. Box 20-1 includes examples of the case manager's legal obligations (CMSA, 2010).

F. This chapter discusses basic legal considerations for sound case management practice. The Legal Standard recognizes that case managers should practice within the scope of their underlying professional licensure and/or certification and in compliance with applicable federal, state, and local laws and regulations.

20-1 | **Legal Obligations of the Case Manager**

- Remain up-to-date about applicable laws and regulations concerning confidentiality, privacy, and protection of client medical information issues.
- Obtain the client's written acknowledgement that he/she has received notice of privacy rights and practices.
- Seek appropriate and informed client consent before implementing case management services and document that client/client's support system has consented.
- Discuss the following with the client/client's support system when obtaining the consent (written or verbal):
  - Case management process and services needed
  - Benefits and costs of the services
  - Alternatives to the proposed services
  - Potential risks and consequences of the proposed services
  - Client's right to refuse care and treatment and consequences of the refusal
- Seek the assistance of legal counsel when unsure about a situation or for support and advice.

 Background

A. Legal basics
1. Understanding the law is much like learning a new language. It is especially important to learn legal terms, because some legal terms are words that have other meanings in common or medical usage.
2. The legal system is divided into two major categories, criminal and civil law. Civil law is the law that applies to private rights, as opposed to the law that applies to criminal matters (Box 20-2).
3. The purpose of tort law is to adjust losses and to compensate one person because of the actions of another. A tort is a civil or personal wrong, as compared with a crime, which is a public wrong.
B. Intentional torts—Intentional torts include assault, battery, false imprisonment, and trespass.
1. These terms are often confused because they also exist in criminal law. When they are used in criminal law, they are defined by statute (laws passed by the legislature) and can vary from state to state.
2. Each intentional tort represents a direct interference with a person's physical integrity or right to property. Personal freedom is a

20-2 | **Civil and Criminal Laws**

Civil law
- The body of law that permits an individual who believes that he or she has been wronged to sue another and recover damages (dollars).

Criminal law
- Public law that deals with crimes and their prosecution. Substantive criminal law defines crimes, and procedural criminal law sets down criminal procedure.

fundamental right. One does not waive a fundamental right, such as personal integrity, automatically, but a person must be aware that he or she possesses the right and can intentionally relinquish it.

   a. Informed consent is a good example of a knowing and voluntary waiver of rights in the medical setting. In the absence of such a waiver of rights, a person touching or keeping another in a clinic, hospital, or any place he or she chooses not to be may be liable for assault, battery, or false imprisonment. Informed consent is a statutorily created right, given to potential recipients of medical treatment.

3. In 2010, as part of the Patient Protection and Affordable Care Act (PPACA), a Federal Patients' Bill of Rights was signed into law and became effective on September 23, 2010; it provided new protections, including but not limited to a prohibition on denying health insurance coverage for those with pre-existing medical conditions (CMSA, 2010).

4. Every person admitted to a general hospital as licensed by the State Department of Health and Senior Services pursuant to P.L. 1971, c. 136 (C. 26:2H-1 et al.) shall have specific rights the hospital and health care providers must respect and meet.

5. Many states have also enacted a "Patient's Bill of Rights" (Box 20-3), which may provide far more comprehensive rights than the federal one. When a law exists, such as a Patient's Bill of Rights in one setting (e.g., the hospital setting), the health practitioner can reasonably assume that the policy established in that law may apply to a setting not articulated specifically.

   a. In other words, if a case manager finds himself or herself in the field setting, on the telephone or communicating electronically and in a decision-making dilemma and, to complicate the matter, the patient is very argumentative and difficult, the case manager must be cognizant of the statutory language that states, "[A patient

BOX 20-3 New Jersey Patient's Bill of Rights

- To considerate and respectful care consistent with sound nursing and medical practices, which shall include being informed of the name and licensure status of a student nurse or facility staff member who examines, observes, or treats the patient.
- To be informed of the name of the physician responsible for coordinating his diagnosis, treatment, and prognosis in terms he can reasonably be expected to understand. When it is not medically advisable to give this information to the patient, it shall be made available to another person designated by the patient on his behalf.
- To receive from the physician information necessary to give informed consent prior to the start of any procedure or treatment and that, except for those emergency situations not requiring an informed consent, shall include as a minimum the specific procedure or treatment, the medically significant risks involved, and the possible duration of incapacitation, if any, as well as an explanation of the significance of the patient's informed consent. The patient shall be advised of any medically significant alternatives for care or treatment; however, this does not include experimental treatments that are not yet accepted by the medical establishment.

continued

BOX 20-3   **New Jersey Patient's Bill of Rights** *continued*

- To refuse treatment to the extent permitted by law and to be informed of the medical consequences of this act.
- To privacy to the extent consistent with providing adequate medical care to the patient. This shall not preclude discussion of a patient's case or examination of a patient by appropriate health care personnel.
- To privacy and confidentiality of all records pertaining to his treatment, except as otherwise provided by law or third-party payment contract, and to access to those records, including receipt of a copy thereof at reasonable cost, upon request, unless his physician states in writing that access by the patient is not medically advisable; to give this information to the patient, it shall be made available to another person designated by the patient on his behalf.
- To expect that within its capacity, the hospital will make reasonable response to his request for services, including the services of an interpreter in a language other than English if 10% or more of the population in the hospital's service area speaks that language.
- To be informed by his physician of any continuing health care requirements, which may follow discharge and to receive assistance from the physician and appropriate hospital staff in arranging for required follow-up care after discharge.
- To be informed by the hospital of the necessity of transfer to another facility prior to the transfer and of any alternatives to it, which may exist, which transfer shall not be effected unless it is determined by the physician to be medically necessary.
- To be informed, upon request, of other health care and educational institutions that the hospital has authorized to participate in his treatment.
- To be advised if the hospital proposes to engage in or perform human research or experimentation and to refuse to participate in these projects. For the purposes of this subsection, "human research" does not include the mere collecting of statistical data.
- To examine and receive an explanation of his bill, regardless of source of payment, and to receive information or be advised on the availability of sources of financial assistance to help pay for the patient's care, as necessary.
- To expect reasonable continuity of care.
- To be advised of the hospital rules and regulations that apply to his conduct as a patient.
- To treatment without discrimination as to race, age, religion, sex, national origin, or source of payment.
- To contract directly with a New Jersey licensed registered professional nurse of the patient's choosing for private professional nursing care during his hospitalization. A registered professional nurse so contracted shall adhere to hospital policies and procedures in regard to treatment protocols and care activities.

N.J.S.A. 26:2H-12.8.

    (client) has a right] to considerate and respectful care consistent with sound ... practices, which shall include being informed of the name and licensure status of a ... staff member who ... observes or treats the patient."

  b. There is no doubt that a case manager is making observations about a patient, whether on the telephone, through electronic communications, or at arm's length. Even if there is no statute directly on point regarding case management practice, you can assume that a court will use existing law as a basis for an alternative practice setting as much as is practical. This is how new laws are developed.

C. Negligence—For a lawsuit to be successful in negligence, there are four required elements. These elements are commonly referred to as duty, breach, cause, and harm.

1. All four of the elements must be proven, and the burden of proof is on the plaintiff (Box 20-4).

   a. A well-established duty and an obvious breach of such duty are not sufficient without also establishing the causal connection to the harm claimed (Keeton & Prosser, 1984). Proof of damages (harm) is an essential element to a negligence case. Negligence is sometimes referred to as simple negligence as compared with malpractice or professional negligence. The standard of proof for a simple negligence case is that of a reasonably prudent person.

   b. The concept of negligence is based on the idea that there can be a generally uniform standard of human behavior. The simplest example of this is that when one drives a car, there is a generally accepted expectation that each person will operate the vehicle in a reasonably prudent and careful manner. Each time that there is a motor vehicle accident, it is likely that one or more persons deviated from the reasonably prudent person's standard and liability may attach. However, state statutes may limit or expand one's ability to bring a cause of action, a lawsuit.

   c. In 12 states, so-called "no fault" insurance is one example of such a limitation, particularly when there is an express limitation on one's ability to sue for certain personal injuries (III, 2014), (N.J.S.A. 39:6B, *et seq*).

D. How cases are decided—What we refer to as "the law" is a combination of legislated rules—statutory law and case law.

1. Case law is the compilation of common law. Common law, with its historical roots dating back to 12-century England, provides the foundation for the collection of decisions, the result of various lawsuits. Such decisions are outcomes of particular cases and are either jury verdicts or judges' decisions.

   a. Judges' decisions may be verbal, on the record, or in the form of a written opinion.

   b. *Res judicata* is the legal term explaining that today's law is based on decisions that came before. Once an issue on a particular set of facts has been decided, there is no reason to relitigate the same issue. For example, it has already been decided that if a surgeon excises the left limb when the informed consent clearly states the right limb, the surgeon is liable and has committed the tort of battery.

BOX 20-4 Four Elements of Negligence

1. A well-established duty
2. An obvious breach of such duty
3. Damages or injuries the client suffered
4. A proximate cause or connection between the breach and the client (evident in the resulting harm)

    c. Whether a new case relates to ears, legs, arms, or breasts, the court will rely on the existing law relating to battery and professional negligence, also known as malpractice. Therefore, today, most cases that are heard in court are not reported.

    d. A reported case is one that can be found in an official reporter. There are state as well as federal reporters. When entered into a reporter, the case is printed and becomes part of the ever-growing body of case law. It is important to remember that what we hear on the news, no matter the source, is simply news (and ofttimes entertainment), not admissible evidence at trial.

E. Professional negligence and malpractice—Each of us comes to case management with education and experience from a profession.

    1. We are typically licensed in that underlying profession. In fact, such licensure is one of the qualifications for a person seeking to become a case manager.

    2. It is critical that the case manager maintains current licensing and/or state certification requirements and updates his or her knowledge each year in both the field of case management and the underlying profession.

    3. The standard by which any case manager will be judged remains one derived from an external authority, such as a governmental standard. If you are a nurse, this standard is derived from the Nurse Practice Act. (Each state has a Nurse Practice Act of one variety or another [N.J.S.A. 45:11–23, *et seq*]). See Additional Resources—States Boards of Nursing and the Nurse Practice Acts.

    4. Nurse Practice Acts provide broad statements defining nursing practice, delineating the educational and other requirements for licensure and renewal, and giving notice to the public of the sort of behaviors that can be expected from a nurse and what unacceptable practices might subject a nurse to disciplinary review or sanctions.

    5. When these laws were drafted, the concept of managed care had not been thought of by the legislatures. For a copy of any state's Nurse Practice Act, contact the board of nursing in that state.

        a. Each profession develops a standard for itself through a complicated process of interaction with other professions, professional journals, meetings, and networking with colleagues and the development and refining of educational programs for the profession.

        b. In the developing world of new names and new roles, the law has not caught up with these rapid changes. Over time, hundreds of separate standards and comments become the "standard practice" (Eddy, 1982). Each profession has an obligation to monitor or "self-police."

        c. Today, although the legal community knows of case management and case managers, that does not mean they have a complete understanding of the role of the case manager, the standard of practice, or the ethical canons that guide practice.

            i. The trend appears to be for inclusion of case managers as potential defendants in malpractice lawsuits. The most prevalent areas are workers' compensation cases where case managers have an active role in service and product selection and in hospital case management.

  ii. That is not to say that there are many successful suits where case managers have been held liable. Such cases are rare. Most malpractice lawsuits settle, prior to trial, in whole or in part.

F. Burden of proof—In the case of professional liability (malpractice), the law requires that an expert witness be engaged to establish the accepted standards of practice; it is not sufficient that such information is available in print.

  1. Experts base their opinions and their testimony on their knowledge, education, and experience. State and federal rules of evidence require that a patient claiming that a professional is responsible for his or her injuries and damages use a "like-kind" expert witness to prove his or her case (Fed. R. Evid. 703,704).

    a. In other words, if the case manager who is being sued is a nurse, then it is necessary for another nurse case manager to act as the expert witness. If the case manager on trial were a social worker by education, the expert would have to be a social worker.

    b. Please note that in recent years, case law has broadened the definition of an expert in a professional case. The variations can be found in state laws.

  2. The plaintiff cannot proceed or be successful in a lawsuit unless a causal relationship is established between the harm claimed, the duty of the case manager, and an alleged breach of such duty.

    a. It is not enough to have a generally experienced nurse testify against a nurse in a unique role; rather, case managers require a nurse case manager expert, utilization review nurses require a utilization review expert, and social workers require a social worker case manager expert.

    b. Expert witnesses must be knowledgeable and up to date in their field and familiar with texts, journals, and the relevant accepted standard of practice and are often published authors.

G. Affidavit of merit—Is designed to provide protection for professionals and reduce the number of frivolous or nonmeritorious suits.

  1. In many states, it is now necessary to file an affidavit of merit upon or within a number of days of the filing of a malpractice lawsuit (N.J.S.A. 2A:53A-27).[1] This is a safeguard for the defendant, the purpose of which is to eliminate lawsuits filed without a genuine cause of action against a professional (licensed) person.

---

[1] Affidavit required in certain actions against licensed persons. In any action for damages for personal injuries, wrongful death, or property damage resulting from an alleged act of malpractice or negligence by a licensed person in his profession or occupation, the plaintiff shall, within 60 days following the date of filing of the answer to the complaint by the defendant, provide each defendant with an affidavit of an appropriate licensed person that there exists a reasonable probability that the care, skill, or knowledge exercised or exhibited in the treatment, practice, or work that is the subject of the complaint fell outside of the acceptable professional or occupational standards or treatment practices. The court may grant no more than one additional period, not to exceed 60 days, to file the affidavit pursuant to this section, on a finding of good cause. The person executing the affidavit shall be licensed in this or any other state and have particular expertise in the general area or specialty involved in the action, as evidenced by board certification or by devotion of the person's practice substantially to the general area or specialty involved in the action for a period of at least five years. The person shall have no financial interest in the outcome of the case under review, but this prohibition shall not exclude the person from being an expert witness in the case (N.J.S.A. 2A:53A-27).

    a. In New Jersey, for example, this was part of major tort reform legislation.

    b. A person who wishes to bring a negligence or malpractice action against a licensed person must submit the affidavit within 60 days from a neutral-licensed person.

    c. This independent person must state that the services were not acceptable, and the law requires that the person providing the affidavit be a qualified expert (N.J.S.A. 2A:53A-27).

2. The only exception to the affidavit requirement is in those cases in which the defendant (licensed professional) failed to provide necessary records that would reveal malpractice (N.J.S.A. 2A:53A-27).

    a. In a recent case, an affidavit prepared by an independent expert was found to be sufficient when the author (expert) submitted his *curriculum vitae*, delineating education, experience specific to the defendant's practice, and scientific presentation and papers he had authored (*Wacht v. Farooqui*, 1998).

    b. In April 2015, this case was reaffirmed with a caveat that a practitioner in one area may be able to testify as an expert in case against a practitioner in another, if those areas of practice have overlapping practice areas, for instance, a podiatrist and an orthopedist who both treat the same area of the body.

3. One interesting variation on the affidavit requirement is in the Commonwealth of Massachusetts, where "Every action for malpractice... against a provider of health care shall be heard by a tribunal consisting of a single justice of the Superior Court [trial court], a physician licensed to practice medicine in the commonwealth ... and an attorney authorized to practice law in the commonwealth, at which hearing the plaintiff shall present an offer of proof and said tribunal shall determine if the evidence presented if properly substantiated is sufficient to raise a legitimate question of liability appropriate for judicial inquiry or whether the plaintiff's case is merely an unfortunate medical result" (Gen. Laws Massachusetts, Part III, Title II, Ch. 231, §60B).

    a. The hearing occurs within fifteen days of the defendant's answer (response to the initiation of a lawsuit). There are similarities and differences between the two approaches.

       i. The affidavit of merit must contain the same offer of proof as the hearing, but must be sworn by a similar practitioner.

       ii. The burden then falls upon the health care provider defendant to challenge the content of the affidavit.

    b. The Massachusetts hearing method places the facts before three professionals, who act as independent and impartial appraisers, and if they are not satisfied that the claim is meritorious, it will be dismissed immediately and end the suit. This system has proven to be effective (Foley, 2010).

    c. These methods are a special protection that modern law provides to health professionals. Their purpose is to avoid dissatisfied or unhappy patients from bringing frivolous lawsuits and ruining a professional's career, where no malpractice has occurred.

H. Liability exposure for case managers—Case managers must be aware of what the law says about case management practice.

1. Because many case managers come from a scientific discipline, with finite rules and measurable answers, it is difficult sometimes to understand the fluid, fact-driven dynamic that is the law. Now case managers have been recognized by some courts as potential defendants.

2. Until there are more reported cases in which case managers have either been found to be liable or relieved from liability, or states create statutes controlling case management practice, the profession must rely on its own developing standards.

   a. In 1995, the New Jersey Supreme Court held that a health maintenance organization (HMO) was liable for the contribution toward the malpractice of a physician they hired as an independent contractor (*Dunn v. Praiss*, 1995).

      i. Logically, it would follow that a case manager performing telephonic or field case management services for an HMO, who deviates from the "accepted standards of practice," could be held liable for his or her actions.

      ii. In addition, the HMO could share in that liability. This is known as *joint* liability.

   b. In an Alabama case, the allegation by a plaintiff/employee, "that the nurse [case manager] was more concerned with saving money than with the employee's recovery," was found to be insufficient to support a claim (*Reid v. Aetna Casualty & Surety Co.*, 1997).

      i. In this case, the client was offered a variety of choices for the treatment of pain management, and the provider chosen was also the least expensive.

      ii. In addition, there was an allegation of fraud on the part of the defendant or insurance carrier, in that they had suppressed the following material information (among other things)—"that the nurse [case manager] was not acting as a registered nurse with the normal professional obligations toward the worker [client]" (*Reid v. Aetna Casualty & Surety Co.*, 1997).

      iii. The court held that even if that were true (and made no finding that it was true), there was no evidence that the actions of the case manager caused any harm to the patient. "It is undisputed that Aetna hired [a case management company] to perform medical case management, that the [case manager] was employed as a registered nurse ... and that she worked on the client's case."

      iv. Although the patient claimed that the case manager "prevented her from undergoing beneficial treatments," she failed to offer proof of such alternative beneficial treatments, and the case was dismissed (*Reid v. Aetna Casualty & Surety Co.*, 1997).

   c. It is very important to note that in the concurring opinion, another judge in this case stated the following—"My objection to this practice is not so much that the insurance carriers are employing these nurses [case managers] but that the [case managers] are usually not forthcoming in revealing the existence, nature, and purpose of their employment. Thus, injured employees are presented with [case managers] who appear to be assisting them, when in actuality the [case manager] might be testifying in court using information gained through the employee's trust in them" (*Reid v. Aetna Casualty & Surety Co.*, 1997). *Author's Note: although the Reid case is nearly 20 years old, it remains the only judicial commentary on case management practice.*

    d. Case managers should recognize this case as a "red flag" and acknowledge it in its historical context. It is one example of a court that had a bad experience with case management. The majority of case managers are forthcoming about who they are, who employs them, and why they are meeting with the client/patient.

    e. This case supports the need for case managers to clarify these issues at the first and subsequent meetings with the patient.

       i. Once the case manager has disclosed this information to the patient, any information obtained by the case manager about the patient's illness, injury, prior history, work history, present income, and source of income can be freely shared with the relevant parties.

      ii. These may include the physician (as is needed for proper treatment), the payer source, and, in some limited circumstances, the employer.

     iii. It is critical that case managers base their assessments and recommendations on the needs of the clients, always keeping the patient's needs and wishes paramount in decision making.

    f. Today, the CMSA Standards of Practice for Case Management, *Rev. 2010* and Commission for Case Manager Certification (CCMC), American Nurses Association (ANA), and National Association of Social Workers (NASW) Ethical Codes provide guidance for ethical practice.

Regulatory Compliance

A. Background—There are regulations and rules (created through statutory authority) in all areas of health care, including licensure, federal and state benefits programs, taxation, etc. The one area that most commonly affects day-to-day health care practice is the Health Insurance Portability and Accountability Act of 1996 (HIPAA), Public Law 104-191, which was enacted on August 21, 1996, a significant piece of civil rights legislation.

  1. HIPAA established a minimum mandatory national standard for privacy protection. "The Privacy Rule" was published on December 28, 2000, with the goal of providing consumers with greater rights for protection of individually identifiable health information, sometimes referred to as Person Health Information (PHI).

    a. In the spring of 2003, there were further modifications to the "Final Privacy Rule." Now that HIPAA has been part of practice for 2 decades, it no longer should be feared.

    b. The key to HIPAA, and all the changes and improvement over time, is meeting educational requirement (at minimum, a yearly update) and demonstrating genuine compliance.

    c. The Privacy Rule is only part of HIPAA compliance requirements. There are complex regulations controlling the use of electronic communications, including telephone, fax, e-mail and text messaging, as well as billing and reporting requirements.

    d. Refer to Codes of Professional Conduct that control your underlying license/profession, policies, and procedures. Authoritative guidance is found at the Office of the Inspector General (OIG), which posts Advisory Opinions on variety of compliance topics, along with links to the full text of the laws and regulations controlling HIPAA compliance (OIG, 2015). See Additional Resources for Office of the Inspector General—Compliance Resources.

2. Since 2003, the U.S. Department of Health and Human Services (HHS) Office for Civil Rights announced two additional updates, in the form of rulemaking by HHS.

   a. The first is the Health Information Technology for Economic and Clinical Health (HITECH) Act, enacted as part of the American Recovery and Reinvestment Act of 2009 and the Omnibus Final Rule (2013) that encompassed the broadest change in requirements since the enactment of HIPAA in 1996.

   b. It codified and strengthened Breach Notification requirements of the HITECH Act (OCR, 2015). See Additional Sources—Department of Health and Human Services—Health Information Privacy.

3. For the most part, changes to HIPAA have added new obligations, supplementing what came before, and do not eliminate prior duties, unless expressly changed or eliminated. Figure 20-1 highlights resources tracing the development of the case manager's duties related to HIPAA its progeny.

HIPAA Compliance Practice Tips

• Professional Case Management. Muller, L.S., Vol.19, No.4, 311–315 (2014)

Integrity and Accountability: The Omnibus Final Rule Part I

• Professional Case Management. Muller, L.S., Vol. 18/No. 4 (2013)

Integrity and Accountability: The Omnibus Final Rule Part II

• Professional Case Management. Muller, L.S., Vol. 6, No. 5 (2013)

Editorial Commentary on HITECH and Portable Devices

• Professional Case Management. Muller, L.S., Vol. 18, No.1, 36 (2013)

To Chat or Not to Chat? That is the Question

• Professional Case Management. Muller, L.S., Vol.16, No.4, 212–214 (2011)

HIPAA: Demonstrating Compliance

• Lippincott's Case Management. Muller, L.S., Vol. 9, No.1, 27–31 (2004)

HIPAA Compliance: Implications for Case Managers

• Lippincott's Case Management. Muller, L.S., Vol.8, No.1, 30–35 (2003)

HIPAA Business Associate Contracts: The Value of Contracts for Case Managers

• Lippincott's Case Management. Muller, L.S., Vol.8, No.1, 3–10 (2003)

FIGURE 20-1. Resources tracing the development of the case manager's duties related to HIPAA.

4. On June 26, 2015, The Supreme Court of the United States (SCOTUS) issued its decision in *Obergefell, et al. vs. Hodges, Director, Ohio Department of Health, et al.* The Court held that "The Fourteenth Amendment requires a State to license a marriage between two people of the same sex and to recognize a marriage between two people of the same sex when their marriage was lawfully licensed and performed out-of-State" (Obergefell v. Hodges, 2015, pp. 3–28).

   a. The question now becomes, how do we as case managers acclimate our practice to comply with the law of the land?

   b. Personal opinions on this topic are just that: personal, and have no place in our professional practice (Muller, 2016).

   c. This significant change in federal law changes the landscape of what a family "looks like."

   d. Tolerance is a good place to start, but as professionals, case managers are called upon to accept the clients/support systems they care for as they find them. Each client and that client's family is unique. A family is where an individual finds love, home, and security and encompasses a broader definition than ever before.

   e. With these changes, legal documents, including Last Will and Testament, Power of Attorney, and Advanced Directives for Health Care are more important than ever.

   f. When conducting a case management assessment, case managers must stay objective and avoid assumptions. It is not for the case managers to judge any client's circumstance, but to use own professional skills, education, and experience to meet the client's needs.

   g. Respecting the gender choice of clients is critical, but to further their health and safety, case managers may have to ask some questions that may be somewhat uncomfortable.

   h. For a complete discussion see *Professional Case Management, May/June 2016, Vol. 21, Issue 3, pp. 149–153 (Muller) and 156–160 (Skehan/Muller).*

Contracts

A. Contract basics—In the discussion of torts and negligence, you learned that a duty is a legally recognized obligation for which a remedy may be sought in the event of breach of that duty. Contract is another example of a source of duty. When a contract is formed, it creates one or many legal obligations for which damages may be available, in the event of a breach of contract. A lawsuit based on contract is a separate and distinct cause of action.

B. Elements of contract—There are three elements to a valid or binding contract: offer, acceptance, and consideration (Box 20-5).

C. The case manager and contract—A simple example of contract creation is the following:

   1. You are an independent case manager.

      a. You receive a telephone call from XYZ Insurance, asking you to provide case management services for Mr. Smith.

      b. In addition, XYZ offers you a fee if you *visit* with Mr. Smith and submit a report with your assessment and make recommendations. There are several ways to bind you to this contract.

         i. The first is to simply say, "Thank you, I'll do it."

         ii. The second is to do what is requested and submit the report.

20-5   Three Elements of a Contract

1. *Offer*—A promise to do or refrain from doing something in exchange for a promise, an action, or refraining from action. An offer is demonstrative of one's (*offeror*— the one who makes the offer) willingness to enter into a contract. The offer must be made known to the *offeree* (one to whom the offer is made) at the time of contract formation.
2. *Acceptance* —Once the offer has been made, acceptance is a voluntary act of the one who is given a contract offer. That person, by his or her action or promise, exercises his or her consent and willingness to enter into agreement and a legal relationship, known as a contract.
3. *Consideration*—Something of value. A contract must be supported by a benefit or believed benefit to the parties.

   c. The problem arises when you make a telephonic contact with Mr. Smith and submit the report anyway, and later, XYZ discovers your "breach." In other words, you failed to perform the entire contract (including an on-site visit to Mr. Smith) as requested and accepted the fee. This is the foundation for contract litigation.
   d. Questions would be asked, such as "Was there a meeting of the minds at the time of contract formation?" "When was the contract formed?" "Was the information contained in the report so complete that the contract was substantially performed, and what is the value of the report and services rendered?" (Williston Contracts, 1957).
2. There are entire courses on this subject. What is important for the case manager to know is that your words and your actions are very important as you perform your day-to-day work. You have entered a phase of your professional life in which your words are central to the creation of obligations.
3. You may be an agent of your employer or the purchaser of case management services, or both. Your actions and your words may effectively bind (obligate) the payer (insurance company, employer, or health benefits provider) to provide disability benefits, medical expenses, and services or any other service or benefit that you include in your verbal or written report.
4. This concept should not intimidate you but rather aid you in your assessment and recommendations.
5. NOTE: In today's case management practice, the relevant contract may exist without you ever seeing it. It is common for payers (either third-party administrators for self-insured companies or insurance carriers themselves) to offer full-service wellness programs. This can occur as part of an employment scenario or as a benefit through a health plan. More and more, case management is a "product" offered in those contracts.
6. Sometimes, liability is raised after a contract has ended or terminated. In this retrospective, liability refers to the time the liability is brought about, but is about an issue or concern that occurred during the time period the contract has been in effect. It is important for case managers to keep records of the care they provide to their clients/patients even after the care has concluded. This is especially necessary to avoid legal concerns and be prepared for the legal defense.

The Case Manager and the Legal Community

A. Throughout your career, you have used a variety of resources to increase your knowledge. Attorneys are another source of valuable information. A case manager is an advocate for the client.[2]

B. When you share a client with his or her lawyer, many of your goals should be the same.

  1. In a personal injury case, the attorney wants his or her client to receive any and all necessary services to improve their medical and physical condition. So do you.

  2. The difference is that the case manager has an obligation to accomplish the delivery of medically necessary services in a cost-effective and efficient manner.

  3. In general, the attorney does not become concerned with the expense to the payer but simply wants the client's needs to be met. These goals are not inconsistent; in fact, there are times when the attorney can be of assistance to the case manager.

  4. If you share a client with a lawyer, and that client is uncooperative in some way, a telephone call or short note to his or her attorney may go a long way.

C. When the case manager learns that a client is represented by a lawyer, the case manager has an obligation to contact that attorney and identify himself or herself and for whom he or she is working, the purpose in wanting to meet or communicate with the client, and generally what the case manager's goals are.[3]

D. If you present yourself by saying, "I represent your client's automobile policy carrier and I'm here to save money," that will be the last conversation you have with the client or the attorney. However, if you say or write, "I am a case manager working for XYZ Insurance, your client's automobile carrier. I have been asked to meet with your client to assess present and future needs and to facilitate the delivery of those services. I plan on meeting with your client on Tuesday. I look forward to communicating with you," the result should be far more to your liking.

  1. Both statements are true, and both statements have the same ultimate goal—cost-effective case management. Remember, there are times when presentation counts.

  2. When the case manager communicates with a lawyer, the telephone call should be outlined in advance (a simple note to yourself will do).

  3. When writing to an attorney or anyone in your professional capacity, such notes, faxes, and e-mails should be presented in a professional manner. The message should remain the same, even when the medium is advanced technology. Attorneys practice the art of persuasion.

  4. Case managers are capable of being persuasive without being combative or confrontational. If you can cultivate the lawyer as an

---

[2]Client—"The recipient of case management services…This individual may be a patient, beneficiary, injured worker, claimant, enrollee, member, college student, resident, or health care consumer of any age group." (CMSA, 2010, p 4).
[3]Note: In some states, particularly in the case of workers' compensation, an attorney cannot keep the case manager from meeting with the patient. Please refer to your practice state for this information.

BOX 20-6 Subpoenas and HIPAA

- The only exception to the HIPAA authorization requirement is a court order, signed by a judge.
- Subpoenas, although they look like and are official court documents, are signed by the clerk of the court (or in most cases, the clerk's name is signed by the lawyer, an approved practice under the rules of court).
- If a subpoena is served upon a case manager and is not accompanied by a HIPAA compliant authorization for release of the concerned client's records, that authorization must be requested and obtained before any records are shared.
- If presented with a subpoena, unless the case manager is in independent practice, the first response to a subpoena should be a call to the company's legal department for further instructions and assistance. In the case of independent practice, seek a private legal counsel for representation.

ally, it can do much to accelerate the progress of your client's case and ultimately contribute to a successful case outcome for all concerned.

E. The case manager and litigation—There are times when the case manager is called as a witness in a patient's case.

1. The case manager will receive a subpoena. There are two types of subpoenas, asking for one of two things—either an appearance by the case manager at a deposition or court *(subpoena ad testificandum)* or the submission of records *(subpoena duces tecum)* kept by the case manager relating to a client—or both.

2. In most jurisdictions (states), interrogatories, which are written questions and answers under oath, are served only on parties to an action, but state rules vary, in an effort to streamline the process, and one could be served with these questions.

3. Federal Rules of discovery rules include interrogatories on nonparties who agents of a named party, where the case manager is an agent of the employer, insurance carrier, etc.[4]

4. In some states, attorneys have been serving "subpoenas" on their own letterhead and failing to name a person to whom the subpoena is directed. These are "fishing expeditions" and are frowned on. In one state, legislation enacted a law sanctioning attorneys for misuse of this tool.

5. A lawful subpoena must relate to an actual case in progress, name an individual (which can be a corporation), request records only, and comply with Health Insurance Portability and Accountability Act (HIPAA) requirements. (It is sufficient for the subpoena to state Custodian of Records, XYZ Hospital, or other entities.)

6. HIPAA and requests for information—With the advent of the HIPAA privacy laws, even a subpoena must be accompanied by a HIPAA-compliant authorization (Box 20-6).

---

[4]CFR§ 12.32 Depositions on written interrogatories. (a) *Notice.* Any party, within the time prescribed by § 12.30(d), may serve on any other party or any officer or agent of a party a notice of the taking of a deposition on written interrogatories.

7. Investigational subpoenas—In the event of an investigation based on a HIPAA complaint, an administrative law judge or the secretary of Health and Human Services (HSS) issues an investigational subpoena.
   a. This document may be very general in nature and not only seeks records but also tries to find to identify individuals.
   b. Once identified, those individuals have a right to counsel (USC §160.504).
   c. Parties in the HIPAA complaint process may request that the administrative law judge issue subpoenas (USC §160.542).

F. The case manager as witness—More and more, the legal community is recognizing the case manager as a valuable source of information. There are two general categories of witness:
   1. The fact witness
      a. In this case, you would simply be asked to speak about things that you had seen or heard. In other words, you might be asked to describe the condition of the patient as you observed her on a particular date and the treatment that you observed and documented and to identify records previously made by you.
      b. Most likely, you would be appearing on behalf of the patient, as plaintiff, in a civil lawsuit. It is also possible that the defendant insurance carrier in a civil case may use the case manager as a fact witness. This is nothing to fear.
      c. Most attorneys will invest time and prepare you before you testify at deposition or trial or both. All you have to do is tell the truth, which you would do without preparation.
      d. In Louisiana, a case manager's determination was used to ascertain whether a claimant's injury was work related. The claimant alleged that the case manager's assessment was not sufficient "investigation of the claim." The case was decided in favor of the employer, who retained the services of the case manager and held that the case manager's visit, assessment, and recommendations did constitute "reasonable effort" to ascertain an employee's exact medical condition [668 So.2d 1161 (La. App. 5 Cir)].
   2. The expert witness
      a. Used when specialized information is required. Case managers are well qualified to provide such information to the court.
      b. In a liability lawsuit, the expert witness does not speak to the specific facts of a case because he or she would not be one of the persons involved in direct care.
      c. An expert witness is expected to be impartial. He or she may discuss issues such as standards of practice, codes of ethical conduct, trends in an industry, educational background, and criteria for entry to a profession and certification.
      d. Case managers have been used to clarify procedure and define case management process and practice. Box 20-7 presents details associated with an unreported case in New York, which demonstrates this point. At any step of the approval process, it would have been simple for a case manager to assess the case and discuss the possibility of giving the patient a hospice classification with the physician. This would have triggered another contract obligation, and 100% of the home care would have been covered without the expense and aggravation of litigation.

20-7   The Case Manager as an Expert Witness

In an unreported New York case, an insurance carrier was joined in a lawsuit initiated by a home care company. After providing more than $65,000 of home care to a cancer patient, the carrier rejected the claim upon the death of the patient. When the home care provider received the case, they immediately and repeatedly contacted the representative of the insurance company. The initial claim was sent to a "nurse approver," a nonmedically trained person, then onto a "nurse reviewer" who was a registered nurse. The reviewer forwarded the claim to the "medical management center," where a nurse would review the claim again, with additional documentation. When the claim was denied at this level, it was sent to a "medical director," a physician, for final determination. Initially, the court dismissed the case. However, a case manager with particular expertise in health benefit contract analysis (Krul, *Personal communication*, 1998) reviewed the contract under which the patient had received home care services. She discovered that the contract required case management and found that the insurance carrier had breached the contract by failing to provide the requisite case management services. The case returned to the New York Superior Court. With the sworn testimony of the case manager expert, the court found in favor of the home care company, thereby relieving the grieving family of the $66,000 burden.

 Frequently Asked Questions

A. *I am a new case manager. My boss gave me a caseload immediately. I've been in the clinical setting for years. How can I be a case manager overnight?*

1. There once was a day when you were a new nurse, social worker, or other health professional. The difference is that as a new case manager, you have been developing the necessary skills from the first day of your education and clinical practice in your primary profession. Unless and until your state has enacted a statute or regulation under your licensing structure, there is no legal restriction regarding representing yourself as a case manager.

2. It is critical that you never forget your professional roots, because the law is slow in developing, and although a case manager, you remain the discipline for which you hold a professional license (or state certification). In the event that you are sued for malpractice, the basis of that allegation would go first to your primary profession, as case management certification (e.g., CCM) is a dependent credential. For example, if you were a nurse, any action brought against you for work as a case manager would be a suit for nursing malpractice.

B. *The insurance carrier who assigned my latest patient wants me to ask the patient questions about "how the accident happened and who might be at fault." Can I do this?*

1. Difficult questions call for complex answers, and this question is actually several questions. When your employer (whether it is an insurance carrier or intermediary) asks you to collect liability information, you are going outside your scope of practice.

2. Your obligation is to collect information relevant to a patient's injuries or illness, along with relevant medical history. A case management

client, sometimes referred to as patient, is "the recipient of case management services. This individual may be a patient, beneficiary, injured worker, claimant, enrollee, member, college student, resident, or health care consumer of any age group" (CMSA, 2010, p. 5).

3. There is nothing contained in the definition of a client that would indicate that your role, as you collaborate with that individual, is to collect facts or evidence pertaining to liability.

4. NOTE: Having been fully informed of your role, including your duty to report relevant information to the carrier, should the patient volunteer information about the accident or onset of the illness; you can and should deliver that information to the appropriate party. It is important that you relate such information accurately and factually, without editorial or judgmental overtones. Using an example of a soccer injury, when that information is reported, it should simply be written, "Client reports playing soccer on the Sunday immediately preceding the reported accident date." This gives the carrier the information it needs to investigate the report further. (See the discussion of the Alabama case in the section on liability exposure for case managers.)

5. Insurance investigators are in the business of delving into the history and details of an injury or illness. They have various resources available to them, such as surveillance, photographs, and telephone and personal canvassing. None of those investigative tools falls within the role of the case manager or your scope of practice.

C. *How can I honestly advise the patient, upon initial contact, whom I represent and why we are meeting (whether in person or by telephone)?*

1. Honesty is always the best policy. If you are an "in-house" case manager, you should tell the patient that you are a case manager from XYZ Insurance, the company handling his or her claim. If you are employed by a case management company, simply modify the answer, "I am a case manager working for ABC Case Management Services, and in your case, we are working for XYZ Insurance, the company handling their claim."

2. The reason why this is so important is seen in the potential conflict between confidential information and the duty of the case manager to disclose information to the insurance company. Both of these obligations can exist simultaneously, but require the case manager to be clear, particularly on the first patient contact, whether in person or telephonic.

D. *What if a patient/client tells me things that may affect his or her coverage under the insurance program through which I was hired?*

1. This is not a new dilemma, merely an old one in a new environment. In your clinical experience, you were required to take patient histories and perform assessments on a regular basis, no matter what your underlying professional background.

2. It is not unusual for a patient in the clinical setting to say, "I'm going to tell you something, but it's just between us." In the clinical setting, the response would be, "I appreciate your feeling comfortable enough to share that information, but I must report it to your physician, because it may affect your diagnosis. Would you prefer telling him yourself?"

3. In the role of case manager, the scenario is much the same. Typically, a patient will say, "I told my boss I fell at work, but I'm telling you that I was injured playing soccer on Sunday. It will be our little secret."

The response is similar to that in the clinical setting. "Remember at our first visit I explained that I was hired by the workers' compensation/automobile/health insurance carrier. I also told you then that I have an obligation to report relevant information to them, and I will be passing this along." Do not apologize. It is your job.

E. *What if the patient asks me to keep something "off the record?"*—Same answer as in D.

F. *What if I observe something that indicates that the patient is working?*— Same answer as in D. Once you have fully informed the patient of who you are, who employs you, and the purpose of your visit/conversation, you can and will report all relevant information that you observe or receive.

G. *What if I see or smell suspected illegal drugs in a patient's home?*
   1. With the advent of lawful marijuana use in many states for medical purposes, this question becomes even more important. In those jurisdictions, marijuana is considered a medication, just like any other prescriptions.
   2. If it is your practice to request to see medication bottles for other medications, you would be acting appropriately to ask to see the prescription for medical marijuana. Remember to apply the medications reconciliation process when reviewing medications with your client/patient. Also, refrain from confusing prescribed controlled substances for illegal drug use.
   3. In those few jurisdictions that lawful use of marijuana is permitted for both medical and recreational uses, you would need to clarify why marijuana is being used by the client, as it may have an impact on symptoms, such as pain management and recovery. The case manager must be very careful not to be judgmental in observations and assessments.
   4. As a case manager, you are not a law enforcement person; however, such substances may impact the potential recovery of the patient. If you observe illegal drug use, you (the case manager) should remove yourself from the situation as quickly as possible and report only true and accurate facts (what you observed) to your supervisor. You would not want to accuse someone of something as serious as drug possession and use and learn later that your olfactory sense had misled you. Do not guess and do not judge; remain objective and stick to the facts.

H. *What if I see my patient abuse a child or parent in my presence?*
   1. Most states now require medical and educational professionals to report actual acts of child or elder abuse that take place in their presence. Know your state's law on the subject. Also, remember to report not just actual but also suspected abuse to the designated agencies in your jurisdiction and follow the required procedures.
   2. Contact your state board of medicine, nursing, social work, or other professional body to obtain such information. Again, do not guess.
   3. When it is necessary to report such information, the result will be an intrusive and long-term investigation by the appropriate state agency. For a complete examination of Mandatory Reporting (Muller, Fink-Samnick), see Professional Case Management Journal, July/Aug. 2015, Volume 20, Issue 4.

I. *What if my patient asks me to change a dressing?*—As a case manager, it is not appropriate to perform "hands-on" care, even if you have the education and training to do so. The case manager's role is to coordinate and facilitate medically necessary treatment; therefore, it would be appropriate to contact the home care provider, physician, or family, depending on the circumstances of the particular case.

J. *What do I do if I walk into a medical emergency in a patient's home?*
   1. You should be familiar with the "Good Samaritan Act" where you practice.[5] All fifty (50) states have enacted a Good Samaritan Act. You must be familiar with the Act in your state, as some include health care practitioners and some do not.
   2. As a licensed health care professional, you are held to a stricter standard of care, unless your state statute states otherwise in the acts of a Good Samaritan.
   3. When you enter someone's home as a case manager, you are not there to act as a "hands-on" practitioner. It would be appropriate to respond to the best of your ability, based on your education and experience. An important approach is calling "911."
   4. A recent revision of one state's law provides that "anyone [including RNs, LVNs (aka: LPNs), MDs, etc.] who in good faith renders emergency care at the scene of an accident or emergency to the victim … shall not be liable for any civil damages as a result of any acts or omissions by such person in rendering the emergency care" (N.J.S.A. 2A:62A-1).
   5. The purpose of such legislation is to encourage knowledgeable licensed persons to act, rather than shy away in fear of being sued. There have been incidents where a client has described symptoms over the telephone that would lead the case manager to believe that a heart attack or other serious medical emergency is in progress; in many cases, the best answer is call "911."

K. *My supervisor edits all my reports. I feel like I'm back in high school. Is that OK?*
   1. It is important that the product—your report—be presented in a clear, concise, and professional manner. Stylistic and grammatical changes are simply a matter of taste and not a problem.
   2. The problem occurs when another changes the substance of your report, particularly if this change is without your knowledge.
      a. Example: You make an observation about a patient and report that he or she has improved significantly since your last contact. You recommend a reduction of services to telephonic case management, with an anticipated closure in 30 to 45 days. The reviewer changes that information to read, "Minimal improvement noted" and changes your recommendation from closing the file to "two to three more visits required to monitor progress."

---

[5]N.J.S.A. 2A:62A-1. Emergency care (commonly known as the Good Samaritan Act)—Any individual, including a person licensed to practice any method of treatment of human ailments, disease, pain, injury, deformity, and mental or physical condition, or licensed to render services ancillary thereto, or any person who is a volunteer member of a duly incorporated first aid and emergency or volunteer ambulance or rescue squad association, who in good faith renders emergency care at the scene of an accident or emergency to the victim or victims thereof, or while transporting the victim or victims thereof to a hospital or other facility where treatment or care is to be rendered, shall not be liable for any civil damages as a result of any acts or omissions by such person in rendering the emergency care.

     b. Several things have happened here:
        i. The report is no longer your professional opinion, based on observation and assessment, but rather is a misrepresentation. It may go so far as to be considered fraud and places you, as well as the employer, in the position of having committed fraud on an insurance company.
        ii. States vary on the consequences of this kind of action, but certainly, the reviewer is risking the company and your presumably good reputation. If the problem is discovered, the company would not hire you again. Not all legal consequences are settled in court. Because litigation is costly, the cost-effective response would be to change case management service providers. Depending on the severity of the fraud, it could result in a lawsuit in which the company would be a named defendant.

L. *What is the significance, if any, of signing my reports?*
   1. If reports are signed, the writer should sign them. It is common practice for the report to be submitted in either a rough form or in some instances entered directly into a company computer network.
   2. All of these methods still permit editing, revision, and the attraction for the editor to fall to the temptation described above in question K.
     a. If you are the last person to review a report before submission to the carrier or another person who has purchased the case management services, then you certainly can sign it.
     b. On the other hand, if you are in a situation in which you do not get to see the final product before mailing, that too should be indicated on the report. Such methods as, "dictated but not read," alert the reader that the author of the report might not have seen the final product.
   3. There is no magic in the signature itself. It is merely another indication that the author is submitting a completed project. In the ideal situation, the report should be submitted, edited, and returned to the author for final review and signature. Should the report end up in a court case, no doubt the author will be held to the contents. Therefore, in a litigious environment, one should diplomatically work toward a policy and procedure that best protects your integrity.

M. *My employer does not pay for continuing education (CE) or make it available in-house. Do I still have to attend CE programs?*
   1. As the field of case management grows and is better recognized by the law, health care providers and case managers are expected to have up-to-date information and current practice-related knowledge and skills.
   2. To reduce your liability exposure, it is important to read, discuss, and earn CE credits.
     a. In most states, your underlying professional license has a mandatory CE requirement for renewal.
     b. It is anticipated that as case management practice becomes codified and as state law regulates professions, CE will be required. If you are to become a certified case manager (CCM) or other certified professional, CE credits are required and necessary to maintain your credential.

3. If you were ever called as a fact or expert witness in a case relating to your case management practice, one of the first questions you would be asked is, "Do you have any special training or certification, and do you have any continuing education in the field of case management?" Continuing education, whether through the university setting or professional CEs, is a valuable addition to your knowledge base and experience.

N. *Is there any value in belonging to a professional organization?*
   1. The benefits of belonging to a professional organization, such as Case Management Society of America (CMSA), are immeasurable.
   2. Such membership becomes a legal issue, as CMSA is your primary source for reliable case management practice information and guidelines.
      a. This is evidenced by the revised standards of practice. CMSA is a leader in the case management industry and works constantly to improve and standardize the practice.
      b. As a member, you will receive educational opportunities; practice updates, policy statements, and opportunities to interact with other members of the profession; and be part of the development of the standards of practice and the profession.
   3. Each licensed profession also has a professional association, such as the American Medical Association, American Nurses Association, and National Association of Social Workers. Each organization works to keep its membership up to date on legal, regulatory, and practice changes.

O. *Can I refuse or decline to see a patient?*
   1. The simple answer is "yes." The real question is "why?"
   2. Patient assignments and services can never have a discriminatory basis. If you sense a potential conflict of interest, this should be reported to your supervisor and a decision should be made as to whether another case manager would be more appropriate for the assignment.
   3. The difficulty occurs when there are personality conflicts or no concrete reason for the refusal or declination. This is best dealt with through consistent professional contacts with the patient and does not become a legal issue.

P. *Do I have to go back to that patient's home?*
   1. Your duty to provide services should never place you in personal or professional danger. If you have been exposed to a danger in a patient's home, the neighborhood, or work environment, there are alternative ways of obtaining necessary information. Such genuine fears should be reported to your supervisor and well documented, if appropriate, as you might be describing a safety issue to yourself, the client, and/or the community.
   2. Do not be judgmental in your report writing. A smart attorney will use this information to demonstrate that you had some prejudice in your decision making in areas in which the patient is concerned.
      a. Describe what you see but do not characterize the information. For example, "The patient was dressed in pajamas when I arrived at his home at 1:30 PM. I asked him three times to turn off the television before I could begin the interview." This description simply tells the reader what you saw and what happened.

  b. In the alternative, "The patient appeared lazy. It was early afternoon; he was still in his pajamas and appeared more interested in the soap opera he was watching than in anything having to do with his recovery." This description is your opinion of why the patient presented in a particular way, which may be based on your life experience and not that of the patient. Be cautious.

Q. *What if I refer a patient to a provider and that provider commits malpractice? Could I be liable?*

 1. Each health (and other) professional is responsible for his or her own actions. Cost-effective, quality, and safe medical/health care is an essential part of case management. Identifying the highest-quality service or product for the lowest price is consistent with one's professional obligations and ethical duty. When, however, price alone dictates your professional decision making, liability may follow.

 2. When you are placed in a position to make a referral, you should not do so blindly. What is the source of your referral? Is it a provider that you or your coworkers have been very pleased with, or is it simply the lowest price you can find? Are you able to procure an identical product or one that performs as well or simply a lesser product?

 3. This problem has become complicated with the increase of hospital case management.

  a. Case managers are finding themselves torn between directives requiring them to stay "in network" or, in some cases, referring only to facilities or vendors owned by large hospital systems rather than identifying the best quality, most cost-effective service.

  b. For the most part, these are ethical dilemmas; however, they can translate into liability exposure for the case manager if the referrals are made without investigation and cost–benefit analysis.

  c. If there is one area where courts have either ruled or given opinions regarding case management practice, it is this. Case managers have an affirmative duty to know the cost and quality of the services before making referrals or obtaining products, such as durable medical equipment (DME).

 4. Make a reasonable inquiry to determine what will be provided for the dollars spent. Sometimes, a dollar saved in the short term can represent long-term expense. It may also expose the decision maker to unnecessary risk. Potential liability rests with whether you acted within the scope of your profession and accepted standards of practice (CMSA, 2010).

R. *I live and work in an east coast state, and my employer requires that I contact clients who live in a west coast state. I'm not licensed in that west coast state. Is that a problem?*

 1. Yes, the law that controls the relationship (or telephonic communication) between the case manager and the patient/client is the law in the state where the client resides, not where the nurse is located or where the employer is based, even in workers' compensation cases.

 2. In the United States today, a professional may practice only in the state or states in which he or she is licensed and in good standing. Therefore, a nurse must be licensed in the state where the patient/

client is. Each nurse's practice is controlled by the law in the state(s) where he/she resides and/or is licensed—typically, by the Nurse Practice Act of that state.

3. The advent of the Nurse Licensure Compact places nurses on notice that interstate or distance practice is only recognized in those states that have passed legislation, rules, and regulations adopting the compact (24 Del. Laws c. 19A, §1901A).

   a. The compact permits nurses whose home state (state of residence) is in the compact to practice in any other compact state. In the absence of such law, a nurse must be licensed in each and every state in which he/she practices.

   b. Twenty-five states are presently included in the compact; the majority of nurses are left having to be licensed in each and every state in which they practice nursing (Table 20-1).

TABLE 20-1 Nurse Licensure Compact States

Compact States (Rev. April 2015)	Implementation Date
Arizona	7/1/2002
Arkansas	7/1/2000
Colorado	10/1/2007
Delaware	7/1/2000
Idaho	7/1/2001
Iowa	7/1/2000
Kentucky	6/1/2007
Maine	7/1/2001
Maryland	7/1/1999
Mississippi	7/1/2001
Missouri	6/1/2010
Montana	10/1/2015
Nebraska	1/1/2001
New Hampshire	1/1/2006
New Mexico	1/1/2004
North Carolina	7/1/2000
North Dakota	1/1/2004
Rhode Island	7/1/2008
South Carolina	2/1/2006
South Dakota	1/1/2001
Tennessee	7/1/2003
Texas	1/1/2000
Utah	1/1/2000
Virginia	1/1/2005
Wisconsin	1/1/2000

Compact states pending implementation:
As of May 2015, Advanced Practice Nurses (APRNs) have been added to the compact. Please check with the licensing board in your state of residence for information on the NLC. Access to all states' boards of nursing is available by selecting your state at https://www.ncsbn.org/index.htm
Source: National Council of State Boards of Nursing, Inc., (NCSBN). Website: http://www.ncsbn.org. Last updated at the time this textbook was written was on September 3, 2015.

4. In December 2005, CMSA took an official position on this issue and incorporated their position in the *CMSA's Standards of Practice for Case Management* (revised 2010), which clearly states that: "The case manager practices in accordance with applicable local, state, and federal laws. The case manager has knowledge of applicable accreditation and regulatory statutes governing sponsoring agencies that specifically pertain to delivery of case management services" (p. 19).

    a. CMSA encourages case managers and case manager employers to work aggressively with the state boards of nursing to encourage compliance and entry into the National Council of State Boards of Nursing (NCSBN) as compact states so that appropriate multistate nursing licensure might continue appropriately and cost-effectively.

    b. Alternatively, CMSA encourages the enactment of federal legislation mandating the recognition of nurse licensure in all states.

    c. CMSA has added its name to the growing list of those organizations supporting and endorsing the nurse compact. See Additional Resources—CMSA Position Paper and CMSA and the Compact.

References

Case Management Society of America (CMSA). (2010). *Standards of practice for case management.* Little Rock, AR: Author.

Cochennic v. Dillard's, 668 So.2d 1161 (La. App. 5 Cir., 1996).

Dunn v. Praiss, 139 N.J. 561 (1995), Rev'd. on other grounds, 193 N.J. 38 (2007).

Eddy, J. (1982). Clinical policies and the quality of clinical practice. *New England Journal of Medicine, 307,* 343.

Fed. R. Evid. 703, 704, N.J.S.A. 2A:84A-2, et seq.

Foley, M. R. (2010, May). *Tribunal system works in Massachusetts.* Retrieved from American Academy of Orthopedic Surgeons: http://www.aaos.org/news/aaosnow/may10/managing6.asp

Keeton, W. P., & Prosser, W. L. (1984). *Prosser and Keeton, the law of torts,* 5th ed. St. Paul: West Publishing.

LAW.COM. (2015). *Search legal terms and definitions.* Retrieved from http://dictionary.law.com/Default.aspx?selected=1771.

Muller, L. S. (2016). Engaging the LBGT Patient: The Medical/Legal Landscape. *Professional Case Management, (21)*3, 149–153.

Obergefell v. Hodges, 576 US 11 (The Supreme Court of the United States June 26, 2015).

OCR. (2015). *Health information privacy.* Retrieved from HHS.Gov: http://www.hhs.gov/ocr/privacy/.

OIG. (2015). *OIG advisory opinions.* Retrieved from Office of the Inspector General: https://oig.hhs.gov/compliance/advisory-opinions/.

N.J.S.A. 2A:53A-27.

N.J.S.A. 2A:62A-1.

N.J.S.A. 39:6B, *et seq.*

N.J.S.A. 45:11–23, *et seq.*

Reid v. Aetna Casualty & Surety Co., et al., 692 So.2d 863 (Alabama App. 1997).

Wacht v. Farooqui, 312 N.J. Super. 184, 711 A.2d 405 (App. Div. 1998).

Williston Contracts §1(3d ed. 1957), Restatement 2d, Contracts §2; See Muller, L. (1998) Provider *contracts:* What case managers need to know. *The Journal of Care Management, The Official Journal of The Case Management Society of America, 4,* 5.

CHAPTER 21

Use of Effective Case Management Plans

Mary Jane McKendry and Teresa M. Treiger

LEARNING OBJECTIVES

Upon completion of this chapter, the reader will be able to:

1. List the components of a case management care plan.
2. Define important terms and concepts related to developing a successful case management care plan.
3. Identify critical multidisciplinary and cross-functional relationships essential for successful execution of a case management care plan.
4. Describe how to identify appropriate, measurable, and achievable case management plan goals and outcomes.

IMPORTANT TERMS AND CONCEPTS

Accountable Care
    Organization (ACO)
Advocacy
Algorithm
Assessment
Care Plan
Care Transitions
Clinical Pathway
CMAG Guidelines
Development
Evaluation

Evidence-Based
    Criteria and/or
    Guidelines
Evidence-Based
    Decision Support
    Criteria
Facilitation
Goal (Measurable)
Implementation
Interdisciplinary
Intervention

Medication
    Reconciliation
Outcome
Patient-Centered Medical
    Home (PCMH)
Patient Empowerment
Patient Protection and
    Affordable Care Act
    (PPACA or ACA)
Planning
Performance Standards

Problem Identification	Resource Consumption	Transition Planning
Problem Statement	Risk Stratification	Utilization
Protocol	Self-management	Management
Quality Standards	SMART Goals	Variance

Introduction

A. Today, in the health care environment, there is an increasing focus on quality and quality-of-care outcomes coupled with an even more intense focus on effectiveness and efficiency of the care received.

   1. In 2010, the Patient Protection and Affordable Care Act (PPACA) was signed into law. Commonly referred to as the Affordable Care Act (ACA), it positions consumers as partners on their health care team.

   2. PPACA put many comprehensive health insurance reforms in place. These were aimed at addressing fragmented care delivery as well as more accessible and affordable preventive care.

   3. The Commission for Case Manager Certification (CCMC) notes that the ACA identified the means to heal an otherwise fragmented health care system through implementation of the Patient-Centered Medical Home (PCMH) and Accountable Care Organization (ACO). Both of these types of organizations rely on care coordination as a central pillar of their success (2015).

   4. Professional care coordination and case management are needed as these activities evolve to fundamental roles driving successful outcomes.

B. As case management roles transform in response to health care changes, many case managers find that some of the traditional goals of case management (CM) seem incongruent with expanding responsibilities.

   1. Patient empowerment, patent-determined goals, patient-agreed-upon care plans, and quality outcomes have always been goals of case management; however, their importance is now front and center. Case managers may feel conflicted as they focus on patient-centered care, quality services, and safety while at the same time attempting to reduce costs and control resource utilization.

   2. The latest Role and Function Study, which captures current knowledge, skills, and activities of case managers, found that "case managers reported an increase in prominence of quality measurement and evaluation functions, likely because of new care models based on value rather than volume. Value-based payment models require quality measures to quantify and reward efficient, effective care delivery" (CCMC, 2014).

C. In reality, case managers are trying to meet the goals of different customers at the same time while ensuring that patient involvement and empowerment leads to supported patient self-management.

   1. Case managers recognize that reducing variation, duplication, and fragmentation of care are all priorities, which must be balanced against keeping care patient-centered.

2. It is imperative that case managers support patient access to appropriate services and resources in order to maintain optimal level of wellness; on the other hand, utilization and costs must be addressed and controlled. Helping patients access appropriate resources at the right time results in cost savings and appropriate utilization of resources.

3. The PPACA drives home these points with the inclusion of various care coordination initiatives highlighting

   a. Use of integrated care approaches to improve quality and reduce health care costs

   b. Establishing quality performance standards for participating providers

   c. Increased demand for professionals with experience coordinating health care services for patients to help them meet goals including those associated with new models of health care delivery

D. Care coordination makes it possible to achieve balance in both the patient-centered and system-centered goals of case management. Recognizing this begins with acknowledging the complexity of a case manager's job and understanding there is a need for tools (e.g., road maps, reports) to support the successful resolution of identified patient needs (e.g., barriers to care, health education).

E. Consider that a case manager must understand the current health care environment and be aware of ongoing transformation at multiple levels (e.g., individual, organizational). Case managers not only need clinical skills and knowledge but also must master business skills and knowledge.

1. System-centered goals may address data gathering and analysis, reducing clinical variation, meeting expectations for time frames, and addressing available resources.

2. Patient-centered goals may address accessing appropriate care in a timely manner, providing education and tools to ensure patient empowerment, and encouraging patient self-management (Pearson, Mattke, Shaw, Ridgely, & Wiseman, 2007).

F. Today, the consumers of case management services demand collaborative, well-defined, and managed plans of care.

1. Care plans must effectively and efficiently address achievable outcomes and appropriate resource utilization/allocation, which ensure access to quality health care products and services.

2. Using collaborative approaches for care planning, a case manager creates a road map in order to meet the goals and responsibilities of his or her job, the needs of the patient, and the needs of other case management customers (e.g., employers, health plans, health care facilities).

3. Generally, a road map supports case management with outcomes and evaluative reports developed for use at the individual, department, and program level.

   a. Reports may vary in scope and content and include a range of available information.

      i. High-level executive summary reports

      ii. Department performance trends

     iii. Individualized patient-specific progress reports

4. Through the use of outcome reports, users are able to determine if, how, and where progress has been made. They also identify where improvement opportunities may exist, especially in meeting care and organizational or case management program goals.

G. This chapter provides an overview of case management plan design, reviews tools available to assist in evidence-based case management plan development, and discusses strategies for developing comprehensive, high-quality, multidisciplinary, patient-centered plans of care.

Descriptions of Key Terms

A. Accountable Care Organization (ACO)—Groups of doctors, hospitals, and other health care providers who come together voluntarily to give coordinated high-quality care to their Medicare patients. The goal of coordinated care is to ensure that patients, especially the chronically ill, get the right care at the right time while avoiding unnecessary duplication of services and preventing medical errors (Centers for Medicare and Medicaid Services [CMS], 2015).

B. Algorithm—A systematic process consisting of an ordered sequence of steps, each step depending on the outcome of the previous one; in clinical management a protocol (MediLexicon.com, 2015) that guides step-by-step assessments and interventions. Algorithms are generally most useful for high-risk groups as they are known for their specificity (very specific) and generally do not allow for provider/patient flexibility. Often utilized to manage a specific process, control care practices, or address an individual problem. Algorithms may incorporate research methodology to measure cause and effect (Wojner, 2001).

C. Care coordination—The deliberative organization of patient care activities between two or more participants (including the patient) involved in a patient's care to facilitate the appropriate delivery of health care services. Organizing care involves the marshalling of personnel and other resources needed to carry out all required patient activities and is often managed by the exchange of information among participants responsible for different aspects of care (McDonald et al., 2014).

D. Case management care plan—A comprehensive plan that includes a statement of problems/needs determined upon assessment, strategies to address the problems/needs, and measurable goals to demonstrate resolution based upon the problem/need, the time frame, the resources available, and the desires/motivation of the client (Case Management Society of America [CMSA], 2010).

E. Clinical pathway—A structured, interdisciplinary care management plan designed to support the implementation of specific clinical guidelines and protocols. Clinical pathways are computational maps or algorithms and are one of the primary tools used to manage health care quality by focusing on the standardization of care processes. Pathways are used to guide the various health care team members on the usual treatment patterns related to common diagnoses, conditions, and/or procedures.

1. Clinical pathways are designed to support clinical management, clinical and nonclinical resource management, clinical audit, and financial management.

2. Clinical pathways are a "process map" utilized to promote quality care and decrease costs by standardizing treatment methods within

clinical processes, while at the same time endeavoring to improve the continuity and coordination of care across different disciplines and ensure successful transitions of care.

3. Clinical pathways are known by many synonyms including care pathways, integrated care paths, multidisciplinary pathways of care, care maps, critical pathways, collaborative pathways, or care paths (Open Clinical, 2015).

F. Clinical practice guidelines (CPGs)—Systematically developed statements designed to assist practitioner and patient decisions about appropriate health care for specific clinical circumstances (Institute of Medicine, 2011).

1. Guidelines commonly apply to a general health condition. To be defensible, guideline development must be able to demonstrate

a. A development process that is open, documented, and reproducible

b. That the resultant product can be of use to both clinicians and patients

c. That the concept of appropriateness of services is well reflected in the guideline

d. That the guideline relates specifically to clearly defined clinical issues (Mulrow & Lohr, 2001)

G. Evidence-based medicine—The definition of evidence-based medicine (EBM) provided in 1996 by Sackett, Rosenburg, Gray, Haynes, and Richardson continues to be relied upon today. EBM is the "integration of the best research evidence with clinical expertise and patient values to make clinical decisions." The evidence being referred to is "patient centered, clinically relevant research found in the medical literature on diagnostic tests, treatment techniques, preventive programs, and prognostic markers" (Steves & Hootman, 2004). EBM injects contemporary research findings into day-to-day clinical practice and patient care.

H. Patient Protection and Affordable Care Act (PPACA or ACA)—A U.S. Federal Statute signed into law on March 23, 2010. Together with the Health Care and Education Reconciliation Act amendment, it represents the most significant regulatory overhaul of the US health care system since the passage of Medicare and Medicaid in 1965. Enacted to increase the quality and affordability of health insurance, lower the uninsured rate by expanding public and private insurance coverage, and reduce the costs of health care for individuals and the government (CMS, 2015).

I. Protocol—Guidelines designed to address specific therapeutic interventions for a given clinical problem. Protocols are less specific than algorithms and do allow for minimal provider flexibility via treatment options. They are multifaceted and therefore can be used to drive practice for more than one discipline. Like algorithms, they may and most often do incorporate research methodology to measure cause and effect. Guidelines are based on examination of current evidence within the paradigm of evidence-based medicine and usually include consensus statements on best practices in health care (Institute of Medicine, 2011; Wojner, 2001).

J. Evidence-based Clinical Decision Support Criteria—Impartial, evidence-based tools used as a lexicon to evaluate the decisions about the appropriateness and quality of care that support integrated care management and utilization management (UM) approaches to evaluate patient care and services (Mitus, 2008).

 ## Applicability to CMSA'S Standards of Practice

A. The Case Management Society of America (CMSA) describes in its standards of practice for case management that case management practice extends across all health care settings, including payer, provider, government, employer, community, and clinic or doctor's office, and that case managers use a variety of tools to ensure effective practice and delivery of safe and quality patient care (CMSA, 2010).

B. This chapter describes various plans, pathways, and protocols, which support the case management roles, functions, and activities described in the CMSA standards including the case management process.

C. According to CMSA, the resource and resource utilization practice standard explains that case managers should incorporate factors related to quality, safety, access to care, and cost-effectiveness in assessing, monitoring, and evaluating resources for the client's care (CMSA, 2010).

D. CMSA standards of practice for case management also state that case management plans should address anticipated resources needed by the client, but case managers must be cognizant of the benefits (health insurance plan) available to provide for these resources (CMSA, 2010).

E. Alternate funding sources serve as added means to secure the resources a client needs.

F. CMSA recommends that resources allocation and consumption should be based on the client's needs as documented in the case management plan of care, evidence-based practice guidelines, care goals, and effective and efficient use of health care and financial resources (CMSA, 2010).

G. This chapter addresses case management practice, which requires knowledge of and proficiency in the following practice standards: Assessment, Problem/Opportunity Identification, Planning, Monitoring, Outcomes, and Facilitation/Coordination and Collaboration.

Case Management Care Planning and Plans of Care

A. Historically, case management was considered a social worker function due to early efforts of settlement houses of the late 1800s and early 1900s. Residents and volunteers of early settlement houses helped create and foster new organizations and social welfare programs, some of which continue to the present time. Settlements were action oriented where programs and services were added as neighborhood needs were discovered. For example, social workers assisted people in the settlements in addressing poverty and health issues in an effort to enhance their quality of life.

B. In the late 1980s, case management care planning became more aligned as a nursing responsibility due to legislative and regulatory requirements. Conceptualizing case management as either social work or nursing is inaccurate; doing so does not effectively capture the spirit of the intervention, nor is it inclusive of an interdisciplinary care team approach.

C. Case managers understand that care planning must include all members of the health care team, especially the patient. Because planning is an essential part of the case manager's work, it has been highlighted as a component of the case management process and identified as a practice standard.

1. Case Management Process
   a. Development of the case management plan
   b. Establish goals of the case management intervention and prioritize client needs by helping to determine types of services and resources required to meet identified needs (CMSA, 2010)
2. Case Management Practice Standard of Planning
   a. Identifies immediate, short-term, long-term, and ongoing needs.
   b. Develops appropriate and necessary case management strategies and goals to address those needs (CMSA, 2010).
   c. The case manager and client are best served when the fundamental components of appropriate case management care planning, as documented in CMSA's Standards of Practice, are applied.

D. Case management care plans are tools to define practice and as guides for patient care activities (Tahan, 2002). Plans should be patient-specific, action-oriented, and time-defined.
   1. The end result of case management care planning is a patient-centered, patient-agreed-upon plan of care that has realistic, achievable goals and focuses on patient self-management and safe, quality outcomes.
   2. Use of SMART methodology to determine or develop goals is an efficient approach.
      a. Goals should be
         i. Specific
         ii. Measurable
         iii. Attainable
         iv. Realistic/Reasonable
         v. Time period specific (Doran, 1981)
   3. One of the most significant responsibilities for a case manager is the development of a case management plan.

E. Tahan (2002) identified a number of characteristics of a case management plans that are helpful for case managers to be aware of and consider when developing and implement case management plans for their patients (Box 21-1).

F. An effective case management plan is a specific document (or electronic equivalent) that delineates
   1. Individual care needs (e.g., diagnostic, therapeutic, social)
   2. Actions required and responsible party (e.g., case manager, patient, caregiver, care team member)
   3. Short- and long-term goals with completion and/or progress time frames for attainment
   4. Anticipated outcomes (e.g., knowledge gained, self-management skill, adherence)

G. The uses of a case management plan include
   1. Cost-effectiveness and reduction in lengths of stay
   2. Improved quality of care and customer satisfaction
   3. Better allocation of resources and coordination of services that result in eliminating redundancy, fragmentation, and duplication of care activities

BOX 21-1 Characteristics of Case Management Plans of Care

- Each plan addresses a specific diagnosis, surgical procedure, or a phase in the care needed.
- The plans represent a time line of patient care activities based on the clinical service. This could be minutes or hours in the emergency department; days in the acute care setting; weeks in the neonatal intensive care unit; months in long-term care facilities; or visit-by-visit in ambulatory or home care settings.
- The plans include well-defined milestones or trigger points that aid in expediting care and indicate an impending change in care activities (i.e., switching from intravenous to oral antibiotics when temperature is within normal range for 24 hours).
- The length of each plan depends on a predetermined length of stay based on the diagnosis/procedure and reimbursement rules, guidelines, and mechanisms.
- The plans clearly delineate the responsibilities of the various health care team members as they relate to each particular department.
- The plans identify the outcome indicators or quality measures used to evaluate the appropriateness and effectiveness of care.
- Each plan may include a specific variance tracking section to evaluate any delays in care activities/processes/outcomes.
- The plans may be used as one strategy to ensure compliance with the standards of care of regulatory and accreditation agencies.
- The plans are interdisciplinary in nature, a mechanism that reinforces a seamless approach to the delivery of care.
- The plans can be used as an educational tool for house staff, student nurses or nurses in training, and newly hired employees.
- The plans help improve performance in the areas of patient and family teaching, coordination of services, collaboration and communication among the health care team members, and discharge planning.

4. Clearly defined plans of care and delineation of responsibilities
5. Improved communication systems among the various disciplines

Case Management Plan Development Begins with Patient Assessment

A. Developing a patient-specific process must follow a logical progression. The format of the care plan (e.g., document, computer, Web-based tool) should not affect the methodology for its intellectual organization. Computer-generated case planning provides a tool, but should not be considered as the end-all-be-all of case management planning.

B. The first step in case management care planning is an accurate and thorough needs assessment. The assessment begins with an accurate capture of the patient's current status in a variety of areas (found in Fig. 21-1).

C. Once a current patient status is determined, the case manager asks fundamental questions in support of identifying the foundation of the case management plan.

   1. What are we trying to accomplish and what are the measurable goals for improvement?

   2. How do we know that an intervention will result in an improvement/goal attainment?

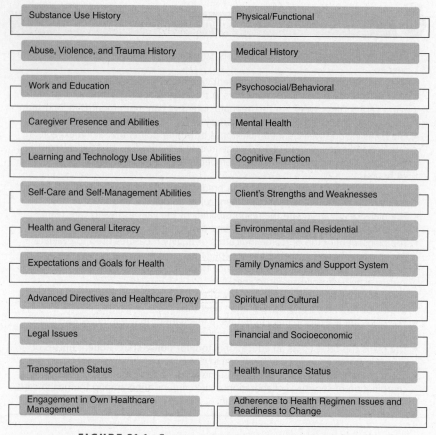

Substance Use History	Physical/Functional
Abuse, Violence, and Trauma History	Medical History
Work and Education	Psychosocial/Behavioral
Caregiver Presence and Abilities	Mental Health
Learning and Technology Use Abilities	Cognitive Function
Self-Care and Self-Management Abilities	Client's Strengths and Weaknesses
Health and General Literacy	Environmental and Residential
Expectations and Goals for Health	Family Dynamics and Support System
Advanced Directives and Healthcare Proxy	Spiritual and Cultural
Legal Issues	Financial and Socioeconomic
Transportation Status	Health Insurance Status
Engagement in Own Healthcare Management	Adherence to Health Regimen Issues and Readiness to Change

FIGURE 21-1. Case management assessment categories.

    3. What intervention will produce a measurable outcome demonstrating the desired improvement and who is responsible to take the necessary intervention(s) (e.g., who, what, why, when, how often)?

D. These answers assist the case manager and client to formulate a plan that is individualized; contains reasonable goals; and has an achievable, specific, measurable, and time-bound quality outcome(s).

E. Questions supporting the formulation of an achievable case management plan include the following:

    1. What are we trying to accomplish? This question may drive one or multiple goals. The case management plan's priorities may begin to emerge, and primary and secondary goals are more easily defined. Examples of goals that may be identified include those described in Box 21-2.

    2. By answering these questions, we obtain useful patient-centered information that allows us to develop specific statements regarding actions (interventions), expected goals, and time frames needed to achieve these goals and determine if the goals are immediate, short term, or long range.

      a. How is each goal measured?

      b. What are the time frames for accomplishment?

21-2 Focus of Goals Targeted in Case Management Plans

- Patient education related to specific aspects of care (e.g., self-management, disease condition/diagnosis, medications)
- Patient empowerment related to self-advocacy, reporting decline or improvement in condition after a treatment change
- Patient self-management of activities of daily living (ADLs)
- Respite care applied when in the right place at the right time
- Transportation established for health care services
- Homemaker services
- Condition-specific guidelines used to monitor treatment and degree of management control (e.g., HgA1c levels)
- Reduction in emergency room utilization
- Healthy family/social support structure engaged in care
- Social, cultural, and spiritual needs addressed
- Access to required nutritional foods, medical care, behavioral health care, and pharmaceutical discount program
- Successful return to work

    c. Are they short-term or long-term goals?
    d. Does the patient/family believe the goals are reasonable?
    e. Will the patient/family need help in meeting some of the goals?
3. It is important to realize that goals contain functional and measurable information such as
    a. A general description of purpose—stating the aim clearly
    b. The specific focus—performed by whom, taking place where, and requiring what
    c. Numerical targets—time frames for completion that are based on measurable data
4. Goals should be considered modifiable targets of achievement based on the individual's circumstance.
    a. Because patients and/or other care team members cannot or do not always conform to care plans, it is essential to formulate flexible and modifiable goals.
5. How do we know that an intervention will result in an improvement?
    a. This question guides the formulation of action items, which are more commonly known as interventions (e.g., case management activities, medical treatments), as well as the identification of problems and the formulation of problem lists.
    b. Basically, this question is asking the case manager to determine what interventions will actually result in improvements or in meeting the defined patient care goal(s). In other words, will the interventions planned actually and positively affect the patient's overall well-being? Does the patient (and family/caregiver) agree with the interventions proposed?
    c. Once goals and priority problems are determined, and interventions are decided upon, the case manager should answer the following additional questions for each problem recognized and intervention established:

      i. Will this problem get better or stabilize?

     ii. Can we make this problem get better or stabilize by the intervention(s) decided on?

    iii. If a problem is not likely to improve or resolve, will the care goal(s) and planned intervention(s) reduce the risk of complications or prevent the problem from getting worse?

    iv. If a problem is not likely to improve and, in fact, deterioration is inevitable, can the care goal(s) and planned intervention(s) provide for optimal safety, quality of life, comfort, and dignity for the patient?

     v. Is each defined intervention both measurable and realistic?

  d. Interventions may address the patient's physical health needs, behavioral health needs, social needs, cultural needs, provider orders, facility protocols, best-practice standards, or accepted critical pathways.

  e. Case management plans of care include interventions that reflect tasks a responsible care team member, including the patient, can actually accomplish.

     i. These interventions should demonstrate the value of case management involvement, such as care coordination and the focus on quality outcomes.

     ii. For example, if a physician orders nutritional supplements, the case management interventions would be focused on understanding the patient's thoughts about nutritional supplements, patient education, strategies for obtaining the nutritional supplements ordered, methods to determine that the patient receives and utilizes the nutritional supplements, etc.

6. What measurable intervention (action) can be made that will result in an improvement in the patient's condition?

  a. This question helps define what the outcomes of the case management plan should be. Just as interventions need to reflect actual tasks that are performed by case managers and/or require case manager involvement, outcomes must be discipline/care team member specific.

  b. The outcomes of a case management plan must objectively measure the patient outcomes that were most influenced by the case manager's involvement, demonstrate the effectiveness of defined interventions, and be variable, depending on many factors such as those described in Figure 21-2.

  c. As these factors demonstrate, outcomes, although needing to be measurable and reportable, need to be realistic, patient specific, and agreed upon by the patient.

7. Recognizing the complexity of care coordination and addressing various care needs together with the diversity of case management practice settings has propelled case managers into utilizing outcomes that are specific to not only their patients' needs but also the environment in which they work. In this way, case managers can best reflect their involvement, directly and indirectly, with patient care plan outcomes. The ultimate purpose of the case management plan is to guide the care team, which consists of everyone involved in the care and management of needs for a specific patient, including the patient, to provide the most appropriate plan to ensure optimal outcomes.

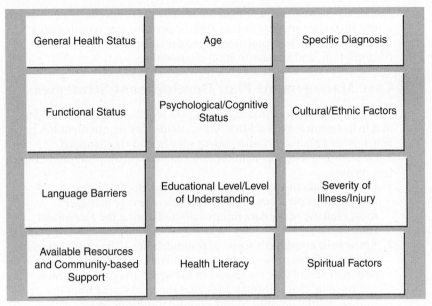

General Health Status	Age	Specific Diagnosis
Functional Status	Psychological/Cognitive Status	Cultural/Ethnic Factors
Language Barriers	Educational Level/Level of Understanding	Severity of Illness/Injury
Available Resources and Community-based Support	Health Literacy	Spiritual Factors

FIGURE 21-2. Case management outcomes variables.

Case Management Plan Development—Data Gathering Format

A. Developing a patient-specific case management plan requires the use of information gathered during the patient assessment; contract-specific performance metrics; and organization-specific protocols, algorithms, or other evidence-based tools.

B. Standardization of case management plans allows for quality and performance outcomes reporting.

C. Outcomes reporting demonstrates both the value of case management and return on investment (ROI) of case manager involvement. This process is accomplished differently across organizations; it may be manual in some while automated in others.

D. It is important that case management software applications and automated care plan development tools allow for patient-specific customization as needed.

1. The use of case management digital tools must allow case managers to easily gather certain data, determine specific patient risk status, and measure outcomes of care interventions and services.

2. Use of proprietary, automated, patient-specific case management plans must also allow for individualization of the tools to meet the needs of the organizations such as the patient population served, industry best-practice recommendations, health insurance plan contract-specific requirements, quality and performance metrics, and regulatory or accreditation standards.

3. Use of templates and workflows to develop individualized case management plans encompassing patient populations, best-practice recommendations, contract-specific requirements, and performance metrics.

E. The ideal case management plan addresses patient-specific needs, patient acuity, insurance and/or contract-specific performance requirements, quality indicators/best-practice recommendations, resource consumption, and standardization methodology.

Case Management Plan Development Strategies

A. Pulling a workable case management plan together requires strategies that help case managers address the contradictory requirement for a case management plan to be both patient specific and standardized.
B. A few strategies that may help the case manager accomplish this complex task include
   1. Focus on patient-specific needs—When developing a case management plan that is patient specific, the case manager must evaluate many data inputs collected during the assessment (Box 21-3).
   2. Know your employer's scope of responsibility—The case manager understands his or her employer organization as well as the scope and intensity of care management for which the organization is responsible. This information is vital for recognizing both the timing and the amount of care coordination is necessary with other organizations to ensure a safe and effective outcome. An example is the case manager of an acute care hospital coordinating transitional care services with the case manager from a home health organization.
   3. Understand patient acuity—Understanding patient acuity helps to determine the types and frequency of interventions performed by the care manager.
      a. With respect to case management plan, the concept of acuity was explored by Huber and Craig in that "acuity represents the level of complexity or difficulty of a CM case in its three primary domains of CM activity: client need-severity, CM intervention-intensity, and healthcare service delivery responsiveness" (2007).
      b. Patient acuity is often determined by some type of identification or stratification process and includes a number of factors according to Huber and Craig (2007, Box 21-4).

BOX
21-3 | **Types of Assessment Data Useful in the Development of Case Management Plans**

- Patient acuity and severity of illness
- Availability of family or other support structures
- Community-based resources, services, and supports
- Functional abilities and limitations
- Cultural, ethnic, and/or spiritual needs and preferences
- Health care and other services required
- Benefits available (health insurance plan)
- Knowledge and skills in self-management
- Health care literacy
- Preferred/desired care goals

21-4 **Factors in Patient Acuity Determination**

- Current illness or injury
- Comorbid conditions
- Complexity of the medical needs
- Care transitions needs
- Medication management/polypharmacy
- Medication reconciliation
- Social support structure
- Behavioral health needs
- Cognitive/educational status
- Complexity and intensity of the health care resources and treatments needed

4. The case manager remains mindful of contractual quality and performance metrics—Recognizing contractually defined performance metrics is essential for the development of effective case management plans of care. Some organizations contract to provide specific services to specific populations. Likewise, individual case managers contract to perform specific services for either individual patients or groups of patients. Health plans and provider groups also have specific quality and performance requirements related to case management and care coordination driving by regulations, accreditation requirements, and other contractual requirements.

    a. Generally, contract requirements are defined as performance measures or metrics. Incorporating these quality and performance metrics into CM plan development helps case managers meet both patient and organizational needs as well as demonstrate the value of CM involvement.

    b. Performance metrics include types of services to be provided, time frame requirements to perform services, guidelines for patient participation in CM, and anticipated outcomes from services provided.

    c. Quality metrics include patient-specific outcomes as well as population outcomes and include health care goals met, reductions in emergency room utilization, reduction in inappropriate admission, and reduction in quality-of-care concern complaints.

5. Quality indicators/best-practice recommendations/protocols—Case managers, by the very nature of their involvement, are uniquely positioned to assess the quality of the health care services provided based on efficiency, effectiveness, and efficacy. Focusing on appropriate quality indicators and best-practice recommendations/ protocols directly aligns with developing appropriate anticipated outcomes. If quality care and services are provided, patients have the optimal chance for the best available outcome.

C. Quality and safety are key—Quality of care is a focus for case manager, and assuring quality and safety supports/demonstrates the need for case management involvement.

    1. Promotion of quality-based outcomes via the use of quality indicators such as improved functional status, improved clinical

status, enhanced quality of life, patient satisfaction, adherence to the medical treatment plans of care, improved patient safety, cost savings, client autonomy, and self-management is important to a CM program.

2. Case managers should engage in strategies to measure improvements in quality of care and services that directly result from CM interventions.

3. Quality indicators and best-practice recommendations/protocols are directly linked to standardization methodology (discussed further in this chapter) and are an important strategy for case management plan development. It is important to remember that CM is regarded as a means to ensure effective quality outcomes and is an area of accountability for case managers.

4. Addressing these expectations can be accomplished by utilizing quality indicators as outcomes measures.

D. Resource consumption—One vital responsibility often overlooked but essential in case management plan development is resource consumption. According to CMSA's Resource and Resource Utilization Practice Standard, the case manager should incorporate factors related to quality, safety, access, and cost-effectiveness in assessing, monitoring, and evaluating resources for the client's care (2010).

1. Case management plans should address anticipated resources needed but also be cognizant of benefits available to provide for these resources. Alternate funding sources serve as added means to obtain resources and should be included as well.

2. CMSA recommends that case managers design case management plans that allow them to carefully document the appropriate allocation and consumption of resources and based on the case management plan. Box 21-5 shares some strategies on this aspect of case management.

3. Be inclusive of all resource needs—But specify the necessary resources to meet the needs. It is imperative to identify anticipated end results, monitor progress toward goals, and adapt the case management plan as necessary.

BOX 21-5   Appropriate Use of Resources and Case Management Plans

- Documentation of the evaluation of safety, effectiveness, cost, and potential outcomes of care when designing care plans to promote the ongoing care needs of the client
- Evidence of follow-through on care plan goals and objectives
- Evidence of utilizing evidence-based practice guidelines
- Demonstration of linking the client and family or caregiver with resources appropriate to the needs and goals identified in the care plan
- Documented communication of the client and other providers, both internal and external, especially during care transitions
- Evidence of promoting the most effective and efficient use of health care and financial resources
- Documentation demonstrating that the intensity of case management services renders corresponds with the needs of the client

E. Standardization methodology—The pressure to demonstrate accountability for care delivered is at the forefront of the health care industry. However, health care quality reporting, at times, presents somewhat of a dilemma.

  1. Metric reports (e.g., report cards, balanced scorecards, regulatory surveys) focus on quality outcomes, but they also include significant detail about systems and processes.

  2. The case manager addresses accountability by utilizing consistent methodology to capture work product and outcomes and

     a. By understanding the quality indicators and/or standards that are applicable indicators of quality and/or are applicable for the case managers' areas of practice

     b. By encompassing the aspects of applicable practice standards that apply to individual care plan interventions

  3. Accreditation standards and outcome expectations that a case manager should be mindful of include

     a. Accreditation standards (e.g., NCQA, URAC, CARF)

     b. Health Plan Employer Data and Information Set (HEDIS)

     c. Medicare Hospital Outcome Survey (HOS)

     d. Minimum Data Set and Care Screening (MDS)

     e. Outcomes and Assessment Information Set (OASIS)

  4. While there are many quality indicators, the important point for a case manager to recognize is to encompass essential components of applicable quality indicators into the case management plan throughout its development and implementation. In this way, the case manager is able to demonstrate the need for case manager involvement, quality outcomes achievement, and compliance with overarching accreditation and certification requirements.

F. In developing a case management plan, the case manager uses all means available in order to create patient-specific, standardized plans with realistic, achievable goals. Reaching consensus/agreement on the case management plan is essential, especially with the client and caregiver. Once defined, the care management plan becomes a road map and provides a means of reporting quality and performance outcomes and demonstrating case manager accountability.

G. By performing a thorough needs assessment, the strength of the case management plan's effective framework is maximized for patient-centered interventions.

Problem List Identification

A. Once an assessment is completed and the framework for the case management plan is in place, a problem list needs to be reviewed and finalized. This list is based on the patient and their support structure's identified needs and may be:

  1. Single focused—Stick to one specific outcome (e.g., return to independent ADL following hip replacement surgery)

  2. Multifocused—Includes more than one issue (e.g., clinical outcome, transportation issue, family/support structure following hip replacement surgery)

B. The problem list may include client strengths and weaknesses; family and relationship issues; cultural concerns; spiritual concerns; behavioral health concerns; psychological and cognitive concerns; clinical needs; and other social, financial, and adherence concerns.

C. When the initial problem list is complete, the case manager reviews it with the client and/or caregiver. Each item is confirmed and adjusted, as necessary. The following discussion points may be helpful cues:

1. Will this problem get better or stabilize? If so, then the intervention(s) and goal(s) for that problem should address the anticipated outcome. Timelines should be incorporated in stages so that evaluation can demonstrate realistic, measurable improvements and outcomes.

a. An example of this type of problem and interventional focus would be self-care deficit related to hip surgery, and the interventions may include rehabilitation therapy services, patient education, and returning to independent ADL status.

2. Will this problem get any worse or develop a complication? If so, then the intervention(s) and goal(s) should focus on the prevention and/or minimization of complications or decline. Again, specific and measurable outcomes should be incorporated that are clearly related to the problem(s).

a. An example of this type of problem and interventional focus would be a patient diagnosed with diabetes. While you cannot make diabetes go away, you can help the patient be able to better self-manage or manage with support to reduce complications of this condition. Interventions may include supporting the patient to better maintain blood glucose levels within acceptable ranges as defined by the attending physician and best-practice recommendations.

3. What can be done to provide optimal quality of life, comfort, and dignity for the patient? If the patient's problems will, most likely, not improve and deterioration is inevitable, then the goal(s) and intervention(s) must reflect the status of the patient and the measures must be appropriate for the types of interventions at hand.

a. An example of this type of problem and interventional focus would be the nutritional needs of a patient with a terminal diagnosis. Interventions may be to maintain nutritional status to the best ability of the patient utilizing supplements that are tolerable to the patient.

D. As the problem list is better defined, the goals, interventions, and outcomes should also be closely aligned to the problem(s) identified. Interventions and approaches to case management include patients' needs and wishes, physician/provider orders, facility/organizational protocols, accepted standards of practice, and defined care paths and algorithms.

Case Management Plan Implementation

A. Implementation of the case management plan requires the involvement and understanding of all who are or will be responsible for certain interventions or activities.

B. The case management plan implementation involves the patient, family/ support structure, facilities, ancillary care providers, physician treatment team, behavioral health agencies, home service providers, transportation agencies, case managers from the various organizations, community-based supports and services, and others as indicated.

C. Once the case management plan is developed, it should be reviewed with and agreed upon with the patient and shared with the primary care providers and any others care team members to whom the patient has granted access. Remember: This is the case management plan for, about, and developed with the patient. Consequently, patients must be in agreement with the plan, interventions, and goals, recognize their role in achieving optimal outcomes, and understand what they need to do to be in support of the defined case management plan and meeting their goals.

D. When working with providers and other members of the health care team, it is important to share that the patient is in agreement with and has helped in the development of the case management plan. Further, by sharing with providers some of the patient's anticipated goals and identifying the providers' role in helping the patient succeed, the providers are able to take a more active role in the successful outcomes defined in the plan.

E. Examples of working with providers and other members of the health care team include
   1. Obtaining laboratory results to evaluate clinical status
   2. Obtaining results of physician visits and changes in orders/medical treatment plans
   3. Coordinating transportation to necessary services
   4. Coordinating nutritional services such as Meals on Wheels
   5. Facilitating home health, durable medical equipment, and other ancillary services

F. For the successful implementation of a patient case management plan, the case manager must involve all who are required to make the plan a success. The purpose of the plan is to guide the case manager and the patient toward actions and interventions that will facilitate problem resolution (or to mitigate the consequences of problems) and goal attainment.

Incorporating Evidence-Based Guidelines in Case Management Practice

A. When performing UM functions, the case manager uses evidence-based clinical practice guidelines and/or decision support criteria; however, it is also the physician's responsibility to practice evidence-based medicine and assure that case management plans of care adhere to best-practice standards.

B. In reality, evidence-based case management tools have subtle differences and therefore should be used differently when developing plans of care.

C. Another important distinction that often is overlooked is that the tools are just that tools to assist case managers in accomplishing their goals. However, they are not, in themselves, case management.

D. Evidence-based medicine (EBM) is the integration of best research-based evidence coupled with clinical expertise and current practice standards. EBM is used as the basis for medical and health decision-making. Medical recommendations based on research evidence can be formed as either guidelines or standards/protocols. Case managers must incorporate evidence into practice at both the departmental or program and patient care levels.

E. Clinical practice guidelines (CPGs)—Systematically developed statements used to assist practitioner and patient decisions about appropriate health care for specific clinical circumstances (Institute of Medicine, 2011). Evidence-based implies that the recommendations are developed using an unbiased process of review, are based on the premise of evidence-based medicine (EBM), and are systematically developed (Field & Lohr, 1990).
   1. As defined, defensible guidelines require four critical concepts:
      a. The development process is open, documented, and reproducible.
      b. The resulting output is of use to both providers and patients.
      c. The concept of appropriateness of services is reflected.
      d. The guideline is related to clearly define clinical issues (Mulrow & Lohr, 2001).
   2. One of the most important attributes of CPG is validity. This means that guidelines should, when followed, lead to the expected clinical, quality, and cost outcomes. Guidelines are considered recommendations for best practices.

F. Clinical standards/protocols—Clinical standards are practices that are medically necessary and services that any practitioner under any circumstances would be required to render. Where guidelines are meant to be flexible, standards are meant to be inflexible and should be followed. In addition, when formulating standards, they require a higher bar than guidelines (Mulrow & Lohr, 2001). Standards or protocols are more specific and define a rigid set of criteria outlining the management steps for a single clinical condition.

G. Case Management Adherence Guidelines (CMAG)—Serves the professional care management community as the standard by which case managers can advance assistance, coaching and monitoring efforts with the goal of ultimately improving care delivery and patient care outcomes (CMSA, 2012).
   1. These adherence guidelines are designed to
      a. Assist case managers in more effectively improving patient adherence to their medication regime and facilitate health behavioral change
      b. Help case managers in the assessment, planning, facilitation, and advocacy of patient adherence to the care plan
      c. Provide an interaction and management algorithm to assess and improve the patient's knowledge and his/her motivation to follow health regimen as prescribed, for example, take medications
      d. Facilitate the patient's ability and comfort in the development of self-management knowledge and skills
   2. Guidelines discuss key areas in which case management has direct impact to assess and improve for adherence:
      a. Motivation
      b. Knowledge
      c. Readiness

3. System of assessment
   a. Classify levels/stages of motivation, readiness, and knowledge
   b. Target strategies for patient-specific interventions
   c. Reassess progress throughout case management intervention
   d. Provides objective goal setting to improve individual adherence
4. CMAG includes
   a. Case Management Adherence Guidelines (CMAG), third revision (2012)
      i. Highlights advances in adherence research and knowledge and the changing landscape of case management practice
      ii. Discusses expanding use of electronic, computer, and Web-based technologies to support adherence efforts
   b. Condition-specific editions
      i. Focus on condition-specific clinical information and strategy
      ii. Workbooks available for breast cancer, COPD, diabetes mellitus, depression, and pain
      iii. Some workbooks translated to Spanish
   c. CMAG live events and webinars
      i. Offered on request or invitation.
      ii. Arranged through sponsor organization representatives.
      iii. Time commitment varies according to module.
H. Some case management programs use the Patient Activation Measure (PAM) to improve patient's adherence and self-management abilities. Evidence has shown that if case managers start their intervention in the area of adherence and lifestyle behavior change at the point where the patient is, case managers are able to achieve greater progress in achieving desired outcomes. The PAM can be used for this purpose.
   1. The Patient Activation Measure (PAM) is a proprietary, evidence-based tool that assesses an individual's knowledge, skill, and confidence levels for managing both own health and health care.
   2. An individual measuring low requires support to improve his/her understanding of managing own health and/or health condition.
   3. The case manager can use this measure to identify barriers and strategies for achieving case management plan goals, including adherence and self-management.
   4. Use of the PAM requires payment of a license fee.
I. Functional independence measure
   1. The functional independence measure (FIM) provides a methodology for uniform measurement for disability. It measures the individual's level disability and indicates how much assistance is required for the individual to carry out activities of daily living.
   2. Although case managers do not routinely perform the FIM assessment, the results of this testing are used as an objective means to measure and track improvement in functional status.
J. Health Status Questionnaire Short Form
   1. The Short Form-36 (SF-36) is one of the most widely used generic measures of health-related quality of life across the health care continuum. The SF-36 is a self-report questionnaire that the patient completes.
   2. The case manager utilizes results derived from the SF-36 to identify individuals who may benefit from case management services and to

identify perceived barriers, which may benefit from additional inquiry and intervention.

K. Patient Health Questionnaire
   1. The Patient Health Questionnaire (PHQ) is copyrighted tool owned by Pfizer, Inc. This is not a diagnostic tool. This screening tool is specific to depression. It is a self-report questionnaire that the patient completes.
   2. There are various lengths of the PHQ based on the number of questions posed. There are also a number of modules pertaining specifically to the anxiety, alcohol, eating, and somatic issues.
   3. The General Anxiety Disorder (GAD-7) is a related Pfizer, Inc. copyrighted tool specific to anxiety.
   4. The case manager utilizes results derived from this screening tool to inquire as to patient self-perception of depression symptoms as well as issues relating to the specialty modules previously noted.

Clinical Pathways

A. Known by a variety of synonyms including care paths, integrated clinical pathways, collaborative care paths, care maps, multidisciplinary action plans, and multidisciplinary pathways of care. Clinical pathways were originally used at New England Medical Center as early as 1985 and created by Karen Zander and Kathleen Bower.
B. Clinical pathways are generally considered to be multidisciplinary tools, which are founded on evidence-based practice specific to a grouping of patients (e.g., health condition, procedure).
C. Members of the care team have sequenced, time-specific interventions pertaining to patient care, diagnostic testing, and treatments. Efforts of the multidisciplinary care team are directly associated with specific outcomes.
D. Clinical pathways may be developed to show current practice parameters, recommended best practices, or a combination of both.
E. Other components of clinical pathways may include target lengths of stay and anticipated alternate levels of care.
F. Clinical pathways incorporate a variety of care needs to be used by members of the interdisciplinary care team (e.g., physicians, nurses, social workers, physical therapists, occupational therapists, nutritionists, pharmacists, respiratory therapists, ethicists, clergy).
G. The four main components of clinical pathways are
   1. A timeline
   2. Identified categories of care and/or activities and their interventions
   3. Immediate, intermediate, and long-term outcome criteria
   4. Some type of allowance for deviations and variances that can be documented and analyzed
H. There are many types of care activities or elements of patient care addressed in clinical pathways. These may vary among health care organizations and settings; however, they generally include those listed in Box 21-6.
I. Clinical pathways do not always address all elements of care shared above. Each organization may decide on its own policy and procedure, format, and content.

21-6 **Key Elements of Clinical Pathways**

- Inclusion and/or exclusion criteria
- Assessment of the patient and monitoring
- Tests and procedures
- Care facilitation/coordination, including important milestones
- Consultations and referrals
- Medications
- Intravenous therapy
- Activity and exercise
- Nutrition
- Patient/family education
- Treatments (e.g., medical, surgical, or nursing interventions)
- Wound care
- Physical and occupational therapy
- Pain management and comfort
- Outcome indicators and projected responses to care/expectations
- Safety
- Discharge planning
- Psychosocial assessment
- Goals of care and expected outcomes
- Variance identification and management

J. These elements of care are not a standardized list of categories. Health care organizations and providers using clinical pathways may decide on their own list; however, it is important to have an organization-specific standard for everyone to follow to eliminate confusion.

K. Clinical pathways may include a preprinted order set, or orders are built into the pathway itself. The pathway may appear on paper or be incorporated into the clinical information system of the facility.

L. While clinical pathways are often viewed as practice guidelines, protocols, or algorithms, they are not the same. Clinical pathway's focus is inclusive of care coordination requirements and the engagement of multidisciplinary care teams.

 Algorithms

A. Algorithms are schematic models used to support clinical decision pathways.
   1. Structured in a yes/no schema, the decision points depend on certain characteristic or diagnostic and treatment options.
   2. Algorithms are straightforward decision trees, and although useful clinical tools, they are not exhaustive, nor do they account for all patient-related variables. Therefore, they are intended as guides for disease states and conditions, clinical settings, insurance issues, or economics of care.

B. Clinical algorithms are flowcharts that represent a sequence of clinical decisions.
   1. Effective algorithms are those that represent the latest scientific evidence and expert consensus and include protocol charts for guiding step-by-step care of a specific health condition, medical procedure, or problem.

2. Organizations (e.g., MD Anderson Cancer Center) share a variety of screening and treatment algorithms on their institutional Web site. This serves to promote transparency in care delivery and consistency in best-practice clinical decision-making.
3. It is important to recognize that although helpful, algorithms serve to guide but not replace informed clinical decision-making and independent medical judgment. Clinical algorithms should never be an excuse to restrict clinical decision-making.
4. Case managers find clinical algorithms helpful in anticipating the trajectory of a patient's care in order to accomplish tasks more effectively (e.g., transition planning). When patient care veers off an algorithm's path, it is important for the case manager to understand the variance. This knowledge supports requests for additional services (e.g., extended length of stay, additional physical therapy).

Evidence-based Decision Support Criteria

A. Evidence-based decision support criteria tools are impartial, evidence-based tools used as a lexicon to evaluate the decisions about the appropriateness and quality of care that support integrated care management and UM approaches to evaluate patient care and services.
B. Evidence-based tools are built on a scientifically valid foundation of medical evidence focused on improving the quality and efficiency of the delivery of health care services by providing a standardized foundation that supports communication and collaboration between providers, payers, and others.
C. The foundation of evidence-based care guidelines is that effective care leads to the best patient outcomes while at the same time avoiding underuse or overuse. These tools are used across the continuum of care and support best-practice transition of care planning.
D. Regardless of the tool(s) used in the case management plan development, it is essential that the case manager use these for guidance only. Consistent use of evidence-based tools are essential for the development of standardized case management plans, which in turn:
1. Allows for uniform data collection and reporting
2. Provides the basis for demonstrating the value of case management services
3. Demonstrates the return on investment of case management intervention

Benefits of Case Management Plans

A. Case management plans, in any form, are known to improve communication among health care providers and with the patient and family/support system; proactively delineate processes of care and services and related expected outcomes; focus on the patient and their family/support; identify performance expectations; ensure quality; define accountability; and improve documentation.
B. Case management plans help define a consistent standard of care for a specific condition, event, or process. This makes it easier for the case manager to support continuity and consistency in care with clear expectations of the roles and responsibilities of the patient, care

manager, various health care providers, and other care team members involved in the provision of care and services.

C. Case management plans function as tools that facilitate the coordination of care across the continuum of care and settings and for collaboration between the case manager and varied providers and practitioners from across the continuum of care.

D. Case management plans also are used as a strategy for ensuring adherence to standards of regulatory and accreditation agencies.

E. Case management plans may be used as tools for training and education of less-experienced health care professionals, students, and newly hired staff.

F. Case management plans may be used in the negotiation of managed care contracts and reimbursement rates.

Case Management and Utilization Management

A. A comprehensive, patient-specific case management plan must address all the applicable aspects of the patient's care. Moreover, case managers have an obligation to manage resources appropriately and effectively in alignment with the Resource and Resource Utilization Standard of Practice.

B. Case management must work hand in hand with other care coordination staff to comprehensively manage patient and family needs and health care resources. Although the integration of UM and case management continues to be a topic of debate, it has been successfully combined in a variety of settings.

C. One of the most significant differences contributing the incongruence of effectively managing UM and case management caseloads is the issue of service intensity, knowledge, and required skill set.

   1. UM activities (e.g., precertification, concurrent review) are driven by the use of criteria. When information given by the provider is compared to evidence-based criterion, it either meets or does not meet requirements. The next step is requesting additional information or forwarding the case to a physician advisor for determination. This caseload can be effectively managed with solid clinical knowledge and ease of using the criteria. The commitment of utilization management usually takes place over a period of hours or days.

   2. Case management requires advanced skills and knowledge. The application of case management intervention requires different skill and knowledge set than that of task-oriented, criteria-supported UM. The commitment of case management resources often takes place over a period of weeks and months.

D. UM is the process of determining whether all aspects of a patient's care, at every level, are both medically necessary and appropriately delivered. Depending on benefit design, a patient's health care services may be subject to one or more of three utilization review (UR) categories. These are

   1. Prospective—Review of a request for services prior to the utilization of those services

   2. Concurrent—Review of services during an episode of care, illness, or injury

   3. Retrospective—Review of services after care has already been completed

E. These three review strategies are important in helping to understand the resources required to meet a patient's care needs for a given episode of care and at a given level of care or setting. Most often, UM uses some type of nationally recognized clinical screening/decision support criteria or critical pathways (discussed earlier) as guidelines for the review process.

F. Generally, UM is a nonphysician function within the health care continuum. However, physicians can get involved in UM activities when the health care team believes that services requested are not appropriate for the patient based on the clinical information available. In such situations, a case manager generally seeks the assistance of a physician to help either validate the request or to deny the request.

G. The understanding of the role of UM is critical for recognizing that although standard processes are in place, even UR needs the flexibility to be patient specific. Physician involvement also supports the flexibility of UM processes as well and can make determinations that are specific for the patients' individual needs.

H. While some case managers perform UM functions and others do not, incorporating some aspects of UM processes into case management and care plan development is a strategy to consider. How can UM become a strategy of case management plan development? The goals of UM can create synergies for case management practice. UM goals may include:
   1. Objectively screening for the most appropriate treatments and services
   2. Documenting the need for requested treatments and services
   3. Assisting in the timely access to care
   4. Ensuring safe transitions to alternate levels of care utilizing objective screening criteria
   5. Allowing early identification of the patient's discharge and/or transfer needs

I. In looking at these goals, synergies begin to emerge. By integrating UM goals into case management planning objectives, case managers can:
   1. Improve communications with care team members
   2. Increase coordination of care and services allowing for a more seamless transition for the patient
   3. Ensure more effective use of health plan benefits
   4. Share resource tools
   5. Coordinate efforts such as transitioning the patient to an alternate level of care or obtaining home care services and products
   6. Reduce/decrease duplication of efforts for approval of certain service requests
   7. Reduce costs associated with the delivery of health care services

J. These synergies can be seen as additional strategies for helping case managers meet the challenges of creating and utilizing patient case management plans that are not only patient specific but also standardized. The process of utilization management can be seen as another tool that case managers may use as a guide to help identify the appropriateness and the timeliness of patient care services.

References

Case Management Society of America. (2010). *CMSA standards of practice for case management.* Little Rock, AR: Author.

Case Management Society of America. (2012). *Case Management Adherence Guidelines (CMAG).* (2012). Little Rock, AR: CMSA.

Centers for Medicare and Medicaid Services (CMS). (2015). *What is an ACO?* Retrieved from https://www.cms.gov/Medicare/Medicare-Fee-for-Service-Payment/ACO/index.html?redirect=/aco, on July 24, 2015.

Commission for Case Manager Certification (CCMC). (2014). *Role & function study key findings.* Rolling Meadows, IL: Author: Written and Produced by Health2Resources; 2011. Retrieved from www.ccmcertification.org, on April, 27, 2015.

Commission for Case Manager Certification (CCMC). (2015). *Center stage in the revolution: A healthcare reform action guide for the professional case manager. Issue Brief Vol. 2(2).* Retrieved from http://ccmcertification.org/sites/default/files/downloads/2011/4.%20Center%20stage%20in%20the%20revolution%20-%20volume%202%2C%20issue%202.pdf, on July 22, 2015.

Doran, G. T. (1981). There's a S.M.A.R.T. way to write management's goals and objectives. *Management Review, 70*(11), 35–36.

Field, M. J., & Lohr, K. N. (1990). *Clinical practice guidelines: Directions for a new program.* Washington, DC: National Academy Press.

Huber, D. L., & Craig, K. (2007). Acuity and case management: A healthy dose of outcomes, Part I. *Professional Case Management, 12*(3), 132–144. Retrieved from http://journals.lww.com/professionalcasemanagementjournal/Fulltext/2007/05000/Acuity_and_Case_Management__A_Healthy_Dose_of.3.aspx, on July 24, 2015.

Institute of Medicine. (2011) *Clinical practice guidelines we can trust.* Washington, DC: Author. Retrieved from https://iom.nationalacademies.org/~/media/Files/Report%20Files/2011/Clinical-Practice-Guidelines-We-Can-Trust/Clinical%20Practice%20Guidelines%202011%20Insert.pdf, on July 24, 2015.

McDonald, K. M., Schultz, E., Albin, L., Pineda, N., Lonhart, J., Sundaram, V., … Malcolm, E. (2014). *Care coordination Atlas version 4 (prepared by Stanford University under subcontract to American Institutes for Research on Contract No. HHSA290-2010-00005I).* Rockville, MD: Agency for Healthcare Research and Quality; AHRQ Publication No. 14-0037-EF. Retrieved from http://www.ahrq.gov/professionals/prevention-chronic-care/improve/coordination/atlas2014/ccm_atlas.pdf, on July 24, 2015.

MediLexicon.com. (2015). *Definition of algorithm.* Retrieved from http://www.medilexicon.com/medicaldictionary.php?t=2189, on July 24, 2015.

Mitus, J. (2008). The birth of InterQual: Evidence-based decision support criteria that helped change healthcare. *Professional Case Management, 13*(4), 228–233.

Mulrow, C. D., & Lohr, K. N. (2001). Proof and policy from medical research evidence. *Journal of Health Politics, Policy and Law, 26*(2), 249–266. Retrieved from http://archive.ahrq.gov/research/findings/evidence-based-reports/jhppl/mulrow.pdf, on July 24, 2015.

Open Clinical. (2015). *Definition of clinical practice guidelines.* Retrieved from http://www.open-clinical.org/guidelines.html, on July 24, 2015.

Pearson, M. L., Mattke, S., Shaw, R., Ridgely, M. S., & Wiseman S. H. (2007). *Patient self-management support programs: An evaluation. Final contract report (prepared by RAND health under Contract No. 282-00-0005).* Rockville, MD: Agency for Healthcare Research and Quality; AHRQ Publication No. 08-0011. Retrieved from http://www.ahrq.gov/research/findings/final-reports/ptmgmt/ptmgmt.pdf, on July 24, 2015.

Sackett, D. L., Rosenburg, W. M., Gray, J. A., Haynes, R. B., & Richardson, W. S. (1996). Evidence-based medicine: What it is and it isn't. *British Medical Journal, 312,* 71–72. Retrieved from http://www.ncbi.nlm.nih.gov/pmc/articles/PMC2349778, on July 24, 2015.

Steves, R., & Hootman, J. M. (2004). Evidence-based medicine: What is it and how does it apply to athletic training? *Journal of Athletic Training, 39*(1), 83–87. Retrieved from http://www.ncbi.nlm.nih.gov/pmc/articles/PMC385266/pdf/attr_39_01_0083.pdf, on July 24, 2015.

Tahan, H. (2002). *A ten-step process to develop case management plans. Lippincott's Case Management*, 7(6), 231–242. Retrieved from http://journals.lww.com/professionalcasemanagementjournal/Fulltext/2002/11000/A_Ten_Step_Process_to_Develop_Case_Management.5.aspx, on July 24, 2015.

Wojner, A. (2001). *Outcomes management: Applications to clinical practice*. St. Louis, MO: Mosby.

CHAPTER 22

Quality and Outcomes Management in Case Management

Michael B. Garrett and Teresa M. Treiger

LEARNING OBJECTIVES

Upon completion of this chapter, the reader will be able to:

1. Define outcomes.
2. List reasons why outcomes management is important in case management practice.
3. Identify frameworks for quality and outcomes measurement.
4. Describe the common categories of outcome indicators.
5. List the characteristics of effective outcome measures.
6. Describe methods of incorporating outcomes measurement into case management practice.
7. Identify key issues in reporting outcomes.
8. Identify case management outcome measures.

IMPORTANT TERMS AND CONCEPTS

Agency for Healthcare Research and Quality (AHRQ)
Clinical Practice Guidelines
Institute for Healthcare Improvement (IHI)

National Quality Forum (NQF)
Outcome Indicator
Outcome Measure
Outcomes
Outcomes Management
Outcomes Measurement
Process

Process Measures
Quality
Reliability
Risk Adjustment
Structure
Structure Measures
The Triple Aim
Variation

Introduction

A. Today's health care consumers are demanding that they receive full value for their health care dollars. Health care executives and other personnel meet customers' expectations by focusing on improving the quality of the services they provide and by ensuring that the customer experience is desirable and rewarding. At the same time, health care executives recognize that a focus on quality care is the best way to ensure that revenues equal or exceed expenses.

B. Health care quality has become a driving force in efforts to improve delivery efficiency and effectiveness along the entire care continuum and health and human services.

1. Leaders in health care quality include organizations and agencies such as the National Quality Forum (NQF), the Institute for Healthcare Improvement (IHI), The Leapfrog Group, and the Agency for Healthcare Research and Quality (AHRQ) that carry the torch for improving the quality of health care for all and serve as resources for professional case managers by providing frameworks on which quality and outcome measures may be built.

2. NQF is a nonprofit organization, leading improvements in health care by building consensus on quality of care indicators and defining standard measures for care quality. When a measure receives an endorsement from NQF, it becomes a gold standard for quality performance. NQF-endorsed measures are evidence based and valid, and in tandem with the delivery of care and payment reform, they help:
   a. Make patient care safer.
   b. Improve maternity care.
   c. Achieve better health outcomes.
   d. Strengthen chronic care management.
   e. Hold down health care costs (NQF, 2015).

3. IHI is an independent not-for-profit organization and a leading innovator and driver of health and health care improvement. IHI's work is focused in five key areas:
   a. Improvement capability
   b. Person- and family-centered care
   c. Patient safety
   d. Quality, cost, and value
   e. Triple aim for populations (IHI, 2015a)

4. The Leapfrog Group is a voluntary program, which focuses the power of employer purchasers of health care by setting the quality bar for specific trouble areas in hospital systems:
   a. Leapfrog encourages transparency and access to health care information.
   b. The Leapfrog survey is the gold standard for comparing hospitals' performance on the national standards of safety, quality, and efficiency that are most relevant to consumers and purchasers of care.

NOTE: This chapter is a revised version of Chapter 25 in the second edition of *CMSA Core Curriculum for Case Management*. The contributors wish to acknowledge Sherry Aliotta, Nancy Claflin, and Patricia M. Pecqueux, as some of the timeless material was retained from the previous version.

    c. The Leapfrog survey makes the only nationally standardized and NQF-endorsed set of measures that captures hospital performance in patient safety, quality, and resource utilization (The Leapfrog Group, 2015).

5. The Agency for Healthcare Research and Quality (AHRQ) exists within the US Department of Health and Human Services (USDHHS or DHHS). Its mission is to produce evidence to make health care safer, higher quality, more accessible, equitable, and affordable and to make sure that the evidence produced is understood and used. A number of resources fall under the AHRQ umbrella including:

    a. National Quality Measures Clearinghouse

    b. TeamSTEPPS

    c. Effective Healthcare Program

    d. National Healthcare Quality and Disparities Reports

    e. National Guideline Clearinghouse (AHRQ, 2015)

C. Case management is in the crosshair of virtually every care coordination initiative launched in the past decade. Case management roles and functions have been recognized in numerous governmental reports focused on health care quality and cited as a means to enact needed changes in the delivery of health care within the United States. While not consistently referred to as case management, the mandate for accountability and improvement in care coordination has been noted to be instrumental for the improvement of health care safety and quality (Treiger & Fink-Samnick, 2013).

D. While it may be unfair to hold the entirety of case management responsible for program success or failure, it is the position in which our practice often finds itself. Our assumed strengths of whole-person care coordination, engaging the client and client's support system in health care improvement, minimizing fragmentation and duplication of care, improving outcomes, collaborating with the interdisciplinary health care team, and supporting excellent care transitions also appear to be weaknesses as the increasing focus on measurable outcomes demonstrate little to no impact from case management interventions.

E. Although there have been numerous anecdotal descriptions of case management outcomes, objective, consistent, and scientific evidence is sparse. What does exist is difficult to compare due to heterogeneity and lack of a priori approach to evaluation. Effective Health Care Program (EHCP) findings for a comparative effectiveness review of outpatient case management programs varied. The very issue of heterogeneity was mentioned as problematic in the research process itself:

1. The most positive findings were that case management improved the quality of care, particularly for patients with serious illnesses that require complex treatments (e.g., cancer, HIV). For a variety of medical conditions, case management improved self-management skills. Case management also improved quality of life in some populations (CHF and cancer) and tended to improve satisfaction with care. For the caregivers of patients with dementia, targeted case management programs improved levels of stress, burden, and depression (Hickam et al., 2013).

2. The same review found a low strength of evidence that case management was effective in improving resource utilization for

BOX 22-1 Contributing Factors to Lack of Reliable Outcomes Data

- Inconsistent definitions of case management and the interventions performed by case managers.
- Inconsistent methods of measurement.
- Organizations maintaining proprietary methods of measuring program and process outcomes.
- Measures are not standardized across organizations or care settings.
- Other confounding variables or practice characteristics are not controlled for and often not communicated in published studies; for example, use of case management associates is not a standard practice across case management programs.
- Rigorous evaluation studies are costly and resource intensive.
- Lack of funding.
- Lack of electronic or automated systems for effective and easy measurement.
- Often, variable measures rely on administrative databases as data sources such as claims data, which leave out important data on specific case management interventions.

patients with congestive heart failure (CHF) and chronic obstructive pulmonary disease (COPD) or in the face of chronic homelessness. In most other cases, case management programs did not demonstrate cost savings. For patients who received case management for multiple chronic diseases, there is a high strength of evidence that the programs did not reduce Medicare expenditures (Hickam et al., 2013).

3. Several issues contribute to the lack of valid, reliable outcomes data; among them are those listed in Box 22-1. The initial purpose of case management was its use as a tool to reduce escalating health care costs. This was accomplished without clear, consistent, or formalized definition, documentation, and measurement of case manager activities except through cost savings.

F. It is essential for case management professionals to scientifically undertake quality practice improvement initiatives, which align with individual and organizational goals. The emphasis on quality performance and outcomes measurement to demonstrate the value of case management interventions and programs has never been more important:

1. It is ineffective to craft carefully worded goals with dubious desired outcomes based on a cursory assessment. Case managers must perform thorough biopsychosocial–spiritual assessments in order to identify real opportunities for improvement.

2. When accurate information is derived through client and care team interactions, the case manager designs a meaningful case management plan of care with achievable goals and client outcomes.

Descriptions of Key Terms

A. Administrative and management processes—The activities performed in the governance and management systems of a health care organization.

B. Benchmark—A standard, or a set of standards, used as a point of reference for evaluating performance or level of quality. Benchmarks may be drawn from a firm's own experience, from the experience of other firms in the industry, or from legal requirements such as environmental regulations (Business Dictionary.com, 2015b).

C. Care delivery processes—The support activities applied by practitioners and all suppliers of care and care products to get the product/service to the patient.

D. Clinical practice guidelines—Systematically developed statements to assist practitioner and patient decisions about appropriate health care for specific clinical circumstances (Institute of Medicine, 1990).

E. Clinical processes—The activities of health care practitioners with and for clients/patients, their families and support systems, and what clients/patients do in response.

F. Direct case management outcomes—The measurement or results of those activities and interventions that are within the scope of the case manager's practice and control. Results of the case management process and interventions executed by the case manager.

G. End health system outcomes—Those performance indicators measured for the health care system overall include the following: cost of care, quality of care, health status and clinical outcomes achieved, and patient/client experience of care.

H. External validity—External validity is related to generalizing the results to settings or people other than those studied. Recall that validity refers to the approximate truth of propositions, inferences, or conclusions. So, *external* validity refers to the approximate truth of conclusions that involve generalizations. Put in more pedestrian terms, external validity is the degree to which the conclusions in your study would hold for other persons in other places and at other times (Research Methods Knowledge Base, 2015a).

I. Information flow—The creating and transporting of facts, knowledge, and data that make for informed decisions. The sharing of data between providers; health care team members, with payers or with patients; and their families.

J. Internal validity—It is the approximate truth about inferences regarding cause–effect or causal relationships. Thus, internal validity is only relevant in studies that try to establish a causal relationship. It's not relevant in most observational or descriptive studies, for instance. But for studies that assess the effects of social programs or interventions, internal validity is perhaps the primary consideration (Research Methods Knowledge Base, 2015b).

K. Materials flow—The movement of equipment and supplies across systems and processes or settings.

L. Outcomes—The end results of care, adverse or beneficial, as well as gradients between the products of one or more processes. Outcomes used as indicators of quality are states or conditions of individuals and populations attributed or attributable to antecedent health care (Donabedian, 1992). Another way of describing an outcome is as a measurable individual, family, or community state, behavior, or perception that is measured along a continuum and is responsive to nursing interventions (Moorhead et al., 2013). Classifications of outcomes include clinical, functional, financial/cost, and experience perceived.

M. Outcomes management—A technology of patient experience designed to help patients, payers, and providers make rational medical care–related choices based on their better insight into the effects of these choices on the patient's life (Ellwood, 1988).

N. Patient flow—The movement of patients from one place to another, from one level of care to another, or from one care setting or provider to another.

O. Process—Sequence of steps, which is taken to achieve a specific goal or end result.

P. Process measure—Used primarily to determine the degree to which the process is being executed as planned. For example, "the number of patients receiving a case management assessment within 24 hours of admission to a hospital setting."

Q. Quality—The definition of quality varies across sectors. The American Society for Quality (ASQ) notes dual meanings of the characteristics of a product or service that bear on its ability to satisfy stated or implied needs or a product or service free of deficiencies (ASQ, 2015).

R. Reliability—Reliability has to do with the quality of measurement. In its everyday sense, reliability is the consistency or repeatability of a measure (Research Methods Knowledge Base, 2015c).

S. Risk adjustment—Risk adjustment is a corrective tool used to level the playing field regarding the reporting of patient outcomes by adjusting for the differences in risk among specific patients. Risk adjustment also makes it possible to compare hospital and doctor performance fairly. Comparing unadjusted event rates for different hospitals would unfairly penalize those performing operations on higher-risk patients (The Society of Thoracic Surgeons, 2015).

T. Standard of care—A diagnostic and treatment process that a clinician should follow for a certain type of patient, illness, or clinical circumstance or, in legal terms, the level at which the average, prudent provider in a given community would practice. It is how similarly qualified practitioners would have managed the patient's care under the same or similar circumstances (Medicinenet.com, 2015).

U. Standard (of practice)—An authoritative statement agreed to and promulgated by the practice by which the quality of practice and service can be judged (Case Management Society of America, 2010).

V. Variation—Inevitable change in the output or result of a system (process) because all systems vary over time. Two major types of variations are either common, which is inherent in a system or special, which is caused by changes in the circumstances or environment (Business Dictionary.com, 2015a).

Applicability to CMSA's Standards of Practice

A. The Case Management Society of America (CMSA) describes in its standards of practice for case management (CMSA, 2010) that case management practice extends across all health care settings, including payer, provider, government, employer, community, and home environment. It also describes that evaluation of the outcomes of case management practice is important in demonstrating its value to various stakeholders including clients/support systems, providers, payers, employers, and regulators.

B. This chapter describes various perspectives on health care quality and outcomes. In striving to maximize outcomes, interventions are delivered within the context of quality case management aimed at achieving client satisfaction, especially in access to and experience of care.

C. This chapter addresses case management practice, which requires knowledge of and proficiency in the following practice standards: problem/opportunity identification, monitoring, outcomes, research, and research utilization.

D. This chapter also provides case managers with an important perspective about how their roles relate to and impact quality, safety, and cost. Additionally, it shares with case managers the requisite knowledge, skills, and competency in the area of quality and safety that are necessary for successful and rewarding practice.

Defining Outcomes Management and Measurement

A. Avedis Donabedian was a physician and is considered founder in the study of quality in health care and medical outcomes research. His model of care described a quality paradigm for examining health services and evaluating quality of health care. (Donabedian, 1966)
   1. His paradigm holds that there are three key factors in determining quality: structure, process, and outcome.
   2. Structure leads to process, which leads to outcome.
   3. These factors represent complex sets of events and factors.
   4. How each relates to the other must be clearly understood before quality measurement and assessment begins.
   5. Causal relationships may be understood between these factors, but they are considered as probabilities, not certainties.

B. When selecting outcome measures, we are attempting to determine in advance the potential effects, side effects, or consequences of our actions.

C. Outcomes measurement can assist in the demonstration of value by validating:
   1. What is effective.
   2. What is ineffective.
   3. What is efficient.
   4. What is inefficient.
   5. What contributes to desirable care quality and patient safety.
   6. The costs of an intervention.
   7. Whether the cost of the intervention is substantiated by the return on the investment.

D. The centerpiece and underlying ingredient of outcomes management is the tracking and measurement of the patient's clinical condition, functional ability, and well-being or quality of life. Today, however, client's safety and experience of care have received major attention in the measurement of quality and the impact of health care services deliver.

E. Outcomes management is a common language of health outcomes that is understood by patients, practitioners, payers, health care administrators, regulators, and other stakeholders.

F. Outcomes management requires a national reference database containing information and analysis on clinical, financial, and health outcomes, estimating:
   1. Relationships between medical interventions and health outcomes
   2. Relationships between health outcomes and money spent/cost of care
G. Outcomes management is dependent on four developing technologies:
   1. Practitioner reliance on standards of care and evidence-based guidelines in selecting appropriate interventions
   2. Routine and systematic measurement of the functioning and well-being of patients along with disease-specific clinical outcomes, at appropriate time intervals
   3. Pooling of clinical and outcome data on a massive scale
   4. Analysis and dissemination of results (outcomes) from the segment of the database pertinent to the concerns of each decision maker
H. One of the typical results from analysis is the detection of variation. Variation is typically measured through an outcomes management program. Variation is neither good nor bad in itself. Further analysis is required to determine what the causation is for the variation. The goal of outcome management is not to eliminate variation but to reduce it in order to produce and sustain stability in processes and practices.
I. There are two types of variation:
   1. Common cause variation—Also referred to as random variation. This is variation due to the process itself. It is produced by interactions of the variables in the process. Process redesign may be required if this type of variation needs to be redesigned through a quality improvement initiative.
   2. Special cause—Variation that is assignable to a specific cause or causes. It is not part of the usual process, but rather is due to particular circumstances. A focused review of the process needs to be conducted in order to conduct root cause analysis and for potential corrective actions to be taken.
J. Once variation is detected, a variety of quality improvement strategies, techniques, and methods can be used to improve outcomes and decrease variation. Examples may include:
   1. Six Sigma—A business strategy focusing on continuous improvement; a disciplined approached in process improvement that addresses the elimination of defects in care or to reduce their occurrence. Often, the Six Sigma improvement process consists of steps that focus on identifying the problem, measuring current state, implementing improvements, testing impacts of these improvements, and controlling or sustaining the realized improvement.
   2. Lean—A methodology focused on reducing lead time by the elimination of waste and non–value-added processes of care.
   3. Human Factors Analysis—A scientific discipline focused on understanding interactions among humans and other system elements in order to optimize human well-being and overall system performance. This form of analysis is fairly new in health care, and its popularity is on the rise, especially in the conduct of root cause analyses.
   4. Plan-Do-Study-Act or PDSA (sometimes called Plan-Do-Check-Act or PDCA)—A quality improvement methodology that is a four-step

model for carrying out change. Often, PDSA is used in small tests of change to expedite improvements.

5. Define-Measure-Analyze-Improve-Control (DMAIC)—a data-driven quality strategy used to improve processes. It is an integral part of a Six Sigma initiative, but in general can be implemented as a stand-alone quality improvement procedure or as part of other process improvement initiatives such as Lean.

Rationale for Outcomes Management

A. Measuring outcomes allows us to base improvement on measurement. Without effective outcome measurements, a health care organization will be unable to objectively track improvements or declines in performance:
   1. Measurement of outcomes provides information that allows us to determine whether the results of the process or intervention yield the desired return on investment.
   2. Measurement also provides a method for demonstrating value of a process to consumers and other stakeholders. With appropriate outcomes data, stakeholders can be educated regarding the value or potential value of the process or intervention.
B. The ability to verify positive outcomes provides a powerful rationale for a service. Outcomes measurement allows us to determine which processes and interventions are effective and which are not, thereby identifying opportunities for improvement.
C. The combination of outcomes management with case management in an overall model (Wojner, 2001) enables providers to improve clinical practice and individual performance by highlighting opportunities to:
   1. Enhance care.
   2. Stimulate the use of science-based interventions and treatment options.
   3. Conduct systematic evaluation of overall program effectiveness.
D. An outcomes measurement program is designed to improve quality by:
   1. Shifting the focus away from anecdotal evidence to objective data
   2. Enhancing our understanding of the variation that exists in a process
   3. Monitoring a process over time
   4. Revealing the effect of a change in a process
   5. Providing a common frame of reference
   6. Providing a more accurate basis for prediction (Lloyd, 2004)
E. The DISMEVAL Consortium (Nolte et al., 2013), when developing and validating disease management evaluation methods for European health care systems, identified a number of reasons for the evaluation of disease management program outcomes, including the following:
   1. Is the program a good investment?
   2. Is the program effective and/or efficient?
   3. What is the longer-term economic impact of the intervention?
   4. Were costs savings such that the intervention yielded a positive return on investment?
   5. Were quality improvement expectations achieved through the structured program (e.g., processes of care, adherence to clinical or practice guidelines, referral rates)?

BOX 22-2   Reasons for Implementation of Outcomes Management Programs

- Understanding and quantifying current performance
- Meeting or exceeding regulatory, accreditation, and contractual requirements
- Meeting or exceeding requirements of standards of care and standards of practice
- Identifying opportunities for improvement
- Improving the accountability of health care providers to patients, families, and other stakeholders
- Improving the financial performance of the organization
- Improving the desirability of the health care organization to employees, peer organizations, payers, and other stakeholders
- Mitigating risk by demonstrating compliance with state-of-the art health care quality guidelines
- Evaluating and improving performance in comparison to peers and national standards
- Meeting or exceeding individual and organizational ethical principles and values and adherence to such related standards

6. Were short-term outcomes such as disease control or satisfaction of participants?
7. What were the health policy implications of the programs?
F. There are a number of clinical and administrative reasons for developing and implementing an outcomes management program (Box 22-2).

Characteristics of Effective Outcome Measures

A. For an outcome measure to be effective, it must be:
   1. Valid—The effect seen is actually related to the intervention and is not a random occurrence.
   2. Reliable—Measuring what it is actually intended to measure.
   3. Not easy to manipulate; as objective and quantifiable as possible.
   4. Comprehensive—Covering most or all aspects of the process being measured.
   5. Dynamic—The measure can change to reflect changes in practice.
   6. Flexible—If an outcome measure can demonstrate outcomes for more than one process or be used to demonstrate multiple outcomes, this is a positive attribute.
   7. Cogent—The outcome measure must make sense to the user.
B. The National Quality Measures Clearinghouse (2015) identified the following desirable attributes of performance measures:
   1. Importance—Relevance to key stakeholders, strategic plan and strategic initiatives, and financial impact
   2. Scientific soundness—Clinical logic and properties of reliability, validity, stratification, and understandability
   3. Feasibility—The explicit specification of the measure, including the numerator and denominator as well as the availability of the data
C. The American Academy of Family Physicians (AAFP) recognized the need for quality, cost-effective health care by delineating the following criteria to evaluate the need, quality, and acceptability of a performance measure: importance, measurability, and achievability (AAFP, 2015).

The AAFP supports the development and application of performance measures that have the following attributes:

1. Focused on improving important processes and outcomes of care in terms that matter to patients
2. Responsive to informed patients' cultures, values, and preferences
3. Based on best evidence and reflect variations in care consistent with appropriate professional judgment
4. Are practical given variations of systems and resources available across practice settings
5. Do not separately evaluate cost of care from quality and appropriateness
6. Take into account the burden of data collection, particularly in the aggregation of multiple measures
7. Provide transparency for methodology used
8. Assess patient well-being, satisfaction, access to care, disparities, and health status
9. Are updated regularly or when new evidence is developed

D. The nursing outcomes classification (Moorhead et al., 2013) identifies three main influences of nursing outcomes:

1. Patient characteristics, such as diagnosis, prognosis, education level, socioeconomic status, and understanding of disease process
2. Nurse characteristics, such as type of licensure, education level, knowledge, skills, and abilities
3. Systems characteristics, such as medical services, community resources, and benefits programs

E. The National Database for Nursing Quality Indicators (NDNQI) is committed to indicator development that is based on empirical research. Those indicators, which are deemed to provide the most value for the effort, are added to the menu of NDNQI nursing-sensitive indicators. The process for developing an indicator includes the following steps:

1. Review of the peer-reviewed literature to determine which indicators have been shown to be nursing sensitive and if there have been reliability studies.
2. Discussions with topic experts to identify measurement issues and additional information that should be collected to support hospital reports or analysis, for example, patient risk level.
3. Develop a plan for data collection and reports.
4. Solicit comments from participating facilities on the feasibility of proposed data collection plan and the utility of the indicators.
5. Conduct pilot studies with volunteer hospitals to test the data collection guidelines and forms.
6. Revise plan for data collection and reports.
7. Develop the Web data collection system, including administrative sections of the database, data entry screens, and tutorial.
8. Announce the availability of the new indicator to member hospitals so that staff may take the tutorial and begin data collection and submission.
9. Conduct data analysis and development of quarterly reports (Montalvo, 2007).

F. When designing an evaluation for the case management program, it is important to describe the goals and objectives before you embark on the evaluation. It is also necessary to write the objectives using the SMART format and define the short-, intermediate-, and long-term objectives. Other aspects of the objectives one must pay close attention to, especially from a case management perspective, is the fact that they may be structure, process, or outcomes oriented and often address Donabedian's quality trilogy.

1. The goal establishes the overall direction and focus of the evaluation program. It is the foundation for developing the objectives of the evaluation and typically consists of a broad general statement that describes what the program plans to accomplish. Sometimes, more than one goal exists.

2. Objectives are the steps or building blocks toward achieving the goal. An objective is a specific and usually quantifiable statement of program achievement. Collectively, objectives represent a quantification of the program goal(s):

   a. Structure objectives are those that measure the characteristics of the program of care provision (e.g., case management program) such as number of staff, educational background, or types of services offered. An example is percentage of case managers who are certified.

   b. Process objectives are those that focus on the systems of care such as the actions and activities of case managers to be completed in a specific time period. They support accountability by setting specific activities to be completed by specific dates and explain what and when they will be completed. For example, brokering postdischarge services for a client before discharge from the acute care setting.

   c. Outcome objectives usually define the expected results or consequences of the structure and process objectives:

      i. They are specific and concise statements that state who will do what, how much, where, and by when.

      ii. Clear, concise outcome objectives clarify program expectations and can be used to determine progress toward achieving the program goal(s).

      iii. Outcome objectives are meant to be realistic targets for a program. In this sense, they represent the expectations and become the yardstick by which real or observed accomplishments will be assessed. For example, achieving a rate of reimbursement denials that is less than 3%.

   d. SMART objectives are specific, measurable, achievable, realistic, and timely (SMART). There is no single correct way to write a SMART objective. The real test is to compare the objective statement to the SMART criteria (Box 22-3).

   e. Developing objectives requires time, orderly thinking, and a clear picture of the results expected from program activities.

      i. Short-term objectives are generally expected immediately or within a short time frame (e.g., months) and occur soon after a program, a care strategy, or an improvement is implemented.

      ii. Intermediate objectives result from and follow short-term outcomes. Intermediate outcomes can be prerequisites to

BOX 22-3 Guide to Writing SMART Objectives

Specific
- Who is the target population?
- What will be accomplished?

Measureable
- Is the objective quantifiable?
- Can the objective be measured?
- How much change or improvement is expected? (target)

Achievable
- Can the objective be accomplished in the proposed time frame with the available resources and support?

Realistic
- Does the objective address the goal?
- Will the objective have an impact on the goal?

Timely
- Does the objective propose a timeline when the objective will be met?

---

long-term outcomes. If unmet, the ultimate objective cannot be met. For example, switching intravenous antibiotics for severe pneumonia to oral medications when a patient is afebrile and free of symptoms.

   iii. Long-term objectives state the ultimate expected impact of a program. Sometimes, they are referred to discharge or end of a care encounter outcomes. For example, discharging a severe pneumonia patient from the acute care setting when free of symptoms after switching to oral antibiotics.

Outcome Measures Selection and Development

A. In order to develop a robust outcomes measurement system or program, it is important to involve stakeholders who are affected by the service being measured because the process should be transparent and pertinent to their needs as much as external requirements (e.g., regulation) or operational goals.

B. The Health Resource and Services Administration (HRSA, 2011) suggests a steps approach to developing performance measures (Box 22-4).

C. In order to better organize and categorize the development and implementation of outcomes indicators, Advocate Health Care developed the Indicator Development Form (Lloyd, 2004), which has been widely used in the measurement field. This form is divided into three major parts (Box 22-5).

   1. Part I—Identification of an indicator. To identify an indicator, one must examine and/or determine the processes and outcomes of interest and why.

   2. Part II—Indicator development and data collection. It is necessary to maintain clarity of the indicator and its use and to prevent confusion from occurring.

BOX 22-4   HRSA's Approach to Performance Measurement

1. Evaluate organizational priorities:
   - Understand organizational goals prior to selecting measures.
   - Select measures, which demonstrate accomplishment of or progress toward organizational goals.
   - Consider organizational and other goals that are relevant to the organization and then what action-oriented steps necessary to achieve them.
2. Choose performance measures and methodology:
   - Measures should reliable, valid, and standardized.
   - Use measures, which have been approved/endorsed by organizations such as NQF or HEDIS.
   - Use data that is readily available to the organization.
   - Determine what constitutes success.
3. Determine baseline performance:
   - Use existing data to determine the baseline for future measurement.
   - This provides a basis for comparison and determination of improvement or decline.
4. Evaluate performance (ongoing):
   - Ways in which to measure may include percent compliance, means, medians, and other rates.
   - Actual versus expected performance.
   - Comparing performance against target(s) and benchmark(s).
5. Report results:
   - Understand the audience and present information in an easy-to-understand format.
   - Share measurement results internally.
   - Explain what results mean and take the opportunity to motivate staff.
   - Release external report(s), as required. Provide context to facilitate understanding of results.
6. Devise and implement a plan to address performance deficiencies.
7. Continue to monitor and measure performance (continuous cycle).

---

      3. Part III—Indicator analysis and interpretation. For effective use and interpretation of findings related to the indicator, one must be proactive in designing the analysis and interpretation processes/activities.

D. Common outcome indicators
    1. There are four broad categories of outcome indicators that are typically used for outcomes. These are:
      a. Clinical—Morbidity, mortality, improvement in clinical signs and symptoms, and absence of complications
      b. Functional—Activities of daily living (ADLs), instrumental activities of daily living (IADLs), ability to return to work or school, and maintaining a healthy life style
      c. Financial—Costs of care, savings, cost per year/per episode/per case, cost of job-related injuries, and recidivism
      d. Satisfaction or care experience—Patient/family, physician, staff, and referral source

E. For the nursing profession, a group of researchers at the University of Iowa (Moorhead et al., 2013) have developed the Nursing Outcomes

22-5 Guide to Advocate Health Care's Indicator Development Form

Part I—Identification of an indicator
- Processes and outcomes the indicator measures
- Rationale for the indicator
- Name of the indicator
- Identification of the teams to which the indicator applies
- Identification of the objectives the indicator satisfies
- Dimensions of excellence the indicator is designed to measure
- Literature references for the indicator

Part II—Indicator development and data collection
- Operational definition
- Description of the data collection plan
- Data collection sampling requirements
- Baseline data for the indicator
- Target or goal for the indicator

Part III—Indicator analysis and interpretation
- The analysis plan, including the statistics to be used (e.g., descriptive, analysis of variance)
- Graphs that will be used
- Data reporting plan, including who will receive the results and how often they will receive the results

Classification (NOC), which is a taxonomy of standardized nursing-sensitive patient/client outcomes.
1. The taxonomy includes outcomes that:
   a. Nursing can affect.
   b. Apply to an individual recipient of nursing care.
   c. Apply to a lay caregiver of an individual.
   d. Describe states and behaviors.
   e. Encompass the entire continuum of care.
   f. Provide a consistent measure of patient/client and lay caregiver status.
2. NOC is a three-level classification system currently composed of 7 domains, 29 outcome classes, and 260 outcomes. The seven health domains in the NOC include:
   a. Functional health
   b. Physiologic health
   c. Psychosocial health
   d. Health knowledge and behaviors
   e. Perceived health
   f. Family health
   g. Community health
F. There have been initial discussions about creating a framework for classifying social work outcomes.
   1. One social work expert (Mullen, 2001) has suggested that the dimensions to be included in a health and mental health social work outcomes measurement framework should include the following variations by:
      a. System level—Clinical, program, and system

  b. Geographical unit—Local, municipality, region, nation, and group of nations

  c. Outcomes measurement questions asked—Efficacy, efficiency, quality, and equity

  d. Effects sought across a continuum of possibilities—Mortality, physiologic, clinical events, generic or specific health-related quality-of-life measures, composite measures of outcomes, and time

 2. The purpose of this outcomes measurement program is performance measurement and management or outcomes research.

G. The Health Enhancement Research Organization (HERO) and Population Health Alliance (PHA) (2015) in their publication, Program Measurement and Evaluation Guide: Core Metrics for Employee Health Management, identified the following categorizes for measurement domains in health management programs delivered to an employer's population, including:

 1. Financial outcomes

 2. Health impact

 3. Participation

 4. Satisfaction

 5. Organizational support

 6. Productivity and performance

 7. Value on investment

H. Cesta and Tahan (2003) broadly classified outcomes into two categories: those that have an effect on the health care organization and those that have an effect on the patient/consumer of health care services:

 1. Outcomes that affect the organization are those that are not directly related to the patient's health. Examples may include patient satisfaction, staff satisfaction, turnaround time of tests and procedures or results, cost per case, length of stay, and interdisciplinary communication.

 2. Outcomes that affect the patient's health tend to be more clinical in nature. They are not directly related to the health care organization. Examples may include prevention of complications in patient's condition, improvement of signs and symptoms of a disease, physical functioning/functional status, and well-being and quality of life.

I. The National Quality Forum (NQF) developed a Framework for Care Coordination that serves as the basis for identifying and organizing NQF-endorsed preferred practices and performance measures based on a set of interrated domains that are applicable to multiple settings, diverse patient populations, and various providers of care (NQF, 2010):

 1. The NQF has endorsed a set of 25 preferred care coordination practices that are suitable for widespread implementation that addresses the domains of the Framework for Care Coordination and the National Priorities Partnership goals.

 2. The preferred care coordination practices were evaluated for their adequacy using NQF-endorsed standard evaluation criteria for all practices, including:

  a. Effectiveness—Clear evidence is presented that indicates that the practice is effective in improving outcomes.

  b. Generalizability—The practice is able to be used in multiple care settings and/or for multiple types of patients.

    c. Benefit—It is clear how the practice improves or increases the likelihood of improving patient outcomes.

    d. Readiness—The training, technology, and staff required for implementation of the practice are available.

Case Management–Specific Outcomes

A. Because case management practice occurs across the health care continuum and is conducted by professionals from a range of health and human services disciplines, it is particularly challenging to develop standardized outcomes metrics. However, there are numerous leading health care organizations and agencies that provide framework for quality health care delivery. These frameworks should be leveraged throughout case management documentation.

B. From a quality perspective, suggested outcome indicators for case management practice include examination of structure, process, and outcomes (Box 22-6).

C. Case managers must also embrace individual accountability and an outcomes-driven ethos. Key elements of outcomes-driven case management include:

    1. Client—The outcomes-driven case manager focuses on maximizing his or her client's health, wellness, and other considerations.

    2. Strategic focus—Working with the client and the care team to establish goals, it is essential to consider the appropriateness of the goal and to what extent moves the client toward optimal function and independence.

BOX 22-6   Examples of Case Management Outcome Indicators/Measures

Structure
- Percentage of certified case managers
- Average caseload per case manager
- Ratio of supervisor to case managers
- Accreditation status of case management program
- Turnover rate for case management staff

Process
- Percentage of clients with documentation of physician collaboration
- Percentage of clients with a written care plan
- Average number of days from referral date to first contact with client
- Average number of days from referral date to care plan
- Average number of case management hours per client
- Percentage of clients with documentation of consent to case management intervention

Outcomes
- Percentage of clients able to assume effective self-management responsibility
- Percentage of clients who are adherent to care/treatment plan
- Percentage of clients who are satisfied or very satisfied with case management intervention
- Percentage of physicians who are satisfied or very satisfied with case management intervention
- Percentage of patients/clients who returned to work

3. Evidence-based practice—Interventions in alignment with IOM-defined, evidence-based practice (e.g., best research evidence, best clinical experience, consistency with client values) leading to better client outcomes and quality care (Treiger & Fink-Samnick, 2015).

D. The NQF-endorsed Framework for Care Coordination serves as a road map for the identification of a set of preferred practices and performance measures:

1. The framework identified five key care coordination domains: health care home, proactive plan of care and follow-up, communication, information systems, and transitions or handoffs (NQF, 2010).

2. The NQF is a partner in the National Priorities Partnership (NPP), a national effort to set national priorities and goals. In November 2008, the NPP deemed care coordination as one of six national priorities and agreed to work toward the following goals, which can be translated into performance measures, such as:

   a. Improve care and achieve quality by facilitating and carefully considering feedback from all patients regarding coordination of their care

   b. Improve communication around medication information

   c. Work to reduce 30-day readmission rates

   d. Work to reduce preventable emergency department visits by 50%

E. AHRQ's Care Coordination Measures Atlas:

1. As care coordination is an essential task of case management, AHRQ's Care Coordination Measures Atlas serves as an objective launching point for selecting meaningful measures of case management intervention. The Atlas aims to support the field of care coordination measurement by:

   a. Providing a list of existing measures of care coordination.

   b. Organizing measures along two dimensions (domain and perspective) in order to facilitate selection of care coordination measures by Atlas users.

   c. Developing a framework for understanding care coordination measurement, incorporating elements from other proposed care coordination frameworks whenever possible. The framework is designed to support current and future development of this field, while remaining flexible so that it may be adapted as the field matures (McDonald et al., 2014).

F. The Council for Case Management Accountability (CCMA) was formed in 1996 by the Case Management Society of America (CMSA) in response to a growing demand for accountability in health care through outcomes reporting. Although no current work has been produced by the CCMA, the accountability perspective must continue to serve as a foundation for development of outcome measures:

1. The CCMA sought opinions from numerous stakeholders regarding case management outcomes and identified the following direct outcomes of case management:

   a. Patient/client knowledge

   b. Patient/client involvement in care

   c. Patient/client empowerment

   d. Improved adherence

   e. Improved coordination of care

2. The CCMA developed the dimensions of accountability, which provide a framework for linking core functions of case management (e.g., assessment, planning, facilitation, evaluation, advocacy) to the direct outcomes of case management and the end outcomes of the health system, including:
   a. Improved health status
   b. Increased quality of care
   c. Decreased costs
G. The IHI Triple Aim:
   1. The IHI Triple Aim is a framework that describes an approach to optimizing health system performance, which encourages designs to simultaneously pursue three dimensions, referred to as the Triple Aim:
      a. Improving the patient experience of care (including quality and satisfaction)
      b. Improving the health of populations
      c. Reducing the per capita cost of health care (IHI, 2015b)
   2. The CCMA dimensions of accountability (noted above) clearly align with the Triple Aim. Program documentation and outcome measurements should also reflect this alignment.
H. Institute of Medicine (IOM):
   1. Crossing the Quality Chasm (Institute of Medicine, 2001) outlines six aims for 21st century health care (Box 22-7).
I. The hospital value-based purchasing (VBP) program, which began in October 2011, impacts the practice of case management and offer an opportunity for case management programs to demonstrate their values to health care executives, clients/support systems, and other stakeholders. The outcome measures included in the VBP:
   1. VBP is a Centers for Medicare and Medicaid Services (CMS) initiative that rewards acute care hospitals with incentive payments for the quality of care they provide to Medicare beneficiaries.
   2. Hospitals are rewarded based on how closely they follow best clinical practices and how well they enhance patients' experiences of care.

BOX 22-7 **IOM's Six Aims of Quality Health Care**

- *Safe*—Avoiding injuries to patients from the care that is intended to help them
- *Effective*—Providing services based on scientific knowledge to all who could benefit and refraining from providing services to those not likely to benefit (avoiding underuse and overuse)
- *Patient centered*—providing care that is respectful of and responsive to individual patient preferences, needs, and values and ensuring that patient values guide all clinical decisions
- *Timely*—Reducing waits and sometimes harmful delays for both those who receive and those who give care
- *Efficient*—Avoiding waste, in particular waste of equipment, supplies, ideas, and energy
- *Equitable*—Providing care that does not vary in quality because of personal characteristics such as gender, ethnicity, geographic location, and socioeconomic status

CMS believes that when hospitals follow proven best practices, patients receive higher-quality care and see better outcomes.

3. In 2015, hospitals were at risk for 1.50% of base operating Diagnosis-Related Group (DRG) reimbursement amounts, as required by the statute. In fiscal year 2016, the percentage rises to 1.75%, and by fiscal year 2017, it reaches 2.00% and stabilizes thereafter.

4. Case management leaders may incorporate the outcome measures included in the VBP in the evaluation of case management as appropriate.

5. In fiscal year 2016 (payment adjustment effective for discharges from October 1, 2015 to September 30, 2016), the VBP program includes a total of 24 measures.

6. The VBP measures are represented in four different domains as follows:
   a. Patient/client experience of care measured using the Hospital Consumer Assessment of Health Care Providers and Systems (HCAHPS)
   b. Outcome of care, which focuses on mortality rates in specific diagnoses including heart failure, pneumonia and myocardial infarction, patient safety, and health care associated infections
   c. Process of care, which focuses on use of specific medications in certain patient populations such as beta-blockers, discharge instructions, and removal of urinary catheters
   d. Efficiency which addresses cost of care (CMS, 2015)

Incorporating Outcomes Measurement into Case Management Practice

A. Build outcome measures into any new intervention, process, or program:
   1. Consider the goals that led to the intervention, process, or program.
   2. List the problems you are trying to solve.
   3. Describe exactly what you want to improve.

B. List the method you will use to determine whether you have reached your goal:
   1. Describe what things will occur when you have achieved the desired outcome (e.g., no patients will be rehospitalized in the first 60 days after discharge for the same or a related diagnosis; or Mrs. Smith will schedule doctor's appointments at least one time per month and keep the scheduled appointments).
   2. Be as specific and as descriptive as possible.

C. Determine how you can measure that achievement using different research designs:
   1. Before-and-after comparison—For example, how many appointments were scheduled and kept before case management; or before case management, 90% of patients returned to the hospital within 60 days past discharge, and after case management, rehospitalization within 60 days occurred with only 20% of patients.
   2. Randomized comparison—For example, a group of patients who are statistically similar is chosen. The group is randomly assigned to one of two groups before the intervention is tested. One group receives the intervention, and the other group does not receive the

intervention. The two groups are compared and the impact of the intervention is evaluated.

3. Comparison groups—For example, compare a group of patients receiving an intervention with a statistically similar group of patients who do not receive the intervention. This differs from the randomized comparison in that the groups may not have been selected in advance of the comparison, and the groups may have differing reasons for why an intervention was not given.

4. Other methods of measuring impact include:
   a. Comparison with established benchmarks (e.g., recommendations for hemoglobin A_1C testing in diabetics).
   b. Progress toward an established goal. (This could include increasing or decreasing a particular measurement. For example, admissions for congestive heart failure patients have declined 15%, and we expect to reach our goal of 45% reduction in 3 months.)

D. Identify the best reporting method:
   1. Use of a database can allow you to report in multiple ways and from multiple perspectives.
   2. Depending on their needs, different perspectives are requested by different people.
   3. If you are unable to show the results in a way that will allow your audience to identify the value of the results to them or to those for whom they are responsible, your results may not receive the attention they deserve.
   4. Identify people who are the stakeholders in the process:
      a. When establishing a report, it is important to know who will be receiving the report and why the report is needed.
      b. Determine what you know or understand about the stakeholders in order to gain insight into the problem from their perspective. For example, physicians may need to know which of their patients have not had a recommended test or treatment in order to ensure that the patient gets the needed service, and the unit manager may want to know the test or treatment that is most frequently missed in order to examine interventions that may be used to remind practitioners to complete the service.
   5. Make sure your report addresses the needs of the stakeholders.
   6. Become familiar with the use of graphs, charts, and diagrams that will provide an interesting and illustrative visual representation of the data.

E. Ask and answer the "so what?" question:
   1. Quantify or describe the impact or final outcome of the process.
   2. If you increased or improved something, what changed other than the process? For example, if the patient keeps all of his or her doctor's appointments, what happens as a result? If readmissions decline, were costs decreased or were patients more satisfied?

F. Think in terms of quantifying and measuring:
   1. Instead of describing and explaining, think of objective ways to count or measure the event.
   2. Collect baseline measurements to use as a comparison for improvement. It is difficult to judge progress without recording your starting point.
   3. Ask yourself how you will know whether your plans or programs are working and how you can demonstrate that success to others.

G. Learn how to use databases and other computer programs:
   1. Databases can store information in a format that allows it to be retrieved in various ways.
   2. This flexibility allows the case manager to look at all of the available information in several ways:
      a. Sorted by different factors such as age, diagnosis, and interventions
      b. Sorted by common factors, such as all those with "x, y, and z"
      c. Sorted by different elements, such as all those with "x, but not y or z."
   3. Looking at the data in different ways can help identify outcomes or suggest other areas for study.
H. Review statistical principles:
   1. Know the key statistical tools to be used in simple comparisons.
   2. Familiarize yourself with the methods of critically reading and evaluating research papers and findings.
I. Review the continuous quality improvement (CQI) processes and tools:
   1. Develop an understanding of key CQI principles.
   2. Be familiar with CQI tools for process improvement.

Common Issues in Outcomes Reporting

A. Varying definitions—For effective comparisons, definitions need to be exact. Even if there are similarities, minute differences can alter the results of a comparison.
   1. For example, compare workers' compensation case management with hospital-based case management. Both are forms of case management, but evaluation would reveal distinct differences.
   2. For case management to compare outcomes across the industry, definitions must be precise.
B. Varying methodologies—In addition to definitions, the methods for calculating and reporting results must be consistent. It is impossible to complete a valid comparison of results if the methodology used to determine the results is different.
C. Sharing of outcomes methodologies—Some organizations believe that the definitions, methodologies, and reporting practices are proprietary to them. For this reason, they do not wish to share these details with the industry at large.
   1. In order to create an opportunity for the growth of outcomes methodology and reporting, organizations on the forefront of case management should gain recognition for setting the standard in outcomes methodology rather than for being the only one with good outcomes methodology.
   2. Case management will only be able to establish its ongoing relevancy in the health care system by having nationally recognized process and outcomes metrics for comparison purposes and for demonstrating its value.

References

Agency for Healthcare Research and Quality (AHRQ). (2015). About AHRQ. Retrieved from http://www.ahrq.gov/cpi/about/index.html, on August 19, 2015.

American Academy of Family Physicians (AAFP). (2015). Criteria for the development and application of performance measures. Accessed on April 25, 2015 from http://www.aafp.org/about/policies/all/performance-measures.html

American Society for Quality (ASQ). (2015). Quality. Retrieved from http://asq.org/glossary/q. html, on August 20, 2015.

Business Dictionary.com. (2015a). Variation. Retrieved from http://www.businessdictionary. com/definition/variation.html, on August 19, 2015.

BusinessDictionary.com. (2015b). Benchmark. Retrieved from http://www.businessdictionary. com/definition/benchmark.html#ixzz3jIfHK1lQ, on August 19, 2015.

Case Management Society of America. (2010). *Standards of practice for case management.* Little Rock, AR: Author.

Centers for Medicare and Medicaid Services (CMS). (2015). Medicare hospital compare: Hospital value-based program. Retrieved from https://www.medicare.gov/hospitalcompare/ Data/hospital-vbp.html, on August 22, 2015.

Cesta, T. G., & Tahan, H. A. (2003). *The case manager's survival guide: Winning strategies for clinical practice* (2nd ed.). St Louis, MO: Mosby.

Donabedian, A. (1966). Evaluating the quality of medical care. *Milbank Memorial Fund Quarterly, 44*(3), 166–206.

Donabedian, A. (1992). The role of outcomes in quality assessment and assurance. *Quality Review Bulletin, 11*, 356–360.

Ellwood, P. M. (1988). Outcomes management: A technology of patient experience. *New England Journal of Medicine, 319*(18), 1549–1556.

Health Enhancement Research Organization (HERO) and Population Health Alliance (PHA) (2015). *Program measurement and evaluation guide: Core metrics for employee health management.* Washington, DC: HERO and PHA.

Health Resources and Service Administration (HRSA). (2011). Performance management and measurement. Retrieved from http://www.hrsa.gov/quality/toolbox/508pdfs/performance-managementandmeasurement.pdf, on August 20, 2015.

Hickam, D. H., Weiss, J. W., Guise, J-M., Buckley, D., Motu'apuaka, M., Graham, E., ... Saha, S. (2013). *Outpatient Case Management for Adults with Medical Illness and Complex Care Needs. Comparative Effectiveness Review No. 99. (Prepared by the Oregon Evidence-based Practice Center under Contract No. 290-2007-10057-I.) AHRQ Publication No.13—EHC031-EF.* Rockville, MD: Agency for Healthcare Research and Quality. Retrieved from www.effectivehealthcare. ahrq.gov/reports/final.cfm, on August 19, 2015.

Institute for Healthcare Improvement (IHI). (2015a). About IHI. Retrieved from http://www. ihi.org/about/Pages/default.aspx, on August 19, 2015.

Institute for Healthcare Improvement (IHI). (2015b). Initiatives—About the triple aim. Retrieved from http://www.ihi.org/engage/initiatives/tripleaim/Pages/default.aspx, on August 21, 2015.

Institute of Medicine. (1990). Medicare: A strategy for quality assurance. Retrieved from http:// www.nap.edu/download.php?record_id=1547, on August 21, 2015.

Institute of Medicine. (2001). Crossing the quality chasm: A new health system for the 21st century. Committee on Quality of Health Care in America, Institute of Medicine. Retrieved from http://www.nap.edu/catalog/10027.html, on August 21, 2015.

The Leapfrog Group. (2015). About leapfrog. Retrieved from http://www.leapfroggroup.org/ about_leapfrog, on August 19, 2015.

Lloyd, R. (2004). *Quality health care: A guide to developing and using indicators* (1st ed.). Burlington, MA: Jones & Bartlett.

McDonald, K. M., Schultz, E., Albin, L., Pineda, N., Lonhart, J., Sundaram, V., ... Davies, S. (2014). Care Coordination Atlas Version 4 (Prepared by Stanford University under subcontract to American Institutes for Research on Contract No. HHSA290-2010-00005I). AHRQ Publication No. 14-0037-EF. Rockville, MD: Agency for Healthcare Research and Quality. Retrieved from http://www.ahrq.gov/sites/default/files/publications/files/ccm_atlas.pdf, on August 20, 2015.

Medicinenet.com. (2015). Standard of Care. Retrieved from http://www.medicinenet.com/ script/main/art.asp?articlekey=33263, on August 19, 2015.

Montalvo, I. (2007). The National Database of Nursing Quality Indicators (NDNQI). *Online Journal of Issues in Nursing, 12*(3), Manuscript 2. Retrieved from http://www.nursingworld. org/mainmenucategories/anamarketplace/anaperiodicals/ojin/tableofcontents/volume122007/no3sept07/nursingqualityindicators.aspx, on August 19, 2015.

Moorhead, S., Johnson, M., Maas, M., & Swanson, E. (Eds.) (2013). *Nursing outcomes classification (NOC)* (5th ed.). St. Louis, MO: Elsevier.

Mullen, E. J. (2001). *Outcomes measurement: A social work framework for health and mental health policy and practice.* New York: Columbia University School of Social Work.

National Quality Forum (NQF). (2010). *Preferred practices and performance measures for measuring and reporting care coordination; A consensus Report.* Washington, DC: National Academies Press.

National Quality Forum (NQF). (2015). About us. Retrieved from http://www.qualityforum.org/story/About_Us.aspx, on August 19, 2015.

National Quality Measures Clearinghouse. (2015). Desirable attributes of a quality measure. Retrieved from http://www.qualitymeasures.ahrq.gov/tutorial/attributes.aspx, on August 19, 2015.

Nolte, E., Conklin, A., Adams, J. L., Brunn, M., Cadier, B., Chevreul, K., ... Vrijhoef, H. (2013). Evaluating chronic disease management: Recommendations for funders and users. Prepared for the European Commission on behalf of the DISMEVAL Consortium. Retrieved from http://www.rand.org/content/dam/rand/pubs/technical_reports/2012/RAND_TR1213.pdf, on August 19, 2015.

Research Methods Knowledge Base. (2015a). External validity. Retrieved from http://www.socialresearchmethods.net/kb/external.php, on August 19, 2015.

Research Methods Knowledge Base. (2015b). Internal validity. Retrieved from http://www.socialresearchmethods.net/kb/intval.php, on August 19, 2015.

Research Methods Knowledge Base. (2015c). Reliability. Retrieved from http://www.socialresearchmethods.net/kb/reliable.php, on August 19, 2015.

The Society of Thoracic Surgeons. (2015). What is risk adjustment. Retrieved from http://www.sts.org/patient-information/what-risk-adjustment, on August 19, 2015.

Treiger, T. M., & Fink-Samnick, E. (2013). COLLABORATE©: A universal, competency-based paradigm for professional case management practice, part I. *Professional Case Management, 18*(3), 122–135. Retrieved from http://www.ncbi.nlm.nih.gov/pubmed/23584522, on August 19, 2015.

Treiger, T. M., & Fink-Samnick, E. (2015). *COLLABORATE© for professional case management: A university competency-based paradigm* (1st ed.). Philadelphia, PA: Wolters Kluwer.

Wojner, A. W. (2001). *Outcomes management: Applications to clinical practice.* St. Louis, MO: Mosby.

Select Specialty Practices in Case Management

CHAPTER 23

Behavioral Health and Integrated Case Management

Rebecca Perez and Deborah Gutteridge

LEARNING OBJECTIVES

Upon completion of this chapter, the reader will be able to:

1. Define the special needs of individuals with behavioral health conditions, mental health disorders, and developmental disabilities.
2. Compare and contrast different behavioral health case management models.
3. Discuss the diagnoses and treatment options of clients commonly referred to case management.
4. Identify and explore challenges in behavioral health case management practice.
5. Discuss briefly behavioral health treatment options.
6. Define Integrated Case Management.
7. Compare and contrast an integrated approach versus a traditional CM approach to working with complex clients or individuals.

IMPORTANT TERMS AND CONCEPTS

Adverse consequences
Assertive Community
  Treatment (ACT)
  Model
Behavioral Health
  Care
Behavioral Health Case
  Management

Behavioral Health
  Home Care
Diagnostic and
  Statistical Manual of
  Mental Disorders, 5th
  edition (DSM-5)
Integrated Case
  Management (ICM)

Self-Neglect
Severe and Persistent
  Mental Illness
  (SPMI)
Strengths Model
Substance-Related and
  Addictive Disorders

Introduction

A. The Case Management Society of America (CMSA) defines case management as "a collaborative process of assessment, planning, facilitation, [care coordination, evaluation,] and advocacy for options and services to meet an individual's [and family's comprehensive] health needs through communication and available resources to promote quality cost-effective outcomes" (CMSA, 2010, p. 6).

B. According to the National Alliance on Mental Illness (NAMI), case managers coordinate needed services and supports so that an individual can successfully live in the community (NAMI, 2015a).

C. Mental health promotion is an integral part of helping individuals with behavioral disorders. Promoting mental health is part of the case manager's duty to advocate for the individual and then to facilitate and coordinate the care and services that will ultimately result in mental health.

D. Mental health is more than just the absence of mental or behavioral disorders but an essential part of health in general. As noted by the World Health Organization (WHO), "There is no health without mental health" (WHO, 2014).

E. Promotion of mental health involves the creation of environments whereby individuals can receive support so that they can adopt healthier lifestyles.

F. Core functions of case management, which are essential when working with individuals who have severe mental health issues, include assessment, treatment planning, linkage, monitoring, and advocacy. Case management plays an integral role in coordination of care, and location and access to needed services and supports.

G. Individuals with mental illness often find it difficult and frustrating to find the right agency or provider. The WHO developed the action plan:
   1. Implementation of this action plan will help persons with mental illnesses find it easier to access services.
   2. Have their care delivered by appropriately skilled health workers in general health settings.
   3. Care will be delivered with treatment that is more responsive to the individual needs.
   4. Improve access to government disability benefits, housing, and employment programs (WHO, 2013).

H. There are many different mental and behavioral disorders that present differently. Generally, the individual will present with abnormal thoughts and abnormal perceptions, emotions, and behaviors (WHO, 2014).

I. Mental disorders include depression, bipolar affective disorder schizophrenia, psychoses, dementia, intellectual disabilities, and developmental disorders including autism spectrum disorders (ASD).

J. There are effective strategies for prevention and effective treatments for mental disorders and ways to help relieve the suffering of others. Depression is one mental disorder that can be prevented.

K. The key is to find health care and social services capable of providing treatment and the necessary support:
1. Serious mental illness is further complicated when chronic medical conditions, social issues, and problems with access to care are present.
    a. This is known as complexity, and approximately 10% of the population is considered complex.
    b. This small percentage of the population can often use more than 70% of health care resources (Kathol, Perez, & Cohen, 2010).
2. Mental conditions are more likely to be treated in the general medical sector.
    a. Primary care physicians give 70% of mental condition treatments, and 85% of mental health patients are seen in the physical health sector; these require an integrated approach, and all health and non–health-related issues need to be addressed.
    b. An integrated approach is very effective in addressing individuals with complex health problems (Kathol, Perez, & Cohen, 2010).
L. ICM may be provided in a variety of settings by nurses, social workers, and licensed behavioral health professionals. These professionals may be trained to provide an integrated approach in the acute care setting, clinics, health plans, and the community (Kathol, Perez, & Cohen, 2010).

Descriptions of Key Terms

A. Behavioral health care—A very broad category often used as an umbrella term for care that addresses behavioral problems bearing on health, including patient activation and health behaviors, mental health conditions, substance use, and other behaviors that bear on health. In this sense, behavioral health care is the job of all kinds of care settings and is done by clinicians and health coaches of various disciplines or training, including but not limited to mental health professionals. It is a competency of clinics, not only of individuals (Peek et al., 2013).
B. Behavioral health case management—It is difficult to find a contemporary definition that is specific to behavioral health case management. Perhaps, this is related to the fact that there is no universally accepted definition of case management in and of itself. For reference purposes, Farnsworth and Bigelow (1997) posited the following definition, a method of providing cost-effective, quality care (cost, process, experience, and outcomes) by managing the holistic health concerns of clients (individuals, families, and groups) who are in need of extensive services. It requires integrating, coordinating, and advocating for complex mental and physical health care services from a variety of health care providers and settings, within the framework of planned behavioral health outcomes (Farnsworth & Bigelow, 1997).
C. Diagnostic and Statistical Manual of Mental Disorders, 5th edition (DSM-5)—The Diagnostic and Statistical Manual of Mental Disorders is now in its fifth edition.

1. This text is used by clinicians and researchers to diagnose and classify mental disorders. It is the product of more than 10 years of effort by hundreds of international experts in all aspects of mental health and is considered an authoritative volume, which defines and classifies mental disorders in order to improve diagnoses, treatment, and research.

2. The criteria are concise and explicit, intended to facilitate an objective assessment of symptom presentations in a variety of clinical settings—inpatient, outpatient, partial hospital, consultation–liaison, clinical, private practice, and primary care. New features and enhancements make DSM-5 easier to use across all settings (American Psychiatric Association, 2013).

D. Self-neglect—Self-neglect is the result of an adult's inability to perform essential self-care tasks due to physical and/or mental impairments or diminished capacity. The tasks may include providing essential food, clothing, shelter, and health care; obtaining goods and services necessary to maintain physical health, mental health, emotional well-being, and general safety, and/or managing financial affairs and adhering to prescribed medications.

E. Severe and persistent mental illness (SPMI)—The term mental health professionals use to refer to mental illnesses with complex symptoms that require ongoing treatment and management, most often requiring varying types and dosages of medication and therapy (University of North Carolina, 2015).

F. Substance-related and addictive disorders—Mind-altering substances all yield three basic types of disorders: substance intoxication, substance withdrawal, and what we now call "substance use disorders." This was formerly referred to as substance dependence and substance abuse (Morrison, 2014).

Behavioral Health Case Management Models

A. The effectiveness of case management intervention in behavioral health and substance use disorder realms is mixed.

1. For behavioral health, outcomes vary across diagnosis grouping. Ziguras and Stuart meta-analysis demonstrated that the case management types that were studied were more effective than what was defined as usual treatment in three outcome domains: family burden, family satisfaction with services, and cost of care (Ziguras & Stuart, 2000).

2. Findings were favorable for intensive case management intervention when applied to patients with severe mental health disorders. Intensive case management compared to standard care was shown to reduce hospitalization and increase retention in care; it also improved social functioning (Dieterich, Park, & Marshall, 2010).

3. For substance use disorder, studies have reported positive effects in terms of the effectiveness of case management as compared with other interventions. Longitudinal effects of case management

intervention remain unclear. It was noted that strengths-based and generalist case management has proven to be relatively effective for substance abusers (Vanderplasschen, Wolf, Rapp, & Broekaert, 2007).

B. Conventional case management has been inconsistent with delivering integrative services located in the community. An assertive model that delivers clinically and cost-effective treatment demonstrates greater reductions in psychiatric rehospitalizations:

1. This model, known as assertive community treatment (ACT), has demonstrated results of lower arrests, jail days, and hospitalizations. One forensic ACT program showed 85% fewer hospital days, saving $917,000 in 1 year and 83% reduction in jail days, saving the cost of incarceration (Lamberti, Weisman & Faden, 2004).

2. ACT is a team-based approach that combines clinical services with care coordination, and case management plays a role in care coordination. When this occurs, outcomes are improved especially for those at most risk.

3. ACT is most effective for individuals with severe symptoms and behavioral impairment, pronounced disability in basic life skills, and/or prolonged course of illness (Bustillo & Weil, 2014). These individuals are not prepared to find the services they need in order to be a functioning member of the community. These services include housing, medical care, medication, and transportation (Bustillo & Weil, 2014).

C. Integrated case/care management is a preferred term pertaining to a parallel approach when there are co-occurring disorders in both medical and mental health realms.

1. Treatment of all disorders by the same clinician, collaborative goal setting with the individual, and demonstrating strength and empathy to develop a trusting relationship are the guiding principles of an integrated approach (Campbell, Caroff, & Mann, 2013).

2. Integrated case/care management means that all treating providers are aware of what the other is ordering. A common treatment plan is created. Communication is facilitated between providers, frequently by a case manager. The response to treatment is monitored and shared, and there is one case manager coordinating and communicating with the member and providers (Campbell, Caroff, & Mann, 2013).

D. Patient Protection and Affordable Care Act of 2010 (PPACA or ACA)—As pertains to behavioral and integrated health care, the ACA created an optional state benefit through Medicaid to coordinate care for individuals with chronic conditions. This whole person approach is known as a health home.

1. Health homes integrate and coordinate primary medical, acute, behavioral, and long-term care and support services, typically within the community. Health homes are for Medicaid recipients who have two or more chronic conditions, those who have one chronic condition but are at risk for another, and those who have one serious mental illness. Health home services include comprehensive care management, care coordination, health promotion, comprehensive transitional care, patient and family support, and referrals to community and social support services.

Applicability to CMSA'S Standards of Practice

A. The Case Management Society of America (CMSA) describes in its standards of practice for case management (CMSA, 2010) that case management practice extends across all health care settings, patient populations, and providers of various professional disciplines. This without a doubt applies to the practice of behavioral health case management.

B. Behavioral health case managers may use the CMSA standards as a guide for the implementation of their roles. All standards are relevant to caring for patients/clients with behavioral and emotional health issues, mental health conditions, and substance use and addiction. The standards include the clinical practice, legal and ethical expectations.

C. Case managers caring for the behavioral health patient population (whether combined with medical conditions or not) and across the various care settings must be aware of the CMSA standards of practice. They also must inform their employers and other professionals they collaborate with when dealing with a client with behavioral health concern about their existence, value, and need to adhere to them.

D. This chapter introduces case managers to the basic concepts of behavioral health case management practice and the role of the case manager in such settings and explains how collaboration may occur between case managers and other providers regardless of the care setting or specialty practice. This collaboration is necessary especially because behavioral health patients seek care not only in behavioral health settings but medical, surgical, and human services as well.

 Behavioral Health Care Conditions and Implications for Case Management

A. Mental health is an integral part of overall health. Health is a state of complete physical, mental, and social well-being and not merely the absence of disease or infirmity. Mental health is a state of well-being in which the individual is aware of his or her own abilities, can cope with the normal stressors of life, can function productively, and can make a contribution to the community (WHO, 2015).

B. Disparities remain as pertains to mental health treatment. For individuals in low- to middle-income countries, between 75% and 85% of people with mental disorders receive no treatment. But interestingly, those in higher-income countries, 36% to 50% receive no treatment (WHO, 2009).

C. Persons with SPMI frequently have physical health problems, in addition to other mental health and substance use disorder problems that require treatment.

1. Comorbid medical, mental health, and substance use present significant challenges. Individuals with these comorbidities need access to treatment, rehabilitation, and often support services that are easily accessible in the community. The case manager is integral in coordination of these often hard to access care and services. Good care coordination by the case manager is the glue that binds together an effective plan of care (De Hert et al., 2011; Scott & Dixon, 1997).

2. There are many mental health disorders and they present differently. Generally, mental disorders present with a combination of symptoms and behavior. These include abnormal thoughts, perceptions, behaviors, and abnormal behavior and relationships with others (National Institutes of Health, 2007).

D. The Diagnostic and Statistical Manual of Mental Disorders (DSM) is the standard classification of mental disorders used by health professionals in the United States.

1. The most recent edition, DSM-5, was published by the American Psychiatric Association (APA) in 2013.

2. The DSM-5 uses three major components in order to make a diagnosis: diagnostic classification, diagnostic criteria sets, and descriptive texts.

3. Some organizations have begun using the DSM-5 for criteria and coding, while others await the ICD-10 release to begin using both. The case manager should be mindful of the edition used for diagnostic coding, as it affects his/her respective job.

E. Depression

1. Depression is a common illness, affecting an estimated 350 million people worldwide. Depression may become a serious health issue when it lasts longer than a brief fluctuation in one's mood, which is a response to day-to-day life challenges. Individuals suffering from depression experience functional difficulties at work, at school, and in the family. At its worst, depression can lead to suicide. Suicide results in an estimated 1 million deaths every year (WHO, 2012).

2. Major depression is a mood disorder manifested by a depressed mood or loss of interest or pleasure in almost all activities for at least 2 weeks.

3. Additional symptoms such as weight changes, disturbances in sleeping pattern, change in psychomotor activity, persistent feelings of guilt or worthlessness, difficulty concentrating or thinking, impairment of social or occupational role expectations, or suicidal ideation may also be present.

4. Despite effective treatments, less than half of people affected receive adequate treatment. This number rises to upward of 90% in some countries (WHO, 2012).

5. Barriers to effective care include a lack of adequate assessment, inaccurate assessment, lack of resources, lack of trained health care providers, and social stigma associated with mental disorders (WHO, 2012). The case manager should be mindful of barriers, which may be addressed as part of the case management plan.

6. The depressed patient may present for evaluation or treatment following a suicide attempt, a past history of suicide attempt along with depression should trigger high risk for suicide. Major depressive disorder can last 6 months or longer if left untreated.

7. Alcohol or other substance abuse can mask symptoms of this disorder. Clients may abuse substances in an attempt to self-medicate symptoms. A careful history of substance use including nicotine should be taken.

8. Depression is diagnosed and treated by trained health professionals delivering primary health care. Once the diagnosis has been

established, management should include psychosocial aspects, including identification of stress triggers such as financial problems, poor work performance, physical or mental abuse, or presence or absence of social support (Box 23-1) (WHO, 2012).

9. Case managers should ask patients if they are considering suicide or self-harm.

   a. Patients may demonstrate increased suicide potential by giving away belongings, making a will, saying goodbye to loved ones, or hoarding medications.

   b. Some patients act on suicidal ideation after initiating treatment for depression, when energy levels begin to improve.

   c. Case managers should be vigilant about the suicide risk in these patients and be watchful of signs that a patient is considering suicide. Refer to Appendix A for additional details on suicide precautions.

F. Alcohol Use Disorder, Substance-related, and Addictive Disorders

   1. Persons exhibiting alcohol abuse show a maladaptive pattern of alcohol use that results in one or more of the following in a 12-month period; DSM-5 defines substance use disorder as core behavior of persons who misuse substances. DSM-5 lists over 300 numbered (in ICD-10) substance-related disorders (Morrison, 2014). Addiction includes behavioral, physiological, and cognitive symptoms.

   2. Alcohol use disorder (AUD) is the medical condition diagnosed when a patient's drinking causes distress or harm. The DSM-5 integrates previously identified separate disorders, alcohol abuse and alcohol dependence, into a single disorder called AUD with mild, moderate, and severe subclassifications (National Institute on Alcohol Abuse and Alcoholism, 2015).

BOX

23-1 **Caring for Patients with Depression**

- Recommended treatment options for moderate–severe depression consist of basic psychosocial support combined with antidepressant medication or psychotherapy, such as cognitive–behavior therapy, interpersonal psychotherapy, or problem-solving treatment.
- Psychosocial treatments are effective and should be the first-line treatment for mild depression. Medicines and psychological treatments are effective in cases of moderate and severe depression.
- Antidepressants along with talking therapies can be very effective for moderate to severe depression. Prescription of an antidepressant should not be the first line of treatment in mild depression. They should not be used for treating depression in children and are not the first-line treatment for adolescents (WHO, 2012).
- Case management services for this patient population focus on the following:
  - Suicide prevention.
  - Referral for psychotherapy and significant other(s) involvement and education. Some clients find the support and structure of group psychotherapy beneficial, especially if social dysfunction has occurred as a result of depression.
  - Supporting antidepressant therapy and monitoring for side effects.
  - Education of family members about the illness, treatment, and signs of recurrence.

3. In 2013, 24.6% of people ages 18 or older reported that they engaged in binge drinking in the past month; 6.8% reported that they engaged in heavy drinking in the past month (Substance Abuse and Mental Health Services Administration, 2013).
4. Case manager must determine the substance involved, resulting problem, and how the substance use impacts the problem behavior.
5. Essential features of substance use disorder fall into three main categories (Box 23-2) according to the US Department of Health and Human Services (MentalHealth.gov, 2015).
6. Substance withdrawal
   a. A physiologic dependence that is characterized by evidence of tolerance (needing more of the substance to produce a desired effect) and withdrawal when administration of the substance is discontinued.
   b. Type of withdrawal dependent on substance used may include alteration in mood (anxiety, irritability, depression), abnormal motor activity (restlessness, immobility), sleep disturbance (insomnia or hypersomnia), or other physical problems (fatigue, changes in appetite) (Morrison, 2014).
   c. Delirium tremens may be considered a more severe form of withdrawal of alcohol and is considered to be a medical emergency.

BOX 23-2) Categories of Substance Use Disorders

- Behavioral
  - Drop in attendance and performance at work or school
  - Frequently getting into trouble (fights, accidents, illegal activities)
  - Using substances in physically hazardous situations such as while driving or operating a machine
  - Engaging in secretive or suspicious behaviors
  - Changes in appetite or sleep patterns
  - Unexplained change in personality or attitude
  - Sudden mood swings, irritability, or angry outbursts
  - Periods of unusual hyperactivity, agitation, or giddiness
  - Lacking of motivation
  - Appearing fearful, anxious, or paranoid, with no reason

- Physical
  - Bloodshot eyes and abnormally sized pupils
  - Sudden weight loss or weight gain
  - Deterioration of physical appearance
  - Unusual smells on breath, body, or clothing
  - Tremors, slurred speech, or impaired coordination

- Social
  - Sudden change in friends, favorite hangouts, and hobbies
  - Legal problems related to substance use
  - Unexplained need for money or financial problems
  - Using substances even though it causes problems in relationships

7. Substance-related and addictive disorders are diagnosed by history, physical examination, and interview. The condition can go undiagnosed if the patient continues to use substances and no withdrawal symptoms are observed. Over time, patients with this disorder may be increasingly unable to fulfill occupational or social expectations, which may cause distress.
8. Treatment of substance-related and addictive disorders is dependent of the substance used and may include the following:
   a. Inpatient hospitalization
   b. Support groups
   c. Individualized psychotherapy
   d. Group psychotherapy
   e. Partial hospitalization/day treatment
   f. Abstinence
9. Treatment should include an integrated team approach, to include person's family and/or available support systems.
10. Care plan development by the case manager should include thorough assessment of available resources to cover potential treatment options, as mental health benefits are often limited.
11. Alcoholism is very common substance disorder. Treatment focuses primarily on alcohol abstinence and 12-step meetings (e.g., Alcoholics Anonymous) or a recovery program (e.g., Rational Recovery, Self-Management and Recovery Training [SMART] Recovery).
12. Case managers support the treatment plan through assessment, monitoring, planning, and resource utilization.
    a. Use of proven screening tools as part of assessing high-risk individuals (e.g., CAGE questionnaire, Alcohol Use Disorder Identification Test [AUDIT]). CAGE refers to the four clinical interview questions (CAGE questions) that have proven useful in helping to make a diagnosis of alcoholism. The questions focus on Cutting down, Annoyance by criticism, Guilty feeling, and Eye-openers. The acronym "CAGE" helps health care professionals recall the questions.
    b. Monitor adherence to medication and treatment program.
    c. Provide resources and encouragement to patients and their significant others (e.g., 12-step programs, private treatment centers).
    d. Remain mindful of the fact that chronic alcohol dependence is associated with social deterioration, decreased tolerance, medical complications of every organ, including liver impairment, which may interfere with the elimination of medications the patient may be on, causing risk for drug toxicity. Monitor for other health-related complications and coordinate care with primary providers (e.g., medical home, behavioral health home).
G. Bipolar disorder
   1. Persons diagnosed with bipolar disorder, a mood disorder, and experience episodes of major depression and mania or hypomania. The individual is either elated and expansive or irritable.
   2. For the diagnosis to be made, a change in mood must be present for at least 1 week (unless the individual is hospitalized with these

symptoms) or three of the following symptoms must be present for a 2-week period: inflated self-esteem or grandiosity, decreased need for sleep, pressured speech, flight of ideas, distractibility, psychomotor agitation, overinvolvement with pleasurable activities to the point of damaging consequences, reckless spending, or reckless behavior.

3. There are no diagnostic tests for bipolar disorder. Diagnosis is made through careful history, interview of client and family or care giver, and observation of both verbal and nonverbal behaviors.

   a. The Young Mania Rating Scale (YMRS) may sometimes be used to quantify the quality and degree of mania (Psychology-Tools.com, 2015).

   b. Brain scans and blood tests may be helpful in ruling out other factors contributing to mood problems such as stroke or brain tumor. Bipolar will worsen if left untreated or undiagnosed.

4. About 50% of clients with bipolar disorder have concurrent substance abuse disorders. There are four basic types of bipolar disorder described in Box 23-3 (National Institute for Mental Health, 2015a).

5. Bipolar disorder usually develops in late teens or early adult years, with at least half of all cases occurring prior to age 25 and usually spans a lifetime.

6. Patients with bipolar disorder tend to be high risk for suicide or self-harm particularly during periods of high impulsivity or when psychotic symptoms develop. Patients are more likely to seek treatment when they are depressed than when experiencing mania.

7. Treatment focuses primarily on suicide prevention, prescription of mood-stabilizing medication and monitoring of blood levels and for side effects of drugs, and psychotherapy.

8. Case managers support the treatment plan through assessment, monitoring, planning, and resource utilization.

   a. Use of proven screening tools as part of assessing high-risk individuals (e.g., CAGE adapted to include drugs [CAGE-AID] questionnaire, drug abuse severity test [DAST]).

   b. Provide support for patients and their significant others who may benefit from support groups (e.g., Narcotics Anonymous, private treatment centers).

BOX 23-3   Types of Bipolar Disorders

- Bipolar I Disorder: Defined by manic or mixed episodes that last at least 1 week or by manic symptoms so severe the person requires immediate hospital care. Depressive episodes occur as well, typically lasting at least 2 weeks.
- Bipolar II Disorder: Defined by a pattern of depressive episodes and hypomanic episodes but no full-blown manic or mixed episodes.
- Bipolar Disorder Not Otherwise Specified (BP-NOS): Diagnosed when symptoms of the illness are present but do not meet diagnostic criteria for either bipolar I or II; however, symptoms are clearly out of normal range of persons' behavior.
- Cyclothymic Disorder or Cyclothymic: A mild form of bipolar disorder wherein people have episodes of hypomania as well as depression for at least 2 years; however, diagnostic criteria for other types of bipolar disorder not met.

    c. Monitor medication and treatment adherence
       i. Patients may not like the loss of euphoria produced when mood is stabilized and may have difficulty adhering to the treatment regimen.
      ii. Coordinate and follow-through on laboratory testing required for mood stabilization medications.
     iii. Monitor for use of herbal and over-the-counter supplements, which may affect prescription medication absorption and efficacy.
     iv. Monitor weight and metabolic changes, which may require referral to nutrition counseling.
    d. The case manager addresses these issues proactively with the client, family/caregiver, and other members of the multidisciplinary team.

H. Schizophrenia
  1. Persons diagnosed with schizophrenia suffer from symptoms that impair functioning and involve disturbances in feelings, thinking, and behavior. Stigma and discrimination often result in a lack of access to care and social services. With appropriate treatment and psychosocial support, individuals can learn to lead a productive life and even recover (WHO, 2014).
  2. Patients may experience delusions, hallucinations, looseness of associations, social withdrawal, absence of motivation, impoverishment of thought, inappropriate affect, agitation, catatonia, and/or disorientation.
  3. This condition is diagnosed through observation, history, and interview.
  4. Treatment consists of symptom control with antipsychotic medications (greatly improved with the advent of atypical antipsychotic medications) and training in social skills and community-based living.
    a. The goals of treatment shall be determined following a comprehensive biological, psychological, social factors, and health system assessments are completed. Interdisciplinary care team discussion as well as client and caregiver input are essential.
    b. Pharmacotherapy once included the use of neuroleptics but was found to be ineffective. Now, the medication of choice is clozapine and other drugs classified as atypical antipsychotics.
    c. Other treatment modalities of interest to case managers consist of those described in Box 23-4.
  5. The case manager uses a strengths model approach to identify and address treatment issues proactively with the client, family/caregiver,

---

BOX 23-4   Treatment Modalities for Patients with Schizophrenia of Special Importance in Case Management

- Modified cognitive–behavioral therapy to reduce the intensity of delusions and hallucinations and reduce the incidence of substance abuse
- Modified motivational enhancement therapy to assist the individual to set goals, encourage an environment that supports sobriety, and develop skills to handle crisis
- Skills training to improve independent living and social interactions
- Assertive community treatment (ACT), which delivers clinical services as well as social services

and other members of the interdisciplinary team in order to mitigate risks for relapse (e.g., nonadherence to treatment, missing outpatient treatment appointments, lack of community-based support, lack of socialization and recreational activity).

   a. The need for ongoing biopsychoeducation for patients and their significant others should also be addressed in the case management plan.

   b. Treatment may involve hospitalization for acute episodes, which require active transition of care.

6. Case managers support the treatment plan of patients with schizophrenia through assessment, monitoring, planning, advocacy, and effective resource utilization (Box 23-5).

7. Case managers are usually members of ACT teams caring for patients with schizophrenia. ACT is a team-based treatment model providing interdisciplinary, flexible support and treatment to people with severe or complex mental illness, including schizophrenia, on a 24-by-7 basis.

   a. Individuals eligible for the ACT team intervention should be referred and assessed for case management intervention, if not already enrolled.

   b. ACT is most beneficial for patients discharging from an inpatient setting who would still benefit from a similar level of care.

   c. The ACT team addresses all aspects of the person's well-being including medication, therapy, social support, employment, and housing.

   d. For those who do not meet ACT criteria, behavioral health home care services should be initiated, as available. Individuals and their significant others may be referred to other support group services.

BOX 23-5 Case Management Activities for Patients with Schizophrenia

- Provide support for patients and their significant others who may benefit from support groups.
- Monitor medication and treatment adherence with special attention to the following aspects of the therapy:
  - Patients may dislike side effects associated with antipsychotic medication and may have difficulty adhering to the treatment regimen (e.g., movement disorders).
  - Coordinate and follow-through on outpatient clinic and laboratory visits (e.g., long-acting antipsychotic injections, required laboratory testing).
  - Assess for use of herbal and over-the-counter supplements, which may affect prescription medication absorption and efficacy.
  - Monitor weight and metabolic changes, which may require referral to nutrition counseling.
- Communicate case management interactions across the care team and in a timely manner.
- Evaluate outcomes of care and facilitate care progression as indicated.
- Prevent delays in care and address resolution when occurred.
- Advocate for activities and programs that promote healthy lifestyles (e.g., exercise, smoking cessation) and prompt health referrals as these patients often suffer from poor generalized health. This may require pursuing extracontractual health plan benefits.

I. Obsessive–Compulsive Disorder

1. Persons suffering from obsessive–compulsive disorder (OCD) experience recurrent intrusive, obsessive thoughts and repetitive, compulsive behavioral patterns. They may also be preoccupied with order and symmetry, have difficulty throwing things out, or hoard unneeded items. If persons attempt to ignore the intrusive thoughts or to curb compulsive behaviors, their anxiety becomes intolerable and gets in the way of daily life.

   a. Obsessions are intrusive, irrational thoughts or impulses that repeatedly occur (e.g., thoughts about harming someone). People with these disorders know these thoughts are irrational but are afraid that somehow they might be true. These thoughts and impulses are upsetting, and people may try to ignore or suppress them (NAMI, 2015b).

   b. Compulsions are repetitive acts that temporarily relieve stress brought on by an obsession (e.g., handwashing, checking door locks). People with compulsive disorders may understand that rituals do not make sense but feel they must perform the act(s) to relieve and/or to prevent something bad from happening (NAMI, 2015b).

2. The disorder is diagnosed through interviews and review of past history.

3. Usually, OCD starts during early childhood or teenage years.

   a. Most people are diagnosed by age 19.

   b. OCD affects approximately 2.2 million American adults (National Institute for Mental Health, 2015b).

   c. OCD affects men and women equally. It may be accompanied by other anxiety disorders, eating disorders, or depression.

4. Generally treated with psychotherapy, medication, or both.

5. Individuals often recognize that their behaviors or obsessions are unreasonable but feel powerless to stop them. Distress occurs when these activities and behaviors become excessively time consuming or interfere with the person's ability to function in role-appropriate situations.

6. Treatment involves medication (typically serotonin reuptake blocking antidepressants or the highly serotonergic tricyclic antidepressant clomipramine).

7. A combination of antidepressants and behavioral therapy is frequently prescribed.

   a. A type of psychotherapy called cognitive–behavioral therapy (CBT) is useful in treating OCD as it teaches the individual different ways of behaving, thinking, and reacting to situations in order to help them feel less anxious or fearful without having obsessive thoughts or acting compulsive (NAMI, 2015b).

   b. Another type of psychotherapy called exposure and response prevention (ERP) has also proven beneficial in reducing compulsive behaviors of OCD (National Institute for Mental Health, 2015b).

8. Case managers support the treatment plan through assessment, monitoring, planning, advocacy, and resource utilization.

> **BOX 23-6**
>
> **Examples of Case Management Activities in the Case of Patients with OCD**
>
> - Monitor medications intake. Patients may dislike side effects associated with medications, which may ultimately contribute to nonadherence.
> - Coordinate and follow-through on outpatient clinic and prescription refills.
> - Assess for use of herbal/homeopathic and over-the-counter supplements, which may affect prescription medication absorption and efficacy.
> - Discuss aerobic activity with treating provider; reinforce recommendations or suggest increased activity level as appropriate and approved by treating provider.
> - Recommend participation in support groups as appropriate.

    a. Case management services focus on the present here and now, supporting medication treatment, significant other(s) involvement in care, and education.

    b. Some patients may find the support and structure of group therapy beneficial, especially if social dysfunction has occurred.

    c. Provide support service referrals for significant others who may benefit.

    d. Monitor adherence to medications and treatments; case managers must keep close attention to the patient's response to treatment and assess the degree of adherence (Box 23-6).

    e. Case managers communicate case management interactions across the care team.

    f. The case manager uses a strengths model approach to identify and address treatment issues proactively with the client, family/caregiver, and other members of the multidisciplinary team in order to mitigate risks for relapse (e.g., nonadherence to treatment, missing outpatient treatment appointments, lack of community-based support, lack of socialization and recreational activity).

    g. The need for ongoing biopsychoeducation for patients and their significant others should also be addressed in a patient-centered way within the case management plan.

    h. Case managers advocate for activities and programs that promote healthy lifestyles (e.g., exercise, smoking cessation) and may be required to pursue extracontractual health plan benefits.

J. Anxiety

    1. Anxiety can be a normal reaction as well as include anxiety disorders. Anxiety associated with an illness may affect the course of treatment.

    2. Anxiety disorders are the most common mental health concern in the United States.

        a. An estimated 40 million adults in the United States, or 18%, have an anxiety disorder.

        b. Approximately 8% of children and teenagers experience the negative impact of an anxiety disorder at school and at home.

        c. Most people develop symptoms of anxiety disorders before age 21, and women are 60% more likely to be diagnosed with an anxiety disorder than men (NAMI, 2015c).

    3. Individuals can react differently to the same diagnosis, prognosis, or treatment of complications.

4. Anxiety disorders are a group of related conditions and each with unique symptoms. However, all anxiety disorders have one thing in common: persistent, excessive fear or worry in situations that are not threatening. Anxiety disorders include phobias, panic disorders, general anxiety disorder, and social anxiety disorder (NAMI, 2015c).
5. Anxiety reactions can include fear of death, fear of pain, fear of loss of control, fear of abandonment, or fear of dependency. Anxiety can also amplify an individual's perception of pain or other aversive reactions.
6. Core symptoms of anxiety include nervousness/tension, panic attacks, and phobias.
7. Treatment of anxiety can vary from in length and approach.
    a. Medication, therapy, and relaxation/stress reduction technique instruction are options, which may be considered. Some forms of psychotherapy include:
        i. Cognitive–behavioral therapy focuses on development of coping skills that should be valuable throughout an individual's life.
        ii. Exposure and response therapy explores and confronts the stimulus for anxiety.
        iii. Dialectical behavioral therapy is a combination of cognitive therapy and meditation (NAMI, 2015c).
    b. Short-term management of anxiety may employ the use of benzodiazepines. Anxiety disorders may require longer-termed treatment with medications such as tricyclic antidepressants, selective serotonin reuptake inhibitors (SSRIs), and serotonin–norepinephrine reuptake inhibitors (SNRIs) (NAMI, 2015c).
8. Similar to care for patients with OCD, case managers support the treatment plan for patients with anxiety disorder through assessment, monitoring, planning, advocacy, and effective resource utilization (Box 23-7).

BOX 23-7 **Examples of Case Management Activities for Patients with Anxiety Disorder**

- Encourage participation in group therapy. Some patients may find the support and structure of group therapy beneficial, especially if social dysfunction has occurred.
- Provide support service referrals for significant others who may benefit from them.
- Monitor medications and treatment adherence
    - Patients may dislike side effects associated with medication, which may contribute to nonadherence.
    - Coordinate and follow-through on outpatient clinic and prescription refills.
    - Assess for use of herbal and over-the-counter supplements, which may affect prescription medication absorption and efficacy.
- Communicate case management interactions and client's progress across the interdisciplinary health care team.
- Provide ongoing biopsychoeducation for patients and their significant others. Offer such services in a patient-centered way and within the case management plan.
- Advocate for activities and programs that promote healthy lifestyles (e.g., exercise, smoking cessation). These may require extracontractual health plan benefits.

K. Dementia
1. Dementia is a chronic, progressive condition in which cognitive function deteriorates more quickly than what can be expected from normal aging. This condition affects thinking, orientation, comprehension, calculation, learning capacity, language, and judgment (WHO, 2015).
2. Dementia can be caused by a variety of illnesses, most commonly known are Alzheimer disease, vascular dementia, dementia with Lewy bodies (abnormal aggregates of protein that develop inside nerve cells), and a group of diseases that contribute to degeneration of the frontal lobe of the brain (WHO, 2015).
3. There is no known curative treatment for dementia or to alter its progressive course. While many treatments are in clinical trials, the best care at present is to provide support to the individual and his or her family (WHO, 2015).

L. Intellectual and Developmental Disorders including Autism Spectrum Disorders
1. Intellectual and developmental disabilities (IDDs) are disorders that are usually present at birth and that negatively affect the trajectory of the individual's physical, intellectual, and/or emotional development. Many of these conditions affect multiple body parts or systems (Eunice Kennedy Shriver National Institute of Child Health and Human Development, 2012).
2. Developmental disorders cover a wide range of intellectual disabilities and pervasive disorders that include ASD. These disorders typically have an onset in childhood but persist through adulthood. The cause of these disorders cannot be generalized so the case manager should pursue further education as to the specific disorder of his/her client.
3. ASD is characterized by the following:
   a. Persistent deficits in social communication and social interaction across multiple contexts.
   b. Restricted, repetitive patterns of behavior, interests, or activities.
   c. Symptoms must be present in the early developmental period (typically recognized in the first 2 years of life).
   d. Symptoms cause clinically significant impairment in social, occupational, or other important areas of current functioning (NIMH, 2015c).
4. Symptoms of these disorders include impaired social behavior, deficits in communication and language, limited range of interests and activities that the individual often perform repetitively, or intellectual delay or disability. Case management interventions are tailored to address the individual's needs.
5. Care of individuals with developmental disabilities requires consistent and committed family or caregiver involvement. Understanding the causes of what distresses the individual as well as what things bring about well-being is essential in the care of the individual. The need for support services for client and caregiver is very important.
6. The environment for these individuals is key to addressing the individual's needs. The environment should be one that is conducive

to learning and is structured by routines that prevent stress like regular times for meals, learning, being with others, and sleeping.

7. Case managers support the treatment plan through assessment, monitoring, planning, advocacy, and resource utilization. Case managers should tailor care planning to each client's specific needs. Addressing the need for a strong support system for client and caregiver will require advocacy for extracontractual benefits. The case manager enlists the caregiver in finding and engaging community resources as well as coordination of care.

 ## Challenges in Behavioral Health Case Management

A. Preventing self-harm and/or suicide. Potentially, all patients with psychiatric and substance-related disorders are at risk for suicide.
   1. The most predictive suicide risk is a past history of a suicide attempt.
   2. The most conservative approach is to admit the patient who is at risk for suicide when there is any doubt about his or her safety.
   3. The implications for case management with these patients are the need to develop an effective support system within the family and community to manage emergency situations and to provide support and safety for the patient. The case manager must also be prepared to ask the patient whether experiencing any thoughts of self-harm as part of the assessment and assessment follow-up.
   4. Behavioral and nonbehavioral health case managers must be aware of the suicide risk factors and incorporate them in their patient assessments (Box 23-8).
   5. Case managers and other health care professionals must apply appropriate procedures in handling individuals with suicide concerns and must listen to the patient/support systems carefully to determine the level of suicide intent.
      a. Does not want to live, does not fear death.
      b. Has active thoughts of harming self.
      c. Has thought of a how to commit suicide but does not have a clear plan.
      d. The individual has a plan for harming himself/herself (Kathol, Perez, & Cohen, 2010).

BOX
23-8 Suicide Risk Factors

- Depression, other mental disorders, or substance abuse disorders
- A prior suicide attempt
- Family history of a mental disorder or substance abuse
- Family history of suicide
- Family violence, including physical or sexual abuse
- Having guns or other firearms in the home
- Incarceration, being in prison or jail
- Being exposed to others' suicidal behavior, such as that of family members, peers, or media figures.

6. The level of concern determines the action(s) taken. Also important to note, action steps may be written into organizational policy. The case manager must be aware of current policy and procedure in this area. Possible action–reaction scenarios include the following:
   a. If the client verbalizes not wanting to live, try to connect the individual with a mental health professional.
   b. If the client has active thoughts, has thought of a plan, or has a plan, the individual should be referred to a mental health professional immediately.
   c. If concerned that a client is imminently going to attempt suicide, call 911 or ask a colleague contact 911 while the client is kept engaged on the phone or face-to-face.
7. The case manager may be trained to utilize an accepted suicide risk tool. The decision as to which tool and who is qualified to administer it should be addressed in organizational policy and procedure.

B. Preventing violence
1. Indications of increased risk for violence include:
   a. A recent violent act
   b. Alcohol or substance intoxication
   c. Verbal or physical threats
   d. Presence of a weapon
   e. Patients responding to psychotic thoughts (i.e., command hallucinations)
2. Patients suffering from disorders that heighten impulsivity (i.e., substance-related disorders, bipolar disorder, disorders affecting the frontal lobe, and clients with personality disorders) may, at times, require crisis intervention in order to protect themselves and others.
   a. The involuntary placement of these patients on locked psychiatric units, when necessary, can increase the patients' anger and aggressive behaviors.
   b. These patients must always be treated in the least restrictive setting necessary to protect themselves and others.
3. It is important that clinicians, including case managers, carefully question patients' significant others regarding domestic violence.
   a. Abused partners should be referred to domestic violence shelters.
   b. Where child abuse is suspected, clinicians are mandated to report observations to authorities.
4. The case manager must be knowledgeable of his/her responsibilities as a mandated reporter. Mandated reporters are individuals who are legally required to report when abuse is observed or suspected.
   a. Specific details vary across jurisdictions.
   b. Reportable abuse may include neglect, financial, physical, sexual, or other types of abuse.

C. Reducing self-neglect
1. Self-neglect is defined as the result of an adult's inability, due to physical and/or mental impairments or diminished capacity, to perform essential self-care tasks including the following:
   a. Providing essential food, clothing, shelter, and health care.
   b. Obtaining goods and services necessary to maintain physical health, mental health, emotional well-being, and general safety.

      c. Managing financial affairs and adhering to prescribed medications.

      d. Nonadherence to treatment may be considered a form of self-neglect (Abrams et al., 2002).

   2. Relapse of symptoms and return to acute care settings most frequently occur when patients are unable to adhere to treatment or manage their self-care activities while in the community. Episodes of relapse can be devastating to patients and their significant other(s) who experience a sense of failure and loss of hope.

   3. The implications for case management are to coordinate and facilitate the care during the acute phase of illness and treatment, monitor adherence, and proactively investigate problems that may contribute to nonadherence (e.g., side effects, ambivalence about taking medications).

   4. Case managers assist the patients and significant others in reframing the relapse and in maintaining hope as well as realistic expectations about recovery and rehabilitation.

   5. For practical case management approaches for clients with low self-care states, refer to Appendix B.

D. Treating clients with psychiatric and substance use-related diagnoses

   1. Assessment and diagnosis of patients with dual diagnosis (psychiatric and substance-related disorders) can be difficult.

   2. A patient who presents for treatment under the influence of mind-altering substances may not be accurately diagnosed until the effects of the substance have been eliminated.

   3. Until the effects of mind-altering substances are managed/overturned, the patient must be treated symptomatically and conservatively, with the health care staff providing a safe environment while observing for symptoms of psychiatric disorders.

   4. Common dual-diagnosis situations include the patient with generalized anxiety disorder or panic who abuses alcohol to reduce feelings of anxiety or the depressed patient who uses cocaine to relieve symptoms of depression.

   5. The patient, once accurately diagnosed, must receive treatment for both disorders concurrently.

   6. Many dual-diagnosis treatment programs have been established in ambulatory settings/clinics to meet the needs of these patients.

   7. The psychiatrist who prescribes anxiolytic medications for a dually diagnosed patient must be aware of the potential for abuse of the medication. Case managers caring for these patients must also be aware of the risk of abuse.

   8. The treating provider must be cognizant of the "normal" sad affect experienced by some patients who are recovering from alcohol or drug dependence, or both, and be able to distinguish this condition from an acute mood disorder that may require pharmacologic intervention.

   9. All treatment practitioners, including the case manager, must be alert to the potential for suicide in this population.

E. Improving the general health of patients/clients requires the acknowledgment that many patients, particularly those with SPMI, suffer from obesity, a general lack of fitness, poor nutrition, and nicotine dependence.

1. Lack of preventive health services, frequent delays in seeking care, unhealthy lifestyles, and general poor health become an even greater concern as patient's age and their chronic illnesses increase.
2. It is vital that case management programs address smoking cessation, health promotion activities, and timely health-related referrals for patients.

F. Improving the social functioning of patients/clients during their daily lives may require that case managers:
   1. Individually tailor treatment plans with the patient/support system to increase sufficiently stimulating, challenging, and interesting daily activities.
   2. Offer educational programs and activities to improve functioning and socialization in all areas, including sexual functioning, that have been underappreciated in case management models.

G. Enhancing the client–case manager relationship and care continuity
   1. Frequent turnover in staff is a significant problem in case management and contributes to poor-quality care, recidivism, and high costs in recruiting and retaining case managers.
   2. Establishing a trusting relationship between the patient and case manager as well as working with families as allies in care are key ingredients for success.
   3. The challenges associated with behavioral health case management are significant but are more than offset by the rewards associated with making a positive impact on the mental, psychological, social, and physical health of individuals with mental health conditions and their associated outcomes.

Treatment Settings and Behavioral Health Case Management

A. Inpatient hospitalization
   1. Used for treatment of acute conditions in which patients are in danger of harming themselves or others.
   2. Also used for the patient who is unable to care for oneself in the community, maintain self-safety, or out of touch with reality.
   3. Hospitalization is the most restrictive type of treatment for behavioral health conditions.
      a. It is occasionally used to initiate new medications when the patient must be observed closely for potentially life-threatening side effects.
      b. Hospitalization is often used for acute detoxification from substances with which the potential for severe withdrawal symptoms exists.
      c. Hospitalization is also used to keep persons with active psychoses safe and to avoid harming oneself or others.
      d. Sometimes, patients are placed in a locked inpatient unit depending on the severity of their condition and the required treatment.

   4. Laws governing involuntary short- or long-term confinement differ
      from state to state, and case managers must be aware of individual
      state laws and restrictions.
   5. The behavioral health case manager's role is to assess the patient's
      overall mental health and to develop a long-term treatment plan to
      align them with mental health professionals in the community for
      afterdischarge care, toward eventual self-management of their own
      mental health. Typically, a case manager is accountable for the welfare
      of the patient during the hospitalization and provides support for the
      client and significant others while moving the client toward a timely
      discharge.
B. Partial hospitalization
   1. This treatment modality involves the patient spending 4 hours or
      more per day in a structured setting. May also be referred to as day
      treatment.
   2. Patients in this setting receive milieu therapy, psychoeducation, and
      individual and group therapies.
   3. Partial hospitalization may be used as an alternative to inpatient
      hospitalization for the patient, who has a strong community
      support system, who is not deemed to be an acute risk, and who
      requires close supervision of medication administration and
      potential effects.
   4. Case management's role in the care of patients who are enrolled
      in a partial hospital program includes knowledge of how to access
      emergency treatment for the patient, support and education of client
      and significant others, and development and implementation of a
      client-centered aftercare plan addressing both mental health and
      physical health barriers to health improvement.
C. Ambulatory care:
   1. Outpatient and intensive outpatient treatment are effective for
      patients whose conditions can be managed outside of a structured
      setting.
   2. Individual, group, family, and couples therapy are delivered in this
      setting.
   3. Patients' medications can be monitored effectively on an ambulatory
      basis once dosages are stabilized.
   4. Case management's role in ambulatory care may be minimal.
      However, it may include patient/family education, counseling,
      encouragement in adherence to regimen, crisis intervention, as well as
      maintenance of follow-up care.
   5. The case manager and patient should be aware and have a
      predetermined plan of how to access emergency services if the
      patient's symptoms should worsen, if he or she experiences suicidal
      thoughts or impulses, or if intolerable or potentially dangerous
      medication side effects occur.
D. Home and community-based settings
   1. Behavioral health home care is a treatment modality for the delivery
      of mental health and related physical care within a patient's home
      setting.
   2. Psychiatric nurses are the major providers of psychiatric home
      care services and function both as direct care clinicians and as case

managers who develop, coordinate, implement, and oversee the interdisciplinary treatment plan.

3. Multidisciplinary team members may include the physician (not required to be a psychiatrist), social worker, physical therapist, occupational therapist, and home health aide.

4. Services are covered by Medicare, as well as other insurances, when the following conditions are met:

   a. The patient has a primary psychiatric diagnosis, has been evaluated by a physician, is re-evaluated by the physician every 60 days, requires skilled nursing intervention by a psychiatric nurse, and meets homebound status.

   b. According to the CMS, a mental health patient is homebound if the person has been diagnosed with a psychiatric condition defined in the DSM-5 and is confined to the home and "their behavioral health condition is manifested in part by a refusal to leave the home, or is of such a nature that it would not be considered safe for the member to leave home unattended even if the member has no physical limitations." Conditions may include agoraphobia, panic disorder, acute depression with severe vegetative symptoms, or disorders of thought processes where hallucinations, delusions, or impaired cognition grossly affects the person's judgment and decision making, thus their safety in the community (2013).

   c. Behavioral health home care services can be particularly effective in settings where there is limited access to behavioral health clinicians, for example, nonambulatory patients and lengthy distances to travel for behavioral health services.

   d. The case manager should check benefits and reimbursement for products and services that a client may need, as well as understand the co-payment and deductible that the client may be responsible for out of pocket.

E. Rural settings

1. To address the limited availability of behavioral health specialists in the rural settings, cognitive–behavioral therapy training has been provided to case managers to an eclectic group of psychiatric nurses and clinicians with social work and psychology backgrounds.

2. Primary care physicians often attempt to deliver behavioral health services due to the lack of available behavioral health specialists.

3. With the expansion of Internet capabilities, behavioral health services are now being delivered via Telehealth in some rural settings. Telehealth can deliver mental health assistance in clinics, schools, nursing homes, and residential programs. Telehealth also enables professional practitioners to receive continuing education training without long-distance travel.

F. Drug courts

1. An innovative model of care that addresses the needs of clients in correctional settings

2. A setting that provides nonviolent offenders with basic access to physical and mental health care as well as intensive case management frequently provided by advanced practice nurses

> **BOX 23-9**
>
> **Core Case Management Activities That Are Important in Behavioral Health**
>
> - Coordination and facilitation of care and treatments
> - Brokerage of services, especially those needed to keep patients in the community
> - Patient and family education regarding health condition and treatment
> - Transitional planning and actual transitioning of patients from one level of care to the next as well as discharge planning that focuses on discharging patients from the hospital/institution setting
> - Assessment, monitoring, and evaluation of the patient's condition and response to treatment
> - Reporting observation findings to other health care providers, especially the psychiatrist and primary care physician
> - Working closely with payers, community agencies (e.g., transportation) in fiscally responsible management of resources, and other health care providers such as physical and occupational therapy, social work, pharmacy, home health, and so on

Roles and Functions of the Behavioral Health Case Manager

A. The roles and functions of behavioral health case managers are similar to those who function in other care settings and care for other patient populations (Box 23-9).

B. Case managers' activities that are more specific to the behavioral health patient population may include those described in Box 23-10.

How Psychological Factors Impact Medical Conditions and Integrated Care Management

A. Medical conditions can be adversely affected by psychological or behavioral factors. Interference by a psychological condition of exacerbation can interfere with treatment and contribute to morbidity and mortality.

B. Almost all physical or medical illnesses can potentially affect the psychological and behavioral factors as well as environmental. Individuals vary in their response to illness so it is important to know what conditions affect each client.

C. Interactions between mind and body affect psychological factors on general medical conditions as well as medical illnesses affect psychological functions (Levenson, 2015).

D. It is difficult to measure the prevalence of psychological factors affecting other medical conditions because disorders may cause many different interactions. Psychological and behavioral factors can influence general medical illnesses by

   1. Promoting known risks for smoking, substance abuse, medication overuse, sedentary lifestyle, poor diet, obesity, poor sleep hygiene, and unsafe sexual practices.

   2. How individuals respond to symptoms and how and whether they seek care.

   3. How the physician decides to diagnose and treat.

BOX 23-10 Specialty Case Management Activities in Behavioral Health

- Patient and family education, support, and encouragement, especially to enhance adherence to treatment regimen and follow-up care.
- Develop and implement of patient-centered aftercare plans.
- Integrate, coordinate, and advocate for complex mental and physical health care services from a variety of health care providers and settings, within the framework of planned health outcomes.
- Develop meaningful, holistic care plans that use evidence-based practice principles for behavioral health.
- Establish trusting relationships with families, caregivers, and guardians to promote families as allies in care.
- Support strategies to improve social functioning.
- Ensure the individual's social functioning improves with tailored interventions.
- Address smoking cessation, health promotion activities, and timely health-related referrals.
- Develop an effective support system within the family and community to manage emergency situations and to provide support and safety for the patient.
- Prevent suicide and homicide risk.
- Monitor any acute phase of illness and treatment and adherence, and proactively investigate problems that may contribute to nonadherence (i.e., side effects to drugs, ambivalence about taking medications).
- Assist patients and their support system in reframing relapse, if it occurs, and in maintaining hope as well as realistic expectations about recovery and rehabilitation.
- Advocate for activities and programs that promote healthy lifestyles such as exercise programs, support groups, and smoking cessation.

---

4. Reduction in compliance with diagnostic recommendations, treatment, and lifestyle changes.
5. Lack of motivation to participate in rehabilitation, low tolerance for pain, and high levels of frustration.
6. Stress has been shown to influence a number of health-related conditions/issues, including myocardial infarction, immune system, wound healing, sleep hygiene, and endocrine function (Levenson, 2015).

 ## Reimbursement Issues

A. Mental Health Parity and Addiction Equity Act of 2008 (MHPAEA).
1. Group health plans and health insurance issuers are to ensure that financial requirements (such as co-pays, deductibles) and treatment limitations (such as visit limits) applicable to mental health (MH) or substance use disorder (SUD) benefits are no more restrictive than the predominant requirements or limitations applied to substantially all medical/surgical benefits.
2. MHPAEA supplements prior provisions under the Mental Health Parity Act of 1996 (MHPA), which required parity with respect to aggregate lifetime and annual dollar limits for mental health benefits.
3. This legislation was enacted because the cost and access to behavioral health care and services was not equal to that of regular medical benefits. The legislation, in theory, has assisted more individuals' access to mental health services, but some private payers have

completely excluded these services from plans of benefits. Access to care is still challenging for those that live in rural areas due to a decidedly low number of mental health providers, especially board-certified psychiatrists.

B. Sources for reimbursement can include government programs, private insurers, and individual contributions.

C. Government programs include Medicaid, Medicare, and school-based health centers (for children and adolescents that already have Medicaid).

D. Medicaid is a joint federal and state program that helps low-income individuals or families pay for the costs associated with long-term medical and custodial care, provided they qualify.

　　1. Although largely funded by the federal government, Medicaid is run by the state where coverage may vary.

　　2. Mental health is one of the services covered under Medicaid. Mental health services can be delivered in a variety of care settings such as the following:

　　　　a. Inpatient hospital

　　　　b. Outpatient hospital

　　　　c. Federally Qualified Health Center (FQHC)

　　　　d. Rural Health Center (RHC) services

　　　　e. Physician services

E. Medicare is the federal health insurance program for people who are 65 or older, certain younger people with disabilities, and people with end-stage renal disease (permanent kidney failure requiring dialysis or a transplant, sometimes called ESRD).

　　1. Individuals with Medicare face challenges when attempting to access care and services, especially outpatient services. Medicare-eligible individuals are used to 20% co-pay for care and services, but depending on the outpatient service, an individual may have as much as 50% co-pay. This poses a financial burden for the individual as well as providers. Many Medicare recipients are poor, so providers know that they will likely be unable to collect any co-pays (Kautz, Mauch, & Smith, 2008).

　　2. These limitations are a disincentive for primary care providers to diagnose and treat mental health problems in Medicare recipients. In addition, Medicare recipients will not bring complaints to the PCP that could be related to behavioral issues because they cannot afford the 50% co-pay (Kautz, Mauch, & Smith, 2008).

F. Other reimbursement sources include private insurance plans, whereby the premium is paid by the individual and employer-sponsored health plans. The employer pays all or part of an employee's health insurance premium. The case manager should understand the specifics about a client's health insurance carrier benefits, cost (e.g., deductible, coinsurance) and out-of-pocket consequences of all treatment options on the client.

Integrated Case Management

A. Traditionally, case management has been separated into disciplines for which the case manager is most comfortable and from which the majority of their clinical experience originates.

　　1. Case managers who come from a medical background focus their practice on individuals with physical illnesses and conditions.

2. Case managers who come from a behavioral health background focus their practice on individuals with mental and behavioral illnesses.
3. Many lessons have been learned in recent years that have led to a change in thinking. Our health care system is fragmented, we better understand and recognize the negative impact behavioral and physical health can have if addressed separately, and we recognize the need for a more patient-centered approach.
4. ICM is designed to collapse the silos that are typically seen in health care. With an integrated approach, case managers, regardless of background, are trained to manage individuals from both the medical and behavioral sectors while working with an interdisciplinary team.
5. Case managers do not diagnose, nor do they prescribe treatment. Case managers facilitate the care and services that a treating provider orders so there is no threat that a case manager would be practicing outside his or her scope of practice.
6. Every individual case must be evaluated for what is of most concern and an assignment made accordingly.
   a. In a majority of situations, mental health case management is managed separately from medical case management. An individual with diabetes and schizophrenia who is the midst of a psychotic break is better served by a behavioral health case manager. Whereas, an individual with depression and excessively high blood sugar is better served by a case manager form the medical sector.
   b. ICM requires assessment of biological, psychological, social, and health system domains within the timeframes of past, present, and future (risk potential).
7. The most important issues reveal themselves through consideration of the individual's global circumstances, rather than simply medical or behavioral health issues. Perspective is creating when considering historical, current, and future risk timeframes.
8. A solid working dynamic and trust relationship develop with the individuals enrolled in ICM. The relationship that builds as a result of one case manager working with the member across medical and mental health contexts, as opposed to being passed from one to the next case manager depending upon whether medical or mental health issues are more urgency, improves adherence and health outcomes.
B. Training Requirements for the Integrated Case Manager.
   1. As discussed in an earlier section, behavioral conditions can further complicate an already behaviorally fragile individual. However, one cannot expect improved outcomes unless all the barriers to health are addressed and addressed by trusted health care professionals. The first requirement for becoming an integrated case manager is the willingness to address both the behavioral and physical aspects of an individual's health. That also includes recognizing social concerns and addressing those as well.
   2. ICM is an advanced practice; in order to be an integrated case manager, the health professional should be proficient in case management knowledge and practice (Box 23-11).
   3. Cross-disciplinary training in the discipline for which the case manager is less familiar: The behavioral case manager will become

23-11   Essential Knowledge and Practices in Integrated Case Management

- Be familiar with CMSA's Standards of Practice for Case Management and those of other key professional organizations such as the National Association of Social Workers (NASW).
- Have strong interpersonal skills or recent training in interpersonal skills.
- Know how to conduct an interview and assessment that results in the development of a relationship; the use of open-ended questions.
- Develop a person-centric care plan from an assessment that covers the physical, psychological, social, and health system challenges.
- Strong organizational skills and ability to prioritize the individual's needs and implement interventions that result in health improvements.
- Knowledge of documentation standards (e.g., accuracy, legally defensible, frequency—as often as required to demonstrate progress).
- Understand HIPAA, individual consent, privacy, mental health regulations in your state or community, and confidentiality.

more familiar with medical conditions and the medical case manager will become more familiar with behavioral conditions.

4. Integrated case managers should work in teams, if at possible, in order to have lacking expertise easy to hand. When this is not feasible, the case manager should have a panel of colleagues, who are subject-matter experts, to call when additional information is needed.

5. Because the development of a relationship is crucial to the success of an ICM program, the case manager must possess skills that will assist with individual engagement. Having been trained in motivational interviewing would be extremely advantageous, if not a requirement.

6. The integrated case manager must have exemplary care planning skills in order to prioritize, what may be an extensive list of problems. The complex individual cannot be given information dropped in the mail and then expected to "pull herself together" to do all the right things. Only a patient and experienced case manager can assist the member and help her eventually move toward self-management.

C. Organizational Implementation of ICM.

1. Before implementing an integrated model of care, an organization must first examine its current practices and then determine what changes need to be put into place in order to transition to an integrated model.

2. The willingness to address both medical and behavioral illnesses in a population must be a clear commitment by the organization. The medical management staff must have the infrastructure to support case managers in work that will probably be different from what they did before. Case managers will be spending more time with their members whether it is on the phone or in person. Caseloads will need to be adapted so that the case manager can provide the member the additional time needed to develop a relationship and work with the member on solving problems and achieving goals.

3. Organizations need to champion the need for improved quality and safe care for all individuals.

Appendix A—Suicide Practice Protocol

Five-Step Evaluation and Triage (SAFE-T) (DHHS, 2009)

I. Identify risk factors
   a. Suicidal behavior: History of prior suicide attempts, aborted suicide attempts, or self-injurious behavior.
   b. Current/past psychiatric disorders: Especially, mood disorders, psychotic disorders, alcohol/substance abuse, ADHD, TBI, PTSD, Cluster B personality disorders, conduct disorders (antisocial behavior, aggression, impulsivity), comorbidity, and recent onset of illness increase risk.
   c. Key symptoms: Anhedonia, impulsivity, hopelessness, anxiety/panic, global insomnia, command hallucinations.
   d. Family history of suicide, attempts, or axis 1 psychiatric disorders requiring hospitalization.
   e. Precipitants/stressors/interpersonal triggering events leading to humiliation, shame, or despair (e.g., loss of relationship, financial, or health status—real or anticipated), ongoing medical illness (especially CNS disorders, pain), intoxication, family turmoil/chaos, history of physical or sexual abuse, social isolation.
   f. Change in treatment: Discharge from psychiatric hospital, provider or treatment change.
   g. Access to firearms.
II. Protective factors (protective factors, even if present, may not counteract significant acute risk)
   a. Internal: Ability to cope with stress, religious beliefs, frustration tolerance
   b. External: Responsibility to children or beloved pets, positive therapeutic relationships, social supports
III. Suicide inquiry (specific questioning about thought, plans, behaviors, intent)
   a. Ideation: Frequency, intensity, duration in last 48 hours, past month, and worst ever
   b. Plan: Timing, location, lethality, availability, preparatory acts
   c. Behaviors: Past attempts, aborted attempts, rehearsals (tying noose, loading gun) versus nonsuicidal self-injurious actions
   d. Intent: Extent to which the patient (1) expects to carry out the plan and (2) believes the plan to be lethal versus self-injurious; explore ambivalence (e.g., reasons to die vs. reasons to live)
IV. Risk level/intervention
   a. Assessment of risk based on clinical judgment, after completing steps 1 to 3
   b. Reassess: As patient or environmental circumstances change
V. Document
   a. Risk level and rationale; treatment plan to address/reduce current risk (e.g., medication, setting, psychotherapy, ECT, contact with significant others, consultation); firearms instructions, if relevant; follow-up plan

 Appendix B—Case Management Approaches for Patients with Low Self-Care States

A. Traditional approaches to clients with low self-care states have shifted from compliance to adherence-focused models.

1. In the era of compliance, it was typical for providers to lecture, impact by fear, and admonish patients for the various self-neglect or abuse symptoms they demonstrated.
2. With the advent of the adherence approach to care, the focus has changed to partnering, communicating therapeutically, negotiating, and planning according to the patient's needs and capabilities.
3. The adherence approach is consistent with the strengths model of case management (Marty, Rapp, & Carlson, 2001).

B. It is important to evaluate the patient globally and consider the accumulation and interaction of medical, psychiatric, social, and physiological aging.
1. Multidisciplinary team meetings are an important means for sharing perceptions, evaluating the treatment plan, and coordinating this plan with the patient and/or the patient's significant others.

C. Persons exhibiting diminished self-care states have risk factors that include the following:
1. Multiple cognitive deficits (e.g., memory impairment, disturbance in executive functioning)
2. Developmental delays
3. Sensory impairments
4. Impaired mobility
5. Social isolation
6. Anxiety, phobias, and depression
7. Psychotic symptoms
8. Long-standing personality traits that lead to the individual's distress or impairment (Abrams et al., 2002)

D. Case management of patients with low self-care states begins by:
1. Assessing the patient's level of self-care using a standardized assessment tool (Sansone & Sansone, 2010).
2. Taking a clear history of the present nonadherence and noting the impact of such behaviors on the patient's quality of life and safety.
3. Questions may include the following:
   a. Section 1
      i. How long has the nonadherence been going on and is it a long-standing or abrupt behavior?
      ii. Is it stemming from medical or hygiene domains or both?
      iii. Is this "assiduous" stemming from young to midadulthood?
      iv. Are there cultural considerations that impact the patient's understanding or behavior?
      v. What is the individual's perception of the condition? Does he or she see a problem or feel uncomfortable?
   b. Section 2
      i. Are the patient's medical needs evident and being addressed?
      ii. Are the patient's activities of daily living (i.e., eating, bathing) and instrumental activities of daily living (i.e., shopping, housekeeping) needs evident? If so, how are they being addressed?
      iii. Is the patient capable of communicating his or her needs and directing care?

      iv. Are there cognitive deficits (e.g., memory deficits), and if so, is the patient responsive to the creation of environmental cues (e.g., calendars and notes) and/or verbal reminders?

      v. Is the case management's philosophy of care consistent with what the patient or his/her health care proxy indicates?

  c. Section 3

      i. What are the etiologies or "host domains?" How many are there?

      ii. Etiologies or host domains many include the following:

        a. Sensory/functional impairments

        b. Mental health problems

        c. Substance abuse problems

        d. Social–legal problems

        e. Medical comorbidity

        f. Health literacy

        g. Environmental domains

        h. Social network

        i. Resource issues

        j. Housing

        k. Transportation

4. For interventions, consider the following:

  a. Create teams for tailored intervention.

  b. Access technology that can improve cognitive functions and optimize medical care.

  c. Address sensory/functional and intellectual impairments.

  d. Identify resources and housing transition.

  e. Negotiate to reduce risks of harm as tolerable to the patient.

  f. Simplify the process whenever possible.

5. For the intractable self-neglecter, consider the following:

  a. Ensure public safety.

  b. Provide nonjudgmental support.

  c. Remember that trust is earned and in little ways first.

  d. Be realistic and be patient.

References

Abrams, R. C., Lachs, M., McAvay, G., Keohane, D. J., & Bruce, M. L. (2002). Predictors of self-neglect in community-dwelling elders. *American Journal of Psychiatry, 159*(10), 1724–1730. Retrieved from http://www.ncbi.nlm.nih.gov/pubmed/12359679, on July 29, 2015.

American Psychiatric Association (APA). (2013). *Diagnostic and statistical manual of mental disorders* (5th ed.). Washington, DC: American Psychiatric Association Press.

Bustillo, J., & Weil, E. (2014). *Psychosocial interventions for severe mental illness.* UpToDate. Retrieved from http://www.uptodate.com/contents/psychosocial-interventions-for-severe-mental-illness, on July 27, 2015.

Campbell, E. C., Caroff, S. N., & Mann, S. C. (2013). *Treatment of co-occurring schizophrenia and substance use disorder.* UpToDate. Retrieved from http://www.uptodate.com/contents/treatment-of-co-occurring-schizophrenia-and-substance-use-disorder, on July 27, 2015.

Case Management Society of America. (2010). *CMSA standards of practice for case management.* Retrieved from http://www.cmsa.org/portals/0/pdf/memberonly/standardsofpractice.pdf, on March 12, 2015.

De Hert, M., Correll, C. U., Bobes, J., Cetkovich-Bakmas, M., Cohen, D., Asai, I., ... Leucht, S. (2011). Physical illness in patients with severe mental disorders. I. Prevalence, impact of medications and disparities in health care. *World Psychiatry, 10,* 52–77. Retrieved from http://www.ncbi.nlm.nih.gov/pmc/articles/PMC3048500, on July 29, 2015.

Department of Health and Human Services (DHHS), Substance Abuse and Mental Health Services Administration (SAMHSA). (2009). *SAFE-T.* Retrieved from http://www.integration.samhsa.gov/clinical-practice/safe-t_card.pdf, on July 29, 2015.

Dieterich, M. C., Park, B., & Marshall, M. (2010). Intensive case management for severe mental illness. *Cochrane Database of Systematic Reviews, 10,* CD007906. doi: 10.1002/14651858. CD007906.pub2. Retrieved from http://www.ncbi.nlm.nih.gov/pmc/articles/PMC4233116/pdf/emss-58195.pdf, on July 27, 2015.

Eunice Kennedy Shriver National Institute of Child Health and Human Development. (2012). What are intellectual and developmental disabilities (IDDs)? Retrieved from http://www.nichd.nih.gov/health/topics/idds/conditioninfo/Pages/default.aspx#f2, on July 29, 2015.

Farnsworth, B. J., & Bigelow, A. S. (1997). Psychiatric case management. In J. Haber, B. Krainorich-Miller, & A. McMahon (Eds.), *Comprehensive psychiatric nursing* (5th ed., pp. 318–331). New York: Mosby Year Book.

Kathol, R. M., Perez, R. R., & Cohen, J. P. (2010). *The integrated case management manual: Assisting complex patients regain physical and mental health.* New York: Springer Publishing Company.

Kautz, C., Mauch, D., & Smith, S. A. (2008). *Reimbursement of mental health services in primary care settings (HHS Pub. No. SMA-08-4324).* Rockville, MD: Center for Mental Health Services, Substance Abuse and Mental Health Services Administration. Retrieved from http://www.nasmhpd.org/sites/default/files/SMA08-4324.pdf, on July 29, 2015.

Lamberti, J. S., Weisman, R., & Faden, D. I. (2004). Forensic assertive community treatment: Preventing incarceration of adults with severe mental illness. *Psychiatric Services, 55*(11), 1285–1293. Retrieved from https://www2.nami.org/Template.cfm?Section=act-ta_center&template=/ContentManagement/ContentDisplay.cfm&ContentID=52382, on July 27, 2015.

Levenson, J. L. (2015). *Psychological factors affecting other medical conditions: Clinical features, assessment, and diagnosis.* Retrieved from http://www.uptodate.com/contents/psychological-factors-affecting-other-medical-conditions-clinical-features-assessment-and-diagnosis, on July 29, 2015.

Marty, D., Rapp, C. A., & Carlson, L. (2001). The experts speak: The critical ingredients of strengths model case management. *Psychiatric Rehabilitation Journal, 24,* 214–221. Retrieved from http://www.ncbi.nlm.nih.gov/pubmed/11315208, on July 29, 2015.

MentalHealth.gov. (2015). *Mental Health and substance use disorder.* Retrieved from http://www.mentalhealth.gov/what-to-look-for/substance-abuse, on July 29, 2015.

Morrison, J. R. (2014). *DSM-5 Made Easy: The Clinician's Guide to Diagnosis.* New York: Guilford Press.

National Alliance for Mental Illness (NAMI). (2015a). *Treatment and services— Case management.* Retrieved from http://www.nami.org/Learn-More/Treatment/Treatment-Settings, on April 26, 2016.

National Alliance for Mental Illness (NAMI). (2015b). *Obsessive-compulsive disorder.* Retrieved from http://www.nami.org/Learn-More/Mental-Health-Conditions/Obsessive-Compulsive-Disorder, on July 28, 2015.

National Alliance for Mental Illness (NAMI). (2015c). *Anxiety disorder.* Retrieved from http://www.nami.org/Learn-More/Mental-Health-Conditions/Anxiety-Disorders, on July 28, 2015.

National Institute on Alcohol Abuse and Alcoholism. (2015). *Alcohol facts and statistics.* Retrieved from http://www.niaaa.nih.gov/alcohol-health/overview-alcohol-consumption/alcohol-facts-and-statistics, on July 28, 2015.

National Institutes of Health; Biological Sciences Curriculum Study. (2007). *NIH curriculum supplement series [Internet].* Bethesda, MD: National Institutes of Health (US); Information about Hearing, Communication, and Understanding. Retrieved from http://www.ncbi.nlm.nih.gov/books/NBK20371/?report=printable, on July 29, 2015.

National Institute for Mental Health. (2015). *Schizophrenia.* Retrieved from http://www.nimh.nih.gov/health/publications/schizophrenia-booklet-12-2015/index.shtml, on July 15, 2015. NIH Publication No. TR 15-3517.

National Institute for Mental Health. (2015a). *Bipolar disorder.* Retrieved from http://www.nimh.nih.gov/health/topics/bipolar-disorder/index.shtml, on July 15, 2015.

National Institute for Mental Health. (2015b). *Obsessive-compulsive disorder, OCD.* Retrieved from http://www.nimh,nih.gov/health/topics/obsessive-compulsive-disorder, on July 15, 2015.

National Institute for Mental Health. (2015c). *Autism spectrum disorders.* Retrieved from http://www.nimh.nih.gov/health/topics/autism-spectrum-disorders-asd/index.shtml, on July 29, 2015.

Peek, C. J.; the National Integration Academy Council. (2013). *Lexicon for behavioral health and primary care integration: Concepts and definitions developed by expert consensus.* Rockville, MD: Agency for Healthcare Research and Quality; AHRQ Publication No.13-IP001-EF. Retrieved from http://integrationacademy.ahrq.gov/sites/default/files/Lexicon.pdf, on July 27, 2015.

Psychology-Tools.com. (2015). *Young mania rating scale.* Retrieved from https://psychology-tools.com/young-mania-rating-scale, on July 29, 2015.

Sansone, R. A., & Sansone, L. A. (2010). Measuring self-harm behavior with the self-harm inventory. *Psychiatry, 7*(4), 16–20. Retrieved from http://www.ncbi.nlm.nih.gov/pmc/articles/PMC2877617, on April 16, 2016.

Scott, J. E., & Dixon, L. B. (1997). *Medscape psychiatry.* Retrieved from Medscape: http://www.medscape.com/viewarticle/430885_print, on July 27, 2015.

Substance Abuse and Mental Health Services Administration (SAMHSA). (2013). *2013 National Survey on Drug Use and Health (NSDUH). Table 2.46B—Alcohol use, binge alcohol use, and heavy alcohol use in the past month among persons aged 18 or older, by demographic characteristics: Percentages, 2012 and 2013.* Retrieved from http://www.samhsa.gov/data/sites/default/files/NSDUH-DetTabsPDFWHTML2013/Web/HTML/NSDUH-DetTabsSect2peTabs43to84-2013.htm#tab2.46b, on July 28, 2015.

World Health Organization (WHO). (2009). *Mental health systems in selected low- and middle-income countries: A WHO-AIMS cross-national analysis.* Retrieved from http://www.who.int/mental_health/evidence/who_aims_report_final.pdf, on July 29, 2015.

World Health Organization (WHO). (2012). *Depression.* Retrieved from http://www.who.int/mediacentre/factsheets/fs369/en/#, on July 29, 2015.

World Health Organization (WHO). (2013). *Mental health action plan 2013–2020.* Retrieved from http://apps.who.int/iris/bitstream/10665/89966/1/9789241506021_eng.pdf?ua=1, on July 29, 2015.

World Health Organization (WHO). (2014). *Mental health: Strengthening our response.* World Health Organization. Retrieved from http://www.who.int/mediacentre/factsheets/fs220/en/, on July 27, 2015.

World Health Organization (WHO). (2015). *Dementia.* Retrieved from http://www.who.int/mediacentre/factsheets/fs362/en/, on July 29, 2015.

University of North Carolina. (2015). *Severe and persistent mental illness.* Retrieved from http://www.med.unc.edu/psych/cecmh/patient-client-information/patient-client-information-and-resources/clients-and-familes-resources/just-what-is-a-severe-and-persistent-mental-illness, on July 27, 2015.

Vanderplasschen, W., Wolf, J., Rapp, R. C., & Broekaert, E. (2007, March). Effectiveness of different models of case management for substance-abusing populations. *Journal of Psychoactive Drugs, 39*(1), 81–95. Retrieved from http://www.ncbi.nlm.nih.gov/pmc/articles/PMC1986794/pdf/nihms29643.pdf, on July 27, 2015.

Ziguras, S. J., & Stuart, G. W. (2000). A meta-analysis of the effectiveness of mental health case management over 20 years. *Psychiatric Services, 51*(11), 1410–1421. Retrieved from http://ps.psychiatryonline.org/doi/abs/10.1176/appi.ps.51.11.1410?url_ver=Z39.88-2003&rfr_id=ori%3Arid%3Acrossref.org&rfr_dat=cr_pub%3Dpubmed, on July 27, 2015.

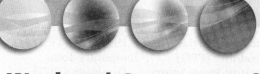

CHAPTER 24

Workers' Compensation Case Management

Hussein M. Tahan and Kathleen Fraser

LEARNING OBJECTIVES

Upon completion of this chapter, the reader will be able to:

1. Define terms and acronyms specific to workers' compensation case management.

2. Identify the primary purpose of workers' compensation for all stakeholders.

3. State the impact of workers' compensation laws on the provision of case management services.

4. Identify how to adapt case management services to adhere to state or federal statutory requirements.

5. Describe the market forces in the cost of workers' compensation programs that produce opportunities for skilled case management.

6. List the types of workers' compensation cases typically assigned for medical management and ways to successfully apply case management skills to them.

7. Understand the burden that medical, legal, and financial factors place on the practice of ethical, advocacy-based workers' compensation case management.

8. Understand the HIPAA ramifications in workers' compensation case management.

NOTE: This chapter is a revised version of Chapter 18 in the second edition of *CMSA Core Curriculum for Case Management*. The contributors wish to acknowledge the work of Deborah V. DiBenedetto, as some of the timeless material was retained from the previous version.

IMPORTANT TERMS AND CONCEPTS

American with
   Disabilities Act (ADA)
Designated Medical
   Evaluation (DME)
Disability
Field Case
   Management (FCM)
First Report of Injury
   (FROI)
Functional Ability
   Testing (FAT)
Functional Capability
   Examination (FCE)
Impairment
Impairment Income
   Benefits (IIBs)
Impairment Rating
Indemnity Payments
Independent Medical
   Evaluation (IME)

Job Analysis
Life Care Plan
Maximum Medical
   Improvement (MMI)
Modified Duty
Modified Work
On-site Case
   Management
Permanent Partial
   Disability (PPD)
Repetitive Stress Injury
   and Cumulative
   Trauma Injuries
Repetitive Strain Injury
Reserves
Return to Work (RTW)
Risk
Scheduled Injury
Second Injury Fund
   (SIF)

Self-insured
Supplemental Income
   Benefit (SIBs)
Temporary Alternate
   Work (TAW)
Temporary Income
   Benefit (TIBs)
Temporary Partial
   Disability (TPD)
Temporary Total
   Disability (TTD)
Third-Party
   Administrator (TPA)
Total and Permanent
   Disability (TPD)
Transitional Work
Vocational Assessment
Vocational
   Rehabilitation (VR)
Work Conditioning

 Introduction

A. Skillful case management in the field of workers' compensation
   demands specialized knowledge, skills, and understanding of pertinent
   terms, practices, and parameters not usually taught in health care
   settings.
B. It is essential for the case manager practicing in the workers'
   compensation field of case management to be familiar with the terms
   used throughout the industry and how to apply them in practice.
C. Review of the history of workers' compensation programs in US business
   leads to an understanding of today's health care delivery and workers'
   compensation systems.
D. The industrial revolution in America that began the transformation of
   the workforce from agrarian to industrial in the late 19th and early 20th
   centuries spawned the workers' compensation system that has taken us
   into the 21st century. In fact, case management began in the workers'
   compensation arena.
   1. Common law practices held that an employer was responsible for
      injuries or death to his or her workers only if they were caused by a
      negligent act.
   2. The injured employees or their survivors had to bring suit to
      establish that there was negligence on the part of employers. This
      process was difficult and out of the reach for most employees or
      family members.
   3. Injured workers' financial, functional, and health needs were
      absorbed by their families or the communities around them.

E. As the workplace became larger and more mechanized, the risk to workers increased. Social reformers recognized the need for legislated standards to protect individual workers and the community as a whole.

F. The first laws passed in the various states merely replaced common law with enacted laws, but the burden remained on the injured worker to prove employer responsibility.

G. In 1911, the first state workers' compensation laws were enacted that established a no-fault system to deal with work-related injuries.

H. Today, all 50 states and several US territories have workers' compensation laws.

I. Federal legislation also has been enacted to cover federal programs for workers' compensation.

J. It is important for case managers directly or indirectly caring for injured workers to be familiar with workers' compensation state and federal laws or how to access such information when needed. Often, case managers in acute or other care settings care for injured workers while collaborating with the workers' compensation claims adjuster or case manager.

 Descriptions of Key Terms

A. Disability—Is a limitation in an activity and/or participation restriction in an individual with a health condition, disorder, injury, or disease.

B. First report of injury (FROI)—This is a formal document completed by the employer—a report of a work-related injury or condition—that begins the process of a workers' compensation claim. The report is filed with the appropriate state jurisdiction and sent to the workers' compensation carrier or third-party administrator (claim handlers for self-insured employers). Workers' compensation systems allow injured workers or their designee to file a report of injury directly with the relevant state or federal workers' compensation board or industrial commission.

C. Functional capacity examination (FCE)—A systematic, objective process of assessing an individual's physical capacities and functional ability to execute tasks (e.g., sedentary, light, medium tasks). The FCE matches human performance levels to the demands of a specific job, work activity, or occupation. The FCE is often used in determining a person's potential for job placement, accommodation, and/or return to work after an injury. A comprehensive FCE also determines the individual's level of effort expended during testing, which can be a critical piece of information to have documented.

D. Impairment—Is a significant deviation, loss, or loss of use of any body structure or body function in an individual with a health condition, disorder, injury, or disease.

E. Impairment rating—The basis for determining the medical outcome of a workers' compensation claim. Many states require an impairment rating to be based on the findings of a licensed physician using an impairment rating system such as the *Guides to the Evaluation of Permanent Impairment*, sixth edition, published by the American Medical Association (AMA).

 1. The guides differentiate between medical impairment and disability and are used in workers' compensation systems, federal systems, automobile casualty, and personal injury cases to rate impairment not disability.

2. The final decision on a disability rating, if contested, rests with the state or federal workers' compensation board or industrial commission.

3. An impairment rating will always be completed; however, there may be a 0% rating. If the injured worker has a medically substantiated permanent change to preinjury health and function, an impairment rating percentage will be assigned. The percentage dictates the final amount of the financial compensation paid to the injured worker.

F. Indemnity payments—Monies paid as wage replacement when the injured worker is determined to be medically unfit to work. Indemnity payments are based on the worker's usual wage, factored by a formula set by the state that has jurisdiction for the claim.

G. Maximum medical improvement (MMI) and maximum medical recovery (MMR)—Terms used to indicate that the injured worker has recovered from injuries to a level at which a physician states that further treatment will not substantively change the medical outcome.

H. Permanent partial disability—The designation used to indicate that there is a presumptive or actual decrease in wage-earning capacity due to injury. A benefit is paid according to the severity of impairment in a formula derived by the state. Most states have *scheduled* injuries (benefit paid by a formula based on loss of, or loss of the use of, specific body members) and *nonscheduled* injuries (a benefit is based on the percentage of impairment in a formula computed by the state).

I. Permanent total disability—This evaluation is based on a medical assertion that the injured worker is precluded by the extent of his or her disability from gainful employment. Each state has guidelines on which this designation and subsequent benefits are paid.

J. Reasonable accommodation—Any change in the work environment or in the way a job is performed that enables a person with a disability to enjoy equal employment opportunities. There are three categories of reasonable accommodations—changes to a job application process, changes to the work environment or to the way a job is usually done, and changes that enable an employee with a disability to enjoy equal benefits and privileges of employment (such as access to training).

K. Reserves—The sum of money the insurance company or self-insured funds set aside to pay all costs associated with a claim.

L. Risk—In the workers' compensation field, risk refers to the extent of loss an organization is able to tolerate or feels comfortable tolerating. The organization usually plans for and manages what is probable or expected and applies a target against which it compares actual occurrences and experiences. The target is determined based on national benchmarks and state or federal laws and regulations.

M. Temporary partial disability—Status in which impairment prevents an injured worker from returning to his or her usual job, but the worker can be employed in some capacity. A benefit is paid when the restrictions to work activity result in a decrease of usual wages.

N. Temporary total disability—Status in which indemnity is paid when an injured worker is unable to work in any capacity while treatment continues, with the expectation of recovery and return to employment.

In most states, the injured receives benefits for the entire time he or she is medically deemed to be unable to work.

O. Vocational rehabilitation—Cost-effective case management services provided by a skilled professional (preferably certified as a vocational rehabilitation professional or counselor) who is knowledgeable about the implications of medical status, functional ability, and vocational services necessary to facilitate an injured workers' expedient return to gainful employment.

Applicability to CMSA's Standards of Practice

A. The Case Management Society of America (CMSA) describes in its standards of practice for case management (CMSA, 2010) that case management practice extends across all health care settings and providers of various professional disciplines. This without a doubt applies to the practice of workers' compensation case management whether in health insurance plans or employer settings.

B. Workers' compensation case managers (as all case managers) should use the CMSA standards as a guide for the implementation of their roles. All standards are relevant to workers' compensation including and perhaps especially the legal and ethical expectations.

C. It is important for case managers in the workers' compensation care settings to be aware of the CMSA standards of practice. When needed, they may inform their employers and other professionals they collaborate with when dealing with a client with a work-related injury or occupational illness about the availability of these standards if appropriate and their value.

D. This chapter introduces case managers to the basic concepts of workers' compensation practice, role of the case manager in such setting, and explains how collaboration may occur between case managers in the workers' compensation and other care settings.

Primary Goals of Workers' Compensation Programs

A. Provide injured workers (or those suffering from an occupational illness) prompt medical care and wage replacement.

B. Establish a single, primary remedy for workplace injuries to decrease the legal costs and relieve the judicial system of heavy caseloads of personal injury cases.

C. Relieve both the public and private sectors from demands on financial, medical, and rehabilitative services.

D. Provide a system for the delivery of workers' compensation benefits, resources, and services.

Understanding the Impact of Workers' Compensation Costs

A. The injuries or occupational illnesses covered under the relevant workers' compensation statute must "arise out of and in the course of employment."

B. Medical costs may represent 60% or a higher portion of workers' compensation expenses. Contributing factors to such costs are as follows:
   1. Obesity
   2. Comorbidities
   3. An aging workforce
   4. The utilization of opioids, which continues to rise at alarming rates
C. Workers' compensation program costs are born by the employers. Whether they "self-fund" or "self-insure" their workers' compensation programs, or make this benefit available through purchased insurance policies, employers must meet state requirements for these types of programs/insurance.
D. The cost of workers' compensation insurance and all costs associated with workplace injuries (or wellness and prevention of injuries) are reflected in the price of goods and services sold by the employer.
E. Besides the direct cost of buying insurance premiums, workers' compensation medical and rehabilitative care, and indemnity payments, there are other indirect costs associated with these programs that are included in the total cost of occupational disability:
   1. Accident investigation
   2. Worker replacement and resultant overtime
   3. Lost productivity
   4. Cost of case management services if assigned and/or required
F. The cost of buying workers' compensation insurance is based on a formula of previous claims, types of workers insured (e.g., clerical personnel have less risk of injury than do truck drivers), and an element calculated by the state based on annual costs (US Chamber of Commerce, 2015). The only factor that can be effectively modified by the employer is the cost associated with the number and severity of workplace injuries.
G. Workers' compensation insurance carriers and self-insured employers have a stake in decreasing costs of claims submitted to them. A competitive marketplace demands that companies sell their products at the lowest possible price; this provides the foundation for managing the cost of risk, and, ultimately, the cost of workers' compensation claims and experience.
H. Many strategies are employed in keeping claims costs low, including loss control, risk or absent management programs, as well as safety and health programs plus managed care arrangements (Box 24-1).

BOX 24-1   Managed Care Arrangements in Workers' Compensation

- Use of preferred providers, physician panels, or networks
- Specialty occupational disability and workers' compensation services
- Use of evidence-based protocols or guidelines
- Medical case management services
- Alternative work programs
- Utilization review services
- Bill review services

Fitting the Pieces Together: Medical Case Management in the Workers' Compensation System

A. Medical management processes have been involved in the periphery of workers' compensation programs for a number of years, both medically and vocationally.

B. Economic changes and escalating medical costs have placed a larger burden on employers required to provide workers' compensation coverage for their employees.

C. Case management strategies, as a component of health insurance and managed care arrangements, can be used as tools to lower workers' compensation and medical costs, improve communication, promote best medical and claim outcomes, and maintain a stable workforce.

D. A workers' compensation claim can be a complicated, often protracted process in which case managers can become involved at any time.

1. The longer the time it takes to assign a case manager to a claim, the potential for financial risk increases and the opportunity for risk mitigation is delayed resulting in the injured worker's potential for suboptimal care. The sooner the workers' compensation case manager becomes involved, the better the outcomes are likely to be. The case manager can then mitigate a progressive and positive claim process and ultimately provide positive outcomes.

2. Case managers assist the injured worker, health care provider, employer, health insurance plan, or third-party administrator (TPA) in understanding the impact of injury, disability, the workers' compensation system, medical care on health, and productivity, which facilitates a quicker yet safer return to work (RTW).

3. Case managers advocate for the client, employer, and the payer to facilitate positive outcomes for all: the client, client's support system, health care team members, employer, and the payer. However, if a conflict arises, the needs of the client must be the priority. A case manager's primary obligation is to the clients.

E. Workers' compensation laws demand the case management process be adapted to work within the workers' compensation and occupational health and safety structure.

Key Stakeholders in Workers' Compensation

A. Case managers working in the workers' compensation field encounter a greater number of stakeholders than in other areas of case management practice (see Box 24-2).

B. Adapting usual case management techniques and practices to the workers' compensation field requires the practitioner to recognize the responsibilities of the various people and organizations with a role in mediating a work-related injury claim (Box 24-3).

C. Due to the large amount of stakeholders, the role of case management is more challenging yet also even more critical.

1. Collaboration and communication with all parties must occur at every segment and level of care in workers' compensation case management.

BOX 24-2   Key Stakeholders in Workers' Compensation Programs

Often Involved
- Employee/injured worker
- Family/significant others
- Health care providers of each level of care or specialty (e.g., medical, rehabilitation, vocational)
- Employer
- Insurance company and claims adjuster
- Attorney or legal advisor
- Third-party administrator (TPA)

Potentially Involved
- Labor union representative (when applicable)
- Worker's immediate supervisor, middle and upper manager, and human resources/labor relations representative
- Occupational health case manager
- Vocational/rehabilitation specialist
- External case managers (e.g., case manager from hospital care setting)
- Social services/community supports
- Employee assistance program representative
- Occupational health and safety representative

2. Case managers are key professionals in maintaining open lines of communication among the stakeholders in the workers' compensation arena and in ensuring the stakeholders are well informed and on the same page at all times.
3. Breakdown in the lines of communication may adversely impact a worker's claim, protract worker disability, delay injured worker access to timely medical care, or delay recovery, return to function, and, ultimately, maximal medical improvement and return to preinjury status.

BOX 24-3   Responsibilities of Key Personnel Involved in a Workers' Compensation Case

- *Employer*—Reports claim and monitors claim; may have a risk manager, human resources manager, occupational health, safety, or other representative to assist with managing or coordinating workers' compensation claims and employee RTW.
- *Claims adjuster/claim examiner*—Has the responsibility of investigating the claim, applying laws, and making the first determination about compensability, paying indemnity, paying medical bills, and directing case management. This is also called adjudicating the claim.
- *Attorney or legal counsel*—The plaintiff if retained by the injured worker; the defense for insurance carrier and employer.
- *Labor union representative*—Can assist in protecting worker's rights and, depending upon negotiated agreements/labor contracts, may also have input regarding RTW, modified duty, or transitional work assignments.
- *State administrative agency*—Body at state level with jurisdiction over workers' compensation claims. These agencies may be called the Workers' Compensation Board, Industrial Commission, or another title.

Workers' Compensation Laws That Directly Affect Case Management Practice

A. Laws governing workers' compensation administration are enacted by each state and territorial legislature and administered by state agencies.

B. The U.S. Congress regulates areas of workers' compensation whose programs are deemed under national commerce. These programs with their own subsets are:
   1. Energy Employees Occupational Illness Compensation Program
   2. Federal Employees Compensation Program
   3. Longshore and Harbor Workers' Compensation Program
   4. Federal Black Lung Benefits Program

C. Laws are written and amended frequently. Because case managers must comply with the laws in order to practice legally and ethically, a source for learning about them is essential. Comprehensive compendia of state and federal laws can be found in:
   1. Annual editions of *Analysis of Workers' Compensation Laws*, prepared and published by the U.S. Chamber of Commerce
   2. U.S. Department of Labor Web site: www.dol.gov/dol/topic/workcomp
   3. The wealth of knowledge of the claims adjuster of the insurance company handling the claims

D. Each state has its own workers' compensation laws, which vary from one state to another; however, the main aspects of workers' compensation case management tend to be similar.

E. The specific workers' compensation laws that are governed federally and cover individuals in certain industries such as railroad workers, longshoremen, and federal employees may be specific to vocational benefits and entitlements of spouses or dependents, especially when the situation involves death.

F. The workers' compensation laws function as "no-fault" laws and protect the employer from civil lawsuits. However, third-party lawsuits can evolve whether due to aspects such as mechanical abnormalities or malfunction that caused the injury. This adds another line of legal contacts.

G. Workers' compensation laws dealing with claim issues may appear to have only a peripheral impact on medical management. However, knowledge of laws affecting the medical system has a direct effect on the case manager's ability to accomplish case management goals and objectives. Some states restrict the contacts with the injured worker up to allowing the injured workers' attorneys to attend provider appointments with the case manager.

H. Workers' compensation case managers have a responsibility to be familiar with applicable laws but must exercise caution to avoid the appearance of giving legal advice or directing care to key stakeholders, especially injured workers, health care providers, employers, and adjusters, among others.

I. Arguably, the most challenging laws for workers' compensation medical managers are those that dictate the selection and use of health care providers. States may mandate the manner in which providers or medical services can be chosen.

1. The initial choice of a health care provider can be made by:
   a. The injured worker without restriction
   b. The employer or insurance company by:
      i. Directly selecting a provider for the injured worker
      ii. Posting a panel of providers from which the injured worker selects
      iii. Belonging to a medical care organization (MCO) with preferred provider (PPO) lists from which the injured worker may choose
2. State laws also control changes of providers during the course of treatment. These guidelines for changes are quite complex in many states, and the claim handler can guide the case manager.[1]
3. State laws may also regulate the use of independent medical examinations (IMEs). These are evaluations generally arranged by the health insurance plan (i.e., workers' compensation benefit plan) or payer to confirm, rebut, or supplement medical findings offered by the injured worker's chosen physician or other provider.
   a. Regulations might limit the number of such examinations.
   b. There may be a specific time interval required between IMEs.
   c. State regulations can limit the type of practitioner who performs IMEs.
   d. Administrative agencies can require the payer and the injured worker to abide by the findings of specific physicians on a "designated provider" list.

J. State regulations pertaining to the use of health care services by injured workers often reflect efforts to contain medical costs. MCOs for workers' compensation health care providers are allowed or required in a few states.

K. Mandated managed care requirements are available from the state workers' compensation administrative agency (see listing of Web sites at the end of this book for relevant state and federal links).

L. Guidelines for case managers working for or with an MCO vary by state.
   1. States that do not allow MCOs often have some mechanism for regulating cost containment efforts by payers.
   2. Use of health care services can be regulated by type of health care provider, number of visits, duration of visits, cost of treatment, utilization and peer review, and medical practice parameters.
   3. Precertification, preauthorization, or utilization review is generally required in some states for:
      a. Nonemergency surgery
      b. High-dollar durable medical equipment, diagnostic tests, and costly or extensive therapies and procedures (such as MRIs, epidural injections, and work-reconditioning programs)
      c. Treatment for specific diagnoses (such as a second opinion for spinal surgery)
   4. Medical bill reviews and repricing services are allowed in most states. State regulations for utilization review and medical payments indicate whether repricing at so-called usual and customary rates (payments are based on a database reflecting standard charges for geographic

---

[1]Information about Official Disability Guidelines, managed care and cost containment strategies in workers' compensation can be accessed at http://www.worklossdata.com/.

area) or a fee schedule (published schedule of reimbursement allowed for charges for health care related to on-the-job injury) is allowed. The repricing is based on uniform databases.

M. States (such as CA) mandate the use of evidence-based medical (EBM) treatment protocols (or in FL, that providers be knowledgeable about relevant EBM guidelines) to direct the medical care of injured workers by their health care providers. The use of EBM tools reduces unnecessary medical care, facilitates positive medical outcomes, and ultimately saves costs.

N. Sources of EBM protocols for workers' compensation medical care and required in most state guidelines include:
   1. American College of Occupational and Environmental Medicine's (ACOEM) *Occupational Medicine Practice Guidelines*, which can be used in the evaluation and management of common occupational health problems, illnesses, and injuries. They also include functional recovery guidelines and are available online at http://www.acoem.org/PracticeGuidelines.aspx.
   2. Medical Disability Advisor (MDA), by Dr. Presley Reed. In-depth disability duration and treatment guidelines are outlined and may be available at http://www.mdguidelines.com/.
   3. Official Disability Guidelines (ODG) *Treatment in Workers' Compensation*, which has been accepted by the Federal Agency for Healthcare Research and Quality (AHRQ) for inclusion in the National Guidelines Clearinghouse, available at http://www.worklossdata.com/.

O. Almost all states and territories set up second injury funds for injured workers. These assist the injured worker and provide a financial offset for the employer. Conditions covered may include:
   1. Previously rated permanent impairment resulting from an on-the-job injury
   2. Medical disability
   3. Diseases that substantially impact recovery from a work-related injury

P. Vocational rehabilitation as provided by workers' compensation regulations is sometimes coordinated concurrently with medical management.
   1. Each state regulates the parameters concerning vocational rehabilitation for injured workers who are unable to return to previous employment. In some states such as Louisiana, the vocational case manager must be certified within that individual state to provide this service.
   2. A complete listing of state and territorial programs is available in the annual *U.S. Chamber of Commerce Analysis and the U.S. Department of Labor*.

Practicing the Case Management Process Within the Workers' Compensation System

A. The entire range of case management practices can be applied in a workers' compensation industry or work setting. The skills, knowledge, and competencies described in other chapters of this book are also critical for case managers in the workers' compensation specialty case management practice.

B. There are customary requirements for employment as a workers' compensation case manager.

C. The settings in which a case manager might practice these processes are varied.

D. The organization or facility paying for case management services often determines the scope and duration of the requested case management service(s).

E. The case management process as described in Chapter 12 and by many other authors can be applied to the most frequently encountered workers' compensation claims. Items F through M below highlight important aspects of the workers' compensation case management process.

F. Case finding and client targeting
   1. "Lost time" or "indemnity" claims (cases in which the injured worker has not returned to work within the time frame that triggers wage replacement benefits) are far more likely to be referred for case management evaluation and service provision than "medical only" cases, implying the injury has not prevented the injured worker from working at his or her usual job.

G. Evaluating and assessing
   1. Case managers in workers' compensation settings assess the needs of the worker who suffers a work-related injury or occupational illness through claim file and medical record review; direct contact with the worker and his or her family, medical providers, employer, and others; and evaluation of current treatment plan and care setting for that treatment.
   2. Part of the assessment process in workers' compensation case management is to evaluate the extent of injuries or occupational illness, probable treatment plan, expectation of complete recovery, impact of the injury or illness on job requirements, and estimated time out of work.
   3. The assessment information is reported to the claims handler so that appropriate reserves can be set.
   4. Reserves may be applied. These are the sum of money the insurance company or self-insured funds set aside to pay all costs associated with a claim. This process is an important one for claims handling, and the case manager's assessment can be critical.

H. Planning, identifying, and solving problems
   1. Case managers in workers' compensation have the special task of recognizing the problems that have resulted from an on-the-job injury or illness and their ramifications.
   2. The payer generally does not address nonoccupational health concerns and/or social problems unless these have a direct impact on the injured worker's recovery from the occupational condition.
   3. Workers' compensation laws proscribe offering benefits for nonrelated care and activity. Case managers can direct injured or ill workers and their families to appropriate agencies and services.
   4. Plans for addressing related problems are written and provided to appropriate parties.

I. Coordinating multiple health care providers
   1. In the current workers' compensation atmosphere, there are likely to be a number of health care providers involved. These depend on the type and severity of injury or occupational illness.

    2. Recognition of state laws governing selection of health care providers, including the use of MCOs, is essential.

    3. Highly developed communication skills are involved in monitoring health care progress, making recommendations based on it, and then assisting the injured or ill worker in receiving the most effective care available.

J. Utilization and peer review

    1. Because workers' compensation laws regulate health care service selection and utilization, the case manager must practice these activities within that framework.

    2. The workers' compensation system contains utilization review (UR) companies, TPAs, and MCOs used by insurance companies, large employers, and self-insureds. Case managers from these settings often have the responsibility of coordinating UR activities with the involved cost containment companies.

    3. UR, case management, and workers' compensation networks may seek to and obtain URAC accreditation in these areas (see www.urac.org). URAC offers health plan, case management, and other specialty accreditation programs.

K. Precertification, preauthorization determinations

    1. In the workers' compensation mosaic of state laws, preauthorization and precertification of procedures, services, assistive devices, and other equipment can be mandatory, allowed, or forbidden. Therefore, it is necessary that the case manager be knowledgeable about these requirements in the state with jurisdiction for the claim.

    2. MCOs and other cost containment companies often have the responsibility for the processes in states with an allowance or requirement for them.

    3. Because providers of health services and durable medical equipment are accustomed to securing preauthorization, a workers' compensation case manager is often requested to make decisions on authorization.

    4. The basic premise in all of workers' compensation health care allowance is that payment will be made for services that are "reasonable and necessary" to treat work-related injuries and illnesses.

       a. The case manager is often called upon to evaluate the reasonableness and necessity of various health care providers' services and charges.

       b. This role may also be a source of ethical conflict for the medical case manager: balancing advocacy, cost, access, and the best solution for the injured worker.

L. Negotiation and contracting

    1. The payment structure in workers' compensation in almost all states is based on a fee schedule or an acceptance of "usual and customary" costs listed in databases. The case manager must be aware of allowable charges before negotiating prices with health care providers or risk negotiating at higher costs.

    2. Some services or equipments that are seen infrequently in dealing with injured workers are considered "off record" and not on fee schedules or in databases. These items must be negotiated on a case-by-case basis or through the use of PPOs.

3. When there is no statutory guidance for regulating charges and the selection of health care providers is strictly the injured worker's choice, there is often little incentive for the providers to negotiate for reduced cost or utilization.

4. Establishing a network of providers is part of most case managers' responsibilities, whether on a formal or informal basis. When provider selection is allowed by the payer, there is an increasing trend toward using established workers' compensation PPOs for both health care services and equipment. It is imperative that the MCO/network providers:

   a. Are familiar with the relevant state workers' compensation laws and requirements

   b. Facilitate maximal medical recovery of the injured worker with return to health and productivity/RTW (i.e., applying a "sports medicine model") in a timely manner

   c. Use EBM tools as recommended by state law and as a best practice in other jurisdictions.

5. Be familiar with established disability duration guidelines to benchmark expected RTW. Popular disability duration guidelines include:

   a. Official Disability Guidelines (ODG).

   b. The Medical Disability Advisor (MDA).

   c. Quoting these guidelines assists in documenting expectations, especially with malingering treatment, without fear of incrimination, for example, "The expected length of disability for this injury is 30 days from date of injury. The injured worker has been off from work for 320 days."

   d. Refrain from subjectivity or judgment in your documentation. Do not give your opinion. Stick to the facts that will give the appropriate message of a red flag, if one exists.

M. Reporting

1. Most case management services in the workers' compensation field are performed at the request of the payer in the system (health insurance company, TPA, employer), and reporting needs to be concise and clear.

2. Reporting of all assessment, planning, intervention, and outcome activities documents the value of case management services in facilitating positive outcomes in workers' compensation such as moving the injured or ill worker toward maximal medical improvement and timely return to function and productivity.

3. All case management reports are part of legal records. In the workers' compensation arena, there is a likelihood that case management reports will appear in litigated cases.

4. HIPAA[2] confidentiality requirements do not apply in workers' compensation, the evaluation of occupational injuries/illnesses, and other agency reporting or medical surveillance/evaluation (such as OSHA and the Department of Transportation [DOT]).

---

[2]Detailed information on HIPAA and workers' compensation may be found at: www.hhs.gov/ocr.

Requirements for Workers' Compensation Case Managers Roles and Employment Settings

A. Although employers of workers' compensation case managers should require a minimum set of qualification for these roles, the requirements do currently vary depending on the employer. Suggested qualifications are:
   1. An educational degree in a health care–related field with a strong clinical background.
   2. Licensure in a relevant professional specialty (e.g., nursing).
   3. National case management and/or rehabilitation certification (a number of certification programs are considered acceptable).
   4. Knowledge of occupational health practice and related laws.
   5. A background in certain clinical specialties such as emergency care, occupational health, rehabilitation, or orthopedics, although not a requirement, is often a preference.
B. Case managers in the workers' compensation arena do not function as lawyers, adjusters, or private investigators. They do not assume responsibility for claims-related activities such as investigation, surveillance, or determination of compensation. However, they are obligated to report acts of fraud, which can add to the frequent gray areas as a patient advocate in this area of case management.
C. Some states may have strict requirements for becoming a workers' compensation case manager, which may include licensure or certification in addition to national credentials.
D. Employment settings for workers' compensation case managers are varied (Box 24-4).

BOX
24-4   **Possible Employment Settings for Workers' Compensation Case Managers**

- Insurance companies and workers' compensation carriers
- Third-party administrators
- Risk management consulting companies
- Independent/private case manager companies
  - National companies
  - Small local companies
  - Individual case managers as contracted independent practitioners
- Employers
- Providers
  - Occupational medicine practices
  - Orthopedic or other medical practices treating large numbers of workers' compensation–injured workers
  - Physical medicine and rehabilitation clinics and facilities
- Government entities
  - State and local government employees
  - Large government institutions such as universities and hospitals
  - State insurance funds
  - Federal government such as case management services conducted through the U.S. Department of Labor
- Managed care organizations

E. Numerous opportunities exist for case managers to choose from when they are pursuing new or a change in employment. Case managers may
   1. Work for both large and small companies with varied workforce sizes
   2. Be part of an integrated disability management, vocational rehabilitation services/teams, or total health management programs
   3. Focus on a nursing-related scope of practice encompassing occupational health nursing
   4. Pursue employment opportunities in state-based workers' compensation agencies

Scope of Medical Management in Workers' Compensation Settings

A. Referrals for most workers' compensation case management services come from the payer (self-insured employer, carrier, or TPA); therefore, the payer generally decides on the scope of services requested or that may be required.
   1. Internal case managers are those working directly for the payer.
   2. External case managers are those, generally in independent case management companies, from whom the payer purchases case management services.
   3. Case managers with providers and MCOs derive their income from the payer.
B. Medical management services may be performed in three different ways:
   1. Telephonic case management (TCM) in workers' compensation is restricted to the three-point contact (injured worker, employer, and physician) via telephone calls, faxes, e-mail, other means of electronic communication, and traditional methods of correspondence, such as letters.
      a. TCM allows a case manager to oversee a high volume of open cases from a single location, seemingly making it a less costly way to apply medical management services.
      b. Relying solely on TCM for catastrophic and serious workplace injures is of limited value to the injured worker.
   2. On-site or field case management, which is the "traditional" method of workers' compensation case management where the injured worker is met in person for an initial assessment, a possible workplace examination, or a job analysis. Often, physician appointments are attended by the case manager as well.
      a. Case selection is an important component in measuring the benefit of on-site case management. In general, the more potentially expensive the claim might be, the more cost-effective on-site case management can be.
      b. On the surface, on-site case management may appear to cost more; however, most claims handled on-site as needed will close faster as a result of more expedient return to work, therefore, less indemnity costs to the file. In these cases, the treating physician's requests and reports are obtained on a "real-time" aspect since the case manager is attending these appointments with the injured worker. Everyone is kept on the same page with a higher instance of positive outcomes.

    c. When on-site case managers have cases in which TCM is appropriate, they are able to influence better outcomes for these cases than case managers who solely perform TCM because the providers' office staff are more responsive and cooperative to the requests for information and reports since they have worked with the CM in person.

3. Case management services in which the same case manager covers both telephonic and on-site activities and services the files accordingly, is the optimal, and offers the most cost-effective services with greater continuity of care providing more positive outcomes. This is the "ideal" but cannot always be possible, due to geographical considerations.

4. Collaborative case management services include an amalgamation of TCM and FCM but with the TCM as the lead case manager working for the insurance carrier and the FCM being contracted with and independent or private company, attending appointments and reporting back to the TCM.

    a. Some insurance carriers and large self-insured employers manage cases in this manner.

    b. The Office of Workers' Compensation for federal employees has been established with the Department of Labor's nursing staff coordinating case management activities with field nurses. Although other factors are involved, case costs decrease dramatically with these programs as opposed to handling the cases with only their telephonic case managers.

Applying the Case Management Process

A. The duration and amount of workers' compensation benefits vary depending on the severity of the injured workers' disability as well as the individual state or federal regulations in which the injury is governed.

1. Most workers' compensation cases do not progress to lost time past the initial waiting period. In some cases, only medical benefits are paid. These cases are referred to as *medical only* cases.

    a. Medical only cases represent a small amount of benefit payments because these injuries are often minor in nature and do not result in lost time from work.

    b. Other cases may involve injured workers with lost work time and cash wage replacement payments. However, the majority of workers' compensation cases are those that receive cash benefits and medical care combined.

2. Most often, it is the lost time indemnity and "catastrophic" cases that are most frequently referred to medical case managers.

B. A workers' compensation claim can be prolonged and complex. A case management referral can occur at any time in that continuum, and the case management process needs to be adapted to meet the needs of the injured worker and the payer at that level. It behooves the payer/insurance carrier/TPA to refer cases as soon as possible for effective case management outcomes.

C. Because relatively few categories of injury cases are referred for case management, the case management process can be modeled to describe the most common types.

1. Catastrophic and serious injury cases may include severe head injuries, spinal cord injuries, severe burns, limb amputation, multiple fractures, and major organ and tissue damage.
   a. These cases are the easiest to identify and are usually referred to case management services soon after notice of the injury is received.
   b. Each referral source may have a different definition of what kinds of injuries are deemed serious, such as potential high-dollar loss or potential for severe impairment.
   c. Goals for case management are to ensure high-quality, effective medical care for the injured worker while containing costs and attempting to limit impairment.
2. The case management process model for catastrophic and serious cases begins with an assessment, which focuses on the activities described in Box 24-5.
3. The next step in the case management process is analyzing the information obtained and planning the workers' compensation case management services (Box 24-6).
4. Next is implementation and coordination of the plan of care and case management services. Services may include medical care, rehabilitation, health instructions, review of benefits, counseling, and communication with stakeholders among other activities. Other activities include those listed in Box 24-7.
5. Monitoring, evaluation, and reporting of outcomes are the next natural activity of the case management process. Here, the case

BOX 24-5 — **The Case Manager's Assessment Activities of Catastrophic Injury Cases**

- Begin the assessment immediately after the referral is received. Discuss expectations for case management with the referral source.
- Identify and contact the facility case manager or discharge planner and establish credentials and responsibility.
- Determine the nature and extent of the injuries, current treatment plan, and prognosis.
- Review the chart and all medical records available.
- Speak to physicians and other caregivers to understand the injured worker's current status.
- Interview the injured worker and family members.
- Determine the injured worker's understanding of the injuries, prognosis, and treatment.
- Identify the strength of the injured worker's support system.
- Identify any critical needs (such as lodging, childcare). The home environment is assessed by establishing where the injured worker lives, with whom, the structure (in case home modification is contemplated), and any safety concerns.
- Question the availability of transportation for injured worker visits when appropriate.
- Contact the employer to identify any source of support by employer and coworkers, including options for the injured worker's RTW. During this contact, a rapport should be developed with the employer that will be maintained throughout the case management process.

BOX
24-6   **The Case Manager's Planning of Care Activities for the Catastrophic Injury Cases**

- Determine whether the current care setting is appropriate for the injured worker's medical and rehabilitation needs and its accessibility for family members. (It is not uncommon for an injured worker to be injured at a remote job site or to be transported to a facility that is a distance from family members.)
- Formulate the expected time frame before discharge. It is best to complete this after assessment of the diagnosis and treatment plan and monitoring of medical progress.
- Establish whether the injured worker can be dismissed directly to home or will need to be admitted to another facility for a different level of care.
- Determine level of care based on knowledge of home environment and support system.
- Determine whether it is more cost-effective and appropriate to offer services at a subacute or skilled care facility. Cost of home care versus institutional care is a strong determining factor. If the injured worker needs multiple health care services or is unable to safely perform activities of daily living (ADL), these needs can often be met more economically at a subacute or skilled nursing facility.
- Develop a case management plan that reflects knowledge of the concurrent plans of medical providers, family members, and the facility case manager. The case management plan must deal with health care needs and optimum recovery of function expected, including RTW.

BOX
24-7   **The Case Manager's Implementation of Care Activities for the Catastrophic Injury Cases**

- Making the facility discharge planner aware of PPOs, special contracts, and other cost containment issues at the outset, especially in states where this is allowed
- If there are no PPOs or other contracts in place, seeking out appropriate providers for needed services and negotiating the best service at the best price with each of them
- Sharing the case management plan with the injured worker, family, claims handler, employer, medical providers, and hospital discharge planner. Adjusting the plan as needed until agreement on the plan is reached
- Coordination with the facility discharge planner and setting up transportation needs, home care providers, durable medical equipment providers, and injured worker appointments for follow-up care
- Coordination with the discharging and the admitting facilities when the injured worker is not yet ready for discharge to home but must be transferred to another facility
- Consulting with the claims manager/payer when needs are identified that seem to be outside the scope of workers' compensation coverage
- Informing the injured worker or the family and the facility discharge planner when it is determined that concurrent medical or social service needs do not arise from the injury and do not significantly impact recovery from injuries
- Assisting in the referral of the injured worker and his family to appropriate providers and agencies

manager receives and reviews reports from all health care providers and maintains contact with the injured worker and family through telephone calls and visits.

    a. If the injured worker is treated in a rehabilitation or another extended stay facility, the case manager attends team conferences.

    b. Physician visits are monitored either by attending appointments when treatment decisions are anticipated or through telephonic management procedures.

    c. Medical services are evaluated, coordinated, and modified or completely changed to meet the goals of recovery of health and function.

    d. The injured worker's recovery is usually monitored until he or she is stated to be at MMI.

    e. Assistance is made to return the injured worker to regular or modified work whenever possible. When a work-related injury results in permanent disability, with ongoing needs for medical care and equipment, the case management plan often includes a life care plan and recommendation for case manager involvement.

D. Injured workers with prolonged treatment, multiple providers, and/or overuse of services are referred for case management often out of the frustration of the injured worker, the claims handler, or the employer over a lack of case resolution. The workers' compensation case manager is likely to receive referrals for such cases later in the claims process (Box 24-8).

    1. These prolonged treatment cases ultimately result in claims handling issues or litigation; often if not already involved, they are imminent.

    2. The goals for case management are to determine appropriate and effective medical care, coordinate timely delivery of that care, communicate goals to all stakeholders, and assist in the injured worker's RTW when possible.

E. Injury claims with known barriers to recovery and rehabilitation are considered "red flag" cases and warrant special attention from the workers' compensation case manager (Box 24-9). The goals for case management for these cases are to address specified problems, identify achievable solutions for problems, coordinate medical care that will

---

BOX 24-8 Examples of Cases with Prolonged Treatment and Overuse of Services

- Prolonged treatment for an injury with unrelated complications
- Development of complex injury sequelae such as regional causalgia (formerly identified as reflex sympathetic dystrophy [RSD]), chronic pain, fibromyalgia, or chronic myofascial syndrome
- Longer-than-expected recovery from injuries without known complications
- Prolonged disability from a minor injury with insufficient medical causation
- Inability to communicate successfully with medical providers or a noted lack of clear diagnosis, treatment plan, or work status
- Multiple treatments with physical therapy, chiropractor, and other practitioners without documented progress

24-9 Examples of Injured Workers with Barriers to Recovery

- Injured workers who have innate or acquired barriers to achieving optimum recovery from injuries and rehabilitation; often referred to case management by claims adjusters.
- Injured workers with concurrent disability or disease that may or may not be associated with a work-related incident.
- Injured workers who do not speak or understand English will have difficulty understanding and complying with medical regimens.
- Injured workers with a perceived lack of incentive to comply with medical treatment and RTW.

help the injured worker recover from injuries, and assist in the injured worker's RTW.

1. Case management process model for cases with prolonged treatment, complications, and complicating factors
   a. Assessment involves discussing case management expectations with the referral source and a review of the claim file thoroughly. Box 24-10 describes the areas of special focus during the assessment.

24-10 Focus of the Assessment of Cases with Prolonged Treatment

- Understand the mechanism and causation of injury.
- Review all medical bills and find matching medical reports.
- Determine the treating physician or other practitioner (such as chiropractor) who is directing care.
- List all health care providers since the injury.
- Identify what medical records are needed to complete a medical record review.
- Interview the employer to gather his or her understanding of injury, treatment, and barriers that are preventing the injured worker from returning to work.
- Interview the injured worker and the family. If the worker is represented by an attorney, permission is sought from the attorney before directly contacting the injured worker or the family. If the worker is represented and contact allowed, the interview might be scheduled in the attorney's office or in other controlled surroundings.
- Determine the injured worker's understanding of the injury; any diagnoses, treatment including medication, and barriers to RTW; and additional treatment that he or she feels might be helpful.
- Determine whether language or culture is a barrier to understanding medical treatment and the RTW process.
- Ask about concurrent medical problems, family dynamics, the home environment, and the potential for job placement if necessary.
- Interview the worker and the family to understand whether the prolonged treatment and time off work is meeting some other needs such as caring for children, other family members, or any other financial disincentives to returning to work.
- The injured worker or his or her attorney might not allow all questions to be answered.

b. Planning and analyzing and focusing the case management plan on the injured worker achieving the goals of return to optimum health and recovery of function, including RTW.
    i. Through the detailed review of medical records, the case manager determines the most appropriate provider to achieve these goals.
    ii. The plan includes suggestions for diagnostic procedures to confirm diagnoses, if appropriate (e.g., if a diagnosis of regional causalgia is suspected, electrodiagnostics, three-phase bone scan, and ganglion blocks are standard procedures in this condition).
c. Implementing and coordinating, which requires the case manager to share the case management plan with all stakeholders and revise it as needed. Examples of workable communication tools for telephone calls and letters can be found in the *Case Manager's Handbook*, 5th Edition (Mullahy, 2014).
    i. Communicate with all medical providers to get the injured worker's updated records, along with current diagnosis, treatment plan, and activity restriction, including restrictions for work.
    ii. Ideally, the injured worker (and attorney) will cooperate in trying to achieve the goals of optimum recovery of health and function, but should an adverse reaction occur, the claims adjuster will be consulted.
    iii. Selecting the appropriate provider to help in achieving goals can be accomplished with the cooperation of the injured worker by scheduling a second opinion or a change of physician. If an adverse situation exists, an IME will be scheduled with approval from the adjuster.
    iv. Determining the availability of modified work to address activity restrictions.
    v. Communication with the employer continues, and efforts are made to assist the injured worker in his or her RTW.
    vi. Coordination of the delivery of appropriate medical care continues until there is a physician-issued MMI date.
d. Monitoring, evaluating, and reporting of outcomes. This requires follow-up with the injured worker and employer to evaluate success of medical and rehabilitation treatment and return to work.
    i. If a full duty release is anticipated soon after the injured worker has returned to work on modified duty or shortened hours, monitoring of status will continue until that release.
    ii. A report of case management activity and outcomes will be given to the adjuster.
F. Workplace violence, a growing concern, results in physical and psychological injuries. Most employers will seek assistance from their employee assistance program (EAP) provider, the occupational health professionals, and, for those employees requiring additional medical care or support, the services of a medical or workers' compensation case manager.
    1. The sources of workplace violence are varied.
        a. Internal conflicts and disruptions such as assaults, fistfights, labor unrest, disgruntled employees or family members, "horseplay," and arson or bomb

    b. External criminal activity such as aggravated robberies, effect of a fellow worker's homicide, and physical assaults outside the workplace (fire personnel, service and delivery employees)

    c. Defense Base Act, which falls under the Longshore Federal Program and covers employees of companies contracted by our armed forces in areas of military activity

2. The workers' compensation aftermath of workplace violence can be very challenging for the case manager.

    a. Physical injuries that result from gunshots, stabbings, and beatings are often complex and require multiple providers for treatment.

    b. Many workplace violence injuries result in some posttraumatic stress symptoms for the injured worker and other personnel.

    c. The aftereffects of violence complicate the RTW process for the injured worker and his or her family, coworkers, and employer.

3. Goals for the case manager are to identify the effects of violence on the injured worker and others; coordinate timely delivery of health care, including psychological support when it is determined to be necessary; and assist in the injured worker's return to work.

4. Case management process model for violence in the workplace—aftermath

    a. Assessment.

        i. Medical records are reviewed and providers consulted to determine nature and extent of the injured worker's injuries, treatment plan, and prognosis.

        ii. Review police and newspaper reports, if available.

        iii. Interview the injured worker and family and determine their understanding of injuries, treatment plan, and prognosis.

           • Understand family structure and support system.

           • Assess the injured worker's ability to remember and discuss the details of the injury.

           • List any preexisting mental and physical health concerns that might affect the injured worker's recovery from injuries.

           • Identify barriers to recovery of health and function, including signs of posttraumatic stress in injured worker or family members or both.

        iv. Interview the employer to discuss the events of the injury and determine plans for the injured worker's return to work.

           • Discuss the impact of the injured worker's injuries on the employer and coworkers.

           • Identify the employer's ability to modify the injured worker's job for RTW, including changes of hours and addressing safety concerns.

        v. Planning and analyzing. Here, the case manager focuses the case management plan on achieving the goals of return to optimum health and recovery of function, including RTW.

           • Determine appropriate health care providers for physical and psychological care.

           • Determine whether posttraumatic stress signs are present; the case management plan includes an opportunity for the

BOX 24-11 Implementation of Care Activities for Workplace Violence Cases

- Whenever possible, attend physician appointments that will include decision-making activity with the injured worker.
- Communicate with the employer.
- Discuss progress of injured worker in return to health and function.
- The employer may identify other workers who are having difficulty coping with the episode of workplace violence. An external case manager can offer services only to an employee who has filed a claim. Therefore, the employer needs to be directed toward other resources such as EAPs for these workers.
- Address concerns in regard to the injured worker's RTW.
- Check on availability for modifications to meet physical restrictions resulting from injuries.
- Implement plan for modification of job duties, task assignments, hours of work, and other workplace concerns in coordination with mental health recommendations if available.
- Facilitate RTW by communicating with appropriate health care providers.

      injured worker to be evaluated by an appropriate mental health care professional.
- Share the case management plan with all stakeholders and modify as needed.

   vi. Implementing and coordinating, which involves gathering the relevant medical records and coordinating all health care provider visits for timely delivery of case management services (Box 24-11).

  b. Monitoring, evaluating, and reporting of outcomes. This requires the case manager to monitor care activities, progress toward achieving goals, and review of all medical records.

     i. Communicate with injured worker, providers, and employer until MMI statement is received and the injured worker has returned to optimum functioning.

    ii. Share the report of case management activities and outcomes with the adjuster.

Workers' Compensation Referrals for Return to Work

A. Workers' compensation case managers may recommend to the adjuster the referral of injured workers to other health care providers and specialists to assist in the RTW activities.

B. Although regaining all functional activities by an injured worker is important, the activity most central to the process is RTW. The longer the treatment and recovery period, the less the chances are that the worker is able to return to work. For example, if a worker is out for 6 months, there is a 50% chance he or she will return to work compared to a worker who is out for 12 months, the likelihood he or she returns to work decreases to about 25% and to virtually no chance of RTW after 2 years (USDOL, 2015a).

1. The case manager integrates RTW in all assigned cases for workers' compensation medical management unless instructed to do so otherwise.
2. Goals of case management are to assess barriers to RTW; communicate with the employer and educate, if necessary, on the positive effects of returning injured worker to work; address medical concerns that may prevent RTW; and coordinate the RTW process.

C. The case management process model for RTW referrals is similar to the general process and that used by workers' compensation case managers.
   1. Assessment the case manager completes for RTW cases focuses on number of activities such as those described in Box 24-12.
   2. Planning and analyzing of the case management plan focusing in particular on barriers to RTW and possible solutions to these identified problems. The case manager shares the case management plan with all stakeholders and modifies it as required.
   3. Implementing and coordinating the case management plan.

BOX 24-12   Case Manager's Assessment for RTW Referred Cases

- Discuss case management expectations with referral source.
- Ascertain whether the assignment includes a need for comprehensive interview with injured worker.
- Identify any claims handling issues involved in the failure of the injured worker to RTW.
  - Extraneous employment issues
  - Plaintiff attorney involvement
- Review the claim file thoroughly.
  - Understand the mechanism and causation of injury.
  - Review all medical records to determine what restrictions on activity have been identified.
  - Determine treating physician or other practitioner (such as chiropractor) directing care.
  - Identify the barriers preventing the injured worker from RTW.
  - Consider the impact of permanent disability and the need to consider reasonable accommodation under the Americans with Disabilities Act (ADA).
- Interview the employer to gather his or her understanding of injury, treatment, and barriers preventing the injured worker from RTW.
- Communicate with the employer about the following:
  - Review of the employer's RTW policy.
  - If no formal policy exists, the case manager will ask about usual practices in allowing an injured worker to RTW before being released for full, unrestricted duties.
  - Modified or "light" duty.
  - Union rules that may affect RTW.
  - Understanding of the injured worker's preinjury position and essential tasks.
  - Application of ADA requirements for permanent disabilities.
- If it is part of the case management assignment, interview the injured worker and the family, if approved by plaintiff attorney of a represented worker.
  - Determine understanding of injuries and treatment.
  - Identify barriers to RTW.

a. The case manager determines whether the treating physician has identified appropriate activity restrictions and, if not, communicates with the physician to determine specific restrictions.

b. The case manager coordinates the medical care identified by the physician as necessary to release the injured worker for work.

c. Communication with the employer about the RTW includes:

   i. Education on the positive effect on both the injured worker and the workers' compensation claim process when the worker returns to work as soon as possible.

   ii. An understanding of modifying usual job duties to meet activity restrictions as stated by the treating physician.

   iii. Discussion of short-term employment in another job for the employer to meet the stated activity restrictions.

   iv. Referral to a claims adjuster to discuss partial temporary payments (PTDs) if wages or hours are less than usual wage.

   v. The case manager derives from communication with the employer an understanding of the physical activity involved to do the injured worker's usual job. The case manager requests the injured worker's job description for analysis and care planning (Box 24-13). If no job description is available or if the physical requirements of the job are not detailed, the case manager may opt to conduct a job analysis that will provide the treating physician with a clear idea of the physical abilities necessary to return the injured worker to his or her usual job.

d. The case manager will recommend using the services of an ergonomic specialist for job analysis and activity recommendations if the physical demands are particularly complex or the RTW issues are critical in the claim handling process.

e. The case manager will communicate with the treating physician and present the completed job analysis for review.

f. If a clear diagnosis is present, appropriate treatment has been rendered, and all barriers for recovery of health and function have been addressed, but the injured worker has not been released

BOX 24-13 **Information Targeted in a Job Description Analysis**

- Job title
- Tools, machines, and equipment used regularly
- The usual work cycle and number of hours worked weekly
- Specific essential physical demands regarding lifting (including amount lifted in pounds), bending, reaching, crawling, climbing, and kneeling
- Hours typically spent sitting, standing, and walking
- The frequency each essential function occurs in a workday
- Repetitive activity, including physical action and duration of activity in a work shift
- Environment (temperature, air quality, uneven surfaces for walking)
- RTW options and modifications available

for work, the case management plan will include a request for a Functional Capacity Evaluation (FCE).

g. The FCE objectively identifies the injured worker's current level of functioning and provides the physician objective testing to assist in determining activity restrictions and possible impairment.

h. The FCE includes testing the work category the injured person is capable of performing, that is, sedentary, light, and medium.

i. Specific validation parameters are taken into consideration and are considered useful in measuring submaximal effort or inconsistencies in work abilities.

j. As a result of the FCE, recommendations for activities, such as work hardening or work conditioning, are determined to increase the injured worker's physical capacity and allow less restrictive functioning.

k. When all activity fails to return the injured worker to work, a referral to vocational rehabilitation may be made in accordance with individual state laws. The case manager's involvement with vocational rehabilitation will be directed by paying source.

4. Monitoring, evaluating, and reporting of outcomes. Here, the case manager follows up with the injured worker and employer to evaluate the success of the medical treatment and RTW plan.

a. If an ultimate full duty release is anticipated, the injured worker may return to work with modified duty first. The case manager soon after the injured worker has returned to work on modified duty or shortened hours monitors the status and will continue to do so until the full release.

b. Vocational rehabilitation is monitored if requested.

c. A report of case management activities and outcomes is given to the adjuster.

D. Cases assigned to a case manager for scheduling of IMEs and second opinions

1. An IME is a frequently used tool to resolve medical issues and questions in a workers' compensation claim.

a. The scope, content, utilization, and provider(s) used may be proscribed by statute in the concerned jurisdiction. Specifically, the frequency and number of IMEs and the practitioner used may be regulated by state workers' compensation laws.

b. Whether the case manager is arranging an IME as a specific task or whether it is part of an ongoing management file, specific guidelines apply (Box 24-14).

c. IMEs are often a claims handling maneuver and are coordinated with the claims adjuster or manager to ensure that appropriate goals are set and met.

d. The final case manager task following an IME is to secure a report and provide it to the claims adjuster for distribution. However, if the IME were directed to the adjuster, the case manager may have to request a copy for her information and case management planning.

24-14 General Guidelines for Use of IMEs

- Because an IME can be viewed as an adversarial action, a careful explanation of the reasons for scheduling the evaluation is made to the injured worker if direct communication is allowed.
- The selection of the practitioner to do the evaluation is key to the outcome.
- The physician selected (or other practitioner required) must be well qualified and credentialed, usually with board certification in the specialty. The American Board of Independent Medical Examiners (ABIME) has developed standards for the delivery of IMEs and certification of IME providers (www.ABIME.org).
- Many physicians do not perform IMEs; the ones who do perform them as part of their practices generally have specific guidelines and requirements they must follow.
- The claims adjuster may have input into selection as part of the overall claim handling process.
- The communication among stakeholders is vital both for the success of resolving medical questions and as a legal responsibility of the case manager.
- It is essential both as a process component and as a legal responsibility that the case manager gets all accumulated medical records, including x-ray studies, to the independent examiner for review.

Ethical Considerations for Workers' Compensation Case Managers

A. Case managers have the responsibility to adhere to established standards of practice and codes of ethics and professional conduct, promote the adherence of ethical standards in the workplace, and sometimes establish ethical standards in their profession.

B. Legal issues in workers' compensation claims challenge both the practice and the professionalism of case managers.

C. Case managers must perform within their professional scope of practice and based on their licensure and/or certifications.

D. Medical case managers (i.e., registered professional and advanced practice nurses) must be licensed in the state in which they deliver medical case management services.

E. In response to interstate practice in today's electronic age and mobile workforces, the National Council of State Boards of Nursing (NCSBN) has developed the "interstate compact." Nurses residing in, and licensed in compact states, have an unrestricted license to practice in states within the compact (see www.ncsbn.org *for more information*).

F. Ethical practice also extends to all members of the health care team involved in the care of an injured worker or the worker suffering from an occupational illness. Case managers act as gatekeepers and function as worker's advocate. In this regard, assuring that the delivery of workers' compensation case management services is an important priority.

G. General ethical principles as defined by a number of ethicists also apply to the practice of workers' compensation case management. The five most commonly referred to are described in Box 24-15.

BOX
24-15

Ethical Principles Applicability in Workers' Compensation Case Management

1. Advocacy and autonomy
   - Goals for advocating for an injured worker include recommending and coordinating the most effective medical care to treat injuries and to lead to an optimum recovery of function.
   - The principle of promoting injured worker autonomy is tempered by state laws and claims considerations. However, the case manager communicates to the injured worker rights and responsibilities of all concerned in the coordination and delivery of medical care.
   - It is imperative that the case manager inform the injured worker when the payer is providing the services and clearly define the expectations of the payer for care activities and reporting.
   - Always represent what is in the best interest of the client/injured worker.
2. Beneficence, maleficence, and malfeasance
   - Promoting good and preventing harm.
   - Medical management systems based on promoting appropriate (preferably EBM) care for the injured worker and working within the laws of the state/ jurisdiction.
   - An example is a positive outcome for the injured worker in achieving maximum medical improvement and a return to the highest possible level of function, including work.
3. Justice
   - Presents one of the most potential ethical dilemmas for a workers' compensation case manager.
   - Focus is on fair treatment of injured workers.
   - A primary goal is to promote safety in the workplace.
   - The injured worker has the right to expect confidentiality in the handling of medical records and other personal information; however, workers' compensation laws give access to the records to a number of stakeholders.
   - Protecting injured worker's privacy and confidentiality when using electronic mail and other Internet-based communication tools.
   - The cost of workers' compensation is borne by the employer and by society as a whole in the price of goods and services. Taxes are used to provide workers' compensation coverage to local, state, and federal government employees. Overuse or abuse of the system by any participant does an injustice to all members of society.
   - Avoiding conflict in the application of the ethical principle of justice. Examples of situations of conflict are:
     - The injured worker has an agenda that does not include recovering from his or her injuries and returning to work.
     - The employer's dealings with the injured worker are not consistent with either the letter or the spirit of employment laws.
     - The claims handler fails to inform the injured worker of pertinent facts and rights that might affect the outcome of his or her injury claim.
     - The medical provider overbills or prolongs medical care, treatment, or management of an injured workers' case unnecessarily.
4. Fairness and equity
   - Treating everyone the same regardless of race, gender, or class.
   - Focus on offering the injured worker equal access to needed health care, services, and resources.
   - No room for bias or prejudice.

continued

BOX

24-15 | **Ethical Principles Applicability in Workers' Compensation Case Management** *continued*

- An example is pursuing the case management services of a consultant or specialist for effective RTW.
5. Veracity and fidelity
    - Telling the truth is an underlying principle in health care, nursing, and other business conduct.
    - Being truthful allows the case manager to gain the trust of the injured worker and others involved. Therefore, cooperation from the injured worker, the employer, the adjuster, and all medical providers increases.
    - Telling the truth is the basis for the case manager as an advocate for the injured worker in a system that has many competing interests.
    - Truthfulness is necessary when medical records are presented to a medical provider for review so that all interests are represented fairly.
    - The case manager should not make promises she or he cannot keep such as benefits for the injured workers, which are actually not covered.

H. Case managers in workers' compensation communicate established ethical standards as developed by their professional societies to guide their practice. Examples of these references or guides for ethical behavior may include but are not limited to the following:
   1. The Case Management Society of America (CMSA) Standards of Practice
   2. American Nurses Credentialing Center (ANCC) Code of Ethics
   3. The Commission for Case Management Certification (CCMC) Professional Conduct for Case Managers
I. Case managers in any practice setting or specialty find themselves in daily struggles to address injured workers' rights while fulfilling responsibilities to the employer or the payer who engages them in a case for which they are paid.
J. Case managers involved in workers' compensation claims practice are in an inherently difficult area because there are many stakeholders, often with sharply competing interests.

 ## Legal Issues for the Workers' Compensation Case Manager

A. The case manager's role, while primarily medically focused, is linked to the legal issues in an injured worker claim.
   1. The case manager has the responsibility of knowing and following state laws dictating medical care providers in a workers' compensation claim.
   2. The case manager cannot contact an injured worker directly when he or she is represented by an attorney without permission and needs to abide by the instructions of the plaintiff attorney in matters concerning communication with the injured worker. The case manager should follow company guidelines/policies when dealing with litigated cases.

3. Laws in some states restrict the flow of information between medical providers and the case manager.
4. Failure to adhere to laws can result in penalties against the payer with substantial fines.

B. The case manager is legally accountable to practice case management within the scope of her or his professional license and laws of the jurisdiction relevant to the place of work.

C. The case manager has the responsibility of knowing about applicable laws dealing with workers' compensation practice; to fail to do so falls below professional standards.

D. Case managers are accountable for referrals to risk management and appropriate health care providers when an unanticipated negative event occurs.

E. The case manager has a responsibility to report accurately on case management activities and provide the report to appropriate parties.

F. Medical case managers must have the relevant state nursing license to provide case management services (see www.ncsbn.org).

Trends in Workers' Compensation Case Management

A. The effort to contain costs in workers' compensation claims continues to promote innovative case management programs.

B. The use of managed care arrangements includes medical case management as an effective means of managing workers' compensation medical care.

C. Outcome-driven quality assessment is a tool for case management practices.

D. The quest for quality and standardization of medical and case management services is evidenced by the development of accreditation programs in workers' compensation and case management (among others), for example, by URAC (see www.urac.org).

E. The mandate for EBM, utilization/peer review, and case management are quality elements in workers' compensation medical care.

F. There is a greater awareness of the impact of technology on practice (i.e., the use of the Internet, telephonic services), mobile/virtual workforces, and globalization.
1. This has moved the NCSBN to initiate the interstate compact form of nursing licensure.
2. This also requires case managers to adhere to ethical and legal standards appropriate to use of Internet-based technology and tools in case management practice.

Medical Cost Containment Programs

A. Managed care companies
1. A number of state legislatures have considered the application of additional managed care principles to their workers' compensation systems.
2. Managed care companies are forming to meet current and anticipated needs in the various states.

3. Case management is a vital part of all managed care practices and legislation.
B. Early intervention by case managers
   1. Historically, claims by injured workers (except for catastrophic or serious cases) have been referred to case management after the worker fails to respond to medical treatment or is unable to return to work.
   2. Today, the trend is to allow both internal and external case managers to become involved soon after the injury is reported to expedite and enhance the chances of RTW.
C. Twenty-four–hour coverage
   1. The concept of 24-hour coverage by combined health and workers' compensation insurance or for self-insured employers has long been considered.
   2. The basic premise is that health insurance would cover all injuries and illnesses to American workers without regard to causation. Therefore, the resources spent in investigating causation and related health care needs would be saved.
   3. Although pilot programs have been tested in several states and by major employers, there is no clear consensus on its applicability for larger populations or how the issue of indemnity is addressed.

Federal Laws Affecting Workers' Compensation Case Management

A. The Americans with Disabilities Act (ADA)
   1. The act went into effect on July 26, 1992.
   2. The intent was to prohibit employers from discrimination against qualified individuals with a disability in many areas of employment.
   3. Nearly 3 years after the law was enforced, the Equal Employment Opportunities Commission (EEOC) reported that 85% of charges received involved existing employees, many of whom reported work-related impairment.
   4. Case managers involved in any part of an injured worker's RTW activities are responsible for knowing the basic tenets of ADA.
   5. The case manager does not give legal advice concerning protection of injured workers' rights in respect to the ADA but refers the employer to his or her employment attorney for that advice.
   6. The Job Accommodation Network (JAN) is a consulting service that provides information about job accommodations and the employability of people with disabilities at no charge. It is an excellent resource in RTW and job accommodation planning (see www.jan.wvu.edu).
B. The Family and Medical Leave Act (FMLA). Case managers in workers' compensation must be familiar with this law to better advocate for their clients.
   1. The FMLA was signed into law in 1993. It only applies to employers who meet certain criteria including private sector employers with 50 or more employees in 20 or more workweeks in current or preceding calendar year; public agency, including a local, state, or federal government agency, regardless of the number of employees it employs; or public or private elementary or secondary school,

regardless of the number of employees it employs (US Department of Labor, 2015b).

2. The intent of the act is to provide employees with an option to take up to 12 weeks of unpaid leave for a serious illness of the worker or a family member with job restoration (or equivalent) guaranteed.

3. Eligible employees are those who work for a covered employer, have worked for the employer for at least 12 months, have accumulated at least 1,250 hours of service for the employer during the 12-month period immediately preceding the leave, and work at a location where the employer has at least 50 employees within 75 miles.

4. Employees are eligible for FMLA in events such as the birth of a child or placement of a child for adoption or foster care; to care for a spouse, child, or parent who has a serious health condition; for a serious health condition that makes the employee unable to perform the essential functions of his or her job; or for any qualifying exigency arising out of the fact that a spouse, child, or parent is a military member on covered active duty or called to covered active duty status.

5. Under some circumstances, employees may take FMLA leave on an intermittent or reduced schedule basis. That means an employee may take leave in separate blocks of time or by reducing the time he or she works each day or week for a single qualifying reason.

6. Most workers' compensation claimants are eligible for FMLA as a result of their work-related injury, if they meet eligibility requirements.

7. Employees are not obligated to return to work on modified or "light duty" when claiming benefits under the FMLA. However, an injured worker might not be eligible for workers' compensation indemnity payments if he or she does not return to work while claiming FMLA benefits, and he or she cannot be dismissed from employment during the 12 weeks of FMLA-sanctioned leave.

8. Upon return from FMLA leave, the employer must restore the employee to his or her original job or to an equivalent job with equivalent pay, benefits, and other terms and conditions of employment. An employee's use of FMLA leave cannot be counted against the employee under a "no-fault" attendance policy.

9. Employers are required to continue group health insurance coverage for an employee on FMLA leave under the same terms and conditions as if the employee had not taken leave (US Department of Labor, 2015b).

 ## Documenting Quality of Services Using Outcome Measurements

A. For legal and ethical protection, the case manager makes referrals to health care providers who offer outcome measurements as proof of their competency. It behooves providers to have the relevant URAC or another accreditation to demonstrate their commitment to excellence and quality.

B. Case managers document the success of their interventions by the outcomes they achieve.

1. Though there is a great deal of anecdotal evidence of the benefit of case management in the workers' compensation system, there are few objective data to confirm it.
2. There is not yet general agreement on what data are measured and what measurements are needed to make comprehensive statements about positive outcomes. Often, measures are limited to time out of duty due to injury and return to work with same or another modified job or duties.
3. Private industry is developing common metrics to define the value and consistency of services in the marketplace. These measures, called the Employers Metrics for Productivity and Quality (EMPAC), are meant to be the beginning of standardized metrics to demonstrate value and return-on-investment for employee benefit and workers' compensation programs. (Weblinks to EMPAC measures are available at the end of this book.)
4. It is estimated that case management activities toward the RTW process may reduce the cost of a claim by 50%.
5. Case managers can demonstrate cost savings on a workers' compensation cases by medical cost avoidance, application of EBM tools and disability duration guidelines, facilitated RTW, saving of lost workdays, and levels of satisfaction among stakeholders (DiBenedetto, 2006).

References

Case Management Society of America (CMSA). (2010). *Standards of practice for case management.* Little Rock, AR: Author.

DiBenedetto, D. V. (2006). *Principles of workers' compensation and disability case management.* Battle Creek, MI: DVD Associates LLC. Available from www.DVDandHaag.com

Mullahy, C. (2014). *The case manager's handbook* (5th ed.). Burlington, MA: Jones and Bartlett Publishers.

United States Chamber of Commerce. (2015). *Analysis of workers' compensation laws.* Washington, DC: Author.

United States Department of Labor (USDOL). (2015a). *Leave benefit: family and medical.* Retrieved from http://www.dol.gov/dol/topic/benefits-leave/fmla.htm, on August 15, 2015.

United States Department of Labor (USDOL). (2015b). *Workers' compensation programs.* Retrieved from http://www.dol.gov/compliance/topics/benefits-comp.htm#overview, on August 15, 2015.

Disability and Occupational Health Case Management

Karen N. Provine

Note: This chapter is a revised version of Chapter 19 in the second edition of *CMSA Core Curriculum for Case Management*. The contributor wishes to acknowledge Lesley Wright, Martha Heath Eggleston, Deborah V. DiBenedetto, and Lewis Vierling as some of the timeless material was retained from the previous versions.

IMPORTANT TERMS AND CONCEPTS

ADA Amendments Act of 2008 (ADAAA)
Americans with Disabilities Act (ADA)
Disability Management
Early Intervention
Employee Assistance Program (EAP)
Ergonomics
Family and Medical Leave Act (FMLA)
Functional Capacity Evaluation (FCE)
Functional Job Analysis
Independent Medical Examinations (IME)
Integrated Benefits
Integrated Disability Management
Long-Term Disability (LTD)
Modified Duty
Occupational Health Case Management
Occupational Injury versus Nonoccupational Disability
Occupational Medicine Practice Guidelines (OMPG)
Paid Time Off (PTO) Arrangements
Reasonable Accommodation
Return-to-Work (RTW) Program
Short-Term Disability (STD)
Third-Party Administrators (TPA)
Time Loss Management
Transitional Work Duty
Treating Physician
Vocational Rehabilitation
Wellness Program
Workers' Compensation (WC)
Workforce Management

 Introduction

A. The current disability management programs evolved from the workers' compensation (WC) practice, laws, and programs.

B. In the 1970s and 1980s, many states reformed their workers' compensation laws because of rising costs. Employers and insurance carriers began to develop cost-effective ways to respond to workers with occupational illnesses and injuries; hence, disability management and occupational health (OH) programs became more common.

C. From the perspective of reducing costs came the implementation of disability management programs, to not only address the needs of those employees, both ill or injured, but also in response to reducing costs and duration of absences from the workplace.

D. By facilitating earlier return-to-work (RTW) activities, the overall cost of disability was not only reduced but there was an increase in productivity as well. Gradually, the disability management programs expanded to include integrated approaches to care delivery and services.

1. Today's integrated disability management programs combine the management of short-term disability (STD), long-term disability (LTD), workers' compensation (WC), and group health benefit programs.

2. Integrated approaches streamline claims handling and reporting, administration, medical management, and RTW activities.

3. Integrated approaches offer single medical management plans focusing on the provision of quality, safe, timely, and cost-effective medical care and successful return to productive activity.

E. The primary mission of disability management programs is to reduce the financial costs associated with all disabilities in a nonadversarial environment of claims administration. This is accomplished through the

BOX

25-1) Employer-Provided Benefit Plans and Services

- WC
- Health care services including 24-hour medical coverage and managed care
- Sick leave
- State disability; STD and LTD
- Salary continuation, pension, and retirement plans
- Union plans
- Medical leaves of absence
- Family leave
- Paid time off (PTO)
- Social Security Disability

development of a coordinated case management program with the focus on the individual's ability rather than disability.

F. Disability management programs include coordinated access to employer-provided benefit plans and services that impact the employee with a disability (Box 25-1).

G. Internal departments that typically have responsibility for the design, administration, and implementation of one or more programs are human resources, risk management, OH, safety, finance, legal, and bargaining units.

H. External sources or departments that may be involved in the disability management program are the WC insurance carriers, health care providers, third-party administrators, life insurance carriers, reinsurers, disability carriers, and managed care providers.

I. The expanding recognition that both nonoccupational and occupational disabilities could be managed effectively and efficiently with the support of employers, supervisors, and caregivers gave rise to the managed integrated disability approach.

J. According to the American Association of Occupational Health Nurses (AAOHN), poor employee health costs about $1 trillion annually, so business executives look to OH nurses and case managers to maximize employee productivity and reduce costs through lowered disability claims, fewer on-the-job injuries, and improved absentee rates.

K. Through their recognized value to business, OH professionals commonly take a seat at the management table, providing input about staffing issues, budgetary considerations, and corporate policies and procedures that positively impact worker health and safety, and thus contribute to a healthier bottom line.

L. The practice of occupational and environmental health focuses on the promotion and restoration of health, prevention of illness and injury, and protection from work-related and environmental hazards.

Descriptions of Key Terms

A. Assistive device—Any tool that is designed, made, or adapted to assist a person in performing a particular task.

B. Assistive technology—Any item, piece of equipment, or product system, whether acquired commercially or off the shelf, modified or customized, that is used to increase, maintain, or improve functional capabilities of individuals with disabilities.

C. Capacity—A construct that indicates the highest probable level of functioning a person may reach. Capacity is measured in a uniform or standard environment and thus reflects the environmentally adjusted ability of the individual.

D. Clinical practice guidelines—Guidelines that summarize based on available evidence and national acceptance recommendations for care of clients with specific conditions. These guidelines are voluntary in nature and may be specific to an institution; some are mandated by state WC laws (e.g., Massachusetts), or they may be voluntary (e.g., New York). There are no nationally promulgated clinical guidelines dictating medical care.

E. Disability—Can be defined in different ways, all referring to a lack of or inability to function in a certain aspect of daily living (Box 25-2).

F. Disability case management—The process of managing occupational and nonoccupational diseases with the aim of returning the employee with a disability to a productive work schedule and employment. It is also known as limiting a disabling event, providing immediate intervention once an injury or illness occurs, and returning the individual to work in a timely manner.

G. Ergonomics—The scientific discipline concerned with the understanding of interactions among humans and other elements of a system. It is the profession that applies theory, principles, data, and methods to environmental design (including work environments) in order to optimize human well-being and overall system performance.

H. Ergonomist—An individual who has (1) a mastery of ergonomics knowledge; (2) a command of the methodologies used by ergonomists in applying that knowledge to the design of a product, process, or environment; and (3) applied his or her knowledge to the analysis, design, test, and evaluation of products, processes, and environments.

I. Functional capacity evaluation (FCE)—A systematic process of assessing an individual's physical capacities and functional abilities. The FCE matches human performance levels to the demands of a specific job or work activity or occupation. It establishes the physical level of

---

BOX 25-2 Definitions of Disability

- A physical or neurological deviation in an individual's makeup. It may refer to a physical, mental, or sensory condition. A disability may or may not be an impairment for an individual, depending on one's adjustment to it.
- A diminished function, based on the anatomic, physiological, or mental impairment that has reduced the individual's activity or presumed ability to engage in any substantial gainful activity.
- Inability or limitation in performing tasks, activities, and roles in the manner or within the range considered typical for a person of the same age, gender, culture, and education.
- Any restriction or lack of ability (resulting from an impairment) to perform an activity in the manner or within the range considered typical for a human being.

work an individual can perform. The FCE is useful in determining job placement, job accommodation, or RTW after injury or illness. FCEs can provide objective information regarding functional work ability in the determination of occupational disability status.

J. Handicapped—Refers to the disadvantage of an individual with a physical or mental impairment resulting in a handicap.

K. Handicap—The functional disadvantage and limitation of potentials based on a physical or mental impairment or disability that substantially limits or prevents the fulfillment of one or more major life activities otherwise considered normal for that individual based on age, sex, and social and cultural factors, such as caring for one's self, performing manual tasks, walking, seeing, hearing, speaking, breathing, learning, working, etc.

L. Impairment—A general term indicating injury, deficiency, or lessening of function. Impairment is a condition that is medically determined and relates to the loss or irregularity of psychological, physiological, or anatomical structure or function. Impairments are disturbances at the level of the organ and include deficiency or loss of limb, organ, or other body structure or mental function, for example, amputation, paralysis, intellectual disability, and psychiatric disturbances as assessed by a physical examination.

M. Injury—Harm a worker encounters while on the job that is subject to treatment and/or compensation under the workers' compensation insurance or laws and regulations. Injury also refers to any wrong or damages done to another, done to his or her person, rights, reputation, or property.

N. Job modification—Altering the work environment to accommodate a person's physical or mental limitations by making changes in equipment, in the methods of completing tasks, or in job duties.

O. LTD income insurance—Insurance issued to an employee, group, or individual to provide a reasonable replacement of a portion of an employee's earned income lost through a serious prolonged illness during the normal work career.

P. Mobility—The ability to move about safely and efficiently within one's environment.

Q. Nondisabling injury—An injury that may require medical care but does not result in loss of working time or income.

R. Nonoccupational disease—Any disease that is not common to or does not occur as a result of a particular occupation of specific work environment.

S. Occupational disease—Any disease that is common to, or occurs as a result of, a particular occupation of specific work environment.

T. Occupational health case management—The process of coordinating the individual employee's health care services to achieve optimal quality care delivered in a cost-effective manner. It may focus on large-loss cases— that is, high-cost, prolonged recovery—or those with multiple providers and fragmented care.

U. Paid time off (PTO) arrangements—A benefit that provides employee with the right to scheduled and unscheduled time off with pay. Full- and part-time regular employees accrue PTO based on years of service. PTO days may be used for vacation, personal time, illness, or time off to care for dependents. It usually does not include jury duty, military duty, bereavement time for an immediate family member, or sabbatical leave.

V. Partial disability—The result of an illness or injury that prevents an insured or injured person from performing one or more of the functions of his or her regular job.

W. Physical disability—A bodily deficiency that interferes with education, development, adjustment, or rehabilitation and generally refers to chronic health problems but usually does not include single sensory impairments such as blindness or deafness.

X. Social Security Disability Income (SSDI)—Federal benefit program sponsored by the Social Security Administration. Primary factor is disability and/or benefits received from deceased or disabled parent; benefit depends on money contributed to the Social Security program by either the individual involved or the parent involved.

Y. STD income insurance—The provision to pay benefits to a covered person/employee with a disability as long as he or she remains disabled up to a specific period not exceeding 2 years.

Z. Time loss management—A proactive process used for the management of employee absenteeism due to sickness and medical leaves. Usually, a time loss management program focuses on ensuring employee's health, productivity, safety, and welfare. It does not aim to prohibit sickness absence; rather, it facilitates a timely return to work.

AA. Vocational assessment—Identifies the individual's strengths, skills, interests, abilities, and rehabilitation needs. Accomplished through on-site situational assessments at local businesses and in community settings.

BB. Vocational evaluation—The comprehensive assessment of vocational aptitudes and potential, using information about a person's past history, medical and psychological status, and information from appropriate vocational testing, which may use paper and pencil instruments, work samples, simulated workstations, or assessments in a real work environment.

CC. Vocational rehabilitation—Cost-effective case management by a skilled professional who understands the implications of the medical and vocational services necessary to facilitate an injured worker's expedient return to suitable gainful employment with a minimal degree of disability.

DD. Vocational rehabilitation counselor—A professional who assists individuals with physical, mental, developmental, cognitive, and emotional disabilities to achieve personal, career, and independent living goals in the most integrated setting possible. Rehabilitation counselors utilize many different techniques and modalities, including assessment, diagnosis and treatment planning, counseling, case management, and advocacy to modify environmental and attitudinal barriers, placement-related services, and utilization of rehabilitation technology.

EE. Vocational rehabilitation counseling process—A process that includes communication, goal setting, and beneficial growth or change through self-advocacy, psychological, vocational, social, and behavioral interventions.

FF. Vocational testing—The measurement of vocational interests, aptitudes, and ability using standardized, professionally accepted psychomotor procedures.

GG. Work adjustment—The use of real or simulated work activity under close supervision at a rehabilitation facility or other work setting to develop appropriate work behaviors, attitudes, or personal characteristics.

HH. Work adjustment training—A program for persons whose disabilities limit them from obtaining competitive employment. It typically includes a system of goal-directed services focusing on improving problem areas such as attendance, work stamina, punctuality, dress and hygiene, and interpersonal relationships with coworkers and supervisors. Services can continue until objectives are met or until there has been noted progress. It may include practical work experience or extended employment.

II. Work conditioning—An intensive, work-related, goal-oriented conditioning program designed specifically to restore systemic neuromusculoskeletal functions (e.g., joint integrity and mobility, muscle performance including strength, power, and endurance), motor function (motor control and motor learning), range of motion (including muscle length), and cardiovascular/pulmonary functions (e.g., aerobic capacity/endurance, circulation, and ventilation and respiration/gas exchange). The objective of the work conditioning program is to restore physical capacity and function to enable the patient/client to RTW.

JJ. Work hardening—A highly structured, goal-oriented, and individualized intervention program that provides clients with a transition between the acute injury stage and a safe, productive RTW. Treatment is designed to maximize each individual's ability to RTW safely with less likelihood of repeat injury. Work hardening programs are multidisciplinary in nature and use real or simulated work activities designed to restore physical, behavioral, and vocational functions. They address the issues of productivity, safety, physical tolerances, and worker behaviors.

KK. Work modification—Altering the work environment to accommodate a person's physical or mental limitations by making changes in equipment, in the methods of completing tasks, or in job duties.

LL. Workers' compensation—An insurance program that provides medical benefits and replacement of lost wages for persons suffering from injury or illness that is caused by or occurs in the workplace. It is an insurance system for industrial and work injury, regulated primarily among the separate states, but regulated in certain specified occupations by the federal government.

Applicability to CMSA's Standards of Practice

A. The Case Management Society of America (CMSA) describes in its standards of practice for case management (CMSA, 2010) that case management practice extends across all health care settings and by providers of various professional disciplines and backgrounds. This without a doubt applies to the practice of disability and occupational health case management.

B. Disability and occupational health case managers may use the CMSA standards as a guide for the implementation of their roles and case management programs. All of the standards are relevant to disability and occupational health case management practices including the case management process, roles and functions, advocacy for the client/support system, and legal and ethical expectations.

C. Case managers in the disability management and occupational health care settings must be knowledgeable about the CMSA standards of practice. They also must inform their employers and other health care professionals they collaborate with when dealing with a client with a work- or non–work-related disability and occupational illness about their existence, value, and need to adhere to them.

D. This chapter introduces case managers to the basic concepts and practices of disability management and occupational health, design of case management programs for this specialized patient population, and role of the case manager in such settings and explains how collaboration may occur between case managers in the medical and rehabilitation work settings and those in private/independent practice or those who work for employers in the occupational health area.

 Perspectives on Disability

A. Disability has been defined in a variety of ways for the purposes of programs, policies, and the law.

B. In a report by the Cherry Engineering Support Services, Inc., Federal Statutory on Definitions of Disability prepared for the Interagency Committee on Disability Research (2003), it was noted there were 67 separate laws defining disability for federal purposes.

C. Section 504 of the Rehabilitation Act of 1973 and the Americans with Disabilities Act (ADA) of 1990 have adopted a definition that takes into consideration the individual, the physical surroundings, and the social environment.

1. The *biopsychosocial approach* to disability emphasizes that a disability arises from a combination of factors at the physical, emotional, and environmental levels.

2. The biopsychosocial approach is in sharp contrast to the *illness model*, which approaches disability from the perspective of diagnosing, treating, and discharge.

3. The biopsychosocial approach focuses on the three interrelated levels cited in one and extends beyond the individual.

D. From a legal, benefit, and social program perspective, disability is often defined on the basis of specific activities of daily living (ADLs), work, and other functions essential to full participation in community-based living.

E. To be found disabled for the purposes of Social Security Disability income benefits, the individual must have a severe disability that has lasted, or is expected to last, at least 12 months and which prevents the individual from working at a "substantial, gainful activity" level.

F. Both Section 504 of the Rehabilitation Act of 1973 and the ADA of 1990 define a person with a disability as someone who:

1. Has a physical or mental impairment that substantially limits one or more "major life activities"

2. Has a record of such an impairment

3. Is regarded as having such an impairment

Components of Disability Case Management Programs

A. The Certification of Disability Management Specialists Commission (CDMSC), the only nationally accredited organization that certifies disability management specialists, recently completed a role and function study tracking the changes in disability management. Four specific practice domains were identified:
   1. Disability and Work Interruption Case Management—Involving ethical performance of necessary activities pertaining to an individual's illness or injury to ensure quality of care, recovery, and cost-effectiveness. This entails planning, managing, and advocating for that individual's return to meaningful work, a process that includes coordination of benefits and services and implementation of return-to-work plans.
   2. Workplace Intervention for Disability Prevention—Involving joint labor/management collaboration in the identification of workplace safety and risk factors. It also covers the recommendation and implementation of prevention, health, and wellness intervention practices and strategies, such as ergonomics, job analyses, and return-to-work programs.
   3. Program Development, Management, and Evaluation—Including identification of, need for, and implementation of comprehensive disability management programs utilizing best practices and metrics.
   4. Employment Leaves and Benefits Administration—Includes management of employment leaves, health and welfare plans, payroll and systems management, and other risks associated with work interruption.
B. Disability and Work Interruption Case Management programs, which consist of functions or activities such as those described in Box 25-3.
C. Workplace Intervention for Disability Prevention consists of activities or functions including those listed in Box 25-4.

BOX 25-3 **Sample Functions and Activities in Disability and Work Interruption Case Management Programs**

- Performing individual case analyses and benefits assessments
- Reviewing disability case management interventions
- Promoting collaboration among stakeholders (e.g., disabled individual, employer, insurer, care provider)
- Performing worksite/job analyses
- Developing individualized RTW and retention plans
- Implementing interventions
- Coordinating benefits, services, and community resources (e.g., prosthetics, independent medical exams [IME], and durable medical equipment)
- Monitoring case progress
- Communicating in compliance with practice standards and regulations
- Developing solutions that optimize health and employment
- Communicating benefits and employment policies

BOX 25-4 Sample Activities and Functions in Workplace Intervention for Disability Prevention Programs

- Implementing disability prevention practices (i.e., risk mitigation procedures including job analysis, job accommodation, ergonomic evaluation, health and wellness initiatives, etc.)
- Developing a transitional work program
- Developing a process for worksite modification, job accommodation, or task reassignment
- Recommending strategies to address ergonomic, safety, and risk factors
- Recommending strategies that integrate benefit plan designs and related services (e.g., EAPs, community resources, and medical services)
- Promoting health and wellness interventions

    D. Box 25-5 includes the essential activities that constitute successful development, management, and evaluation of disability management programs.

    E. Employment Leaves and Benefits Administration is accountable for the following activities:

      1. Managing employment leaves

      2. Administering health and welfare plans

      3. Managing payroll and systems data

      4. Identifying risks associated with interruptions and leaves

    F. Disability case management not only is an important workplace productivity program but also addresses more advanced workplace productivity concepts. These include:

      1. *Absence management,* which entails addressing unscheduled absences by workers due to illnesses, disability, personal, or other issues.

      2. *Improving the productivity of employees* who are on the job but may not be performing at their maximum potential. This deficient performance can be related to a variety of health, personal, or other issues.

BOX 25-5 Activities of Successful Disability Management Programs

1. Establishing program goals
2. Designing the program
3. Designing a financial plan
4. Developing staff
5. Selecting metrics for program evaluation
6. Implementing cross-functional processes
7. Offering health education and training
8. Managing program's operational and financial performance
9. Integrating data from all relevant sources
10. Procuring internal and external services
11. Managing service providers
12. Managing access to care and services including wellness and prevention
13. Assessment, monitoring, and evaluation of the program
14. Continuous quality improvement and management

G. Disability managers are a part of an interdisciplinary team involved in integrated benefit practice, productivity enhancement, and health and wellness programs.

H. Increased emphasis on early intervention and job accommodation reduces disability-related costs.

   1. Combined direct and indirect costs of disability and absences, according to recent research, often exceed 20% of a company's payroll—or more than $40 million in annual absence costs for a company employing 5,000 people at an average salary of $40,000 per year.

Challenges to Disability Case Management

A. It is important to recognize that from a disability case management perspective, the number of workers 55 years of age and older is expected to grow 38% by the year 2020. The incidence of disability increases with age; the number of employees with work-limiting disabilities is usually much higher in the 50- to 59-year age group.

B. The U.S. Census Bureau of Americans with Disabilities reported that in 2010, approximately one out of ten persons with disabilities has a severe disability. In the prime employable years of 21 to 64, over 30% of those individuals with severe disabilities are employed (US Census Bureau of Americans With Disabilities, 2012).

C. According to the U.S. Department of Labor's Office of Disability Employment Policy, every seven seconds, a baby boomer turns 60.

   1. Given generational shifts and the current economic environment, many will try to postpone retirement for as long as they are able to work. This works out well for employers because the cost of recruiting and training new workers can be significant.

   2. As a result, it's often in an employer's best interest to keep mature workers on the job for as long as they wish to work. However, this aging workforce is more likely to acquire hearing, vision, or mobility disabilities or chronic health conditions.

   3. The key to being able to keep these experienced workers may be through right job accommodations and flexible work arrangements. The aging workforce will demand more services, especially because of the increasing number of people with disabilities.

   4. This trend positions disability case management to be a key strategy in prevention and wellness programs (US Bureau of Labor Statistics, 2012).

D. The Society for Human Resource Management (SHRM) released the results of a recent survey related to employers' incentives for hiring individuals with disabilities.

   1. The primary focus of the survey was to determine how knowledgeable human resource professionals were regarding various governmental incentives for hiring individuals with disabilities.

   2. Of the human resource personnel surveyed, 77% reported not using any incentive program for hiring persons with disabilities.

   3. It should be noted that seven different tax credits are available to companies who hire workers with a disability. However, fewer than 20% of human resource personnel surveyed reported being "very familiar with any of these tax credits" (SHRM, 2014).

4. Research findings from the John J. Heldrich Center for Workforce Development at Rutgers University, New Jersey, indicate that many employers do not provide any training to their employees regarding working with people with disabilities.[1]
5. Less than half (40%) of employers surveyed provided training of any kind to their employees regarding working with or providing accommodations to people with disabilities.
6. The employment environment for people with disabilities has a direct effect on disability management programs.
7. As the population ages and experiences more disabilities, the number of chronic conditions also increases and is associated with higher health care costs. All work places are affected.

The Americans with Disabilities Act (ADA)

A. The ADA is both a challenge and a resource in disability case management. The ADA was originally enacted in 1990. The ADA Amendments Act of 2008 (ADAAA) became effective on January 1, 2009. The ADAAA overturns a series of Supreme Court decisions that interpreted the Americans with Disabilities Act of 1990 in a way that made it difficult to prove that an impairment is a "disability." The ADAAA made significant changes to the ADA's definition of "disability" that broadens the scope of coverage under both the ADA and Section 503 of the Rehabilitation Act.
B. The ADA took effect on July 26, 1992. Title I of the ADA prohibits private employers, state and local governments, employment agencies, and labor unions from discriminating against qualified individuals with disabilities in job application procedures, hiring, firing, advancement, compensation, job training, and other terms, conditions, and privileges of employment. Title II has similar prohibition in public entities.
C. The overall goal of ADA is to extend maximum opportunities for full community integration to people with disabilities in both public and private sectors of our society.
D. The law was enacted to provide a clear and comprehensive national mandate for the elimination of discrimination against individuals with disabilities.
E. The goals of the ADA are as follows:
1. Equality of opportunity
2. Full participation
3. Independent living
4. Economic self-sufficiency
F. According to the Supreme Court:
1. An *employer* is a "person engaged in an industry affecting commerce who has 15 or more employees for each working day in each of twenty or more calendar weeks in the current or preceding calendar year."
2. An *employee* is defined as "an individual employed by an employer."
G. The Supreme Court has not recognized just any impairment to be a per se disability.

---

[1]See http://www.heldrich.rutgers.edu (John J. Heldrich Center for Workforce Development).

1. A per se disability or condition, by its very nature, presumably would qualify as a disability.
2. It is no longer enough for an individual to submit evidence of a medical diagnosis of impairment. The individual must have a case-by-case assessment to prove that a particular or specific impairment is protected under the ADA.
3. Under the ADA, individuals are protected, not specific disabilities.

H. To be a qualified individual with a disability, the individual must possess the requisite skills, education, experience, and training for the position and be able to perform the essential job functions with or without reasonable accommodation.
  1. Under the definition of disability, the impairment must substantially limit a major life activity.
  2. The impairment may be so severe that the individual with or without reasonable accommodation is unable to participate in the covered activity or, in the case of employment, is not able to perform all the essential job functions.
  3. Another challenge for the employer and employee with impairment may be that individuals with impairment are considered to be a direct threat to either themselves or others in the workplace.
  4. The individual with impairment may not be qualified under the ADA if it can be shown that the individual poses a direct threat to the health and safety of others and to himself or herself and that the threat cannot be eliminated by modification of policies, practices, procedures, or by the provision of auxiliary aids or services.

I. The Supreme Court has noted that employers are justified in their desire to avoid losing time as a result of sickness; WC claims; excessive turnover from medical, retirement, or death; and the threat of litigation, under state law.
  1. Employers are not required to hire individuals who are unable to carry out the essential functions of the job without incurring risk to the health and safety of others and to themselves.
  2. The Supreme Court included a provision in its decision that requires employers to assess the individual's current or prospective ability to safely perform the essential functions of the job.
    a. The assessment must be individualized and based on reasonable medical judgment that relies on the most current medical knowledge and the best available objective evidence.
    b. The imminence of risk and severity of harm to the individual also must be assessed.
  3. The following four factors are to be considered in deciding whether an individual poses a direct threat:
    a. Duration of the risk
    b. Nature and severity of the potential harm
    c. Likelihood that the potential harm will occur
    d. Imminence of the potential harm
  4. The Supreme Court has held that employers must gather substantial information about the employee's work history and medical status.

     a. Employer's requiring that an employee must be "100% healed" before returning to work is considered an ADA violation.

     b. The emphasis should not be whether or not the individuals are 100% healed but rather whether they pose a direct threat to themselves or others in the workplace.

5. The Supreme Court has also held that an employer is free to decide that physical characteristics or mental conditions that do not rise to the level of a disability are preferable to others. The Court has noted that the employer is free to decide that some limiting, but not substantially limiting impairments, make individuals less suited for a job.

6. Generally speaking, the ADA permits qualification standards that are "job related" and "consistent with business necessity."

7. In October 2002, the Equal Employment Opportunity Commission (EEOC) issued enforcement guidelines on reasonable accommodation and undue hardship under the ADA (EEOC, 2002).

     a. The updated guidelines revised the standards for "reasonableness" of an accommodation. Reasonableness is now evaluated on whether or not it is considered not only effective but also "feasible or plausible" for the typical employer.

     b. Requests for accommodation can be made either verbally or in writing (Box 25-6).

     c. Situations may arise in which the employer will need additional information regarding the disability and the employee's level of functioning.

       i. The employee may need to undergo an evaluation by a health care professional.

BOX 25-6   Requests for Accommodation

- In most cases, the employee must request the accommodation before the employer is obligated to respond.
- Requests for accommodation may be made at any time during the employment application process or at different intervals during an individual's employment with the company.
- The employer is obligated to consider each request and engage in an "interactive process" to investigate, assess, and provide reasonable accommodations.
- If the employer is aware that an employee with a disability is experiencing problems in the workplace or is unable to request an accommodation because of mental impairment, the employer is obliged to initiate the process. However, each situation requires a case-by-case assessment.
- Reasonable accommodation may include job restructuring, leave of absence, modified or part-time schedules, and reassignment to a vacant position.
- Unreasonable accommodation may include reducing production or performance standards that are not uniformly applied, providing personal use items, changing supervisors, monitoring medications, unwarranted promotion, or eliminating the essential functions of the job.
- If the problem an employee is experiencing as a result of the disability is not related to the actual performance on the job, reasonable accommodation may not be required. For example, a request to transfer to a different work shift may not be considered a reasonable accommodation.

      ii. In order to be protected under the ADA, the employee is obligated to cooperate with this aspect of the interactive process.

      iii. The employer has the final discretion to choose a reasonable accommodation.

      iv. If an employee refuses to accept the employer's offer of reasonable accommodation, the employee then may not be qualified to remain in the job.

      v. The employee first bears the burden of proof that an accommodation would be considered reasonable. That burden then shifts to the employer to prove that the accommodation would cause an undue hardship (EEOC, 2002).

8. Almost all federal courts, as well as the EEOC, are in agreement that an employer must consider reassigning an employee who is no longer able to perform his or her job because of impairment. There is general agreement on the following points:

    a. Reassignment is available only to employees and not to job applicants.

    b. Employees on probationary status who have been performing the job satisfactorily may be entitled to reassignment.

    c. An employer is not required to create a new position by "bumping" another employee.

    d. An employer is not required to promote an employee as a reassignment. This includes promoting an individual with impairment from a part-time position to a full-time position or hourly to a salaried position.

    e. Employees may only be reassigned to a job that they are qualified to perform and the EEOC and courts agree that reassignment should be considered as a "last resort."

J. The Job Accommodation Network (JAN) is a service of the Office of Disability Employment Policy of the U.S. Department of Labor. JAN's mission is to facilitate the employment and retention of workers with disabilities by providing employers, employment providers, people with disabilities, family members, and other interested parties such as case managers with information on job accommodations (JAN, 2014).

K. Often, most accommodations needed by employees and job applicants with disabilities result in no cost to the employer. Employers experienced multiple direct and indirect benefits after making the accommodations. The top three most frequently experienced direct benefits are:

    a. Retaining qualified employees

    b. Eliminating the cost of training a new employee

    c. Increase in the workers' productivity (JAN, 2014)

L. Case managers are oftentimes confronted with how to handle circumstances surrounding the employment of individuals who have a drug and/or alcohol (substance) addiction.

1. A frequent question case managers raise is "if the individual has been terminated because of conduct related to drug or alcohol addiction, do they have rehire rights under the ADA?" Another issue is "can the organization refuse to rehire the individual following successful rehabilitation?"

2. The ADA protects qualified individuals with drug addiction if they have been rehabilitated. However, the ADA does not protect employees currently engaging in drug and/or alcohol use.
3. If an employer has a neutral no-rehire policy, one that refuses to rehire an employee who was terminated for violating workplace conduct rules, then the policy is considered legitimate and nondiscriminatory.
4. While the ADA does not protect an employee or applicant who is currently engaging in drug use, it protects qualified individuals with a drug addiction who have been successfully rehabilitated.

M. The role of mitigating and/or corrective measures
1. The Supreme Court has ruled that the use of mitigating measures, such as medications, corrective lenses, prosthetic devices, and the body's ability to compensate for impairment, is to be a part of determining whether an individual has a disability under the ADA.
2. When assessing an individual, the case manager must consider whether or not the individual is using any mitigating and/or corrective measures. The individual's actual circumstances must be assessed in this process.
3. The case manager needs to understand that mitigating measures may lessen or eliminate limitations caused by impairment. Both the positive and negative effects of mitigating or corrective measures need to be considered in the assessment process.

N. Social Security Benefits and the ADA
1. In a disability case management program, the case manager may be confronted with a situation in which an employee on Social Security Disability Income (SSDI) may seek protection under the ADA.
2. The Supreme Court has declared that because the qualification standards for social security benefits and the ADA are not the same, that application for receiving social security benefits is not inconsistent with being a qualified individual with a disability under ADA.
3. The implications of this may be when individuals on SSDI seek to RTW and identify themselves as qualified to do the essential functions of the job. The conflict is that they have stated in the social security application that they are not gainfully employable.
4. The Courts have ruled that this is not inconsistent and that the individual may still be able to perform the essential functions of the job with or without reasonable accommodation.
5. The case manager should be aware that there is a possibility that an individual receiving social security benefits would still be protected under the ADA and would require reasonable accommodation to RTW especially if they are qualified to perform the essential functions of the job.

Resources for Disability Case Management Programs

A. The Disability Management Employers Coalition, Inc. (DMEC), is a national organization that focuses on education and training of employers.

- *Section 501, Rehabilitation Act 1973:* Requires affirmative action and nondiscrimination in employment by federal agencies of the executive branch
- *Section 503, Rehabilitation Act:* Requires affirmative action and prohibits employment discrimination by federal government contractors and subcontractors with contracts of more than $10,000
- *Section 188, Workforce Investment Act:* Prohibits discrimination against people with disabilities in employment service centers funded by the federal government
- *Americans with Disabilities Act, Title II:* Prohibits discrimination in the provision of public benefits and services (e.g., public education, employment, transportation, recreation, health care, social services, courts, voting, and town meetings).
- *Section 504, Rehabilitation Act:* Requires that buildings and facilities that are designed, constructed, or altered with federal funds, or leased by a federal agency, comply with federal standards for physical accessibility.

1. DMEC promotes an integrated approach to employer programs in disability and health management, absence, and productivity management.
2. DMEC has developed, in association with the Insurance Education Association (IEA), the Certified Professional in Disability Management (CPDM) Program. This program provides training to industry-specific personnel who are involved in the integrated process.
B. The Integrated Benefits Institute, located in San Francisco, California, provides research, discussion and analysis, and date of services to improve integrated benefit programs.
C. The Washington Business Group on Health (WBGH) has taken an active role in educating the industry on disability management. WBGH coordinates an annual national conference on disability management topics.
D. The American Association of Occupational Health Nurses (AAOHN) and the American College of Occupational and Environmental Medicine (ACOEM) provide disability management and RTW services in addition to OH programs for employers.
E. Box 25-7 lists some employment laws that are helpful for the disability case manager.

Integrated Disability Case Management Strategies

A. Disability case management should encompass both occupational and nonoccupational disabilities and be fully integrated with STD, LTD, and WC programs.
B. Often, the first groups of benefits to be integrated are STD and WC.
C. The disability case management process should involve establishing clinical guidelines and expectations that can assist with the medical management of disabilities.
D. Employing a managed care network minimizes time lost accessing specialty physicians and treatment providers.

E. Using one source to provide medical equipment, pharmaceuticals, and other supplies can promote efficiency of delivery and cost containment.

F. Having on-site wellness programs benefits all areas of health and disability management.

G. Qualified professionals can create therapeutic RTW protocols as a part of the program. Use of these protocols ensures quality and cost-effectiveness.

H. Transitional work and modified duty programs are essential components of disability case management programs. They are especially effective in returning employees to work and add to the productivity of the workforce.

I. Integrated disability case management strategies ensure that injured employees have timely intervention, medical, disability, and RTW management. Integrated disability case management programs often include OH case management as a fundamental component.

Occupational Health Case Management

A. According to AAOHN, occupational and environmental health nursing is the specialty practice that provides for and delivers health and safety programs and services to workers, workers' families, worker populations, and community groups (AAOHN, 2012a).

B. Whenever case management services are provided to workers, worker populations, or persons whose care is financed by an employer's benefit program, the implications for the individuals' health status and functional recovery must be coordinated with OH and RTW goals and objectives.

C. OH case management involves the management of occupational (WC) disability, nonoccupational disability, and incidental absence from work.

D. OH case management is designed to prevent fragmented care and delayed recovery while facilitating the employee's recovery and appropriate RTW in a full-duty or modified work capacity.

E. OH case management includes the development of preventive systems and the mobilization of appropriate resources for care over the course of the health event.

F. OH case management and medical care are delivered with the ultimate goal of returning the worker to preillness or preinjury function or to the highest level of functioning achievable in the most cost-effective and time-efficient manner.

G. Standards of practice for OH nurses have been established by AAOHN.[2]

Role of OH Case Managers

A. The scope and role of the OH case manager providing services vary depending on the nature of the business setting, expectations of the employer, role assignments, and philosophy of the OH program.

B. OH case managers, in collaboration with other providers, such as physicians, play an integral role in determining, facilitating, and

---

[2]Standards of practice may be obtained by contacting AAOHN at www.aaohn.org or by calling (800) 241-8014.

expediting the appropriate RTW of employees who are absent from work due to occupational or nonoccupational injuries or illnesses, or both. This also may include the delivery of case management services to the worker's dependents.

C. Case management has generally been an integral component of OH programs but is becoming more formalized as a specialty within the field of practice. The OH scope of practice has expanded today to include:
   1. Health promotion
   2. Emergency preparedness in response to natural, technological, and human hazards to work and community environments

D. In addition to assessing, planning, directing, coordinating, implementing, managing, monitoring, and evaluating care, the OH case manager establishes or qualifies a provider network, recommends treatment plans, monitors outcomes, and maintains a strong communication link among all the parties (AAOHN, 2012b).

E. OH case managers coordinate the proactive efforts of the multidisciplinary health care team to facilitate an individual's health care services from the onset of injury or illness to a safe RTW or an optimal alternative. This may include:
   1. Coordinating treatment, follow-up, and referrals, as well as emergency care for job-related injuries and illnesses
   2. Gatekeeping for health services, rehabilitation, RTW, and case management issues
   3. Influencing employers' health care quality and cost containment
   4. Providing counseling and crisis intervention, developing health education programs, and working with employers to comply with workplace laws and regulations (AAOHN, 2012b)

F. OH case managers may conduct research on effects of workplace exposures, gathering health data, and using this information to prevent injury and illness.

G. OH case managers are most often registered professional nurses or vocational rehabilitation counselors. Employers in the OH areas of case management practice are increasingly requiring a certification in case management as a prerequisite credential for hiring (Box 25-8).

H. OH case managers generally belong to the AAOHN, the Case Management Society of America (CMSA), or a similarly oriented professional organization.

BOX
25-8   Certification in Occupational Health Case Management

- Certified Case Manager (CCM)
- Certified OH Nurse (COHN)
- Certified OH Nurse Specialist (COHN-S)
- Certified OH Nurse Case Manager (COHN/CM)
- Certified OH Nurse Specialist/Case Manager (COHN-S/CM)
- Certified Disability Management Specialist (CDMS)
- Certified Rehabilitation Counselor (CRC)

Key Concepts of OH Case Management

A. Goals of OH case management programs are many. DiBenedetto (2000) articulated a comprehensive list of goals, which included those listed in Box 25-9.

B. The American College of Occupational and Environmental Medicine (ACOEM) has developed clinical practice guidelines for potentially work-related health problems in worker populations, entitled *Occupational Medicine Practice Guidelines: Evaluation and Management of Common Health Problems and Functional Recovery in Workers*, 3rd Edition (ACOEM, 2011).

C. The Occupational Medicine Practice Guidelines (OMPGs):
   1. Are based on the injured workers' presenting complaints
   2. Emphasize prevention
   3. Emphasize proper clinical evaluation
   4. Provide guidance for medical and disability management

D. Guidelines are invaluable as a frame of reference when used in conjunction with other factors of disability, work requirements, values and belief systems, and so forth.

E. Guidelines that are important for OH case management, other than the OMPGs, include the disability duration guidelines (DDGs) and specified recovery guidelines (SRGs).
   1. The DDGs help the provider and OH case manager to determine a person's potential for RTW within a given time frame.
      a. A variety of DDGs are available for determining the potential length of a worker's absence due to injury or illness; examples include:
         i. The Medical Disability Advisor
         ii. Occupational Disability Guidelines
         iii. Milliman Care Guidelines
   2. The SRGs assist by establishing a benchmark or expected time frame during which a worker recovers from his or her disability or injury.

BOX 25-9   Goals of Occupational Health Case Management

- Facilitating the employee's RTW in a timely manner
- Assisting employees in navigating the benefit and medical care arenas
- Minimizing lost time in the workplace
- Decreasing the cost of lost-time benefit programs such as STD and LTD, salary continuation, and WC
- Facilitating employers' control of disability issues
- Improving corporate competitiveness
- Maximizing use of employer resources
- Reducing the cost of disability
- Enhancing employees' morale by valuing their physical and cultural diversity
- Protecting the employability of the worker
- Ensuring compliance with relevant laws and organizations, such as the ADA, FMLA, OSHA, and Department of Transportation (DOT)
- Ensuring the delivery of quality services

3. Persons with the same diagnosis or medical condition will recover at different rates and be able to RTW within a general time frame; however, recovery is as variable as a person's individuality.

F. Disability and ability to RTW are dependent on the worker's healing or response to illness or injury and the scope of his or her job functions.

G. Functional capacity evaluations (FCEs) are used in OH case management programs and by OH case managers to directly measure a person's functional ability to perform specific work-related tasks.

1. An FCE may be requested by the OH professional/case manager, human resources, provider, adjustor, or other key stakeholder.

2. The FCE involves examining an individual as he or she performs activities in a structured setting. It does not necessarily reflect what the person should be able to do, rather what he or she can do or is willing to do at the time of the evaluation.

3. The FCE depends on motivation, cognitive awareness, behavioral factors, and sincerity of effort, all of which have a major impact on the FCE (AMA, 2009).

H. There are three primary tools used in OH case management programs that assist in returning individuals to work and in planning the care and necessary treatments. These are:

1. Functional job analysis that is used to help return the injured worker to his or her preinjury occupation or job. The job analysis defines job requirements and lists and describes the job's essential and nonessential functions. It should be current and representative of the employee's job responsibilities and should always be shared with the treating physician or provider and the OH case manager to aid in RTW planning.

2. Independent medical examination (IME) that is used to confirm a person's diagnosis, current medical treatment and care, the scope and nature of disability, the potential for permanent disability and impairment, ability to RTW, and medical information and testing outcomes. The IME provider never becomes the treating physician.

3. Second opinion examination (SOE) that also is used to confirm a person's diagnosis, provide more information, and make recommendations for potential treatment options. Often, the employee may choose to be treated by the SOE provider.

I. Occupational or vocational rehabilitation services are often used in OH case management in addition to the usual medical and physical rehabilitation. The main goal is to restore the employee's function and return him or her to the preinjury state.

J. Work hardening is also used in OH case management. It is therapy that mimics actual work demands and includes exercises and work-simulated activities that are monitored by professionals to allow the injured worker to gradually build up his or her work task tolerance. Work hardening activities may be provided at the work site under the supervision of physical therapists and the OH case manager (DiBenedetto, 2000).

Success Factors for OH Case Management Programs

A. Know the organization's employee benefits program.[3]
   1. In addition to WC, STD, LTD, and sick pay programs, monetary benefits often can be obtained through life insurance programs, pension programs, retirement, and union and state disability benefits.
   2. This information usually can be accessed through the human resources or benefit departments, which is why members from these disciplines make good RTW program team members.
B. Know the organization's most commonly occurring illnesses and disabilities. Identifying these is beneficial for the safety or OH case manager so that clinical pathways/guidelines or established modified jobs can focus on these frequent disabilities.
   1. If the in-house case manager does not have a medical background, this information can be sought from a medical case manager, OH nurse/case manager, or established primary treating physician.
C. Selecting vendors
   1. Select a network of providers that not only covers tertiary care but that specializes in the core area that the organization predominantly needs.
   2. Maintain a provider database that lists both their addresses and specialties.
   3. Select vendors who are invested in the employees and will assist in the implementation of the RTW program.
   4. If possible, implement a software program that will enhance communications between the organization and its vendors.
D. Education: The case manager, in collaboration with the employer's representative or team, will need to educate all parties involved in the RTW program.
   1. Education should begin before implementation so that all divisions associated with the program have become thoroughly acquainted with it and understand their role in its success and purpose.
   2. Education should also include the case manager who is managing individuals' care both proactively and after disability.
   3. Providing employees with information on the organization's policies and procedures can prepare them in the event of a disability or disease.
   4. Proactively providing the access channels, corporate policy, and structure can minimize many of the traditional obstacles that prevent people with a disability from returning to gainful activity.
E. Accessibility: The OH case manager must remain accessible to both the employees and employers.
   1. Delegation is an important skill the case manager can learn. He or she should be prepared to guide employees to the appropriate division to obtain the information they are seeking.

[3]Adapted from Wright, L., Eggleston, M. H., & DiBenedetto, D. V. (2000). *Disability case management.* In S. K. Powell & D. Ignatavicius (Eds.), *CMSA core curriculum for case management* (pp. 181–194). Philadelphia, PA: Lippincott Williams & Wilkins.

2. State and federal laws and statutes often have minute changes that can affect individuals' benefits significantly. Although informed OH case managers are aware of much of this information, it is usually best if it is provided by an individual in that discipline—that is, benefits, human resources, or bargaining union.

F. Modified or transitional duty team may be used to expedite return to work.

1. Productivity management is the goal driving the RTW program. To maximize productivity management, an organization needs to minimize costs associated with it.

2. From a disability perspective, costs can encompass "hard dollar" savings by minimizing loss time, training time, and medical costs or "soft dollar" savings by improving employee morale.

3. The OH case management team should meet routinely and should be led by the OH case manager.

   a. The OH case manager may often be the primary coordinator of the RTW program.

   b. In other cases, the team may be chaired by representatives of the organization (e.g., human resources and OH).

G. Clinical aspects

1. The OH case management program may benefit from an assigned precertification program.

2. Thorough clinical communication and documentation should be made so that administrative personnel can make informed decisions.

3. An OH case manager with related credentials and experience in occupational illness or injuries and RTW clinical, vocational, and psychological aspects of injury, disability, and disease would likely be best suited for this position.

4. An RTW support group would provide avenues for shared experiences and peer assistance.

5. Make available an early intervention program with clear access method.

   a. Many employers have adopted a call-in telephone number or reporting line.

   b. Timely access through one source can minimize lost and delayed reported claims.

   c. It may be of benefit to standardize the intake format so the emergency or treating physicians become familiar with the specific information needed to document the claim appropriately.

6. Implementation of a communication protocol.

   a. Often, losing or displacing employees arises from a lack of communication between the employer and the injured employee.

   b. Traditional WC field case managers have reported that one of their primary obstacles in returning an injured worker back to his or her place of employment is the worker's perception that the employer lacks interest in the worker and does not wish for his or her return—that he or she may somehow now be "labeled."

   c. In-house OH case management programs facilitate effective communication skills and can accomplish this goal.

7. Employee Assistance Programs (EAPs) are excellent resources for OH case managers and can provide confidential counseling services for a variety of needs.
   a. OH case managers need to be aware of other problems that can arise from an individual's disability such as financial difficulties (e.g., reduced income), dependency difficulties (e.g., single parent), or addiction (e.g., prescription drugs).
   b. With the OH case manager's trained ear, the ill or injured employee can be referred to an EAP should concerns arise about his or her emotional well-being.
8. If the organization has the capability, establish an employee wellness program. This program can be in house or can be in partnership with a local facility. Such programs have the capacity to:
   a. Facilitate on-site extended physical and occupational therapy services
   b. Allow a specially devised program to combine both therapy and job functions in the RTW processes
   c. Implement proactive wellness incentives and programs
   d. Coordinate with the wellness program's routine health screens and education on routine aging illnesses and concerns (e.g., high-cholesterol diets, high blood pressure)
   e. Encourage corporate physical activities (e.g., walks, aerobics, softball team) that are designed to provide employees with the recommended weekly exercise regimens.
H. Coordination of program: The OH case manager is ultimately the RTW coordinator in the absence of an RTW coordinator at the employer's site. As the RTW coordinator, the case manager maintains regular contact with all key stakeholders (Box 25-10).
   1. Establishing workflow procedures. These may include:
      a. The OH case manager must be immediately advised that a claim has been filed.
      b. If the claim warrants specialty care, the case manager can advise of the referral and submit to the treating physician a description of the worker's job functions.

BOX 25-10 Stakeholders of Occupational Health Case Management

- Injured or sick worker and family
- Treating physician
- Other treatment providers
- Employer
- Worker's supervisor and management
- Medical, occupational health, and wellness departments
- Human resources and employee benefits
- External case management (as appropriate)
- Claims adjuster or third-party administrator
- Modified or transitional duty team
- Employee Assist Program (as appropriate)

    c. The case manager should expect from the physician time frames for medical or rehabilitation intervention and estimates on the duration of the worker's treatment and rehabilitation plans and what, if any, physical limitations may be permanent.

    d. Important information should be provided to the members of the case management team.

2. The OH case manager may assume a number of responsibilities that are similar to those of the general or medical case manager (Box 25-11).

3. The OH case manager's knowledge is instrumental in reporting satisfaction with the providers of service.

4. The OH case manager has an ethical and professional obligation to ensure that the client—the injured or ill person—receives appropriate, quality medical intervention and is not placed at risk for further injury. Continuity of medical care and its proper sequencing is necessary for promoting the patient's early RTW.

5. Cost-contained quality medical care can be afforded to all employees who require it by systematically streamlining access to quality care and monitoring standards and progress of care or service provided.

I. Corporate policy and other pressures are frequently focused on productivity and finance. In this regard, the OH case manager must sensitively meet the needs of both the employer and the employee when coordinating the RTW program.

1. Juggling personalities and problems is what effective OH case managers are often recognized for, despite their intensive training within their own discipline.

2. For example, accessing ergonomic specialists who can make worksite accommodations for modified duty or injury prevention programs is an excellent tool for combining productivity management with employee needs.

BOX 25-11 Responsibilities of Occupational Health Case Managers

- Provide the treating physician with a description of a modified duty/job and for authorization to release the employee back to work on a limited, part-time, or full-time basis.
- Communicate the treating physician's projections to the benefits division so that benefit providers can be informed.
- Coordinate with the team all activities of the RTW process and plan of care.
- Implement, supervise, document, and monitor the plan of care.
- Communicate the plan of care and progress to key stakeholders.
- Document progress, address pitfalls, and consult with administration, precertification, managed care, health care, or any other outside provider who is not part of the internal modified duty team.
- Assist in the availability of quality care for all people by eliminating providers or participants recognized for acts of abuse or fraud. Having access to all medical files improves the chances that fraudulent or "laissez-faire" practices are identified.
- Promote effective, intensive medical care to bring about healthy outcomes.

Maximizing Workforce Health and Productivity

A. Proactive education of the employee in the organization's total benefits program can enhance employee morale; reduce lost time, malingering, litigated costs, and training and production costs; and foster a supportive work environment.

B. Workforce management centers on the concept of managing all aspects of occupational disability and proactive health and safety information and training, aggressive management (including case management) of occupational and nonoccupational lost-time cases, and effective RTW within the regulatory arena specific to the employer.

C. Many aspects of workforce management are important for OH case management (Box 25-12). Case managers must be well aware of this value and use workforce management information effectively in their roles and when creating or improving their OH case management programs.

D. Transitional work duty (TWD) programs are progressive, individualized, time-limited programs that focus on returning the employee with an injury and/or disability to the original employment site, however, with some restrictions.

E. Transitional work allows the injured worker to perform productive work at the workplace under the direction of rehabilitation professionals. The program may include progressive conditioning, on-site work activities, education for safe work practices, work readjustment, and job modification. The costs associated to a transitional work program are rehab costs charged to the surplus fund.

 1. TWD programs use structured protocols of "value-added temporary positions" that are focused on RTW. The protocols are carefully designed to be appropriate for the skills, knowledge, and capabilities of the recovering employee so that the work can be accomplished safely.

 2. A TWD assignment is temporary in nature and complies with all medical restrictions indicated by the employee's treating physician. It may involve modification of the injured employee's job duties, that is, tailoring work duties to the injured employee's medical limitations and vocational abilities to maximize recovery, or alternate work that is compatible with the employee's job skills and experience.

BOX
25-12 **Aspects of Workforce Management of Value in OH Case Management**

- Demographics of the employer's worker populations
- OH and non-OH management
- Health and productivity programs, metrics, and outcomes
- Benefit plan design that augments the needs of the worker population
- Consideration of work, life, and family impacts on the worker population and the impact on their ability to be at work
- Integrating benefit programs such as integrated disability management, OH case management, and coordinated RTW programs

25-13   Benefits of Formal Transitional Work Duty Programs

- Return of injured employees to work sooner than those not provided with transitional work duty opportunities.
- Claims costs can be reduced.
- Employees recover faster than those that attempt recovery while at home.
- Reduced malpractice litigation.
- Avoidance of the time and expense involved in hiring and training replacement workers.
- Maintaining productivity of injured employee while paying for actual work.
- Reduction in fraud.
- Increased employee morale.

3. TWD programs cover all compensable disabling conditions insured under Workers' Compensation and are limited to employees with temporary impairments.

4. The TWD assignment is documented by a Transitional Work Plan that is written for a specific period of time (90 calendar days on average). The Plan is signed by the injured employee and the department supervisor or representative.

5. Employees with temporary partial disabilities are eligible for transitional work if they are anticipated to progress in their recovery from an industrial injury or illness and require temporary, short-term modification of their job duties.

6. Employees with restrictions that would permanently prevent them from returning to the job and hours worked at the time of their injury are not eligible for participation in the TWD programs.

7. Employees who participate in TWD programs obtain written medical documentation from their treating physician or health care professional indicating their specific work restrictions.

8. There are many benefits to formalized TWD programs such as those listed in Box 25-13.

Models of OH Case Management

A. OH case management is generally provided by OH case managers and physicians who are familiar with the employee's job tasks, conditions of work, work processes, benefit programs, supervisors, and community providers.[4]

B. OH case managers possess knowledge of medical and vocational aspects of disability, OH and safety practices, relevant work conditions, health promotion, regulatory issues, benefit programs, and RTW requirements.

C. OH case management service delivery may include on-site, telephonic, or field models (Box 25-14).

D. OH case management settings include acute care hospitals and systems; corporations; social insurance programs; public and private

[4]Adapted from DiBenedetto, D. V. (2000). Occupational health case management. In S. K. Powell & D. Ignatavicius (Eds.), *CMSA core curriculum for case management* (pp. 195–212). Philadelphia, PA: Lippincott Williams & Wilkins.

25-14 Models of Occupational Health Case Management

On-site OH case management models
- Services are provided by the employer's own staff or designee (i.e., vendor) at the actual workplace.
- The services may involve actual client contact in the workplace, by phone, or through field visits.

Telephonic OH case management models
- Services are coordinated through electronic communication.
- The services may be provided on an interstate or intrastate basis.

Field case management models—also known as offsite models
- Services are provided outside of the employer's workplace, generally by a TPA, insurance company, or OH case management vendor.
- In some cases, the employer's OH case managers may conduct field visits to the employee, provider, or carrier to facilitate appropriate case management services and RTW.

insurance sectors; fee-for-service, managed care, and case management organizations; government, military, and government-sponsored programs; and provider agencies and facilities.
E. OH case managers follow the same case management process similar to those in other case management settings. However, they apply the OH concepts and purposes into the process and the activities they are involved in when caring for an employee (Box 25-15) (ABOHN, 2012).

25-15 Occupational Health Case Management Process (ABOHN, 2012)

Assessment
- Establish criteria and use case finding and screening to identify workers who are appropriate candidates for OH or disability case management.
- Conduct comprehensive assessment of employees.
- Assess employee's and organization's informal and formal support systems.
- Assess community, workplace, and vendor resources.
- Assess essential functions of job (physical and mental demands) to facilitate hiring, proper placement, and RTW activities.
- Identify gaps that exist in the service continuum.
- Periodically reassess the health status of the worker.
- Assess the need for health-risk appraisals, for safety, accident prevention, wellness, and health promotion programs.
- Conduct comprehensive assessment of all disability-related expenses and benefit utilization.
- Assess workplace policies on RTW and job accommodations.
- Identify legal, labor, and regulatory implications.
- Assess disability plans, policies, procedures, and communication links.
- Identify roles and responsibilities of the worker, supervisor or manager, case manager, benefit–risk manager, health care providers, TPAs and insurers, and others as needed.
- Recognize challenges to successful outcomes.

25-15 Occupational Health Case Management Process *countinued*

Planning
- Review worker's goals.
- Review employer's and corporate goals for integrated health management team approach.
- Prepare analysis and synthesis of all data to formulate an appropriate plan of care.
- Use appropriate components of employee benefits plan(s).
- Analyze and synthesize data to formulate appropriate diagnoses and interdisciplinary problem statements.
- Plan and balance the needs of the worker's RTW.
- Coordinate service providers responsible for furnishing services.
- Participate in special provider arrangements, for example, preferred provider organizations (PPOs), health maintenance organizations (HMOs), point-of-service organizations (POSs), and managed care contractors.
- Collaborate with community, workplace, and vendor personnel.
- Develop a plan of care or an RTW plan, including health care and medical treatment goals, through an interdisciplinary and collaborative group process, which includes the employee and his or her caregivers.
- Participate in development of programs for safety, accident prevention, and health promotion to prevent future occurrence of injury and illness cases.
- Coordinate administration of case management services among benefit plans, including WC and OH.
- Apply principles consistent with the ADA in preplacement and ongoing job placement activities.
- Participate in disability plan design and policy and procedure development.

Implementation
- Link the worker with the most appropriate community resources.
- Act as a liaison with health care providers.
- Coordinate access to quality, cost-effective care, and services.
- Coordinate clinical and medical management of cases.
- Implement early RTW/modified duty programs.
- Facilitate rehabilitation and job accommodation for WC and nonoccupational disabilities and/or injuries.
- Provide appropriate education for the worker, family, providers, and community resources.
- Assist the worker in negotiating the health care system.
- Develop and maintain standards, policies, and protocols to support the case management process.
- Participate with interagency groups and community agencies to support or represent the case management program.
- Prepare for legal proceedings.
- Provide testimony during legal proceedings.
- Assure confidentiality and comply with established codes of ethics and legal or regulatory requirements.
- Document case management activities and outcomes.
- Participate in public speaking and marketing related to case management services and the programs involved.
- Function as an employee advocate and balance the needs of the workplace with the needs of the worker.

Evaluation
- Manage data and information systems for the purposes of research, trend analysis, program modification and evaluation, and continuous quality/performance improvement.

continued

25-15 Occupational Health Case Management Process *countinued*

- Evaluate quality of management efforts, teamwork, and workflow design.
- Monitor and modify the RTW plan.
- Monitor the worker and others to ensure a smooth transition to work and continued progress.
- Evaluate and monitor the plan of care/RTW plan to ensure its quality, efficiency, timeliness, and effectiveness.
- Ensure that services are appropriate, cost effective, and supportive of worker independence.
- Monitor the worker's decision-making abilities regarding choices, utilization of resources, and consequences.
- Evaluate worker's outcomes to determine case disposition.
- Evaluate the effectiveness of safety, accident prevention, and wellness/health promotion programs.
- Evaluate disability-related expenses and programs for program or benefit enhancement and refinement, as well as for areas of duplication.
- Track and evaluate program outcomes periodically for success of case management activities (e.g., reduced cost, reduced accidents, reduced severity, efficiency of process, and customer satisfaction).
- Evaluate due diligence of providers and provider networks.
- Participate in public speaking, marketing, and research related to case management services and the programs provided.

The Knowledge Base Required for OH and Disability Case Managers

A. It is necessary for OH and/or disability case managers to be familiar with the federal regulatory programs in the area of occupational health. This is necessary for success in the role and advocating for the employees they serve. Examples of these laws are:
   1. Family and Medical Leave Act (FMLA)
   2. Employee Retirement Income Security Act (ERISA)
   3. Americans with Disabilities Act (ADA)
   4. Social Security Insurance (SSI)
   5. Consolidated Omnibus Budget Reconciliation Act (COBRA)
   6. Department of Transportation (DOT)
   7. Occupational Safety and Health Administration (OSHA)
B. Aside from laws and regulations, OH and disability case managers must also demonstrate they possess key knowledge, skills, competencies, and abilities that are necessary to function effectively in their roles. ABOHN identified a comprehensive list of these requirements (ABOHN, 2012), presented in Box 25-16.
C. OH and disability case managers are not expected to know or be an expert in every law and knowledge topic. However, they are expected to seek the support of other experts or be familiar where to obtain the information needed.

BOX 25-16 Essential Knowledge, Skills, and Competency Areas for OH and Disability Case Managers

- Process of case management
- Rehabilitation principles, for example, work hardening/conditioning, functional capacity evaluation, worker, and workplace
- Fitness for duty and vocational rehabilitation, for example, labor market survey, transferable skills analysis
- Prevention and wellness promotion
- State regulatory programs, for example, WC, statutory disability
- Liability issues in case management
- Legal/ethical issues, for example, confidentiality, privacy (e.g., HIPAA [United States] and the protection of health information, PIDA [Canada])
- Community/governmental agencies and resources
- Life-care planning concepts
- Statistical/data analysis, benchmarking, incidence, prevalence, trending, economic analysis
- Tracking/measuring costs, cost–benefit, return on investment, trends analysis
- Conflict management skills
- Employee advocacy, balancing worker/workplace issues, negotiating skills, benchmarking, cost–benefit analysis
- Oral and written communication skills
- Decision-making ability
- Problem-solving ability
- Adult learning principles
- Principles of teaching
- Marketing internal/external
- Principles of quality improvement, for example, continuous quality improvement (CQI), total quality management (TQM), International Standards Organization (ISO) 9000, ISO 14,001
- Protocol development/utilization
- Understanding of the role and function of case management participants, that is, human resource personnel, benefits managers, insurance carriers, TPAs, risk managers, safety professionals, line managers, external providers, labor relations, and legal counsel
- Use of information technology
- Sociocultural influences
- Principles of utilization review and precertification
- Alternative treatment modalities
- Job analysis
- Principles of management/utilization of resources
- System abuse, for example, fraudulent practices by worker, employer, or vendor
- Health care delivery systems, for example, health insurance, managed care models (HMO, PPO, POS)
- Trends in case management, that is, disability, WC, rehabilitation, integrated models, etc.
- Disability plan designs, for example, STD, LTD, WC
- Disability terminology and concepts, for example, IME, second opinion, impairment ratings, deductibles, co-pays, indemnity, reserves
- Contractual agreements, that is, with workers, employers, vendors, TPAs, unions
- Clinical guidelines, clinical pathways, algorithms, standards of care
- Screening tools, for example, CAGE, health-risk appraisals, depression screening
- Role of the case managers on the interdisciplinary team

Return-to-Work Programs

A. In OH case management, case managers are not only concerned about ensuring appropriate medical care but must also address, from the initial assessment on the date of injury or illness, the goal of returning an individual to productive work at the earliest possible time in a transitional, modified, or full-duty capacity.[5]

B. The ultimate goal of OH case management is to assist the ill or injured person to achieve the highest level of medical improvement and to facilitate his or her successful RTW in the most cost-effective and efficient manner.

C. Companies should have in place formal RTW policies and procedures to expedite the injured worker's effective RTW in a timely manner.

D. Employer RTW programs should allow for the following types of work assignments:
   1. Full duty
   2. Temporary, alternative, or transitional work
   3. Modified duty assignments

E. RTW assignments that focus on "other than full duty" must be reviewed on a regular basis by both the OH case manager and company to ensure the employee is progressing as planned.

References

American Association of Occupational Health Nurses (AAOHN). (2012a). *Position statement: The occupational and environmental health nurse role.* Pensacola, FL: AAOHN.

American Association of Occupational Health Nurses (AAOHN). (2012b). *Occupational and environmental health nursing profession information sheet.* Retrieved from http:www.aaohn.org.

American Board for Occupational Health Nursing (ABOHN). (2012). *Case management candidate handbook.* Hinsdale, IL: ABOHN.

American College of Occupational and Environmental Medicine (ACOEM). (2011). *Occupational medicine practice guidelines: Evaluation and management of common health problems and functional recovery in workers* (3rd ed.). Elk Grove Village, IL: ACOEM.

American Medical Association (AMA). (2009). *Guide to the evaluation of permanent impairment* (6th ed.). Chicago, IL: AMA.

Americans with Disabilities Act of 1990, 41 U.S.C., section 12101 *et seq.*

Cherry Engineering Support Services, Inc. (2003). *Federal statutory definitions of disability prepared for the Interagency Committee on Disability Research.* Washington, DC: United States Department of Health & Human Services.

Case Management Society of America (CMSA). (2010). *Standards of practice for case management.* Little Rock, AR: Author.

DiBenedetto, D. V. (2000). *Principles of workers' compensation and disability case management course.* Yonkers, NY: DV DiBenedetto & Associates.

Job Accommodation Network (JAN). (2014). workplace accommodations: Low cost, high impact, annually updated research findings address the cost and benefits of job accommodation for people with disabilities. *Accommodation and Compliance Series.* Retrieved from https://askjan.org/, on August 20, 2015.

Society of Human Resource Managers (SHRM). (2014, October). *Executive summary: Total financial impact of employee absences in the U.S.* Retrieved from http://www.shrm.org/Research/

---

[5]Adapted from DiBenedetto, D. V. (2000). Occupational health case management. In S. K. Powell & D. Ignatavicius (Eds.), *CMSA core curriculum for case management* (pp. 195–212). Philadelphia, PA: Lippincott Williams & Wilkins.

SurveyFindings/Documents/Kronos_US_Executive_Summary_Final.pdf, on August 20, 2015.

The U.S. Equal Employment Opportunity Commission (EEOC). (2002, October 17). *Enforcement guidance: Reasonable accommodation and undue hardship under the Americans with Disabilities Act. EEOC, notice number 915.002.* Retrieved from http://www.eeoc.gov/policy/docs/accommodation.html, on August 20, 2015.

United States Bureau of Labor Statistics. (2012). *Employment Outlook: 2010–2020 Labor force projections to 2020: a more slowly growing workforce.* Retrieved from http://www.bls.gov/opub/mlr/2012/01/art3full.pdf, on August 20, 2015.

United States Census Bureau of Americans With Disabilities. (2012). *2010: Current population reports household economic studies.* Retrieved from http://www.census.gov/prod/2012pubs/p70-131.pdf, on August 20, 2015.

United States Department of Labor, Office of Disability Employment Policy. Retrieved from http://www.dol.gov/odep/return-to-work/, on August 20, 2015.

CHAPTER 26

Life Care Planning and Case Management

Hussein M. Tahan

LEARNING OBJECTIVES

Upon completion of this chapter, the reader will be able to:

1. Define life care planning.
2. Develop a life care plan.
3. Describe the role of the life care planner.
4. List five activities included in the life care planning process.
5. List three applications for use of a life care plan.
6. Discuss three phases of development of a life care plan.
7. Describe five categories of assessment in the life care planning process.
8. Compare the components of a life care plan with those of a case management plan.

IMPORTANT TERMS AND CONCEPTS

Accessible
Actionable Tort
Assessment
Clinical Practice
   Guidelines
Deposition

Efficacy of Care
Expert Witness
Exposure
Life Care Plan
Life Care Planner
Life Care Planning

Medicare Set Asides
   (MSA)
Medicare Secondary
   Payer (MSP)

Note: This chapter is a revised version of Chapter 17 in the second edition of *CMSA Core Curriculum for Case Management*. The contributor wishes to acknowledge the work of the late Patricia McCollom, as some of the timeless material was retained from the previous version.

Introduction

A. Life care planning is a program established for the management of the care, resources, and services required by the catastrophically injured or disabled or the person suffering from a complex chronic health condition.

B. Life care planning focuses on promoting the client's independence and empowerment, as well as the enhancement of the quality of care to ensure safety and a meaningful life for the chronically or catastrophically ill.

C. According to the International Academy of Life Care Planners (IALCP), life care planning is defined as an advanced and collaborative transdisciplinary practice that includes the patient (client), family (client's support system), varied health care providers, and other parties who are concerned in coordinating, accessing, evaluating, and monitoring the necessary services required for the care of a catastrophically injured or chronically ill client.

D. The American Association of Nurse Life Care Planners (AANLCP) defines life care planning specialty in nursing practice as "the protection, promotion, and optimization of health and abilities for individuals and families affected by catastrophic injuries, and chronic and complex health conditions" (AANLCP, 2014, p. 5).

E. Deutsch describes life care planning as "a consistent methodology for analyzing all of the needs dictated by the onset of a catastrophic disability through to the end of life expectancy. Consistency means that the methods of analysis remain the same from case to case and does not mean that the same services are provided to like disabilities" (Deutsch, 2010, pp. 4–5). Case managers and/or life care planners:

1. Deliberately and methodically organize, evaluate, and interpret the client/patient-specific information they gather and manage systematically, resulting in comprehensively understanding the client's situation. Case managers then effectively prevent potential complications, incongruences in care including use of equipment and other resources, and unrealistic rehabilitation programs.

2. Recommend a life care plan that is specific to the assessed needs and limitations of the client. Case managers identify care goals, interventions, and desired outcomes based on available evidence and what historically have been found to be effective (Deutsch, 2010).

F. Life care planning is a transdisciplinary specialty practice. Each professional, including rehabilitation specialists, nurses, case managers, physicians, social workers, and other allied health personnel, involved in life care planning brings his or her expertise and specialization to the life care planning process and to the life care plan for the ultimate benefit of the client/patient.

G. Life care planning has experienced tremendous growth in the last three decades. This growth is due to the use and benefit of life care plans within the rehabilitation, insurance, and legal professions. It has primarily emerged from combining case management and catastrophic disability.

H. The standards of practice for life care planning are developed based on the standards of practice of the individual disciplines that constitute the life care planning team such as nursing, medicine, case management, and rehabilitation.

I. The International Academy of Life Care Planners (IALCP) is the professional organization responsible for the development, maintenance, and promotion of life care planning standards. IALCP is sponsored and supported by the International Association of Rehabilitation Professionals (IARP). AANLCP also is involved in the development and promotion of life care planning standards; however, these apply only to nurses who function as life care planners.

J. When as a health care professional and case manager you find yourself wondering about the extent of the client's injury or disability and the cost of future care, it is time to consider a life care plan for the client:
   1. The time to get a life care planner involved is as soon as possible.
   2. Starting early in addressing the life care planning needs of the client allows time for necessary assessments to take place, which ultimately allows for effective and comprehensive care planning.

K. The life care plan is a team effort that uses the opinions of the client's physicians, therapists, counselors, specialty providers, other involved health care professionals, and client's support system.

L. According to Deutsch (2010), life care planning has its philosophical roots in three distinct fields of practice: experimental analysis of behavior, developmental psychology, and case management (Box 26-1). With catastrophic injuries, complex illnesses, and long-term disabilities, clients experience behavioral changes and limitations in function, coupled with the complex needs based on the developmental life stage of the client. These factors make life care planning a beneficial option. It then assures the delivery of quality and cost-effective care and facilitates improvement in condition.

BOX
26-1   Philosophical Roots of Life Care Planning

Life care planning is the integration of three fields of practice. These are:

1. *Experimental analysis of behavior*: applies the study of behavior and how it changes over time, principles of learning theory and behavior psychology, and techniques used in behavioral analysis
2. *Developmental psychology*: involves the study of social, cognitive, and physical changes that occur throughout the developmental stages of life
3. *Case management*: focuses on the importance of integrated and coordinated services for those with long-term medical, support care, and rehabilitation needs

INTEGRATION: the practices and basic principles inherent within rehabilitation counseling, rehabilitation nursing, rehabilitation psychology, and case management culminate in the establishment of the standards, tenets, and methodologies of life care planning.

From Deutsch, P. M. (2010). *Life care planning.* In J. H. Stone & M. Blouin (Eds.), *International encyclopedia of rehabilitation.* Available online: http://cirrie.buffalo.edu/encyclopedia/en/article/18.

Descriptions of Key Terms

A. Accessible—A term used to denote buildings/environments that are barrier free, thus allowing all members of society safe entry and exit.

B. Actionable tort—A legal duty imposed by statute or otherwise, owing by a defendant to the person injured.

C. Assessment—The process of collecting in-depth information about a person's situation, family, and functioning to identify an individual's needs in order to develop a comprehensive life care plan. Information should be gathered from all relevant sources (patient, family, caregivers, employers, medical records, etc.).

D. Clinical practice guidelines—Systematically developed statements on medical or nursing practices that assist a practitioner in making decisions about appropriate diagnostic and therapeutic health care services. Practice guidelines are usually developed by authoritative professional societies and organizations.

E. Deposition—The testimony of an individual taken under oath, but not in open court, on the subject at hand, reduced to writing, and authenticated, which may be used in court.

F. Efficacy of care—The potential, capacity, or capability to produce the desired outcome through evidence-based findings.

G. Expert witness—An expert qualified to provide court testimony by virtue of knowledge, skill, experience, training, or education.

H. Exposure—The amount of money for goods, care, and services an insurance company owes, when there is liability for the injured/ill person.

I. Life care plan—A dynamic document based on published standards of practice, comprehensive assessment, research, and data analysis, which provides an organized, concise plan for current and future needs, with associated costs, for individuals who have experienced catastrophic injury or have chronic health care needs (IALCP, 2009).

J. Life care planner—A health care professional specifically educated regarding the methodology for life care planning. Professionals engaged in this specialty practice may be nurses, vocational rehabilitation counselors, rehabilitation psychologists, disability management specialists, physicians, occupational therapists, social workers, physical therapists, and speech/language pathologists.

K. Outcome—The result and consequence of a health care process. In life care planning, an outcome is used to describe the result of the expected care or services.

 Applicability to CMSA'S Standards of Practice

A. The Case Management Society of America (CMSA) describes in its standards of practice for case management that case management practice extends across all health care settings, including payer, provider, government, employer, community, and home environment (CMSA, 2010):

1. Life care planning is practiced directly or indirectly in most of these settings where a client with a complex injury, illness, or disability is cared for.

  2. Life care planners practice in a variety of settings for diverse entities, such as legal practices, government agencies, insurance companies, banks, private companies, or, most commonly, in private practice as self-employed consultants.

  3. Life care planners interact with injured or chronically ill clients and their associated support systems, legal representatives, health care providers, insurance companies/payers, employers, other public or private agencies, and the community at large.

B. Case managers as life care planners are embedded in life care planning programs. They apply the CMSA standards of practice, in addition to the life care planning standards, in their work settings and as appropriate to the client population they serve.

C. In some organizations, case managers are the life care planners for their clients; in some others, they are not. Regardless, however, they collaborate with life care planners as part of their professional roles. Therefore, being knowledgeable of the CMSA standards of practice and how they relate to life care planning is essential. It is also necessary for case managers who are not life care planners to understand this specialty practice to facilitate timely access to care and services and the achievement of desired outcomes for both the clients and providers of care.

D. The case management process described in the CMSA standards of practice for case management is similar in focus and purpose to the life care planning process. These two processes align well. Although, in life care planning, the case manager or life care planner is often involved in testimony about the client's care and actual or projected cost of interventions and needed resources included the life care plan, such involvement is an uncommon practice in other work settings or specialties.

Aims of Life Care Planning

A. The aims of life care planning are similar to those of case management and focus on meeting the client's/support system's needs, interests, and care preferences while addressing the client's health condition, disability, or complex illness and coordinating the life care plan (Box 26-2).

B. Life care planners assist clients and their support systems in achieving optimal outcomes by developing appropriate life care plans. These plans include prevention of complications and restoration of health and well-being while assuring client safety and cost-effectiveness. The plans also recommend evaluations, interventions, services, and treatments that contribute to the client's level of wellness and restoration of function and provide information regarding care and resource requirements.

C. Life care planners communicate the plan of care. Goals and objectives of the treatment and interventions and expected outcomes to their clients, support systems, and involved members of the health care team. They also use comprehensive assessment tools to monitor and evaluate the client's condition, progress toward achieving the goals, and identify situations where modification of the life care plan are necessary.

BOX 26-2   Aims of Life Care Planning

- Assist clients in achieving optimal health outcomes for clients/support systems.
- Provide health education to client and other interested or involved parties.
- Ensure the appropriate allocation of resources and timely access to necessary and specialty services. This may include the development of alternate care plans.
- Communicate accurate and timely cost information for ease of utilization by clients, support systems, and members of the life care planning team.
- Develop measurement tools for the evaluation of outcomes.
- Ensure that all parties involved, including the client/support system and other health care professionals, are well aware of the life care plan, including the goals, milestones, and expected outcomes.
- Provide care and services that are cost effective and produce the best possible outcomes.
- Promote teamwork and collaboration among the varied health care providers involved in the care of the client; external parties such as employers, lawyers, and community agencies; and insurers or payers.

From International Academy of Life Care Planners (IALCP). *Life care planning guidelines: Standards of practice, goals.* Accessed on July 22, 2015; Available at http://ialcp.org/#goals.

D. Initially, life care planning was known as a specialty within rehabilitation. However, as its "standards and methods gained acceptance outside of the general rehabilitation circle, insurance carriers, worker's compensation judges, circuit...[and] federal court judges, attorneys, and others involved in litigation have called upon life care planners as experts in long-term disability management... [As a result, life care planners are sought after for their] specialized knowledge... to understand the long-term effects of catastrophic injuries and the associated economic damages of such cases" (Deutsch, 2010, p. 4).

The Process of Life Care Planning

A. The life care planning process is similar to that of case management. IALCP describes the process based on the functions of the life care planner, which include the following (IALCP, 2009):
   1. Assessment—Collection and analysis of data about the client's health condition, injury, finances, and social network. Assessment focuses on the client's medical, health, biopsychosocial, financial, educational, and vocational status and needs.
   2. Life care plan development and research—Determination of the content of the life care plan and researching the associated potential cost. The life care planner pays special attention in this activity of available evidence-based clinical practice guidelines and current standards of care.
   3. Data analysis—Deciding on the patient's care needs and ensuring that the recommended care activities are consistent with national standards. The life care planner also assesses the need for further consultation with or need for experts opinions of specialty care providers or allied health professionals.
   4. Planning—Organizing the data and content of the life care plan. It also involves the creation of reports including cost projections.

5. Collaboration—Developing effective relationships with other professionals and sharing relevant information with the health care team to formulate care recommendation.
6. Facilitation—Expediting care and resolving disagreements. Also eliciting cooperation and partnerships and keeping all involved aware of the life care plan.
7. Evaluation—Reviewing and revising the life care plan, monitoring use of resources, and ensuring completeness and consistency with standards. Providing follow-up consultation to ensure the life care plan is well understood and discrepancies are resolved for the benefit of the client.
8. Testimony—Participation in legal matters, such as expert sworn testimony, or acting as a consultant to legal proceedings related to determining care needs and costs.

Role of the Case Manager as a Life Care Planner

A. Case managers in a life care planning program are called *life care planners*. Those who are nurses are referred to as *nurse life care planners*. They use tools such as the life care plan to provide individualized and comprehensive life care services for clients with catastrophic illnesses and/or disabilities. In their roles, they project current and future long-term care needs and potential costs that are congruent with the level of disability evident in the condition of the catastrophically injured or chronically ill individual.
B. Life care planners must possess appropriate educational and licensure requirements and knowledge as defined by their professional discipline and its associated standards and scope of practice.
C. Life care planners must have a foundation of knowledge and appropriate experience in a specialty such as rehabilitation and/or nursing. According to IALCP (2009), they:
   1. Possess specialized knowledge and skills in researching and critically analyzing health care data and resources.
   2. Manage and interpret large volumes of information related to the care of an individual patient.
   3. Work autonomously.
   4. Attend to details and communicate effectively (both written and verbal communication).
   5. Develop positive relationships and partnerships with clients and other health care professionals.
   6. Create and use networks for gathering necessary information.
   7. Participate in professional, community, and national organizations.
   8. Demonstrate professional demeanor.
D. With its foundation in rehabilitation, it is natural that health professionals interested in the role of a life care planner are those from rehabilitation-related clinical specialty (Box 26-3).
E. Health professionals who function as life care planners are usually licensed or certified in a primary health discipline such as rehabilitation counseling. Many also hold either of the following certifications:
   1. The certified in life care planning (CLCP), which is offered by the Commission on Health Care Certification

BOX 26-3 Professional Backgrounds of Those Involved in Life Care Planning

- Rehabilitation counseling
- Rehabilitation nursing
- Rehabilitation psychology
- Physiatry
- Case management
- Nursing
- Vocational rehabilitation
- Workers' compensation
- Other allied health professions (e.g., physical therapy, occupational therapy)

    2. The certified nurse life care planner, which is offered to registered nurses by the American Association of Nurse Life Care Planners (CNLCP)

F. The American Association of Nurse Life Care Planners (AANLCP) and the Certified Nurse Life Care Planner (CNLCP) recognize life care planning as a nursing specialty practice. They describe the primary role of the nurse life care planner to be the development of a client-specific lifetime plan of care applying the nursing process. They also recognize the American Nurses Association's scope and standards of nursing practice and apply them to life care planning (AANLCP and CNLCP, 2014).

G. The AANLCP states that nurse life care planners apply advocacy, judgment, and critical thinking skills and use the nursing process in their practice and when caring for clients/support systems or developing long-term (lifetime) plans of care for these clients (AANLCP, 2014).

H. Nurses in life care planning use a holistic framework of practice, which recognizes the biological, psychological, social, and spiritual factors associated with and affected by a client's disability and chronic health conditions (AANLCP, 2014):

    1. Nurse life care planning is enriched, strengthened, and diversified by elements of case management, rehabilitation nursing, community health, public health, and legal nurse consulting.

    2. Nurse life care planning requires a working knowledge of economic trends, health care policy, funding sources, medical coding, and reimbursement issues (AANLCP, 2014).

I. Nurse life care planners apply their expertise in many ways, expanding beyond litigation-based traditional life care planning practices (Box 26-4).

J. A case manager who is a nurse life care planner may perform a broad range of activities and apply highly specialized skills and advanced knowledge (Box 26-5). In a typical day, it is quite possible for the case manager (nurse life care planner) to engage in a variety of interventions such as the following:

    1. Research changing wheelchair needs over a person's lifetime.

    2. Determine hours of care required for a client with a particular level of spinal cord injury.

    3. Work with a contractor on an individual's specific accessible housing requirements and plans for home modification (AANLCP, 2014).

26-4 Aspects of Practice of Nurse Life Care Planners

- Complex rehabilitation discharge planning
- Complex utilization review
- Independent nursing assessments
- Lien investigations
- Medical cost projections
- Medicare set-aside arrangements
- Reasonableness of past medical bills
- Setting insurance reserves

From American Association of Nurse Life Care Planners (AANLCP). (2014, September 19). *Nurse life care planning: Scope and standards of practice.* Salt Lake City, UT: Author.

K. Life care planners rely on the skills, knowledge, and contributions of other health care professionals to determine the immediate and future needs of their clients. They collaborate with these experts, who come from various disciplines, through consultation, and interact with the client's treating physician(s) and allied health team members and use of both clinical practice guidelines as well as the research literature in the development of life care plans and the management of the client's care.

L. Life care planners may testify as experts in particular cases. In this regard, they provide testimony on disability and function, safety, health care, reasonable and necessary future care, and associated costs. They also may provide the judge, jury, mediator, or arbitrator involved in a case with facts about the identified needs of a concerned client and share evidence regarding the life care plan's foundation, contents, recommendations, and outcomes.

26-5 Functions of Life Care Planners

- Assess and diagnose the individual client's response to the disability or illness.
- Anticipate the effects of disability or illness and future needs as the client ages and throughout the stages of life.
- Collaborate with health care providers when possible and applicable.
- Consider risk minimization and the promotion of function over the lifetime.
- Research and document the costs necessary to implement the care plan.
- Identify desired outcomes of plan elements.
- Incorporate information and opinions from other health providers and involved stakeholders.
- Identify available community, public, and insurance funding and how to access those resources.
- Initiate aspects of the life care plan during its development.
- Educate the client and client's support system (family, caregiver, or guardian) on the life care plan initiatives.
- Provide for the life care plan to be implemented by other health professionals including case managers (choice depends on jurisdiction).
- Update the life care plan based on the findings of the monitoring and evaluation of client's condition and responses to care.

From American Association of Nurse Life Care Planners (AANLCP). (2014, September 19). *Nurse life care planning: Scope and standards of practice.* Salt Lake City, UT: Author.

M. In the event case managers do not also function as life care planners, the case manager may then collaborate with the life care planer and contribute to the life care plan development process and offer opinions on expected needs for the client/family over the life expectancy. In this case, life care planners also may make provisions for case management services; the collaboration is often mutual.

The Life Care Plan

A. The term *life care plan* was introduced into the health care literature in 1981 by Paul Deutsch and Fred Raffa in a legal publication entitled *Damages in Tort Action*. The publication described how damages could be identified in civil litigation.

B. In 1987, the life care plan was introduced into the field of rehabilitation in *Guide to Rehabilitation* (Deutsch & Sawyer, 1987). The life care plan was identified as part of a rehabilitation evaluation to project the impact of catastrophic injury on an individual's future and was differentiated from a *discharge* plan by its specification of costs for long-term services to meet the needs of the catastrophically injured patient.

C. Communicated in 2000 and revised in 2006, the IALCP published the following definition of the life care plan: "A life care plan is a dynamic document based upon published standards of practice, comprehensive assessment, research and data analysis, which provides an organized, concise plan for current and future needs with associated costs, for individuals who have experienced catastrophic injury or have chronic health care needs" (IALCP, 2009, p. 4).

D. The life care plan has been used in a variety of health care settings, including the legal and ethical domains, to provide information regarding the cost of services needed for the catastrophic and long-term care of an individual. Life care plans focus mainly on rehabilitation planning, services implementation, management of health care costs and funds, transitional/discharge planning, and patient and family education (IALCP, 2009). An example of a life care plan is shown in Table 26-1.

E. The American Association of Nurse Life Care Planners (AANLCP) describes the life care plan as an important document that:
   1. Includes the future cost of identified interventions and associated costs for health maintenance, health promotion, and optimization of physical and psychological abilities for the life expectancy of the individual.
   2. Contains an organized, comprehensive, and evidence-based approach that estimates current and future health care needs.
   3. The associated costs and frequencies of interventions, resources, and services can be used as a guide in various applicable health care practices including private, medical–legal, and case management (AANLCP and CNLCP, 2014).

F. A life care plan is also used as a tool in the administration and litigation of catastrophic injury claims of persons who have long-term health care needs related to a chronic illness. In this case, it:
   1. Provides a comprehensive assessment of the current and future medical and rehabilitative needs of a person over his or her lifetime
   2. Assists in determining the long-term financial exposure to a carrier or to help evaluate a claim for settlement value

TABLE 26-1 Example of a Life Care Plan for Mr. Jameson, a Client with a Severe Spinal Cord Injury

CONCLUSION NO. 1: Due to health status, Mr. Jameson will require various medications throughout his life, as prescribed by his treating physicians.*

Current Prescription	Frequency	Outcome	Current Cost†	Comments	Resource/Reference
Levaquin	250 mg daily	Urinary tract infection controlled/resolved	$263.95/30 tablets $1,583.70/year (anticipate 6 prescriptions per year)	This was a current prescription, 12/2015	3, 7

NOTE: All the other medications will be listed in the life care plan, including information similar to that described for Levaquin.

CONCLUSION NO. 2: Due to functional limitations associated with injury, Mr. Jameson requires specific durable medical equipment to maintain his health, functioning, and safety for the remainder of his life.

Care/Need	Frequency	Outcome	Current Cost	Comments	Resource/Reference
Manual lightweight wheelchair	Current prescription; replace every 5–7 y	Mobility throughout the home and community	$2,895–$3,400	Currently uses this prescribed equipment	1, 2, 3, 9, 13
Wheelchair maintenance	Annual, beginning 2016	Prolong functioning of equipment	$350	Annual cost of manual chair maintenance, beginning 1 y after purchase	10, 13
Tire replacement (manual chair)	Minimum annual, beginning 2016	Mobility	$42 each	4 tires must be replaced	10, 12
Inner tubes (manual chair)	Minimum annual, beginning 2016	Mobility	$12 each	4 inner tubes must be replaced, depending on tire prescribed	10, 12
Jay II low-pressure cushion	Replace every 2–4 y, after wheelchair purchase	Prevent skin breakdown.	$294–$350	Currently uses a Roho and has had skin breakdown	2, 8, 10, 11

continued

TABLE 26-1 Example of a Life Care Plan for Mr. Jameson, a Client with a Severe Spinal Cord Injury, *continued*

Care/Need	Frequency	Outcome	Current Cost	Comments	Resource/Reference
Cushion covers	Replace annually		$75/cover (2 covers needed)	Cushion covers are additional cost but are necessary due to incontinence	2, 8, 10, 12
Power wheelchair	Purchase once at age 60	Mobility throughout the community	$12,000–$15,000 $350–$500 (annual maintenance)	Due to endurance and a shoulder injury, a power chair is anticipated	1, 2, 5, 9, 10
Handheld shower	Replace every 10 y	Ease in personal hygiene	$28.40	Bathroom must be accessible	1, 9
Shower chair	Replace every 7–10 y	Ease in personal hygiene	$695–$972 (list price)	This item can only be used with an accessible bathroom	1, 11
Reacher	Replace annually	Independent retrieval of items	$57	This item would promote independence	6, 11
Sliding board	Replace annually	Ease in transfers	$49	Current prescription	1, 3, 11
Standing frame	Daily use; one time purchase	Promote circulation, cardiac/respiratory/renal function	$2,075	Not able to use in current residence	1, 6, 11

CONCLUSION NO. 3: Due to medical diagnosis of a spinal cord injury, Mr. Jameson will require specific medical supplies to maintain health, functioning, and well-being.

Care/Need	Frequency	Outcome	Current Cost	Comments	Resource/Reference
Intermittent catheter	8 times daily	Bladder drainage	$29/30 catheters	Currently uses this item. Note: At assessment, he stated self-catheterization 4–5 times daily; 12/21/2015, he stated "every 2 h"	3, 11
Lubricating jelly	One tube per month	Ease in catheterization and bowel program	$348/year $14/each	Currently uses this item	3, 11
Bed drainage collection bag	Once per week	Urine collection	$168/year $91/20	Currently uses this item	3, 11
Chux	Daily	Bed protection	$273/year $37/200	Currently uses this item	3, 11
Depend	Daily 3–4	Clothing protection from incontinence	$135/year $13.79/16 $1,101/year	Currently uses this item	3, 7

Note: This life care plan is neither thorough nor comprehensive. It includes three conclusions as examples for clarification purposes. Ideally, the life care plan addresses all conclusion/problems as well as presents a summary of the patient's medical history, the acute or subacute treatment and progression prior to the involvement of the life care planner, and a report on the injury if applicable.
*Mr. Jameson is a construction worker who sustained a spinal cord injury while on the job after a fall from the roof of a building. Mr. Jameson's treating physician prescribed him multiple medications for anticoagulation prophylaxis, diabetes, hypertension, and hyperlipidemia. It is reasonable to anticipate that with appropriate rehabilitation intervention, additional medications relating to improved health with spinal cord injury will be prescribed.
*Costs are based on rates at the time this chapter was written. They vary based on insurance agency, state of patient's residency, and cost of living.

G. Characteristics that differentiate life care plans from other plans of care including case management plans are as follows:
   1. Life care plans are projections for care and resource *needs* into the future, rather than planned *actions* related to an acute health/illness episode. They describe the specific need for intervention.
   2. Life care plans include recommendations supported by the literature, research, and evidence-based clinical practice guidelines that meet legal requirement and court-imposed parameters.
   3. Life care plans are preventive in their approach, relating recommendations to prevention of high-cost complications, high-cost equipment, replacement costs, and uncontrolled, unmanaged purchases.
   4. Life care plans delineate options for maintaining care and needed goods and services within a managed care environment and within a realistic framework for individual needs, family structure and dynamics, and geographic location.
   5. Life care plans demonstrate researched costs for care, equipment, supplies, and services, as well as alternate resources to meet individual needs.
H. As life care planning has evolved over the past almost four decades, it has been influenced by extensive research and has become recognized that life care plans must reflect four critical aspects of a client's condition as appropriate. These are:
   1. Medical
   2. Rehabilitation
   3. Case management
   4. Psychological (Deutsch, 2010)
I. Benefits of a life care plan may include the following:
   1. The life care plan is a tool for case management.
   2. It may be used to educate patients and families regarding the need for and outcomes of ongoing monitoring and care.
   3. The plan may be used to collaborate among health care providers when providing case managements services in complex cases.
   4. The life care plan offers a mechanism to serve as an information management tool for the complex information generated in catastrophic cases or individuals with chronic illness.
   5. The life care plan specifies long-term medical, psychological, rehabilitation, and quality needs for the individual's life.
J. Applications for a life care plan are multiple. The life care plan is a preventive plan used for:
   1. Disability management
   2. Elder care management
   3. Discharge planning from health care facilities
   4. Long-term care for children or adults with disabilities
K. A life care plan may be used in litigation to:
   1. Establish long-term needs.
   2. Specify costs.
L. A life care plan may be used in insurance settings to:
   1. Determine cost exposure.
   2. Identify a profile for long-term needs.

M. Life care plans include specific information. They must be consistent with the clinical needs of the individual. The life care plan must:
1. Reflect risk factors for complications that may lead to higher costs.
2. Include the quality-of-life needs.
3. Identify the impact of aging on needs.

 Development of the Life Care Plan

A. Health care professionals in various disciplines may prepare the life care plans. Case managers may prepare the life care plans due to their role in referral, purchase of goods and services, knowledge of psychosocial status, health plans and other insurance carriers, and local resources.
B. Professionals involved in life care planning must:
1. Have a thorough understanding of the diagnoses, treatment protocols, factors affecting the diagnoses, psychological implications, rehabilitation relating to disability or complex illness, psychosocial implications, family dynamics, reimbursement structures and methods, and legal requirements or implications.
2. Possess knowledge of available community resources.
3. Be creative in the development of alternative plans and in maintaining fiscal accountability to meet the patient's and family's needs.
4. Develop a life care plan that integrates available resources and is preventive, rehabilitative, and curative, if possible, for the individual with catastrophic injury and/or long-term health care needs.
C. Review of records is an initial activity in the development of the life care plan. The review usually includes the following:
1. *Medical records*, both pre- and postinjury, disability, or illness, to provide background in diagnosing and treating and to identify the expected outcomes of care for the individual.
2. *School records* to clarify the individual's cognitive and social abilities and behaviors. These may be especially helpful in working with a child or a teenager.
3. *Military records* may define work tasks assigned, performance, and physical capabilities.
4. *Depositions*, if available or appropriate to the case, to provide insight into the patient and family understanding of their situation and perception of their condition and needs.
5. *Rehabilitation records* to understand the rehabilitation consultation and services provided, client's response to these services, and plan for continued rehabilitation.
D. An assessment interview with the client/patient and family must also be completed so that the life care plan is comprehensive, individualized, and specific to the patient and family needs:
1. If the patient is nonverbal, assessment and observation periods of care and outcomes are critical to accurate understanding of his or her needs.
2. Care providers and/or family members must be included in the interview to clarify needs, define roles and role reversals, and identify stresses and their reasons.

3. Data gathering for the development of the life care plan is necessary and must be comprehensive. It focuses on various aspects of the client's condition and may include those shared in Box 26-6.
4. Observations made during assessments may include the patient's mood, willingness to respond, patient's and family's behavior, voice characteristics, and manner.

BOX 26-6   Elements of a Life Care Planning Assessment/Data Gathering

- History of injury and health, including past medical history and consumption of medications
- Complications
- Current diagnoses:
  - Patient understanding of the diagnoses
  - Family understanding of the diagnoses
- Treatment plan:
  - Current care
  - Future potential care
  - Patient and family understanding of the treatment plan
- Current status
- Functional skills and abilities:
  - Self-care
  - Communication
  - Cognition
  - Behavior
  - Mobility and physical functioning
  - Safety
  - Community reintegration
  - Household management and safe environment
- Risk factors:
  - Psychosocial dynamics
  - Health condition related
  - Financial/insurance related
- Psychosocial impact:
  - Viability of the family unit
  - Family of choice involvement
- Education:
  - Formal/degree(s) held
  - Military
  - Experiential
- Vocational background:
  - Financial status
  - Social Security benefits obtained
  - Eligibility for Medicaid or Medicare benefits
  - Current or previous health insurance plan if any
- Medications:
  - Confirm knowledge of why prescribed, schedule of medications intake
  - Confirm knowledge of side effects
  - Confirm knowledge of proper medications administration and adherence
- Medical supplies
- Durable medical equipment
- Adaptive equipment
- Accessibility needs
- Home care/facility care
- Personal care attendant

E. Collaboration with a treatment team when possible helps to determine projected treatment and potential associated cost, actual or potential needs, frequency of care or services, and the probability of future therapeutic or diagnostic interventions.

F. A life care planner/physician team may assess a patient for the collaborative development of the life care plan.

G. Clinical practice guidelines and other types of literature may serve to supplement medical records when a treatment team is not immediately accessible.

H. Community resources and geographically accessible services may be identified through collaboration with community-based programs.

I. Data analysis must be completed to develop recommendations for long-term needs:
1. The life care planner must analyze all the data collected through the assessment and monitoring of the patient's condition, interactions with the patient's family, and collaboration with the treatment team.
2. The life care planner must use the results of the analysis in the development of the treatment plan or life care plan, which includes goals, priorities, and expected outcomes.
3. The life care planner must have a strong clinical knowledge base as well as ability to collect and analyze relevant data to provide for accurate projections of the patient's needs.
4. Data analysis produces a clear presentation of the patient's needs, the necessary goods and services, and the outcomes of implementation of the recommendations.

J. Research in life care planning improves patient care outcomes and allows the provision of quality health care services and treatments.
1. Recommendations for management of the patient's condition as included in the life care plan must be supported by the evidence-based literature, clinical practice guidelines, and/or physician recommendation.
2. Cost research for the purpose of cost-effectiveness may be completed by the life care planner through contacting other care providers and health care agencies, bill review, or search of computer databases for durable medical equipment or supplies.
3. Current published data on length of stay, frequency of complications or services, and outcomes of care may be used as adjunct research.

Components of the Life Care Plan

A. The life care plan should initially specify the records reviewed as a foundation for the plan.
1. A brief summary of the patient's history and injury/illness identifies diagnostics and treatment.
2. Current status defines the patient's ability to participate in routine life activities, functional skills, medications, activities of daily living, complications, and perception of status.
3. The family status should also be addressed, as well as family stressors.

B. Projections within the life care plan are important.
1. Projected medical care identifies both periodic and episodic care activities, both diagnostic and therapeutic, that may be necessary and consistent with the patient's and family's needs and interests.

2. Projected interventions specify necessary treatment or services that are designed to maintain or improve the patient's status, prevent complications, or minimize risk factors.

C. Diagnostic testing may relate to monitoring the patient's condition medically, psychologically, socially, and cognitively. These may include neuropsychological evaluation or vocational assessment.

D. Durable medical equipment and maintenance address mobility needs, physical functioning, community reintegration, and socialization.

E. Supplies are identified to meet individual needs to maintain health.

F. Adaptive equipment and assistive devices promote independence and well-being. Certain equipment and assistive technologies may be essential to enhance the patient's ability to be socially interactive.

G. Medications that are currently prescribed and risks for additional medication use may be noted.

H. Home care or facility care must be included, noting the impact and ability of the family to be involved in care.

I. Transportation needs must also be included. The plan, in this way, provides for the patient's accessibility to the community, medical care and services, recreation, and vocational needs.

J. Accessibility issues and the barrier-free environmental needs of the patient must be noted within the life care plan. Types of necessary home furnishings and accessories may be specified.

K. Vocational needs and services must be addressed, as appropriate, within the plan. Community resources for evaluation, training, and job placement should also be included.

L. Health maintenance services such as counseling, recreation, occupational therapy, and community involvement should be defined within the life care plan.

Medicare Set Asides: a Life Care Planning Specialty

A. Medicare Set Asides (MSA) has been mandatory for workers' compensation claims since 2001. It requires documentation that shows the amount of dollars that must be "set aside" for a workers' compensation liability case. These set-aside funds are used for coverage of future medical expenses:
   1. Workers' compensation MSA arrangement is a financial agreement that allocates a portion of a workers' compensation settlement to pay for future medical services related to the workers' compensation injury, illness, or disease. These funds must be depleted before Medicare will pay for treatment related to the workers' compensation injury, illness, or disease.

B. An MSA is a document that specifies future injury-related care needs and associated costs. Only Medicare-covered expenses are identified in this document and may include:
   1. Costs based upon Medicare payments within the beneficiary's state of jurisdiction
   2. Part of a settlement award "set aside" to pay for future costs that Medicare would have paid

C. MSA was legislated to protect Medicare from being placed in a role as the primary payer, when it should be in the role as secondary payer and when the primary payer should be the responsibility of another entity:
   1. The Medicare Secondary Payer (MSP) statute was created in 1980, to ensure that other insurance carriers covering the individual for payment of medical expenses would be primary payers.
   2. The statute was created to prevent shifting of the burden of future expenses for injury-related care from workers' compensation insurance companies or others with responsibility for payment to Medicare:
      a. An MSA considers Medicare's interest when agreement is reached for the future medical needs of the injured individual.
      b. The Center for Medicare and Medicaid Services (CMS) is to be contacted if a workers' compensation claim is going to settlement.
      c. The arrangement for an MSA document is necessary when there is an expectation of enrollment within 30 months of a settlement date on a claim.
      d. The arrangement for an MSA document is necessary when there is anticipation of a greater than $250,000 settlement.
D. Development of an MSA:
   1. Review of records, which may include the following:
      a. Medical
      b. Billing records
   2. Verify eligibility for benefits:
      a. Social Security
      b. Medicare
   3. Secure a rated age
   4. Obtain medical recommendation for ongoing care:
      a. Research applicable standards of care
      b. Research clinical practice guidelines
      c. Research evidence-based literature and health outcomes
   5. Research a Medicare lien
   6. Identify future medical needs:
      a. Medicare-covered goods and services
      b. Medicare costs specific to the individual's geographic region
E. Consequences for noncompliance with the statute:
   1. Denial of payment for future medical care.
   2. Medicare may designate its own allocation.
   3. Lawsuit filed against the injured individual, attorney, and/or the insurance carrier.
F. The life care planners/case managers may be best to assume responsibility for MSA:
   1. They analyze services rendered compared to the patient's medical diagnosis eliminating any unnecessary costs associated with a claim. By compiling, analyzing, and summarizing extensive amounts of medical data, case managers are able to reduce the amount of time and money spent preparing for the application process of an MSA.
   2. They provide a standardized, objective, organized, and concise projection of current and long-term medical and nonmedical needs and associated costs for individuals who have experienced catastrophic injury or significant chronic or long-term medical impairment.

3. They ensure that the MSA includes a complete file review, execution of appropriate medical releases, projection of future medical needs, and submission and tracking of the MSA to the appropriate CMS regional office.
4. They ensure that the MSA also provides a complete and accurate picture of Medicare's expected future medical exposure, by utilizing Medicare's current reimbursement guidelines in determining eligibility and coverage for future medical treatment.

Health and Disability Insurance

A. Case managers and/or life care planners who work for health and disability insurance companies help claims personnel set annual reserves on high-cost members. They possess working knowledge of insurance terminology, regulations, and applicable laws and are sought by other professionals for guidance as needed:
   1. They may apply the case management and life care planning processes to determine future medical care needs and costs.
   2. They provide the gathered information to actuaries, who calculate reserves to be set aside according to state or federal requirements to pay for the following year's health care needs. This position also requires working knowledge of insurance terminology, regulations, and applicable laws.

References

American Association of Nurse Life Care Planners (AANLCP). (2014, September 19). *Nurse life care planning: Scope and standards of practice.* Salt Lake City, UT: Author.

American Association of Nurse Life Care Planners (AANLCP) and Certified Nurse Life Care Planner (CNLCP) Certification Board. (2014, June 6). *Position statement: Education and certification for nurse life care planners.* Authors. Retrieved from http://cnlcp.org/wp-content/uploads/2014/08/Joint-Statement-Approved-6-6-142.pdf, on May 1, 2016.

Case Management Society of America. (2010). *Standards of Practice for Case Management.* Little Rock, AR: Author.

Deutsch, P. M. (2010). *Life care planning.* In J. H. Stone & M. Blouin (Eds.), *International encyclopedia of rehabilitation.* Available online: http://cirrie.buffalo.edu/encyclopedia/en/article/18

Deutsch, P., & Sawyer, H. (1987). *Guide to rehabilitation.* New York, NY: Matthew Bender and Co., Inc.

International Academy of Life Care Planners (IALCP). (2009). *Standards of practice for life care planners.* Glenview, IL: International Association of Rehabilitation Professionals. Accessed from http://www.rehabpro.org/sections/ialcp/focus/standards/ialcpSOP_pdf, on July 20, 2015.

CHAPTER 27

Suggested Resources and Readings in Case Management

Teresa M. Treiger and Hussein M. Tahan

IMPORTANT TERMS AND CONCEPTS

Accreditation
Certificate
Certification
Credentials

Credentialing
Professional
Development

Scholarly
Activities
Scholarship

 Introduction

A. Although it is challenging to maintain a current case management resource list, an attempt to do so herein has been undertaken. These resources are intended to facilitate the continuous pursuit of knowledge, which is a hallmark of professional case management practice.

B. The resources available to case managers and other health professionals are constantly changing. New textbooks are often published by experts in the field and competing publishers, while other existing textbooks are updated to reflect current or future anticipated practices. Additionally, some textbooks are left untouched, which makes them outdated and no longer appropriate for application in practice. Moreover, some authors and publishers may decide to sunset certain textbooks, and therefore, these textbooks disappear from the industry altogether. These constant changes make it necessary for case management professionals to remain up to date on the knowledge available for practice.

C. Journal articles (or periodicals) generally are more current in their content compared to textbooks; however, periodicals are often not comprehensive enough in addressing a particular topic compared to textbooks, and sometimes, they share one expert's experience or philosophical opinion instead of innovative, common practices and generalizable knowledge.

D. Despite the existing advantages and disadvantages to textbooks and periodicals, it is advisable for case management professionals to review both textbooks and periodicals available on a phenomenon of interest to gain a broader and more comprehensive perspective on the practice.

E. It is essential for case management professionals to conduct literature searches on topics or phenomena of interest and refrain from assuming that what is listed in this chapter is what they need or a comprehensive review of literature and the best available knowledge on the topic. The resources provided herein are but the proverbial tip-of-the-iceberg and intended as a first step in your lifelong learning quest as a case management professional.

F. No specific criteria (e.g., quality, credibility, accuracy, currency, or evidence rating scales) were applied in the selection of the resources (i.e., textbooks, periodicals, and Web sites) listed in this chapter.

   1. In most cases, the textbook and journal references shared in this chapter are contemporary (2010 or more recent). Other resources are included when found to be the most current resource on the topic, a historically significant reference, or if it is otherwise regarded as classic or seminal work.

   2. Regarding Internet sites, all Web site URL addresses were verified as valid and functional as of September 2015. If an address is no longer valid, the editors kindly suggest locating the host Web site's home page and searching for the content from that point. Unfortunately, Web site content and locations change constantly. Also, keep in mind that content may no longer be freely accessible at the time you search for it. You may be required to register on a Web site in order to obtain the desired resource information or pay a nominal fee for accessing the resource.

G. It is likely that a textbook included in the resource list is an older edition from what is Retrieved from the time you are interested in it. Therefore, the editors suggest that you take the time and check first if a more recent edition is available before you access it. You may do this by checking the publisher's Web site or any other commonly used sales site you may be routinely accessing when you purchase your textbooks.

H. The resources included in this chapter are in no way meant to constitute an "exhaustive," "comprehensive," or a "systematic" review of the literature on case management. These resources are a starting point to get you going with your quest for key resources in case management. You may then locate other resources that are of greater interest to you in your specialty area (e.g., practice setting, professional discipline, or patient population you care for).

Descriptions of Key Terms

A. Accreditation—A program that is designed based on nationally recognized standards and reflective of the latest quality and safety practices in a particular specialty or health care organization type. The program is usually offered by a nongovernment agency, which acts as an independent reviewer of the interested health care organization. Based on defined standards, the accreditation agency makes a determination whether the organization meets the nationally recognized standards (also referred to as accreditation criteria). Based on the review findings, a decision is rendered. The organization is then referred to as accredited by that organization.

B. Certificate—A document awarded to affirm that an individual participated or attended a given educational program. It can be provided by any professional agency (private or public, for profit and not for profit), university, or college. Usually, a certificate is not nationally recognized in any form other than an evidence of educational credit. In cases where continuing education credit (CE) or units are offered, the CE certificate then reflects that a professional body, other than the agent offering the educational program, has reviewed the offering and deemed it appropriate for CE.

C. Certification—Use of this term varies based on its reference to an individual professional or to an organization or a program within an organization.

1. Certification (individual)—An official form of credential that is provided by a nationally recognized governmental or nongovernmental certifying agency (i.e., credentialing body) to a professional who meets a set of predetermined eligibility criteria and requirements of a particular field, practice, or specialty. It usually signifies the achievement of a passing score on an examination prepared by the certifying agency for that purpose. It also denotes an advanced degree of competence.

2. Certification (organization or program)—An official form of accreditation that is provided by a nationally recognized governmental or nongovernmental agency to an organization or a program within an organization (e.g., center of excellence) that meets nationally recognized requirements or standards of quality and safe performance.

D. Credentialing—Similar to certification, the use of this term varies based on whether it refers to an individual professional or to an organization, program, or service within an organization.
   1. Credentialing (individual)—The process used to protect the consumer and to ensure that individuals hired to practice case management are providing quality case management services. This involves a review of the provider's licensure; certification; insurance; evidence of malpractice insurance (if applicable); performance; knowledge, skills, and competencies; and history of lawsuits/malpractices.
   2. Credentialing (organization, program, or service)—The process used in the review of a case management program or organization to ensure that it meets nationally recognized industry standards of quality. This is necessary for the provision of quality case management services and to protect the consumer.
E. Credentials—Evidence of competence, current and relevant licensure, certification, education, and experience.
F. Professional development—The process of ongoing learning and advancement of one's specialty-based practice knowledge, skills, and abilities. It encompasses a variety of formal, informal, and ongoing job-embedded and facilitated learning opportunities. Examples of learning activities are academic degrees, coursework, attendance at conferences, on-the-job training, reading textbooks and journal articles, and formal coaching or mentoring.
G. Scholarly activities—The professional actions taken to disseminate knowledge and innovations. The main purpose is the sharing of information with others including one's peers in a written, oral, or performance presentation using multimedia technology, which ultimately subjects the knowledge to critique or review for its utility and value in practice.
H. Scholarship—The development of new knowledge or enhancement of existing knowledge in a specific area or specialty. This may entail the discovery of new practices or insights about a phenomenon through research, application of the new discoveries into practice (translation of evidence into practice), or teaching others about, and the use of, the new discoveries in one's practice.

Applicability to CMSA's Standards of Practice

A. In its standards of practice for case management, CMSA describes the requirements for the case manager role including education, licensure or certification, and other qualifications. The standards also emphasize that case managers should maintain knowledge, skills, and competence in their area of practice (CMSA, 2010).
B. Case managers and other involved professionals are able to maintain and advance their knowledge, skills, and competence through professional development, scholarship, and scholarly activities.
C. Case managers have a primary obligation toward the field of case management: advancement of the practice. They can achieve this by engaging in research activities and sharing of their discoveries and

innovations with others either via presentations at conferences or publishing their work in the form of textbooks or journal articles.

D. Case managers can also contribute to the field through volunteer activities, which may include membership in professional organizations (e.g., CMSA), assuming positions on association boards, and engaging in local, regional, or national taskforces about some aspects of case management practice (i.e., health and public policy).

E. Through scholarship and scholarly activities, case managers are able to contribute to the standards of practice so that these standards remain current and appropriate for guiding the practice.

Case Management Standards of Practice

A. Often, professional organizations or associations develop standards of practice in their area of specialization to guide their membership about the expected practice in that area.

B. There are many professional organizations that are directly or indirectly related to case management. These have developed and published standards either about the general or specialty practice of case management. Some also have published about case management practice in a particular patient population. Case managers must be familiar with the standards advocated for and published by the professional organizations in their case management specialty practice whether based on care settings, patient population, or professional discipline.

C. Here are some examples of widely used standards in case management practice:
   1. Case Management Society of America, CMSA Standards of Practice for Case Management, revised 2010. Available at http://www.cmsa.org/portals/0/pdf/memberonly/StandardsOfPractice.pdf
   2. Department of Veteran Affairs, Case Management Standards of Practice. Available at http://www1.va.gov/optometry/docs/VHA_Handbook_1110-04_Case_Management_Standards_of_Practice.pdf
   3. National Association of Social Workers (NASW), 2013 NASW Standards for Social Work Case Management. Available at https://www.socialworkers.org/practice/naswstandards/CaseManagementStandards2013.pdf
   4. Commission for Case Manager Certification (CCMC), Case Management Body of Knowledge (CMBOK). Available at http://www.cmbodyofknowledge.com
   5. Commission for Case Manager Certification (CCMC), Code of Professional Conduct for Case Managers with Standards, Rules, Procedures, and Penalties, revised 2015. Available at http://ccmcertification.org/content/ccm-exam-portal/code-professional-conduct-case-managers

Case Management Textbooks

A. The case management textbooks available vary based on the target audience or the basis of the core subject matter they address. They vary across work settings, practice sites, professional disciplines, and patient populations.

B. Below is a select list of available textbooks that case managers may find helpful in their quest for ongoing professional development and advancement.

1. Birmingham, J. (2010). *Discharge planning guide: Tools for compliance* (3rd ed.). Danvers, MA: HC Pro.

2. Bond, C. P., & Coleman, E. A. (2010). *Reducing readmissions: A blueprint for improving care transitions.* Danvers, MA: HC Pro.

3. Cesta, T. G., & Cunningham, B. A. (2009). *Core skills for hospital case managers, a training tool for effective outcomes.* Marblehead, MA: HCPro.

4. Cesta, T. G., & Tahan, H. A. (2016). *The case manager's survival guide: Winning strategies in the new healthcare environment* (3rd ed.). Lancaster, PA: DEStech Publications, Inc.

5. Cohen, E. L. & Cesta, T. (2004). *Nursing case management: From essentials to advanced practice applications* (4th ed.). Maryland Heights, MO: Mosby.

6. Daniels, S., & Ramey, M. (2005). *The leader's guide to hospital case management.* Sudbury, MA: Jones and Bartlett.

7. Eack, S. M., Anderson, C. M., & Greeno, C. G. (2011). *Mental health case management: A practical guide.* Thousand Oaks, CA: Sage Publications.

8. Finkelman, A. (2011). *Case management for nurses.* Upper Saddle River, NJ: Prentice Hall.

9. Huber, D. L. (Ed.). (2013). *Leadership and nursing care management* (5th ed.). Maryland Heights, MO: Saunders Elsevier.

10. Kathol, R. M., Perez, R. R., & Cohen, J. P. (2010). *The integrated case management manual: Assisting complex patients regain physical and mental health.* New York: Springer.

11. Mullahy, C. M. (2014). *The case manager's handbook* (5th ed.). Burlington, MA: Jones & Bartlett Learning, LLC.

12. Powell, S. K., & Tahan, H. A. (2009). *Case management: A practical guide for education and practice* (3rd ed.). Philadelphia, PA: Wolters Kluwer.

13. Rossi, P. (2014). *The hospital case management orientation manual.* Danvers, MA: HC Pro.

14. Summers, N. (2015). *Fundamentals of case management practice* (5th ed.). Boston, MA: Cengage Learning.

15. Treiger, T. M., & Fink-Samnick, E. (2015). *COLLABORATE® for professional case management: A universal competency-based paradigm.* Philadelphia, PA: Wolters Kluwer.

16. Walsh, K., & Zander, K. (2007). *Emergency department case management: Strategies for creating and sustaining a successful program.* Danvers, MA: HC Pro.

17. Weil, M., Karls, J. M., & Associates. (1985). *Case management in human service practice.* San Francisco, CA: Jossey-Bass.

18. Woodside, M., & McClam, T. (2013). *Generalist case management (SAB 125 substance abuse case management)* (4th ed.). Boston, MA: Brooks/Cole.

19. Zander, K. (2008). *Hospital case management models: Evidence for connecting the boardroom to the bedside.* Danvers, MA: HC Pro.

Case Management Journals

A. Journal articles about the practice of case management are as important as textbooks for professional development. Case managers must be familiar with available journals in case management. Accessing case management journals and reviewing their content help keep case managers up to date in their knowledge of the practice. It is a way of maintaining one's knowledge, skills, and competencies, which ultimately enhance one's image and identity as a professional.

B. Below is a list of select case management journals. Case managers may use these journals, and others, to publish their work and innovations and to remain abreast of others' work and innovations.
   1. Care Management Journals: Journal of Case Management; Journal of Long-Term Home Health Care; published by Springer Publishing Company.
   2. Care Management: Official Journal of the Academy of Certified Case Managers and Commission for Case Manager Certification; published by the Academy.
   3. Case in Point; published by Dorland Healthcare.
   4. CMSA Today: The Official Voice of the Case Management Society of America; published by Naylor, LLC.
   5. Geriatric Nursing; published by Elsevier.
   6. Journal of the American Geriatrics Society; published by Wiley.
   7. Population Health Management; the Official Journal of the Population Health Alliance; published by the Alliance.
   8. Professional Case Management: The official journal of CMSA; published by Wolters Kluwer.

History and Evolution of Case Management

A. Select Periodicals, Books, and Other Sources:
   1. Buhler-Wilkerson, K. (1993). Bringing care to the people: Lillian Wald's legacy to public health nursing. *American Journal of Public Health, 83*(12), 1778–1786.
   2. Education for All Handicapped Children Act of 1975. 20 U.S.C. §1401 (1975). Retrieved from http://www.gpo.gov/fdsys/pkg/STATUTE-89/pdf/STATUTE-89-Pg773.pdf
   3. Feld, M. N. (2008). *Lillian Wald: A biography*. New York: The University of North Carolina Press.
   4. Fulmer, H. (1902). History of visiting nurse work in America. *American Journal of Nursing, 2*(6), 411–425.
   5. Johnson, M. A. (2005). *Hull house. The electronic encyclopedia of Chicago.* Retrieved from www.encyclopedia.chicagohistory.org/pages/615.html
   6. Lane, L. C. (1963). Jane Addams as social worker, the early years at Hull House. (Doctoral dissertation). Retrieved from ProQuest Dissertations and Theses. Accession No. AAI6307514
   7. Lewis, L. (2008). Discussion and recommendations: Nurses and social workers supporting family caregivers. *Journal of Social Work Education, 44*(3), 129–136.

8. Linn, J. W. (1935). *Jane Addams: A biography.* [*Kindle version*]. Retrieved from http://www.amazon.com/Jane-Addams-James-Weber-Linn-ebook/dp/B00CIX2USC/ref=tmm_kin_title_popover

9. Lundblad, K. S. (1995). Jane Addams and social reform: A role model for the 1990s. *Social Work, 40*(5), 661–669.

10. Murdach, A. D. (2011). Mary Richmond and the image of social work. *Social Work, 56*(1), 92–94.

11. Netting, F. E. (1992). Case management: Service or symptom? *Social Work, 37*(2), 160–164.

12. Older Americans Act of 1965, 42 U.S.C. 3056. Retrieved from http://www.gpo.gov/fdsys/pkg/STATUTE-79/pdf/STATUTE-79-Pg218.pdf

13. Social Security Act of 1935 Legislative History. (2013). Retrieved from http://www.ssa.gov/history/35act.html

14. Social Welfare History Archives. (n.d.). *Henry street settlement records.* Retrieved from http://special.lib.umn.edu/findaid/xml/sw0058.xml

15. Tahan, H. A. (1998). Case management: A heritage more than a century old. *Nursing Case Management, 3*(2), 55–60.

16. The Social Welfare History Project. (n.d.). *Mary Ellen Richmond (1861–1928). Social work pioneer, administrator, researcher and author.* Retrieved from http://www.socialwelfarehistory.com/people/richmond-mary

17. Treiger, T. M., & Fink-Samnick, E. (May/June, 2013). COLLABORATE: A universal competency-based paradigm for professional case management, Part I: Introduction, historical validation, and competency presentation. *Professional Case Management, 18*(3), 122–135. doi:10.1097/NCM.0b013e31828562c0

18. U.S. Department of Health and Human Services. (2011). *Historical evolution of programs for older Americans. Administration on Aging.* Retrieved from www.aoa.gov/AoARoot/AoA_Programs/OAA/resources/History.aspx

19. Wade, L. (1967). The heritage from Chicago's early settlement houses. *Journal of the Illinois State Historical Society, 60*(4), 411–441. Retrieved from http://www.jstor.org/stable/40190170

20. Wald, L. D. (1991). *The house of Henry Street.* New Brunswick, CA: Transaction Publishers.

Healthcare Benefits, Payment, and Reimbursement Systems

A. Select Periodicals, Books, and Other Sources:

1. Ball, R. M. (1973). Social Security Amendments of 1972: Summary and Legislative History. *Social Security Bulletin, 36*(3), 3–25.

2. Bodenheimer, T., & Grumbach, K. (2009). *Understanding health policy: A clinical approach* (6th ed.). New York: McGraw Hill Medical.

3. Buchmueller, T. C., & Monheit, A. C. (2009). Employer-sponsored health insurance and the promise of health insurance reform. *National Bureau of Economic Research. Working Paper 14839.* Retrieved from http://www.nber.org/papers/w14839

4. Cohen, W. J., & Ball, R. M. (1965). Social Security Amendments of 1965: Summary and legislative history. *Social Security Bulletin, 28*(9), 3–21.

5. Fuchs, B. (1997). Managed health care: Federal and State Regulation. *Library of Congress—Congressional Research Service, Series 97-938 EPW.* Retrieved from http://research.policyarchive.org/485.pdf

6. Health Insurance Association of America. (1997). *Fundamentals of health insurance: Part A.* Washington, DC: Health Insurance Association of America.

7. Health Insurance Association of America. (1997). *Fundamentals of health insurance: Part B.* Washington, DC: Health Insurance Association of America.

8. Wrightson, C. W. (2002). *Financial strategy for managed care organizations: Rate setting, risk adjustment, and competitive advantage. [ACHE Management Series].* Chicago, IL: HealthAdministration Press.

Case Management Practice Settings and Throughput

A. Select Web sites:
1. Care Transitions Intervention Program: http://www.caretransitions.org
2. Community-Based Care Transitions Program: http://innovation.cms.gov/initiatives/CCTP/
3. National Transitions of Care Coalition: http://www.ntocc.org
4. Project RED (Re-Engineering Discharge): https://www.bu.edu/fammed/projectred/
5. Project BOOST (Better Outcomes for Older adult Safe Transitions): http://www.hospitalmedicine.org
6. Transitional Care Model: http://www.transitionalcare.info

B. Select Periodicals, Books, and Other Sources:
1. AHC Media. (2013). *Barrier reduction teams smooth throughput.* Retrieved from http://www.ahcmedia.com/articles/65235-barrier-reduction-teams-smooth-throughput, on August 31, 2015
2. HCPro. (2011). *Work with bed flow coordinators to improve throughput.* Retrieved from http://www.hcpro.com/CAS-259559-2311/Work-with-bed-flow-coordinators-to-improve-throughput.html, on August 31, 2015
3. KPMG. (2015). *Capacity management: Patient throughput and case management improvement.* Retrieved from http://www.floridahfma.org/regional-presentations2.lib/items/capacity-management/KPMG%20Capacity%20Management%20Presentation_Final_022515.pdf, on August 31, 2015
4. Rossheim, J. (2012). The key to ED patient throughput. *Curaspan Blog.* Retrieved from https://connect.curaspan.com/blog/key-ed-patient-throughput/, on August 31, 2015
5. Turtle, D. (2007). Create virtual beds with aggressive throughout management. *QHR White Paper.* Retrieved from http://healthleadersmedia.com/content/89062.pdf, on August 31, 2015

Case Management in the Acute Care Setting

A. Select Periodicals, Books, and Other Sources:
1. Daniels, S. (2009). Advocacy and the hospital case manager. *Professional Case Management, 14*(1), 48–51.

2. Daniels, S. (2011). Introducing HCM v3.0: A standard model for hospital case management practice. *Professional Case Management, 16*(3), 109–125.

3. Eramo, L. A. (2013). *Case managers show their worth.* Retrieved from http://www.fortherecordmag.com/archives/1113p26.shtml, on August 31, 2015.

4. Fink-Samnick, E., Owen, M., & Rasmussen, T. (2013). 5 ways case managers contribute to a hospital's bottom line. *Becker's Infection Control & Clinical Quality.* Retrieved from http://www.beckershospitalreview.com/quality/5-ways-case-managers-contribute-to-a-hospitals-bottom-line.html, on August 31, 2015.

5. Reynolds, J. J. (2013). Another look at roles and functions: Has hospital case management lost its way? *Professional Case Management, 18*(5), 246–254.

Case Management in the Community and Postacute Care Settings

A. Select Periodicals, Books, and Other Sources:

1. Glendenning-Napoli, A., Dowling, B., Pulvino, J., Baillargeon, G., & Raimer, B. G. (2012). Community-based case management for uninsured patients with chronic diseases: Effects on acute care utilization and costs. *Professional Case Management, 17*(6), 267–275.

2. Holland, D. E., Vanderboom, C. E., Lohse, C. M., Mandrekar, J., Targonski, P. V., Madigan, E., & Powell, S. K. (2015). Exploring indicators of use of costly health services in community-dwelling adults with multiple chronic conditions. *Professional Case Management, 20*(1), 3–11.

3. Jacobs, B. (2011). Reducing heart failure hospital readmissions from skilled nursing facilities. *Professional Case Management, 16*(1), 18–24.

4. Joo, J. Y., & Huber, D. L. (2014). Evidence-based nurse case management practice in community health. *Professional Case Management, 19*(6), 265–273.

5. Kulbok, P. A., Thatcher, E., Park, E., & Meszaros, P. S. (2012). Evolving public health nursing roles: Focus on community participatory health promotion and prevention. *Online Journal of Issues in Nursing, 17*(2), Manuscript 1.

6. Treadwell, J., & Giardino, A. (2014). Collaborating for care: Initial experience of embedded case managers across five medical homes. *Professional Case Management, 19*(2), 86–92.

Case Management in the Home Care Setting

A. Select Web sites:

1. American Association for Homecare: https://www.aahomecare.org/
2. Home Care Association of America: http://www.hcaoa.org/
3. National Association for Home Care and Hospice: http://www.nahc.org

B. Select Periodicals, Books, and Other Sources:

1. Kelly, M. M., & Penney, E. D. (2011). Collaboration of hospital case managers and home care liaisons when transitioning patients. *Professional Case Management, 16*(3), 128–136.

2. Watkins, L., Hall, C., & Kring, D. (2012). Hospital to home: A transition program for frail older adults. *Professional Case Management.* *17*(3), 117–123.

Case Management in Palliative and Hospice Care Settings

A. Select Web sites:
 1. Death With Dignity National Center: http://www.deathwithdignity.org
 2. Family Caregiver Alliance: https://caregiver.org
 3. The Hastings Center Guidelines on End-of-Life Care: http://www. thehastingscenter.org/Research/Detail.aspx?id=1202
 4. National Association for Home Care and Hospice: http://www.nahc. org
 5. National Hospice and Palliative Care Organization: http://www. nhpco.org
 6. National Hospice Foundation: http://www. nationalhospicefoundation.org
B. Select Periodicals, Books, and Other Sources:
 1. Head, B. A., LaJoie, S., Augustine-Smith, L., et al. (2010). Palliative care case management: Increasing access to community-based palliative care for Medicaid recipients. *Professional Case Management,* *15*(4), 206–217.
 2. Rome, R. B., Lumunais, H. H., Bourgeois, D. A., & Blais, C. M. (2011). The role of palliative care at the end of life. *The Ochsner Journal, 11,* 348–352.

Case Management in Remote and Rural Care Settings

A. Select Periodicals, Books, and Other Sources:
 1. Fink-Samnick, E., & Muller, L. S. (2015). Case management practice: Is technology helping or hindering practice? *Professional Case Management, 20*(2), 98–102.
 2. Health Affairs. (2014). Early evidence, future promise of connected health. *Health Affairs, 33*(2). (Entire issue devoted to discussion of connected health).
 3. Klobucar, T. F., Hibbs, R., Jans, P., & Adams, M. R. (2012). Evaluating the effectiveness of an aggressive case management and home telehealth monitoring program for long-term control of A1C. *Professional Case Management, 17*(2), 51–58.
 4. Powell, S. K., & Fink-Samnick, E. (2013). To boldly go where no case manager has gone before: Remote patient monitoring and beyond. *Professional Case Management, 18*(1), 1–2.
 5. Smith, M. A., Smith, W. T., & Stanton, M. (2015). Universal postoperative hip instruction protocol for rehabilitation in rural skilled nursing facilities. *Professional Case Management, 20*(5), 241–247.
 6. Snell, A. (2014). The role of remote care management in population health. *Health Affairs.* [blog]. http://healthaffairs.org/blog/2014/04/04/ the-role-of-remote-care-management-in-population-health/

Case Management and Transitional Care

A. Select Web sites:
1. Community-Based Care Transitions Program (CCTP): http://innovation.cms.gov/initiatives/CCTP/
2. National Transitions of Care Coalition: http://www.ntocc.org
3. The Joint Commission, Transitions of Care Portal: http://www.jointcommission.org/toc.aspx
4. The Society for Post-Acute and Long-Term Care Medicine (formerly AMDA): https://www.amda.com/tools/clinical/Transitions%20of%20Care%20Models.pdf

B. Select Periodicals, Books, and Other Sources:
1. Bisiani, M. A., & Jurgens, C. Y. (2015). Do collaborative case management models decrease hospital readmission rates among high-risk patients? *Professional Case Management, 20*(4), 188–196.
2. Bowles, K. H., Hanlon, A., Holland, D., Potashnik, S. L., & Topaz, M. (2014). Impact of discharge planning decision support on time to readmission among older adult medical patients. *Professional Case Management, 19*(1), 29–38.
3. Breslin, S. E., Hamilton, K. M., & Paynter, J. (2014). Deployment of lean six sigma in care coordination: An improved discharge process. *Professional Case Management, 19*(2), 77–83.
4. Delisle, D. R. (2013). Care transitions programs: A review of hospital-based programs targeted to reduce readmissions. *Professional Case Management, 18*(6), 273–283.
5. Granata, R. L., & Hamilton, K. (2015). Exploring the effect of at-risk case management compensation on hospital pay-for-performance outcomes: Tools for change. *Professional Case Management, 20*(1), 14–27.
6. Rutherford, P., Nielsen G. A., Taylor J., Bradke P., & Coleman E. (2013). *How-to guide: Improving transitions from the hospital to community settings to reduce avoidable rehospitalizations.* Cambridge, MA: Institute for Healthcare Improvement. Retrieved from http://www.ihi.org/resources/pages/tools/howtoguideimprovingtransitionstoreduceavoidablerehospitalizations.aspx
7. Smith, S. B., & Alexander, J. W. (2012). Nursing perception of patient transitions from hospitals to home with home health. *Professional Case Management, 17*(4), 175–185.
8. Watkins, L., Hall, C., & Kring, D. (2012). Hospital to home: A transition program for frail older adults. *Professional Case Management, 17*(3), 117–123.

 The Roles, Functions, and Activities of Case Management

A. Select Web sites:
1. Commission for Case Manager Certification. Roles and functions research: http://ccmcertification.org/media/media-kit/role-function-key-findings.

2. American Nurses Credentialing Center. (2013). *Nursing Case Management Board Certification: Test content outline.* Silver Springs, MD: ANCC.

B. Select Periodicals, Books, and Other Sources:

1. Gray, F. C., White, A., & Brooks-Buck, J. (2013). Exploring role confusion in nurse case management. *Professional Case Management, 18*(2), 66–76.

2. Reynolds, J. J. (2013). Another look at roles and functions: Has hospital case management lost its way? *Professional Case Management, 18*(5), 246–254.

3. Smith, A. C. (2011). Role ambiguity and role conflict in nurse case managers: An integrative review. *Professional Case Management, 16*(4), 182–196.

4. Tahan, H., & Huber, D. (2006). The CCMC's national study of case manager job descriptions: An understanding of the activities, role relationships, knowledge, skills, and abilities. *Lippincott's Case Management, 11*(3), 127–144.

5. Tahan, H. M., Watson, A. C., & Sminkey, P. V. (2015). What case managers should know about their roles and functions: A national study from the Commission for Case Manager Certification-Part I. *Lippincott's Case Management, 20*(6), 271–296.

6. Tahan, H. M., Watson, A. C., & Sminkey, P. V. (2016). Informing the content and composition of the CCM certification examination: A national study from the Commission for Case Manager Certification-Part II. *Lippincott's Case Management, 21*(1), 3–21.

7. Tahan, H. A., & Campagna, V. (2010). Case management roles and functions across various settings and professional disciplines. *Professional Case Management, 15*(5), 245–277.

 ## The Case Management Process

A. Select Periodicals, Books, and Other Sources:

1. Commission for Case Manager Certification. (2015). Case management process. Retrieved from http://www.cmbodyofknowledge.com/content/case-management-knowledge-2

Transitions of Care and Case Management Practice

A. Select Web sites:

1. Care Transitions Intervention Program: http://www.caretransitions.org

2. Community-Based Care Transitions Program (CCTP): http://innovation.cms.gov/initiatives/CCTP/

3. National Transitions of Care Coalition: http://www.ntocc.org

4. Project BOOST (Better Outcomes for Older adult Safe Transitions): http://www.hospitalmedicine.org

5. Project RED (Re-Engineering Discharge): https://www.bu.edu/fammed/projectred/

6. The Joint Commission, Transitions of Care Portal: http://www.jointcommission.org/toc.aspx

7. The Society for Post-Acute and Long-Term Care Medicine (formerly AMDA): https://www.amda.com/tools/clinical/Transitions%20of%20Care%20Models.pdf

8. Transitional Care Model: http://www.transitionalcare.info

B. Select Periodicals, Books, and Other Sources:
1. Delisle, D. R. (2013). Care transitions programs: A review of hospital-based programs targeted to reduce readmissions. *Professional Case Management, 18*(6), 273–283.
2. Rutherford P., Nielsen G. A., Taylor J., Bradke P., & Coleman E. (2013). *How-to guide: Improving transitions from the hospital to community settings to reduce avoidable rehospitalizations.* Cambridge, MA: Institute for Healthcare Improvement. Retrieved from http://www.ihi.org/resources/pages/tools/howtoguideimprovingtransitionstoreduceavoidablerehospitalizations.aspx

 ## Resource and Utilization Management

A. Select Web sites:
1. Health Resources and Services Administration (HRSA): http://www.hrsa.gov/index.html
2. MCG (formerly Milliman): https://www.mcg.com
3. McKesson InterQual Decision Management: http://www.mckesson.com/payers/decision-management/decision-management-interqual/interqual-criteria/
4. National Committee for Quality Assurance—Health Plan Accreditation Program: http://www.ncqa.org/Programs/Accreditation/HealthPlanHP.aspx
5. URAC—Health Utilization Management Accreditation Program: https://www.urac.org/accreditation-and-measurement/accreditation-programs/all-programs/health-utilization-management/

 ## Case Management and Use of Technology

A. Select Web sites:
1. American Health Information Management Association (AHIMA): http://www.ahima.org
2. American Medical Informatics Association (AMIA): http://www.amia.org
3. American National Standards Institute (ANSI): http://www.ansi.org
4. American Telemedicine Association (ATA): http://www.americantelemed.org
5. Certification Commission for Health Information Technology (CCHIT): http://www.cchit.org/
6. College of Healthcare Information Management Executives (CHIME): http://www.cio-chime.org/index.asp
7. eHealth Initiative: http://www.ehealthinitiative.org
8. Healthcare Information and Management Systems Society (HIMSS): http://www.himss.org
9. Health Insurance Portability and Accountability Act of 1996 (HIPAA): http://www.cms.hhs.gov/hipaa/
10. Medical Records Institute: http://www.medrecinst.com/
11. National Alliance for Health Information Technology (NAHIT): http://www.nahit.org

12. National Health Information Infrastructure: http://aspe.hhs.gov/sp/nhii/index.html
13. Systematized Nomenclature of Human Medicine and Systematized Nomenclature of Medicine (SNOMED): http://www.snomed.org

B. Periodicals, Books, and Other Sources:
1. Cudney, A. (2010). How case management leaders can succeed with information technology. *Professional Case Management, 15*(6), 330–332.
2. Fink-Samnick, E., & Muller, L. S. (2015). Case management practice: Is technology helping or hindering practice? *Professional Case Management, 20*(2), 98–102.

Case Manager's Role Leadership and Accountability

A. Select Web sites:
1. American Association of Colleges of Nursing (AACN), Leadership for Academic Nursing: http://www.aacn.nche.edu/lanp
2. American Nurses Association (ANA), Program offerings: http://www.ana-leadershipinstitute.org/Main-Menu-Category/Offerings
3. American Nurses Credentialing Center (ANCC), Magnet recognition program model: http://www.nursecredentialing.org/Magnet/ProgramOverview/New-Magnet-Model
4. American Organization of Nurse Executives (AONE), Nurse executive competencies: http://www.aone.org/resources/leadership%20tools/nursecomp.shtml
5. Council on Social Work Education (CSWE), Leadership Institute: http://www.cswe.org/CentersInitiatives/CSWELeadershipInst.aspx
6. National League for Nursing (NLN), Leadership Institute: http://www.nln.org/facultyprograms/leadershipinstitute.htm
7. National Transitions of Care Coalition, Improving Transitions of Care: Model for Accountable Communication. White paper Retrieved from http://www.ntocc.org/Portals/0/PDF/Resources/PolicyPaper.pdf
8. Network for Social Work Management (NSWM), Human services management competencies: https://socialworkmanager.org/competencies
9. Society for Social Work Leadership in Health Care (SSWLHC): http://www.sswlhc.org/html/publications.php

B. Select Periodicals, Books, and Other Sources:
1. Badshah, S. (2012). Historical study of leadership theories. *Journal of Strategic Human Resource Management, 1*(1), 49–59.
2. Bankston White, C., & Birmingham, J. (2015). Case management directors: How to manage in a transition-focused world: Part 1. *Professional Case Management, 20*(2), 63–78.
3. Bankston White, C., & Birmingham, J. (2015). Case management directors: How to manage in a transition-focused world: Part 2. *Professional Case Management, 20*(3), 115–127.
4. Busse, R. (2014). Comprehensive leadership review—Literature, theories and research. *Advances in Management, 7*(5), 52–66.
5. Gardner, H. E. (2011). *Leading minds: An anatomy of leadership.* New York: Basic Books.

6. Health Resources and Services Administration (HRSA). (September 2010). *The registered nurse population: Findings from the 2008 national sample survey of registered nurses.* Washington, DC: U.S. Department of Health and Human Services.

7. Institutes of Medicine. (2011). *The future of nursing: Leading change, advancing health.* Washington, DC: The National Academies Press.

8. Kotter, J. (2011). *Change management vs. change leadership: What's the difference?* Retrieved from http://www.forbes.com/sites/johnkotter/2011/07/12/change-management-vs-changeleadership-whats-the-difference

9. Porter-O'Grady, T., & Malloch, K. (2011). *Quantum leadership: Advancing innovation, transforming health care* (3rd ed.). Burlington, MA: Jones & Bartlett Learning.

10. Treiger, T. M., & Fink-Samnick, E. (2015). *COLLABORATE for professional case management: A universal competency-based paradigm.* Philadelphia, PA: Wolters Kluwer. (Chapter on Leadership).

11. Treiger, T. M. (2014). The importance of leadership followership. *Professional Case Management, 19*(2), 93–94.

12. Treiger, T. M., & Fink-Samnick, E. (2013). COLLABORATE: A universal competency-based paradigm for professional case management, Part II: Competency clarification. *Professional Case Management, 18*(5), 219–243. doi:10.1097/NCM.0b013e31829c8a3a

Certification and Accreditation in Case Management

A. Select Web sites on Certification:
   1. American Association of Occupational Health Nurses (AAOHN): http://www.aaohn.org
   2. American Association of Managed Care Nurses (AAMCN): http://www.aamcn.org
   3. American Board of Disability Analysts (ABDA): http://www.americandisability.org
   4. American Board of Quality Assurance/Utilization Review Physicians (ABQAURP): http://www.abqaurp.org
   5. American Case Management Association (ACMA): https://www.acmaweb.org
   6. American Health Insurance Professionals (AHIP), Academy for Healthcare Management: http://www.ahip.org/ciepd/ahm
   7. American Nurses Credentialing Center (ANCC): http://www.nursecredentialing.org
   8. Association of Rehabilitation Nurses (ARN): http://www.rehabnurse.org/certification/content/Index.html
   9. Association of Social Work Boards (ASWB): http://www.aswb.org
   10. Center for Case Management: http://www.cfcm.com/wordpress1
   11. Certified Disability Management Specialists: http://www.cdms.org
   12. Commission for Case Manager Certification: http://ccmcertification.org
   13. Commission on Rehabilitation Counselor Certification: http://www.crccertification.com

14. Institute on Credentialing Excellence: http://www.credentialingexcellence.org
15. National Association for Health Care Quality: http://www.nahq.org/certify/content/index.html
16. National Academy of Certified Care Managers: http://www.naccm.net
17. National Association of Social Workers: http://www.socialworkers.org

B. Select Web sites on Accreditation:
1. Commission on Accreditation of Rehabilitation Facilities (CARF) International: http://www.carf.org/home/
2. The Joint Commission: http://www.jointcommission.org/
3. National Committee for Quality Assurance: http://www.ncqa.org/
4. URAC: https://www.urac.org/

Professional Development and Academic Programs in Case Management

A. Select Academic Case Management Programs:
1. Rutgers School of Social Work, Certificate Program in Case Management: http://socialwork.rutgers.edu/continuingeducation/ce/certificateprograms/certcasemanagement.aspx
2. Saint Peter's University, School of Nursing, Master's of Science in Nursing Case Management: http://www.saintpeters.edu/school-of-nursing/curriculum/graduate-programs/master-of-science-in-nursing/
3. Samuel Merritt University, Post Professional MSN Case Management: https://www.samuelmerritt.edu/nursing/cm_nursing/curriculum
4. Seton Hall University College of Nursing, Certificate in Case Management: http://www.shu.edu/academics/nursing/case-management-certificate.cfm
5. University of Alabama, Capstone College of Nursing—Master's of Science in Nursing Case Management: http://nursing.ua.edu
6. University of California San Diego Extension, Case Management Certificate (see Healthcare, Behavioral Sciences and Safety): http://extension.ucsd.edu
7. University of California Riverside, Professional Certificate in Medical Case Management (see Healthcare): http://www.extension.ucr.edu
8. University of Florida, Geriatric Care Management Graduate Certificate: http://bsch.phhp.ufl.edu/distance-learning/geriatric-care-management-online
9. University of Southern Indiana, Case Management/Care Coordination Certificate: https://www.usi.edu/health/certificate-programs/case-managementcare-coordination-certificate-program
10. University of Southern Maine, Professional Development Programs, Certificate Program in Case Management: https://usm.maine.edu/pdp/certificate-program-case-management

B. Select Continuing Education Programs:
1. American Case Management Association (ACMA), Annual Conference: https://www.acmaweb.org
2. Case Management Society of America, Annual Conference: http://www.cmsa.org/

3. Commission for Case Manager Certification, Annual Conference: http://ccmcertification.org
4. Contemporary Forum: http://contemporaryforums.com/

 ## Ethics and General Case Management Practice

A. Select Web sites:
   1. American Nurses Association (ANA), Ethics: http://www.nursingworld.org/MainMenuCategories/EthicsStandards
   2. Commission for Case Manager Certification (CCMC), Code of Professional Conduct for Case Managers: http://www.ccmcertification.org
   3. National Association of Social Workers (NASW), Code of Ethics: http://www.socialworkers.org/pubs/code/default.asp
B. Select Periodicals, Books, and Other Sources:
   1. Banja, J. D., & Craig, K. (2010). Speaking up in case management, Part II: Implementing speaking up behaviors. *Professional Case Management, 15*(5), 237–242.
   2. Craig, K., & Banja, J. D. (2010). Speaking up in case management. Part I: Ethical and professional considerations. *Professional Case Management, 15*(4), 179–185.
   3. Fink-Samnick, E. (2015). E-ACTS: A framework for difficult decision-making. *Professional Case Management, 20*(4), 206–210.
   4. Moffat, M. (2014). Reducing moral distress in case managers. *Professional Case Management, 19*(4), 173–186.
   5. Muller, L. S. (2013). Advocacy and organ and tissue donation. *Professional Case Management, 18*(2), 89–94.
   6. Smith, A. C. (2011). Role ambiguity and role conflict in nurse case managers: An integrative review. *Professional Case Management, 16*(4), 182–196.
   7. Terra, S. M., & Powell, S. K. (2012). Is a determination of medical futility ethical? *Professional Case Management, 17*(3), 103–106.
   8. Treiger, T. M., & Fink-Samnick, E. (2015). *COLLABORATE for professional case management: A universal competency-based paradigm.* Philadelphia, PA: Wolters Kluwer. (Chapter on Ethical-Legal practice).

Ethical Use of Case Management Technology

A. Select Web sites:
   1. American Telemedicine Association: http://www.americantelemed.org
   2. Center for Telehealth and e-Health Law: http://www.ctel.org
   3. National Conference of State Legislatures: http://www.ncsl.org
B. Select Periodicals, Books, and Other Sources:
   1. Cudney, A. (2010). How case management leaders can succeed with information technology. *Professional Case Management, 15*(6), 330–332.
   2. Fink-Samnick, E., & Muller, L. S. (2015). Case management practice: Is technology helping or hindering practice? *Professional Case Management, 20*(2), 98–102.

3. Muller, L. S., & Fink-Samnick, E. (2012). Legal & regulatory issues. *Professional Case Management, 17*(4), 191–195.

 Legal Considerations in Case Management

A. Select Web sites:
1. Case Management Society of America, Multistate Licensure Position Paper: http://www.cmsa.org/Portals/0/PDF/MultistateRNLicensurePositionStatement.pdf and http://www.cmsa.org/Chapter/LocalInvolvement/MultiStateNursingLicensure/tabid/161/Default.aspx
2. Department of Health and Human Services, Health Information Privacy: http://www.hhs.gov/ocr/privacy and http://www.hhs.gov/ocr/privacy/hipaa/understanding/coveredentities/contractprov.html
3. National Council of State Boards of Nursing, Boards of Nursing Contacts: https://www.ncsbn.org/contact-bon.htm
4. National Council of State Boards of Nursing, Licensure Compacts: https://www.ncsbn.org/compacts.htm
5. Office of the Inspector General, Compliance Opinions and Resources: https://oig.hhs.gov/compliance/advisory-opinions/ and https://oig.hhs.gov/compliance/provider-compliance-training/files/ListofComplianceResourcesHandoutBR508r1.pdf
B. Select Periodicals, Books and Other Sources:
1. Muller, L. S., & Fink-Samnick, E. (2015). Mandatory reporting: Let's clear up the confusion. *Professional Case Management, 20*(4), 199–203.
2. Muller, L. S. (2014). A case management briefing on domestic violence. *Professional Case Management, 19*(5), 237–240.
3. Muller, L. S. (2014). HIPAA compliance practice tips. *Professional Case Management, 19*(4), 191–193.
4. Treiger, T. M., & Fink-Samnick, E. (2015). *COLLABORATE for professional case management: a universal competency-based paradigm.* Philadelphia, PA: Wolters Kluwer. (Chapter on Ethical-Legal practice).

 Use of Effective Case Management Plans

A. Select Web sites:
1. Adult Medication, Improving Medication Adherence in Older Adults: http://adultmeducation.com
2. Agency for Healthcare Research and Quality: http://www.guideline.gov
3. American College of Physicians Clinical Practice Guidelines: http://www.acponline.org
4. Careplans.com (for nursing care plans): http://www.careplans.com
5. Case Management Society of America, Case Management Adherence Guidelines: http://www.cmsa.org/cmag
6. Comprehensive Interdisciplinary Patient Assessment Tool: https://www.annanurse.org/advocacy/resources/comprehensive-interdisciplinary-patient-assessment-tool
7. Modified Morisky Scale (MMS): http://www.healthpointpathways.co.nz/assets/AtRiskIndividuals/modified%20morisky%20scale.pdf

8. National Guidelines Clearinghouse: http://www.ngc.gov
9. National Institutes of Health (NIH): http://www.health.nih.gov
10. Patient Activation Measure: http://www.insigniahealth.com
11. Patient Health Questionnaire (PHQ): http://www.phqscreeners.com
12. Patient Safety Assessment Tool (PSAT): http://www.patientsafety.va.gov/professionals/onthejob/assessment.asp
13. SAMHSA-HRSA Center for Integrated Health Solutions: http://www.integration.samhsa.gov/clinical-practice/screening-tools

Quality and Outcomes Management in Case Management Practice

A. Select Web sites:
   1. Agency for Healthcare Research and Quality: http://www.ahrq.gov
   2. Effective Health Care Program: http://effectivehealthcare.ahrq.gov
   3. Case Management Society of America, Award for Case Management Research, http://www.cmsa.org/Individual/MemberResources/AwardsRecognition/AwardforCaseManagementResearch/tabid/557/Default.aspx; Award for Excellence in Adherence Management, http://www.cmsa.org/Individual/MemberResources/AwardsRecognition/AEAMAwardforExcellenceinAdherenceMgmt/tabid/246/Default.aspx; and Award for Case Management Practice Improvement, http://www.cmsa.org/Individual/MemberResources/AwardsRecognition/AwardforCaseManagementPracticeImprovement/tabid/556/Default.aspx
   4. Effective Health Care Program: http://effectivehealthcare.ahrq.gov
   5. Health Resources and Services Administration: http://www.hrsa.gov/index.html
   6. Institute for Healthcare Improvement: http://www.ihi.org/Pages/default.aspx
   7. The Leapfrog Group: http://www.leapfroggroup.org
   8. National Commission for Quality Assurance: http://www.ncqa.org
   9. National Quality Forum: http://www.ihi.org/Pages/default.aspx
   10. URAC: http://www.urac.org
B. Select Periodicals, Books, and Other Sources:
   1. Hickam, D. H., Weiss, J. W., Guise, J-M, Buckley, D., Motu'apuaka, M., Graham, E., ... Saha, S. (2013). *Outpatient case management for adults with medical illness and complex care needs.* Comparative Effectiveness Review No. 99. (Prepared by the Oregon Evidence-based Practice Center under Contract No. 290-2007-10057-I.) AHRQ Publication No. 13-EHC031-EF. Rockville, MD: Agency for Healthcare Research and Quality.
   2. Holland, D. E., Vanderboom, C. E., Lohse, C. M., Mandrekar, J., Targonski, P. V., Madigan, E., & Powell, S. K. (2015). Exploring indicators of use of costly health services in community-dwelling adults with multiple chronic conditions. *Professional Case Management, 20*(1), 3–11.
   3. Sterling, Y. M., & Linville, L. J. (2015). A qualitative study of case management of children with asthma. *Professional Case Management, 20*(1), 30–39.

Behavioral Health, Substance Use, and Integrated Case Management

A. Select Web sites:
  1. Agency for Healthcare Research and Quality (AHRQ): http://www.ahrq.gov
  2. American Association of Health Plans (AAHP): http://www.aahp.org
  3. American Managed Behavioral Healthcare Association: http://www.ambha.org
  4. American Psychiatric Nurses Association: http://www.arpna.org
  5. Case Management Society of America, Integrated Case Management: http://www.cmsa.org/icm
  6. Institute for Behavioral Healthcare: http://www.ibh.com
  7. Mental Health Parity Act of 2008: http://www.dol.gov/ebsa/newsroom/fsmhpaea.html
  8. National Alliance for the Mentally Ill (NAMI): http://www.nami.org
  9. Rural Assistance Center: https://wwwraconline.org/topics/healthcare-access#barriers
  10. Psychotherapy Finances and Managed Care Strategies: http://www.psyfin.com
  11. Substance Abuse and Mental Health Services Administration (SAMHSA): http://www.samhsa.gov
B. Select Periodicals, Books, and Other Sources:
  1. Duncan, B. L., Miller, S. D., & Sparks, J. A. (2000). *The heroic client.* San Francisco, CA: Jossey-Bass.
  2. Miller, W. R., & Rollnick, S. (2013). *Motivational interviewing: Helping people change* (3rd ed.). New York: The Guilford Press.

Workers' Compensation Case Management

A. Select Web sites:
  1. Cornell University Law School, Workers' Compensation: https://www.law.cornell.edu/wex/workers_compensation
  2. Department of Labor—Worker's Compensation: http://www.dol.gov/dol/topic/workcomp/
B. Select Periodicals, Books, and Other Sources:
  1. Borchers, C. E. (2011). Practical tips for the new workers' compensation case manager. *Professional Case Management, 16*(3), 158–160.
  2. Carter, J., Watson, A. C., & Sminkey, P. V. (2014). Pain management: Screening and assessment of pain as part of a comprehensive case management process. *Professional Case Management, 19*(3), 126–134.
  3. Carter, J. (2011). Workers' comp case management being an advocate amid complexity. *Professional Case Management, 16*(2), 95–97.
  4. Commons, D., & Borchers, C. (2012). Documentation in workers' compensation case management: RU@RISK? *Professional Case Management, 17*(6), 296–298.
  5. Commons, D. S. (2011). The value of medical recovery guidelines in workers compensation case management. *Professional Case Management, 16*(5), 269–271.

6. Fairnot, D. C. (2012). *A guide to successful workers compensation case management*. Alpharetta, GA: BookLogix.
7. Jensen, S. (2013). A "return" to best practice basics: Establishing rapport in workers' compensation cases. *Professional Case Management, 18*(5), 264–265.
8. Langstaff, M. A. (2011). Case managers take "whole person" approach to workers' compensation cases. *Professional Case Management, 16*(5), 267–269.
9. Lowe, J. (2013). Functional testing: When is it appropriate? *Professional Case Management, 18*(1), 46–47.
10. Zawalski, S. (2015). Taking a multidisciplinary approach to workers' compensation case management. *Professional Case Management, 20*(1), 50–51.

 ## Disability and Occupational Health Case Management

A. Select Web sites:
1. Centers for Disease Control, Disability & Health: http://www.cdc.gov/ncbddd/disabilityandhealth
2. Disability.gov: https://www.disability.gov
3. Disability History Museum: http://www.disabilitymuseum.org/dhm/index.html
4. Disability Rights Education and Defense Fund: http://dredf.org
5. Law, Health Policy, and Disability Center: http://disability.law.uiowa.edu/index.htm
6. Social Security, Disability Benefits: http://www.ssa.gov/disabilityssi
B. Select Periodicals, Books, and Other Sources:
1. Hercules-Doerr, K. (2013). Looking into the disability "crystal ball." *Professional Case Management, 18*(3), 157–159.
2. National Public Radio. Unfit for work: The startling rise of disability in America. Retrieved from http://apps.npr.org/unfit-for-work/
3. Pederson, I. (2012). Insight into evidence-based return to work guidelines. *Professional Case Management, 17*(2), 96–98.
4. Tugman-Swanson, K., & Brimrose, H. (2011). Transitional return to work: It works, but how? *Professional Case Management, 16*(2), 97–99.
5. Vierling, L. E., & Vierling, D. J. (2012). What every case manager needs to know about the ADAAA! *Professional Case Management, 17*(1), 39–42.

 ## Life Care Planning and Case Management

A. Select Web sites:
1. American Association of Nurse Life Care Planners: http://www.aanlcp.org
2. Foundation for Life Care Planning Research: http://www.flcpr.org
3. International Association of Rehabilitation Professionals, Life Care Planning Section-IALCP: http://www.rehabpro.org/sections/ialcp
4. Life Care Planning Law Firms Association: https://www.lcplfa.org
B. Select Periodicals, Books, and Other Sources:
1. Apuna-Grummer, D., & Howland, W. A. (2013). *A core curriculum for nurse life care planning*. Bloomington, IN: iUniverse.

2. Deutsch, P. *Life care planning*. Retrieved from http://cirrie.buffalo.edu/encyclopedia/en/article/18/, on September 29, 2015.

3. International Association of Rehabilitation Professionals, International Academy of Life Care Planners, Standards of Practice, Retrieved from http://www.rehabpro.org/sections/ialcp/focus/standards/ialcpSOP_pdf

4. Life Care Planning, Frequently Asked Questions (FAQs), Retrieved from http://www.paulmdeutsch.com/FAQs-life-care-planning.htm

5. Riddick-Grisham, S., & Deming, L. (2011). *Pediatric life care planning and case management* (2nd ed.). Boca Raton, FL: CRC Press.

6. Weed, R. O., & Berens, D. E. (2009). *Life care planning and case management handbook* (3rd ed.). Boca Raton, FL: CRC Press.

Reference

Case Management Society of America (CMSA). (2010). *CMSA standards of practice for case managers*. Little Rock, AR: Author.

Index

Note: Page numbers followed by "*f*" indicate figures; those followed by "*t*" indicate tables.

A

Absence management, 648
Acceptance, 506
Accessibility, 660–661, 675
Accident insurance, 44
Accommodation
    reasonable, 608, 651
    requests for, 652
Accountability, 394, 396–397
Accountable Care Organization (ACO),
        38, 79, 139–141, 246, 256, 263,
        521, 523
Accreditation, 247, 262–263, 419, 420, 694
    CMSA's standards of practice, 421–422
    NCQA, 449–452
    organizational, 453
    organizations performing, 443–448
    resources, 707–708
    standards for, 445, 535
Actionable tort, 675
Activities of daily living (ADL), 24, 130
Activity, 270
Acuity, 532, 533
Acute care case management, 100–124,
        700–701
Acute care hospitals, 321–323
Acute level of care, 315
ADA. *See* Americans with Disabilities Act
        (ADA)
Addictive disorders, 575, 579–581
Adjudicating the claim, 612
Administrative and management
        processes, 550
Admission certification, 350–351
Admitting department case management,
        79–82
Adult day care facilities (ADCFs), 157
Advance care planning, 197
Advance directive, 197
Advance request payment, 181
Adverse determination, 351, 358, 359
Advice, patient request for, *vs.* case
        manager role, 512
Advocacy, 538
    in case management process, 309

definition, 295, 458, 466
    ethical issues in, 458, 466
    injured worker, 633
Advocate, 277, 458, 492
Affidavit of merit, 501–502
Affordable Care Act (ACA), 38–39, 253,
        521, 522, 524
Agency for Healthcare Research and
        Quality (AHRQ), 137, 549
Agent, 492
Aggregated data, 369
Aging in place, 130, 158–159
Alcohol issues, in Americans with
        Disabilities Act, 653–654
Alcohol use disorder (AUD), 579–581
Alcoholism, 581
Algorithms, 369
    case management care plan, 523,
        541–542
Alternative level of care, 351
Ambulatory case management, 77–78, 593
Ambulatory payment classification (APC),
        43
American Academy of Family Physicians
        (AAFP), 556–557
American Association of Nurse Life Care
        Planners (AANLCP), 673, 674,
        679, 681
American Association of Occupational
        Health Nurses (AAOHN), 642, 655
American Association of Retired Persons
        (AARP), 165
American Board of Independent Medical
        Examiners (ABIME), 632
American Board of Quality Assurance and
        Utilization Review Physicians
        (ABQAURP), 439
American College of Occupational
        and Environmental Medicine
        (ACOEM), 615, 655, 658
American Nurses Association (ANA), 28
American Nurses Credentialing Center
        (ANCC), 32, 288–289
American Recovery and Reinvestment Act
        (ARRA), 389

American Society for Quality (ASQ), 552
Americans with Disabilities Act (ADA),
    325, 646, 650–654, 668
  definitions of, 650
  disability and occupational health,
    650–654
  drug and alcohol issues in, 653–654
  employer's rights and responsibilities
    in, 650
  goals of, 650
  history of, 649
  impairments in, 650
  Job Accommodation Network in, 653
  qualified individual with disability in,
    650
  reassignment in, 653
  Title II, 650, 655
  in workers' compensation, 636
Anxiety disorder, 586–587
App, 369
Appeal, 351
  Medicare, 361–362
  standard, 360
  in utilization management, 360–363
Application program, 369
Appropriateness
  of services criteria, 58
  of setting, 353
Area Agency on Aging (AAA), 165
Assertive community treatment (ACT),
    576, 583, 584
Assessment, 24. See also specific areas
  case management care plan, 527–531,
    528
  in case management process, 301
  comprehensive geriatric, 174–175
  definition of, 295
  of elderly, 63
  in life care planning, 675, 686–687
  in occupational health case manage-
    ment, 666
  in outcome and assessment informa-
    tion set, 181, 187–188
  outcome-driven quality, in workers'
    compensation, 635
  patient assessment instrument, 43
  for placement, of geriatric patient,
    175–177
  reassessment in, 310
  screening vs., 173–174
  vocational, 644
  workplace violence process model,
    627–628
Assisted living, 130
Assisted living facility (ALF), 156–157,
    335–336

Assistive device, 641
Assistive technology, 641–642
Association of Rehabilitation Nurses
    (ARN), 28
Associations, professional, 31
Attorneys, 508, 612
Audit trail, 369
Authorization, 351
Autism spectrum disorders (ASD),
    588–589
Autonomy, 24, 458, 463
  injured worker, 633

B
Balanced Budget Act (BBA), 42, 192, 385
Battery, 492
Behavioral health care, 574
  addictive disorders, 579–581
  alcohol use disorder, 579–581
  anxiety disorder, 586–587
  bipolar disorder, 581–583, 582
  conditions and implications, 577–589
  dementia, 588
  depression, 578–579
  intellectual and developmental dis-
    abilities, 588–589
  obsessive–compulsive disorder,
    585–586
  schizophrenia, 583–584, 583, 584
  substance use disorder, 579–581, 580
Behavioral health case management,
    574. See also Integrated case
    management (ICM)
  activities in, 596
  ambulatory care, 593
  challenges in, 589–592
  community-based settings, 593–594
  CMSA's standards of practice, 577
  drug courts, 594
  home care, 593–594
  inpatient hospitalization, 592–593
  with low self-care states, 600–602
  models of, 575–576
  overview of, 573–574
  partial hospitalization, 593
  reimbursement issues, 596–597
  resources, 712
  roles and functions of, 595
  rural settings, 594
  suicide practice protocol, 600
  suicide risk factors, 589
  treatment settings in, 592–595
Benchmarks, 551
Beneficence, 458, 463
  in workers' compensation, 633
Benefits programs, employee, 660

Best evidence, 352
Best-practice recommendations, 531, 533, 534
Beyond-the-walls case management, 64
Bill of Rights, 497
Biometric identification, 369
Bipolar disorder, 581–583, 582
Blogs, 473
Bluetooth, 369
Board certification (BC), 437–438
Boarding, 64
Boundary, 473
Boundary crossing, 473
Boundary violation, 473
Breach, 492
Breach of contract, 492
Bridge model, 255
Burden of proof, 501
Business associate agreement, 492

C
Capacity, 642
Capitation, 39, 52
Care coordination, 4, 247, 275, 523
Care coordinators, 5, 182
Care delivery processes, 551
Care management, 34, 273, 274
Care plans. *See* Case management care plans; *specific areas*
Care setting, 4
Care team, 247
    responsibilities, 249
Care transitions, 533, 534
Care transitions intervention (CTI), 254
Carve-out services, 53
Case law, 492
    on workers' compensation, 635
Case management (CM), 4–5, 47. *See also specific areas*
    academic programs, 708–709
    accreditation in, 419, 420
        NCQA, 449–452
        organizations performing, 443–448
    activities of, 703–704
    certification in, 419, 420, 707–708
        ABQAURP, 439
        contact information, 440t
        differentiating individual from organization, 452–453
        nursing, 437–438
        oldest, 436–437
        overview of, 434–436
    certifications and sponsoring organizations, 29t
    competency, 429
    conventional, 576
    core curriculum to, 6–7
    core functions of, 573
    credentials in, 419, 420, 431–434, 441t–443t
    definition, 10–13, 273, 274
    in disease management, 64
    domains in, 33
    education, 30–31
    education and training for, 425
        approaches to, 429–431
        classification, 430
        consensus areas for, 425–426, 426t–428t, 429
    effective plans, 710–711
    essential activity domains of, 279–281
    ethical use, 709–710
    ethics and general practice, 707
    financial/cost–benefit analysis, 408–410
    functions, 703–704
    functions and activities, 278–283
    goals of, 32, 521, 563
    growth of, factors for, 26–28
    guiding principles, 15–17
    health care settings, 19–20
    healthcare benefits, 699–700
    historical perspective, 7–10
    history and evolution of, 698–699
    history of, 22–24
    home care setting, 701–702
    integration and coordination of health care in, 63, 64
    interdisciplinary health care team, 19
    journals and publications in, 30
    knowledge and skills, 288–290
    knowledge area domains, 284–285
    legal considerations in, 710
    main characteristics of, 63
    model legislation on, 29
    organizations, accreditation sources for, 29
    outcomes, 410–411, 549, 563–566, 563
    outpatient, 64
    for patient safety, 64
    payment, 699–700
    in patient-centered medical home, 78–79
    philosophical tenets of, 32–33
    philosophy of, 6, 13–15, 432–433
    practice and qualifications knowledge, 283–288
    primary care, 34
    professional associations for, 31
    professional development, 708–709
    professional recognition awards, 31
    programs/models, 63
    purpose of, 31–32, 550

Case management (CM), (*Continued*)
  reasons for implementation of, 62
  recipient of, 5
  resources in, 692–714
  roles, 703–704
  roles and functions, 549
  rural areas
    programs and services, 225–229
    projects and research, 234t–240t
  scope of, 62–63
  social work, 30
  standards of practice for, 318
  standards of professional practice in, 28
  substance use, 712
  target populations, 33
  team, 18
  technology use, 705–706
  variability of, 63
  within the walls and beyond the walls, 64
  workers' compensation, 606 (*See also*
    Workers' compensation)
Case Management Adherence Guidelines
    (CMAG), 538–539
Case management care plans, 247, 520–544
  algorithms, 541–542
  assessment categories, 527, 528
  characteristics, 527
  clinical pathways, 540–541
  CMSA's standards of practice, 525
  collaborative approaches, 522
  computer-generated case planning, 527
  data gathering format, 531–532
  definition, 523
  development strategies, 532–535
  effective, 526
  evaluation of, 534, 536
  evidence-based decision support
    criteria, 542
  evidence-based guidelines in, 537–540
  evidence-based medicine in, 352
  goals, 521, 522, 526, 529
  implementation, 536–537
  intervention, 528–531
  nursing responsibility, 525
  outcomes variables, 530, 531
  overview of, 521–523
  patient assessment in, 527–531
  plans of care, 525–527
  problem list identification, 535–536
  purpose of, 530
  road map, 522
  settlement houses, 525
  software applications, 531
  standardization, 531
  uses, 526–527
  and utilization management, 543–544

Case management information systems
    (CMISs)
  accountable care organization, 376
  assessments, 372
  automated tracking, 374
  communication tools, 373
  cost-benefit analysis, 383
  double-data entry, 374
  electronic transfer, 373
  evaluation of, 381
  functional capabilities of, 372
  goal setting, 373
  goals, 374–376
  gut factor, 377
  health information technology and,
    372–374, 389–390
  hospital, 376
  identification of problems, 380
  information gathering, 368
  lack of standardization, 379
  limitations, 377–379
  long-term postacute, 376
  measuring effectiveness of outcomes, 383
  measuring patient care outcomes,
    381–382
  medication reconciliation, 390
  milestones, 373
  monitoring, 380–381
  organizational benefits, 377
  patient assessment, 379–380
  patient assignment, 379
  patient care benefits, 377
  patient identification, 379
  patient selection, 379
  patient-centered data/information, 375
  patient-centered medical home, 376
  payer, 376
  planning, 380
  plans of care, 372
  population-level system, 374, 375
  problems, 373
  risk stratification software, 379
  rule-based systems, 373
  sharing of key documents, 373
  telehealth
    barriers, 386–388
    interventions, 383–384
    legislation, 385–386
  traditional individual-level system, 374
  usability and, 368, 374
  utilization management, 373–374
  Web sites evaluation, 388–389
  worker's compensation and disability, 376
  workflow benefits, 376–377
Case management practice standard of
    planning, 526

Case management process, 293–310, 526, 704
  advocacy in, 309
  assessment and problem identification in, 299–301
  client identification/selection in, 297–299
  CMSA's standards of practice, 296–297
  continuous monitoring in, 294
  discharge/transition plan in, 307
  documentation and record keeping in, 310
  implementation and coordination of care in, 304
  interventions to meet treatment goals in, 304–305
  monitoring in, 309–310
  overview of, 293–295
  plan development in, 301–304
  plan evaluation and follow-up in, 305–306
  reassessment in, 309–310
  reevaluation in, 309–310
  systematic approach, 297
  termination of, 307–308
Case Management Society of America (CMSA), 26, 40–41, 66–67
Case Management Society of America (CMSA) standards of practice, 6–10, 26, 40–41
  acute care setting, 103–104
  behavioral health and integrated case management, 577
  case management care plan, 525
  case management process, 296–297
  case manager's role leadership and accountability, 395–396
  disability and occupational health case management, 645–646
  ethical uses, 476
  ethics and general practice, 460
  health care insurance, benefits, and reimbursement systems, 40–41
  home care setting, 182
  legal issues, 495
  life care planning, 675–676
  palliative and hospice care settings, 198–199
  postacute care settings, 133–134
  practice settings, 66–67
  professional development, certification, and accreditation, 421–422
  quality and outcomes management, 552–553
  remote and rural care settings, 218–219
  resource and utilization management, 353–354
  resources, 695–696
  roles, functions, and activities, 270–272
  technology use, 371–372
  transitional care, 245–246
  transitional planning and transitions of care, 317
  workers' compensation, 609
Case managers, 5, 24, 33. *See also* Legal issues
  accreditation of, 419, 420
  activities based job descriptions, 282–283
  business skills, 522
  career opportunities, 368
  certifications in, 419, 420
  as change agents, 411–412, 413*t*
  client information, 374
  common skills for, 287–288
  credentialing in, 419, 420
  definition, 270, 420
  design case management plans, 534
  diversity of roles assumed by, 276
  education and training of, 422–425
    core components, 423
    foundation for, 424
    programs for, 422–423
  educational preparation of, 419
  employer's scope of responsibility, 532
  essential knowledge areas and skills for, 271
  health care informatics principles, 368
  in health care reimbursement, 39
  in home care
    community-based, 193
    hospital-based, 192–193
  insurance-based, 58
  interventions and care contributions, 246
  knowledge necessary for, 56–57
  as leadership and accountability, 395–396, 706–707
  liability exposure for, 502–503
  licensure concerns, 389
  as life care planner, 674, 676, 678–681, 686 (*See also* Life care plan; Life care planning)
  medication reconciliation, 390
  and motivational interviewing, 413–416
  patient acuity, 532
  patient self-management, 521–522
  patient-specific needs, 532
  payer-based, 338
  provider-based, 338–340
  roles and functions, 67, 269, 272
    vs. patient request for advice, 512
  roles of, 142–143, 395–396
  transitional planning, 343–344

Case mix group (CMG), 43
Case rate, 351
Catastrophic injury cases, 24
  in life care plan, 677
  in workers' compensation, 622–624
Causal connection, 492
Centers for Medicare and Medicaid
        Services (CMS), 37, 289, 690
Centers of excellence, 50
Certificate, 694
Certification, 29, 29t, 247, 262–263, 419,
        420
  ABQAURP, 439
  case management and sponsoring orga-
        nizations, 29t
  CMSA's standards of practice, 421–422
  contact information, 440t
  definition, 420
  differentiating individual from organi-
        zation, 452–453
  employment experience, 437
  individual, 420, 452, 694
  nursing, 437–438
  in occupational health case manage-
        ment, 657
  oldest, 436–437
  organization or program, 420, 694
  organizational, 453
  overview of, 434–436
  requirements for, 436–437
  resources, 707–708
Certification of Disability Management
        Specialists Commission
        (CDMSC), on case management
        practice, 647
Certified Case Management Administrator
        (CCMA), 438–439
Certified Case Manager (CCM),
        262–263
Certified home healthcare agency
        (CHHA), 181, 183
Certified in life care planning (CLCP), 678
Certified Nurse Life Care Planner
        (CNLCP), 679
Certified Professional in Disability
        Management (CPDM) Program,
        655
Certified Professional Utilization
        Management (CPUM), 365
Certified Professional Utilization Review
        (CPUR), 365
Child abuse, by patient, 513
Civil law, 492
Claims adjuster/examiner, 612
Client, 458
  identification, 297–298

  selection, 33, 298
  support system, 5
Clinic case management, 77–78
Clinical decision support system (CDSS),
        369, 370
Clinical information system (CIS),
        369–370
Clinical nurse specialist (CNS), 233
Clinical pathway, case management care
        plan, 523–524, 540–541
Clinical practice guidelines (CPGs), 351,
        524, 538, 551, 642, 675
Clinical processes, 551
Clinical review criteria, 351
Clinical standards, 538
Clinician, 277
Cloned medical records, 473
CM. See Case management (CM)
CMISs. See Case management information
        systems (CMISs)
Code of Professional Conduct for Case
        Managers, 458, 461, 462
Codes of ethics, 458
Codify (codification), 493
Cognitive–behavioral therapy (CBT), 585,
        587
Coinsurance, 39
Collaboration, 295
  hospice care, 202, 212
  life care planning, 678
  palliative care, 200, 212
Collaborative team, 20
Collaborator, 276–277
Commercial insurance, 39
Commercial payers, on reimbursement
        systems, 41–42
Commission for Case Management
        Certification (CCMC), 29,
        262–263, 521
  conduct rules of, 466
  ethical principles, 465–466
  values in, 465
Commission for Case Manager Certification
        (CCMC), 14, 15, 273, 320, 458,
        504, 521, 696, 698, 703, 704
Committee for Nursing Practice
        Information Infrastructure
        (CNPII), 378
Common cause variation, 554
Common law, 493
Communication
  electronic, 478–479, 484t–485t
  skills, 404–406
Communicator, 276
Community care case management,
        76–77, 701

Community Health Center (CHC), 133
Community Mental Health Act, 22
Community-based case manager, in home care, 193
Community-based settings, 593–594
Comparison groups, 567
Compensable, 493
Competence (competency), 459
Comprehensive outpatient rehabilitation facilities (CORFs), 130, 152
Comprehensive primary care (CPC) initiatives, 256
Computerized Provider Order Entry (CPOE), 370
Concurrent review, 49, 351, 543
Conditioning, work, 645
Conditions of participation, 314
Conduct, CCMC rules of, 466
Confidentiality, 459
  and insurance coverage, 512–513
Conflict of interest, 459, 473, 493
Congestive heart failure (CHF), 233, 241
Consensus, 420
Consolidated Omnibus Budget Reconciliation Act (COBRA), 55, 668
Constipation, 171
Consumer driven, 44
Context, 270
Continued stay review, 49, 351–352, 543
Continuing care retirement community (CCRC), 130
Continuing education, 515–516
Continuity of care, 314
Continuous monitoring, 309
Continuum of care, 24, 47, 65, 295, 352
  case management models of, 67–68
  major settings for, 68
  patient safety and medical errors and, 95–98
Contracts, 493, 506–507
  breach of, 492
  requirement, 533
  in workers' compensation, 617
Contract-specific performance requirements, 531, 533
Contractualism, 459, 462
Contribution, 493
Coordination, 25, 295
  in hospice care, 197, 202, 213
  in palliative care, 197, 202, 213
  of program in OH case manager, 662–663
Coordinator, 276

Co-pay/co-payment, 39
Core curriculum, 3–4
  applicability, 6–7
Cost containment, in workers' compensation, 635–636
Cost of health care, 27
Cost–benefit analysis, 383, 408–410, 425, 517
Council for Case Management Accountability (CCMA), 564–565
Credentialing, 47. *See also* Certification
  individual, 695
  organization or program/service, 695
Credentials, 420, 695
  individual, 420
  organization program, or service, 420
Criminal law, 496
Critical Access Hospital (CAH), 330
Critical thinking
  and decision-making, 406–407
  definition, 394
Cross-disciplinary training, integrated case management, 598–599
Crowding, 64–65
Crowdsourcing, 473
Current Procedural Terminology (CPT) codes, 261
Custodial care, 130, 159, 181
Custodial care facility, 130
Custodial services, 145

D
Damages, 493
Data analysis, of life care planning, 677, 688
Data mining, 370
Data warehouse, 370
Databases, 370
  in outcomes measurement, 568
Day rehabilitation services, 152–153
Decision, 493
Decision making
  about legal cases, 497, 499–500
  ethical issues in, 460–461
  ethical principles and, 462–466
Decision support system (DSS), 370
Deductible, 39
Defendant, 493
Defense Base Act, 627
Define-Measure-Analyze-Improve-Control (DMAIC), 555
Delegation
  definition, 394
  skills, 403–404
Demand management, 72
Dementia care, 157, 588

Denials, 352
    admissions, 358
    payment, 41, 54
    services, 358
Dental health care, 221
Deontologism, 459, 462
Department of Transportation (DOT), 668
Deposition, 493, 509, 675
Depression, 578–579
Description of services, 466
Development, of case management
        plan, 301–303. *See also* Case
        management care plans
Developmental disability, 25
Diagnosis-related groups (DRGs), 39, 52,
        316, 352
Diagnosis-specific benefit, 44
Diagnostic and Statistical Manual of
        Mental Disorders, 5th edition
        (DSM-5), 574–575, 578
Digital health, 473
Dignity, 459
Direct case management outcomes, 551
Disability, 642, 644
    biopsychosocial approach to, 646
    definitions of, 642, 650
    developmental, 25
    illness model of, 646
    perspectives on, 646
    prevention of, 647, 648
    severity of, in workers' compensation,
        621
Disability and occupational health,
        611, 640–670. *See also* Workers'
        compensation
    Americans with Disabilities Act (ADA)
        in, 636, 646, 650–654 (*See also*
        Americans with Disabilities Act
        (ADA))
    case management programs in, 642,
        647–650 (*See also* Disability case
        management)
    CMSA's standards of practice, 645–646
    Disability Management Employers'
        Coalition in, 654–655
    history and overview of, 640–641
    integrated case management strategies
        in, 655–656
    key definitions in, 641–645
    knowledge base for case managers in,
        668, 669
    occupational health case manage-
        ment in, 656–669 (*See also*
        Occupational health case
        management)
    resources, 713

return to work programs in, 640, 659,
        670
    workforce health and productivity in,
        maximizing, 664–665
Disability case management, 25, 640–650
    challenges to, 649–650
    definitions of, 642
    early intervention and job accommoda-
        tion in, 649
    employer-provided benefit plans and
        services, 641
    employment laws, 655
    evaluations in, 648
    functions and activities in, 647, 648
    interdisciplinary teams in, 649
    practice domains in, 647
    prevention and workplace intervention
        in, 647, 648
    workplace productivity in, 648
Disability duration guidelines (DDGs), 658
Disability Management Employers'
        Coalition (DMEC), 654–655
Discharge, 314
Discharge criteria, 352
Discharge planners, 182
Discharge planning, 25, 49, 247, 295,
        314, 320, 352
Disclosure, 467
Discounted fee for service, 51
Discovery, 493
Disease management (DM), 25, 47
DISMEVAL Consortium, 555
Distance counseling, 473
Diversion, 65
Documentation, 310
    professional objectivity in, 469
Domains, 269
    of case management, 33
DRG/case rate, 52
Drug abuse
    Americans with Disabilities Act on,
        653–654
    patient, 513
Drug courts, 594
Dual relationships, 473–474
Durable medical equipment (DME),
        190–191, 336–337
Duty, 462, 493

E
E-ACTS, 486
Early intervention
    in disability case management, 649
    in occupational health, 661
Editorial control, by case manager
        supervisor, 514–515

Education and training, 30, 425. *See also* Certification; Credentialing
  approaches to, 429–431
  of case managers, 511
  classification, 430
  consensus areas for, 425–426, 426*t*–428*t*, 429
  occupational health case management, 660
Educator, 276
Effective Health Care Program (EHCP), 549
Effective rural case management, 226
Efficacy of care, 675
Eight-Stage Change Process, 412, 413*t*
Elder abuse, 130
Elder depression, 170–171
Elder neglect, 131
Electronic communication, 478–479, 484*t*–485*t*
Electronic health record (EHR), 370
Electronic medical record (EMR), 371
Electronic technology, 474
Emergency department case management, 86–88
Emergent, 72
Emotional intelligence, 394
Employee, 650
Employee assistance program (EAP), 626, 662
Employee benefits program, 660
Employee Retirement Income Security Act (ERISA), 54–55, 668
Employer, 650
  workers' compensation, 612
Employers Metrics for Productivity and Quality (EMPAC), 638
Employment Leaves and Benefits Administration, 648
Employment network, 655
Empowerment, 394
Encryption, 474
End health system outcomes, 551
End-of-life care, 197
End-stage disease, indicators of, 204–205
Ensuring anonymity and confidentiality, 230
Environmental health nursing, 656
Equal Employment Opportunity Commission (EEOC), 636, 652–653
Equity, in workers' compensation, 633
Ergonomics, 642
Ergonomist, 642
Errors, medical, case manager role in, 95–98
Ethical ambiguity, 457
Ethical Assessment Screen (EAS), 486

Ethical conflicts, 457
Ethical dilemma, 459
Ethical issues
  resources, 707, 709–710
  in workers' compensation, 632–634
Ethical principles, 457
  CCMC, 465–466
  CMSA, 465
  decision making and, 462–466
  in workers' compensation, 633–634
Ethical Principles Screen (EPS), 486
Ethical Rules Screen (ERS), 486
Ethical theories, 462
Ethical uses
  of case management practice, 472
  challenges, with technology proficiency, 477
  CMSA's standards of practice, 476
  electronic communication, 478–479
  formal decision-making models, 483
  professional interaction, 476–477
  social media, 479–483, 482*f*, 482*t*
  transition in, modes of patient, 476–477
Ethics, 457–469, 459
  advocacy in, 458
  case manager responsibilities in, 466–467
  CMSA's standards of practice, 460
  committees, 467
  decision making, 407–408, 460–466
    CCMC rules of conduct in, 466
    CCMC values in, 465
    CMSA ethical principles in, 465
    ethical theory *vs.*, 462–463
    four ethical principles in, 463–464
    Four-Quadrant model in, 464–465
  ethical conflicts in, 467
  ethical groups/committees in, 467
  justification in, 468
  law *vs.*, 457–458
  moral feelings and, 468
  overview of, 457–458
  record keeping in, 467
  scope of practice in, 469
  strategies for ethical behavior in, 467–469
  theories in, 462
Evaluation, 295–296
  of case management plan, 306
  in disability case management, 648
  functional capacity, 642–643
  of life care planning, 678
  medical, left before, 65
  in occupational health, 667–668
  vocational, 644

Evidence, best, 352
Evidence-based Clinical Decision Support Criteria, 524–525
Evidence-based decision support criteria, 542
Evidence-based guidelines, in case management care plan, 537–540
Evidence-based medicine (EBM), 352, 524, 538
    in case management care plans, 352
    in workers' compensation, 615
Examination
    functional capacity, 607, 642–643, 659
    independent medical
        in disability case management, 647
        in occupational health, 659
        in workers' compensation, 614, 631, 632
    second opinion, 659
Exchange visitor visa. See J-1 visa
Expert witness, 493, 510, 675
Exposure, 675
Exposure and response prevention (ERP), 585, 587
External case management, 84–85
External validity, 551

F
Facilitation, 296, 538, 541
    in life care planning, 678
Facility urban, rural, or highly rural (URH) classification, 222
Fact witness, 510
Fairness, in workers' compensation, 633
Family and Medical Leave Act (FMLA), 668
    in workers' compensation, 636–637
Federally Qualified Health Centers (FQHCs), 79, 133–136
Fee for service (FFS), 51
    in Medicare, 361–362
Fidelity, in workers' compensation, 634
Field case management (FCM), 621
First report of injury (FROI), 607
Focused utilization management, 358
Follow-up care, 252
Formal ethical decision-making models, 483
Formal leadership, 393
Foundation for Rehabilitation Education Research (FRER), 273–274
Four-Quadrant model, 464–465
FQHC Look-Alike (FQHC LA), 133
Friend, 474
Function, 269, 270
Functional ability, 607, 609

Functional capacity evaluation/examination (FCE), 607, 631, 642–643
    occupational health case management, 659
Functional independence measure (FIM), 539
Functional job analysis, 659
Functional status, 315
Fundamental right, 493
Futile care, 197

G
Gatekeeper, 39
General Anxiety Disorder (GAD-7), 540
Geographic HPSA, 221
Global payment and package pricing, 53
Goals. See also specific topics
    Americans with Disabilities Act, 650
    of case management, 32, 521, 522, 526, 529
    case management information systems, 374–376
    occupational health case management, 658
    outcomes management, 553–555
    palliative care, 206–208
    system-centered, 522
    utilization management, 354
    workers' compensation, 609
Good death, 197
Good Samaritan Act, 514
Government payers, 39, 42, 54
Green houses, 158
Group homes, 157
Group medical, 44
Guided care model, 255
Guiding principles, 5, 15–17

H
Handicap, 643
Handicapped, 643
Handoff, 65, 95–98, 315
Handover, 247–248
Hard savings, 394
Harm, 493
Health and disability insurance, 691
Health and human services, 215
Health care continuum, 65. See also Continuum of care
Health care delivery systems, 39, 50–51. See also specific systems
Health care informatics, 371
Health care provider engagement, 252
Health care proxy, 197, 209
Health Care Quality Management Board Certification (HCQM), 439

Health care reimbursement, 39. *See also*
  Reimbursement, health care
Health home, 576
Health Improvement Protection and
  Accountability Act (HIPAA),
  323–324
Health information exchange (HIE), 371
Health Information Portability and
  Accountability Act (HIPAA), 55,
  504, 509
Health information technology (HIT),
  368, 371
  and CMISs, 372–374, 389–390
Health Information Technology for
  Economic and Clinical Health
  (HITECH) Act in 2009, 368
Health insurance, 44
Health insurance marketplaces, 215,
  231–232
Health Insurance Portability and
  Accountability Act (HIPAA), 23,
  379
Health Level Seven International (HL7)
  facilitates standardization, 377–378
Health literacy, 248
Health Maintenance Act, 23
Health maintenance organization (HMO),
  50–51
Health On the Net (HON) Foundation, 388
Health Plan Employer Data Information
  Set (HEDIS), 49
Health professional shortage areas
  (HPSAs), 216, 217, 220–221
Health Resource and Services
  Administration (HRSA), 559, 560
Health Status Questionnaire Short Form,
  539–540
History, of case management, 22–24
Home care, 180
  behavioral health case management,
  593–594
  CMSA's standards of practice, 182
  functions of, 179–180
  history of, 180
  nursing services, 188–189
  patients eligible for, 180, 183–184
  rehabilitation services, 189–190
Home care case management, 179–194
  community-based case manager role
  in, 193
  demand for, 180
  durable medical equipment and other
  services in, 190–191
  home health care visits, 184–187
  hospital-based case manager role in,
  192–193

hospital-based interdisciplinary team
  in, 182–184
  nursing services in, 188–189
  overview of, 179–180
  patient safety in, 194
  rehabilitation services in, 189–190
  reimbursement for services in, 187–188
  resources, 701–702
  satisfaction with, 194
  savings from, 194
  social work services in, 191
Home health agency, 334
Home health aide (attendant), 187, 189
Home health care services, 315–316
Home health care visits, 184–187
Home health resource groups (HHRGs),
  181, 316
Home visits, to patient, 516–517
Homebound, 181
Hospice care, 189, 196–213, 316, 334–335
  advance directives and health care
  proxies in, 209–211
  barriers to, 202
  case management services in, 211–213
  CMSA's standards of practice, 198–199
  definitions and functions of, 197, 200f,
  201–206
  guidelines for, 202
  identification of patients for, 202
  indicators of end-stage disease and,
  204–205
  Karnofsky performance status scale
  and, 203
  overview of, 196
  primary, 198
  principles and goals of, 206–208
  resources, 702
  scope of, 208–209
  specialty, 198
Hospital case management (HCM), 101,
  102, 104–106, 109, 110, 114, 116,
  117, 119
Hospital-based case manager, in home
  care, 192–193
Hospital-based interdisciplinary team, in
  home care, 182–184
HRSA. *See* Health Resource and Services
  Administration (HRSA)
Human Factors Analysis, 554

I

ICM. *See* Integrated case management
  (ICM)
IHI Triple Aim, 565
IME. *See* Independent medical
  examination (IME)

Impairment, 607, 643
Impairment rating, 607–608
Impartiality, 459
Implementation, 25, 296
case management care plan, 536–537
Improving Medicare Post-Acute Care
Transformation Act of 2014
(IMPACT), 327–328
Indemnity, 44
Indemnity claims, 616, 621
Indemnity payments, 608, 610, 612, 637
Independent case management, 84–86
Independent living, 131
Independent medical examination (IME)
disability case management, 647
occupational health, 659
workers' compensation, 614, 631, 632
Index of Medical Underservice (IMU), 217
Indicator Development Form, 559, 561
Individual certification, 452, 453
Individual factors, 19
Informal leadership, 393
Informatics, 368, 379–383. See also Case
management information systems
(CMISs)
Information flow, 551
Information system (IS), 372. See also
Case management information
systems (CMISs)
Information technology (IT), 474. See also
Case management information
systems (CMISs)
Information transfer, 251–252
Informed consent, 493, 497
Infusion therapy, 335
Injured worker advocacy and autonomy,
633
Injury, 643
first report of, 607
nondisabling, 643
nonscheduled, 608
scheduled, 608
second, fund for, 615
serious, in workers' compensation,
622–624
Inpatient hospitalization, 592–593
Inpatient rehabilitation facility (IRF), 131,
331, 331t–332t
Input, 65
Input-throughput-output model, 92
Institute for Healthcare Improvement
(IHI), 548
Institute of Medicine (IOM), 14, 27, 104,
565
clinical practice guidelines, 351
patient-centered care, 248

Institution certification, 452
Instrumental activities of daily living
(IADLs), 131
Insurance
accident, 44
commercial, 39
health, 44
liability, 43
workers' compensation, 44
Insurance carrier requests, for questioning
patients, 511
Insurance case management, 73
Insurance Company, of North America, 22
Insurance Education Association (IEA),
655
Insurance plans, 43–44
Insurance-based case manager, 58
Integrated benefits, 649, 655
Integrated Benefits Institute, 655
Integrated case management (ICM),
597–599. See also Behavioral
health case management
CMSA's standards of practice, 577
cross-disciplinary training, 598–599
essential knowledge and practices in,
599
impact of psychological factors,
595–596
organizational implementation, 599
overview of, 573–574
reimbursement issues, 596–597
resources, 712
training requirements for, 598–599
Integrated delivery system (IDS), 25, 51
Integrated disability management,
655–656
Intellectual and developmental disabilities
(IDDs), 588–589
Intellectual disability, 25
Intentional tort, 493
Interdisciplinary team
care management plan, 523, 525, 540
in home care, hospital-based, 182–183
in palliative and hospice care, 199, 208,
212
Intermediate objectives, 558
Intermediate rehabilitation facilities
(IRFs), 152
Intermittent services, 181
Internal case management, 84
Internal validity, 551
International Academy of Life Care
Planners (IALCP), 673, 674, 678
International Association of
Rehabilitation Professionals
(IARP), 674

Internet, 474. *See also* World Wide Web (WWW)
Internet of Things, 474
Interprofessional collaborative practice (IPEC) competencies, 249
Interprofessional practice (IPP), 248
Interrogatories, 493, 509
Interstate compact, 632, 635
Interventions, 296. *See also specific interventions*
  case management care plan, 528–531
Investigational subpoenas, 510

J

J-1 visa, 222
Jimmo v. Sebelius, 325–326
Job accommodation, 649
Job Accommodation Network (JAN), 636, 653
Job description, 270
Job modification, 643
Joint liability, 494, 503
Journals, 30, 693, 698
Justice, 459
  in workers' compensation, 633

K

Karnofsky performance status scale, 203
Knowledge, 270
  for case managers, 56–57, 668, 669
  integrated case management, 599
Kotter's change process, 412, 413t

L

Labor union representative, 612
Lack of certification, 358
Language therapy, 190
Law, 494
  case, 492
  civil, 492
  common, 493
  criminal, 496
  ethics *vs.*, 457–458
  statutory, 494, 499
Lawyers, 494
  case managers and, 508
Leader, 277
Leadership
  core components of, 393
  definition, 393, 394
  formal and informal, 393
  skills, 400–401
  styles, 397–400, 399t
Lean, 554
Leapfrog Group, 548
Leaving Against Medical Advice (LAMA), 314

Left before medical evaluation, 65
Legal counsel, 612
Legal issues, 492–519
  affidavit of merit in, 501–502
  attorneys in, 508
  burden of proof in, 501
  child or parental abuse in, patient, 513
  CMSA's standards of practice, 495
  confidentiality in
    patient, and coverage, 512–513
    patient requests for, 513
  continuing education in, 515–516
  contracts in, 506–507
  drug abuse in, patient, 513
  emergency care at patient's home in, 514
  how cases are decided in, 499–500
  insurance carrier requests in, 511–512
  intentional torts in, 496–499
  legal basics in, 496
  legal community in, 508–511
  liability exposure for case managers in, 502–504
  licensing across states in, 517–519, 518t
  litigation in, 509–510
  malpractice in, professional, 500–501
    referred provider, 517
  on managed care, 54–55
  negligence, 499
  overview of, 492
  patient advice *vs.* role in, 512
  patient home visits in, 516–517
  Patient's Bill of Rights in, 496–499
  patient's work status in, observations on, 513
  professional organizations in, 516
  questioning patients in, 511–512
  refusal to *see* patients in, 516
  resources, 710
  signing reports in, 515
  subpoenas in, 508–509
  supervisor editorial control in, 514–515
  in workers' compensation, 634–635
Legislation, 28, 29, 252–253
Length of stay (LOS), 352
Level of care (LOC), 5, 65, 315–316, 329, 352
  alternative, 351
  long-term care (*See* Long-term care)
  nonmedical, 156–159
  rehabilitation, 146, 147t, 148–150, 150t–151t
Level of service, 65
Liability, 494
  case manager exposure in, 501–502
  joint, 494, 503, 507
  several, 494

Liability insurance, 43
Liable, 494
Licensing, nursing, across states, 517–519, 518t
Licensure, 420–421, 436
    nurse licensure compact states in, 517–519, 518t
Life care plan, 673–691
    applications of, 685
    benefits of, 685
    in catastrophic injury claims, 677
    characteristics of, 685
    components of, 688–689
    definition and overview of, 673–674
    development of, 686–688
        assessment interview in, 686–687
        clinical practice guidelines in, 688
        community resources and services in, 688
        data analysis in, 688
        professionals in, 686
        records review in, 686
        research in, 688
        team approach in, 688
    example of, 681, 682t–684t
    health and disability insurance, 691
    history of, 681
    in insurance, 685
    in litigation, 685
    Medicare Set Asides in, 689–691
    specific information in, 686
    use of, 685
Life care planner, 675. *See also* Life care planning
    aspects of practice of nurse life, 680
    case manager role as, 678–681
    CMSA's standards of practice, 675–676
    critical aspect of, 685
    development of, 676
    functions of, 680
Life care planning, 673–674. *See also* Life care plan
    aims of, 676–677
    assessment in, 677
    collaboration in, 678
    data analysis, 677, 688
    definition and overview of, 673–674
    development of, 677
    evaluation of, 678
    facilitation in, 678
    Medicare Set Asides in, 689–691
    philosophical roots of, 674
    planning in, 678
    process of, 677–678
    resources, 713–714
    testimony of, 678

Lifetime maximum, 44, 56
Limitation of activity, 131
Limits, 46
Litigation, 509
Loan forgiveness, 221–222
Long-term acute care, 155
Long-Term Acute Care Hospital (LTACH), 330
Long-term care, 143–146
    case management roles in, 162–165, 163f, 164t
    conditions, 143
    custodial care, 144, 145
    definition, 131
    financial aspects of, 161–162
    at home, 189
    insurance, 131
    nursing homes, 156
    postacute care settings, 143–146
    skilled care, 144, 145
    skilled nursing facilities, 155
Long-term disability (LTD) income insurance, 643
Long-term objectives, 559
Lost time claims, 616, 621. *See also* Indemnity payments
Low-income population HPSA, 221
Low-utilization payment, 188

M
Maleficence, 633
Malfeasance, 633
Malpractice, 494
    professional, 500–501
    by referred provider, 517
Managed care, 37–39
    strategies in, 55–56
Managed Care Appropriateness Program (MCAP), 351, 357
Managed care case management, 73
Managed care health plans, 37
Managed government plans, 53
Managed Medicaid, 45–46
Managed Medicare, 41, 45
Materials flow, 551
Maximum medical improvement (MMI), 608
Maximum medical recovery (MMR), 608
Meaningful use, 371, 389
Media sharing sites, 474
Medicaid, 22, 37, 45–46, 576, 597
Medical care organization (MCO), 614
Medical condition case management, 595–596

Medical Disability Advisor (MDA), 615
Medical errors, case manager role in,
   95–98
Medical malpractice, 494
Medical management, 47
Medical Marijuana, 494
Medical necessity, 56, 58
Medical review outcomes, 359–360
Medically Underserved Area (MUA), 217
Medically Underserved Population
   (MUP), 217
Medical–Surgical Nursing Certification
   Board (MSNCB), 263
Medicare, 37, 45, 594, 597
   home care nursing services reimburse-
      ment by, 188
   managed, 41, 45
   payment for home care services
      by, 188
MEDicare Act of 2013, 385
Medicare appeals, 361–362
Medicare bonus, 221
Medicare demonstration projects, 22
Medicare Secondary Payer (MSP), 690
Medicare Set Asides (MSA), 689–691
Medicare Shared Savings Program (MSSP),
   39–40
Medication management, 251
Medication reconciliation, 390, 533
Mental disorders, 573
Mental health care, 221
Mental Health Parity and Addiction
   Equity Act (MHPAEA), 596–597
Mental health promotion, 573
Mental retardation, 25
Merit, affidavit of, 501–502
Metric reports, 535
Micropolitan statistical area (MSA), 217
Military insurance, 46
Milliman care guidelines, 351
Minimum data set (MDS), 40, 43
Misconduct, reporting, 466
Mobile device, 474
Mobility, 643
Modified duty, 612, 626, 631, 656, 663
Modified duty team, 661
Modified work, 624, 626
Monitoring, 25, 296
   continuous, 309
Moral character, 459
Moral distress, 474
Moral feelings, personal, 468
Morality, 459
Motivational interviewing (MI)
   achieving and sustaining lifestyle, 416
   characteristics of, 415

comprehensive assessment of, 413
concept and strategy, 414
definition, 394
skills and principles, 414–415
Multiple providers, in workers'
   compensation, 624

N
National Academy of Certified Care
   Managers, 438
National Alliance on Mental Illness
   (NAMI), 573
National Association of Social Workers
   (NASW), 17, 28
National Committee for Quality
   Assurance (NCQA), 42, 56, 263,
   364, 449
National Council on Aging (NCOA),
   28
National Database for Nursing Quality
   Indicators (NDNQI), 557
National Long Term Care Channeling
   Demonstration Projects, 23
National Quality Forum (NQF), 275, 548,
   562–564
National Quality Measures Clearinghouse,
   556
National Transitions of Care Coalition
   (NTOCC), 245, 250–252
Necessity, medical, 58
Negligence, 494
Negotiation
   definition, 394
   skills, 401–403
Negotiator, 277
Netiquette, 474
Network model, 40
Noncertifications. See Denials
Noncovered services, 131
Nondisabling injury, 643
Nonmaleficence, 459–460
Nonmedical custodial services, 337
Nonoccupational disease, 643
Nonscheduled injury, 608
Nonskilled services, 181
Nonurgent, 72
Normative guidelines, 460
Notice of hospital discharge, 325
Nurse licensure compact states, 517–519,
   518t
Nurse Practice Act, 500
Nursing homes, 131
   without walls, 189
Nursing Information and Data Set
   Evaluation Center (NIDSEC),
   378

Nursing Outcomes Classification (NOC), 557, 560–561
Nursing services, at home, 188–189

O

Objectivity, 466–467
Obsessive–compulsive disorder (OCD), 585–586
Occupational and environmental health nursing, 656
Occupational disease, 643
Occupational health. *See* Disability and occupational health
Occupational health case management, 643, 656–669
  accessibility in, 660–661
  assessment in, 666
  case manager role and functions in, 656–657
  certification in, 657
  clinical aspects of, 661
  clinical practice guidelines for, 658
  common illnesses and disabilities in, 660
  communication protocol, implementation of, 661
  definitions in, 656
  education in, 660
  Employee Assistance Programs, 662
  employee benefits programs in, 660
  evaluation in, 667–668
  functional capacity evaluations, 659
  functional job analysis in, 659
  goals of, 658
  implementation of, 667
  independent medical examination in, 659
  key concepts of, 658–659
  knowledge base for case managers in, 668, 669
  models of, 665–666
  modified or transitional duty team in, 661
  occupational or vocational rehabilitation services in, 659
  planning in, 667
  process in, 666–668
  program coordination in, 662–663
  responsibilities of, 663
  scope and role of, 656
  second opinion examination in, 659
  selecting vendors in, 660
  stakeholders of, 662
  success factors for, 660–663
  work hardening in, 659
  workforce health and productivity in, maximizing, 664–665
  workforce management of, 664

Occupational Medicine Practice Guidelines (OMPGs), 658
Occupational rehabilitation services, 659
Occupational Safety and Health Administration (OSHA), 668
Occupational therapy (OT), 131, 189
Offer, 506
Offeree, 507
Offeror, 507
Office of Rural Health (ORH), 222
Office of Rural Health Policy (ORHP), 220
Official Disability Guidelines (ODG), 615
Older Americans Act, 23
Ongoing long-term care, 143
Online, 474
Onsite case management, 75
Opinion, 494
Organizational certification/accreditation, 453
Organizational factors, 20
Outcome and assessment information set (OASIS), 181, 187–188
Outcome indicators, 25
Outcome measurement, 25
Outcome-driven quality assessment, in workers' compensation, 635
Outcomes and outcome analysis, 551–552
  in case management care plans, 530, 531 (*See also* Case management care plans)
  definition of, 65, 296, 675
  objectives, 558
  specific, 563–566
  in throughput, 88–93
Outcomes indicators, 559–560, 563
Outcomes management, 547–555
  definitions in, 553–555
  disease management programs for, 555–556
  overview of, 548–550
  rationale for, 555–556
  reporting of, 568
  resources, 711
  scope and goals of, 553–555
Outcomes measurement
  in case management, 563–568
    goals in, 563
    incorporation of, 566–568
    specific outcomes in, 563–566
  CMSA's standards of practice, 552–553
  continuous quality improvement, 568
  databases and computer programs in, 568
  definition, 553–555
  documenting quality of services by, in workers' compensation, 637–638

effective, characteristics of, 556–559
effective measures in, 556–559
implementation, 556
quantification and measurement in, 567
rationale for, 555–556
reporting methods in, 567
research designs in, 566–567
scope and goals of, 553–555
selection and development of, 559–563
    categories of, 562
    Cesta and Tahan's classification of, 562
    Health Resource and Services Administration, 559
    Indicator Development Form in, 561
    National Quality Forum, 562–563
    Nursing Outcomes Classification in, 560–561
    social work outcomes classification in, 561–562
statistical principles in, 568
value-based purchasing program, 565–566
Outcomes reporting, 49
    key issues in, 568
Outlier payment, 188
Out-of-pocket, 40
Outpatient care, 132
Outpatient case management, 77–78
Outpatient clinics or centers, 336
Output, 65
Overuse of service cases, in workers' compensation, 624
Overutilization review, 353

P
Paid time off (PTO) arrangements, 643–644
Palliative care, 196–213, 335
    advance directives and health care proxies in, 209–211
    case management services in, 211–213
    CMSA's standards of practice, 198–199
    definitions and functions of, 200f, 209–211
    identification of patients for, 202
    indicators of end-stage disease in, 204–205
    Karnofsky performance status scale and, 203
    overview of, 196
    primary, 198
    principles and goals of, 206–208
    resources, 702
    scope of, 208–209
    specialty, 198

Partial disability, 644
Partial hospitalization, 593
Partial permanent disability, 608
Partial temporary disability, 608, 630
Partial-episode payment, 188
Part-time care, 183
Pathway, clinical, 523–524
Patient Activation Measure (PAM), 539
Patient acuity, 532, 533
Patient and family/caregiver engagement/ education, 251
Patient assessment, CMISs, 379–380
Patient assessment instrument (PAI), 43
Patient empowerment, 521, 522, 529
Patient flow, 65–66, 88–93, 552
Patient Health Questionnaire (PHQ), 540
Patient or client system factors, 20
Patient portal, 371
Patient Protection and Affordable Care Act (PPACA), 24, 215, 230–233, 241, 275, 341, 576
Patient RUCA classification, 223
Patient self-determination, 198
Patient URH classification, 222–223
Patient-centered care, 248
Patient-centered goals, 522
Patient-centered medical home (PCMH), 78–79, 136–137, 248, 256–257, 521
Patient's Bill of Rights, 496–499
Patient-specific needs, 532
Payer, 5
    source, 38
Payer-based case management, 75
Pay-for-performance, 53
Payment case management, 699–700
Payment structures, 37
Peer review, in workers' compensation, 617
Peer review organizations (PROs), 46
Peer-to-peer conversation, 356
Peer-to-peer discussion, 360
Per diem, 51
Percent of charges, 51–52
Performance metrics, contract-specific, 531, 533
Performance reporting, in utilization management, 363
Performance standards, 522
Perioperative services case management, 82–84
Permanent partial disability, 608
Permanent total disability, 608
Personal care services, 132
Personal health information (PHI), 55
Personal health record (PHR), 371

Pharmaceutical services, 50
Philosophical tenets, of case management, 32–33
Philosophy, 6
of case management, 6, 13–15
Physical disability, 644
Physical therapy (PT), 132, 190
Physician Quality Reporting System (PQRS), 40
Plaintiff, 494
Plan-Do-Study-Act (PDSA), 554–555
Planning, 25, 296. *See also* Case management care plans
case management care, 525–527
in life care planning, 678
in occupational health case management, 667
Podcast, 475
Point of service (POS), 51
Polypharmacy, 171–172
Postacute care
Accountable Care Organizations, 139–143
CMSA's standards of practice, 133–134
comprehensive geriatric assessment, 174–175
Federally Qualified Health Centers, 134–136, 142–143
geriatric and older adult patient, 165–172
geriatric assessment, for placement, 175–177
high-risk geriatric patients, identification of, 172–174
long-term care, 143–146
non–inpatient, rehabilitation services in, 152–156
nonmedical levels of care, 156–159
overview of, 127–130, 128*f*
patient-centered medical home, 136–139, 142–143
rehabilitation levels of care, 146, 147*t*, 148–150, 150*t*–151*t*
resources, 701
resources for, care of elderly, 165
respite care, 159–160
Potential savings. *See* Soft savings
Practice Acts, 28
Practice, representation of, 466
Practice settings, 4, 67–70, 269
acute, 68, 69
admitting department, 79–82
ambulatory or clinic/outpatient, 77–78
CMSA's standards of practice, 66–67
community care, 76–77
emergency department, 86–88

fundamentals of, 66
independent/private, 84–86
insurance/managed care, 73
onsite, 75
payer-based, 75
perioperative services, 82–84
post-acute, 68, 69
pre-acute, 68, 69
resources, 700
telephonic case management, 70–72, 75
Practice site, 4
Preadmission certification, 353, 543
Preadmission Screening and Resident Review (PASRR), 324
Preauthorization, in workers' compensation, 617
Precertification, 49
review, 353
in workers' compensation, 617
Predictive modeling, 40
Predictor of repeat admissions (PRA), 132
Preferred provider organization (PPO), 51, 614, 617
Prevention, disability, 647, 648
Primary care, 25
Primary care case management, 34
Primary health care, 221
Primary hospice care, 198
Primary palliative care, 198
Prior authorization, 49
Privacy, 460
The Privacy Rule, 504
Privacy setting, 475
Private case management, 84–86
Private sector, 28
Problem identification, 296
Problem list identification, 535–536
Problem statement, 523
Process, 66, 89, 552, 563
case management, 307–308 (*See also* Case management process)
objectives, 558
Process measure, 552
Productivity, workforce
maximizing, 664–665
in return to work, 661
Productivity, workplace, 648
Professional associations, 31
Professional development, 421–422, 695
Professional negligence, 494, 500
Professional networking, 475
Professional organizations, on legal issues, 516
Professional Standards Review Organization (PSRO), 321

Project BOOST, 255–256
Project RED (reengineered discharge), 255
Prolonged treatment, in workers'
    compensation, 624, 625
  with complications and complicating
    factors, 625–626
Proof, burden of, 501
Prospective payment system (PPS), 37, 40,
    43, 316, 353
Prospective review, 353, 543
Protocol, case management care plan,
    524, 533, 534, 538
Provider, 25
Proximate cause, 494
Public awareness, 27
Public sector, 28
Publicity, 460
Purposes, of case management, 31–32

Q

Qualified DRG, 316
Quality, 547–568. *See also* Outcomes
    management
  definition, 552
  resources, 711
Quality improvement organization
    (QIO), 46, 350, 353, 362–363
Quality indicators, 533, 534
Quality management program/model,
    46–47
Quality manager, 277
Quality metrics, 533
Quality of care, 533–534
Quality of services, in workers'
    compensation, 637–638
Quality standards, 531
Questioning patients, legal issues with,
    511–512

R

Random variation, 554
Randomized comparison, 567–568
Rapid and significant changes, 27
Readmission, 316
Reasonable accommodation, 608, 651
Reasonable and necessary care, 132
Reasonable services, 181
Reassessment, 309–310
Reassignment, 653
Recertification, 435
Reconsideration, 356
Record keeping, 310
  professional objectivity in, 467
Records
  ethics and, 467
  submission of, 509

Recovery, barriers to, in workers'
    compensation, 624–626
Recredentialing, 434
Red flags, in workers' compensation,
    624–626
Re-evaluation, 310
Referral, 316
Referred provider, malpractice by, 517
Refusal, to see patients, 516
Regulations, 28, 494
Rehabilitation, 132
  barriers to, in workers' compensation,
    624–626
  occupational or vocational services in,
    659
  vocational, 26
  work, 646
Rehabilitation Act
  Section 501, 655
  Section 503, 655
  Section 504, 646, 655
Rehabilitation care settings
  case management roles in, 162–165,
    163f, 164t
  financial aspects of, 161–162
Rehabilitation levels of care, 146, 147t,
    148–150, 150t–151t
Rehabilitation prospective payment
    system, 43
Rehabilitation services, at home, 189–190
Reimbursement
  behavioral health and integrated case
    management, 596–597
  health care, 37, 40–41
    challenges with, 54
    components of, 46–50
  for home care services, 188
  mechanism, 46
  resources, 699–700
Reimbursement methods, 37, 51–54. *See
    also specific methods*
Reinsurance, 40
Reliability, 552
Remedy, 494
Remote care, 218–219, 702
Reported case, 500
Reporting
  misconduct, 466
  in workers' compensation, 618
Reports
  signing of, 515
  supervisor editing of, 514–515
Representation of practice, 466
Res judicata, 494
Researcher, 278
Reserves, 608

Residents, 157
Resource consumption, 534
Resource management (RM), 353–354, 705. *See also* Utilization management (UM)
Resource utilization groups (RUGs), 40, 316
Resources, 521, 525, 534
Respite care, 132, 159–160
Responsibility, health care, 38
Restorative nursing services (NRS), 132
Retrospective review, 49, 353, 543
Return on investment (ROI), 368, 531
Return to work (RTW), 611, 640, 659
    activity referrals, in workers' compensation, 628–631
    coordinator, 662–663
    programs, 640, 659–661, 670
        productivity management in, 661
        success factors for, 660–663
Rights
    Bill of, patient's, 496–499
    fundamental, 493
Risk, 608
    adjustment, 552
    manager, 278
    sharing, 47
    stratification, 532
Role, 269, 270. *See also specific areas* of case manager, 67
Role and Function Study, 521
Rules of conduct, CCMC, 466
Rural area, 218, 230
Rural area health care settings
    abuse of alcohol, 216
    accidents, 216
    acute myocardial infarction, 216
    behavioral health care in, 229–230, 229f
    case management
        programs and services, 225–229
        projects and research, 234t–240t
    culture health care considerations, 223–225
    health insurance marketplaces, 215
    hypertension, 216
    Medicaid benefits, 215
    Medicare payments, 216
    Patient Protection and Affordable Care Act, 230–233, 241
    smokeless tobacco use, 216
    suicide rate, 216
Rural behavioral health interventions, 231
Rural care
    behavioral health case management, 594
    CMSA's standards of practice, 218–219
    resources, 702

Rural case management programs, strategies and interventions, 227
Rural community case management model, 229f
Rural homeless, 225
Rural residents, 216
Rural–Urban Commuting Area (RUCA), 218

S
Safety issues, 168–170
Safety, patient, 95–98
Scheduled injury, 608
Schizophrenia, 583–584
Scholarly activities, 695
Scholarship, 695
Second injury fund, 615
Second opinion examination (SOE), 659
Second opinions, 631
Section 188, Workforce Investment Act, 655
Section 501, Rehabilitation Act of 1973, 655
Section 503, Rehabilitation Act, 655
Section 504, Rehabilitation Act, 646, 655
Security, 475
Select management, 82–84
Selective serotonin reuptake inhibitors (SSRIs), 587
Self-determination, patient, 198
Self-funding, for workers' compensation, 610
Self-insuring, for workers' compensation, 610
Self-management, 521, 526, 529
Self-neglect, 575, 590–591
Self-reliance *vs.* dependency, 230
Serious injury cases, in workers' compensation, 622–624
Serotonin–norepinephrine reuptake inhibitors (SNRIs), 587
Settings. *See* Practice settings
Several liability, 494
Severe and persistent mental illness (SPMI), 575, 577
Shared accountability, across providers and organizations, 252
Short-term disability (STD) income insurance, 644
Short-term objectives, 558
Significant change in condition payment, 188
Signing reports, 515
Six Sigma, 554
Skilled care, 132
Skilled nursing care, 132

Skilled nursing facility (SNF), 132–133, 153–155, 315, 322, 332–334
Skilled services, 145, 181
Skype, 475
SMART goals, 526
SMART objectives, 558, 559
SNF coinsurance, 133
Social media, 475, 484*t*–485*t*
Social network, 475
Social Security Act, 22, 134
Social Security Disability Income (SSDI), 644, 646, 654
Social Security Insurance (SSI), 668
Social work, 25–26
Social work services, at home, 191
Society for Human Resource Management (SHRM), 649–650
Soft savings, 394
Solicitation, 467
Special cause variation, 554
Specialty hospice care, 198
Specialty palliative care, 198
Specialty population HPSA, 221
Specified recovery guidelines (SRGs), 658–659
Speech and language pathology (SLP), 133
Speech therapy, 189
Standard
    individual, 421
    organization, 421
Standard of care, 421, 494, 552
Standard of practice, 421, 503
    authoritative statements, 6
    Case Management Society of America, 6–10, 26, 40–41
    acute care setting, 103–104
    behavioral health and integrated case management, 577
    case management care plan, 525
    case management process, 296–297
    case manager's role leadership and accountability, 395–396
    disability and occupational health case management, 645–646
    ethical uses, 476
    ethics and general practice, 460
    health care insurance, benefits, and reimbursement systems, 40–41
    home care setting, 182
    legal issues, 495
    life care planning, 675–676
    palliative and hospice care settings, 198–199
    postacute care settings, 133–134

practice settings, 66–67
professional development, certification, and accreditation, 421–422
quality and outcomes management, 552–553
remote and rural care settings, 218–219
resource and utilization management, 353–354
resources, 695–696
roles, functions, and activities, 270–272
technology use, 371–372
transitional care, 245–246
transitional planning and transitions of care, 317
workers' compensation, 609
definition, 26, 552
resources, 696
Standardization methodology, 535
Standards of Practice for Case Management, 519
State administrative agency, 612
Statutory law, 494
Stop loss, 53
Stop loss insurance, 44
Strategies, in managed care, 55–56
Stratification, 532
Structure, 66, 89, 553
    objectives, 558
Subacute level of care, 315
Submission of records, 509
Subpoenas, 494, 509
    investigational, 510
    requests for information in, 509
Substance use disorders, 575, 576, 579–581
Substance-related disorders, 575
Successful interdisciplinary case management teams, 20
Succession planning, 394–395
Supervisor, editorial control by, 514–515
Support system factors, 20
Supreme Court of the United States (SCOTUS), 24, 506
Systematized Nomenclature of Medicine (SNOMED), 378
System-centered goals, 522

T
Target populations, 33
Tax Equity and Fiscal Responsibility Act (TEFRA), 272
Tax-qualified policies, 131

Team factors, 20
Technology, 371–372, 475, 705–706
Telehealth (TH), 241, 371
    barriers to, 386–388
    cost, 387
    digital divide, 387
    interventions, 383–384
    legislation, 385–386
    licensure concerns, 389
    reimbursement for services, 387
    security and privacy, 386, 387
    standard of care issues, 389
Telemedicine (TM), 371
Telemental health (TMH), 384
Telephone triage, 72
Telephonic case management (TCM),
        70–72, 75
    in workers' compensation, 620, 621
Temporary long-term care, 143
Temporary partial disability, 608, 630
Temporary total disability, 608–609
Termination of services, 466
Terminologies, and classifications,
        378
Testimony, life care planning, 678
Text message, 475
Textbooks, 693, 696–697
TH. *See* Telehealth (TH)
The Joint Commission (TJC), 364
Third party administrator/administration
        (TPA), 54
    in workers' compensation insurance,
        611, 641
Throughput, 66, 88–93, 700
Time loss management, 644
Tort, 494
    actionable, 675
    intentional, 493
Total permanent disability, 608
Total temporary disability, 608–609
Training. *See* Education and training
Transfer, 316
Transfer DRG, 316
Transition of care, 66
    certification and accreditation in,
        262–263
    conceptual model for, 259*f*
    definition, 249, 250, 317
    essential intervention categories,
        250–252
    hallmark of patient-centered, 313
    and implications for case management
        practice, 257
    legislative and regulatory consider-
        ations pertaining to, 252–254,
        254*t*

models and delivery systems,
        254–257
    Patient Protection and Affordable Care
        Act, 245
    professional case managers, 246
    reimbursement issues, 261–262
    roles and functions associated with,
        257–259
Transition planner, 277
Transition planning, 26, 251, 542
Transitional care, 245–246, 317, 703
Transitional care model (TCM), 254–255
Transitional care unit (TCU), 315
Transitional duty, team for, 661
Transitional planning, 49
    case manager and managing care,
        343–344
    case manager role, 337–341
    CMSA's standards of practice, 317
    continuity of care, 318–320
    cross-setting measures management,
        327–328
    definition, 316–317
    Federal rules, 323–327
    four-stage process, 322
    importance of, 313
    influence transitional care, 321–323
    levels of care, 329–337
    overview of, 313
    transition management and readmis-
        sions, impact on, 341–343
    value-based purchasing, 341–343
Transitional work, 612, 656, 664, 665
Transitional work duty (TWD) programs,
        664–665
Transitions, 93–95
    case manager role in, 94
    fundamentals of, 93
    HMO Workgroup on Care Management
        on, 94
    National Quality Forum on care transi-
        tion on, 94–95
    patient safety and medical errors in,
        95–98
Transitions of care, 6, 317
Treating physician, in disability and
        occupational health, 659–663, 665
Treatment, prolonged, in workers'
        compensation, 624, 625
    with complications and complicating
        factors, 625–626
Triage, telephone, 72
Tricare, 46
Truth, in workers' compensation, 634
Tweet, 475
Twenty-four–hour coverage, 636

U

Underinsured patients, 54
United States Department of Agriculture (USDA), 220
Unprofessional behavior, 460
Urban clusters, 218
Urbanized area, 218
Urgent, 72
Urinary incontinence, 167
US Census Bureau, 219
U.S. Department of Labor's Office of Disability Employment Policy, 649
Usability, and CMISs, 368, 374
Utilitarianism, 460
Utilization management (UM), 49, 350–365
    adverse review determination in, 359
    appeal process in, 360–363
    case management and, 543–544
    certification programs, 365
    certifications related to, 357
    clinical review criteria and guidelines for, 357
    CMSA's standards of practice, 353–354
    criteria and strategies, 357
    definition, 353
    denials of admissions and services in, 358
    focused, 358
    key regulatory and accreditation bodies in, 363–364
    medical review outcomes, 359–360
    Milliman care guidelines in, 351
    overview of, 350
    performance reporting, 363
    program and goals in, 354
    regulatory and accreditation processes, 364–365
    resources, 705
    review process and types in, 354–356
    team, 356
Utilization manager, 277
Utilization review (UR), 26, 57, 321
    categories, 543
    certification programs in, 357
    definition, 353
    in workers' compensation, 617
Utilization Review Accreditation Commission (URAC), 263, 359
    in workers' compensation, 617, 637

V

Value-based payment models, 521
Value-based purchasing (VBP), 40, 565–566

Values, 460
Variances, case management care, 540, 541
Variation, 552
    common cause, 554
    random, 554
    special cause, 554
Veracity, 460
    in workers' compensation, 634
Verdict, 494
Veteran Administration, 46
Veterans Health Administration (VHA), 222
Videoconference, 475
Violence, behavioral health case management, 590
Violence, workplace, 626–628
    process model for, 627–628
    sources of, 626–627
Virtual relationship, 475
Virtue ethics, 460
Visa waiver, 222
Visual acuity, 177
Vocational assessment, 644
Vocational evaluation, 644
Vocational rehabilitation (VR), 26, 609, 615, 631, 644
Vocational rehabilitation counseling process, 644
Vocational rehabilitation counselor, 644
Vocational rehabilitation services, 659
Vocational testing, 645

W

Waiver, 495
Washington Business Group on Health (WBGH), 655
Wellness programs, employee, 656, 662
Wiki, 476
Within-the-walls case management, 64, 66
Witness, 495
    case manager as, 510
    expert, 493, 509–510, 675
    fact, 510
Work adjustment, 645
Work adjustment training, 645
Work conditioning, 645
Work hardening, 645, 659
Work modification, 645
Work setting, 4
Work status, observations on, 513

Workers' compensation, 44, 605–638
  Americans with Disabilities Act in, 636
  applying case management process to,
    621–628
    case management referral in, 621
    catastrophic and serious injury cases
      in, 622–624
    known barriers to recovery/rehab
      and "red flag" cases in, 624–626
    prolonged treatment, multiple
      providers, and overuse of service
      cases in, 624
    prolonged treatment with complica-
      tions and complicating factors in,
      625–626
    severity of disability in, 621
  case management processes in, 615–618
  CMSA's standards of practice, 609
  cost impact of, 609–610
  cost-containment programs in,
    635–636
  definitions of, 645
  documenting quality of services by out-
    comes measures in, 637–638
  employment settings for case managers
    in, 619–620
  ethical considerations in, 632–634
  federal laws in, 636–637
  goals of, 609
  key stakeholders in, 611–612
  laws on, 613–615

  legal issues in, 634–635
  managed care arrangements, 610
  medical case management in, 611
  overview of, 606–607
  practicing case management in,
    615–618
  prolonged treatment, multiple provid-
    ers, and overuse of service cases
    in, 624, 625
  reform of, 640
  requirements for case managers in,
    619–620
  resources, 712–713
  RTW activity referrals in, 628–631
  scope of medical management in,
    620–621
  self-fund or self-insure, 610
  trends in, 635
  utilization and peer review, 617
  workplace violence in, 626–628
  workplace violence process model in,
    627–628
Workforce health, maximizing, 664–665
Workforce Investment Act, 655
Workforce management, 664
Workforce productivity
  maximizing, 664–665
  in return to work, 661
Workplace intervention, 647, 648
Workplace productivity, 648
World Wide Web (WWW), 476